PULMONARY/ RESPIRATORY THERAPY

PULMONARY/ RESPIRATORY THERAPY

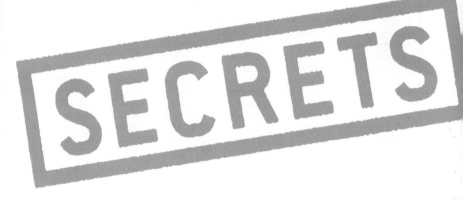

Third Edition

Polly E. Parsons, MD
Professor, Department of Medicine
University of Vermont College of Medicine
Chief, Critical Care Service
Fletcher Allen Health Care
Burlington, Vermont

John E. Heffner, MD
Professor of Medicine
Executive Medical Director
Medical University of South Carolina
Charleston, South Carolina

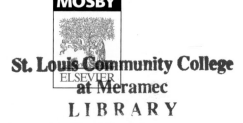

1600 John F. Kennedy Boulevard
Suite 1800
Philadelphia, PA 19103-2899

Pulmonary/Respiratory Therapy Secrets
Third Edition

ISBN-13: 978-0-323-03586-6
ISBN-10: 0-323-03586-8

NOTICE

Knowledge and best practice in this field are constantly changing. As new research and
experience broaden our knowledge, changes in practice, treatment and drug therapy
may become necessary or appropriate. Readers are advised to check the most current
information provided (i) on procedures featured or (ii) by the manufacturer of each
product to be administered, to verify the recommended dose or formula, the method
and duration of administration, and contraindications. It is the responsibility of the
practitioner, relying on his or her own experience and knowledge of the patient, to make
diagnoses, to determine dosages and the best treatment for each individual patient,
and to take all appropriate safety precautions. To the fullest extent of the law, neither the
Publisher nor the Editor assumes any liability for any injury and/or damage to persons
or property arising out or related to any use of the material contained in this book.

Library of Congress Cataloging-in-Publication Data

Pulmonary/respiratory therapy secrets / [edited by] Polly E. Parsons, John E. Heffner.–3rd ed.
    p.; cm. – (The secrets series)
  Includes bibliographical references and index.
  ISBN-13: 978-0-323-03586-6
  ISBN-10: 0-323-03586-8
    1. Lungs–Diseases–Examinations, questions, etc. 2. Respiratory therapy–Examinations,
questions, etc. I. Parsons, Polly E., 1954– II. Heffner, John E. III. Series.
    [DNLM: 1. Respiratory Tract Diseases–Examination Questions. WF 18.2 P982 2006]
  RC756.P84 2006
  616.2'0076–dc22
        2005057665

Vice President, Medical Student Publishing: Linda Belfus
Developmental Editor: Stan Ward
Senior Project Manager: Cecelia Bayruns
Marketing Manager: Kate Rubin

Working together to grow
libraries in developing countries

www.elsevier.com | www.bookaid.org | www.sabre.org

Printed in China.

ELSEVIER   BOOK AID International   Sabre Foundation

Last digit is the print number: 9 8 7 6 5 4 3 2 1

DEDICATION

To our spouses, Jim Jacobson and Ann Heffner, for their support and understanding, and to our children, Alec and Chandler Jacobson and John and Jim Heffner, for their inspiration and patience.

CONTENTS

CONTRIBUTORS

Elizabeth L. Aronsen, MD
Division of Pulmonary Sciences and Critical Care Medicine, University of Colorado Health Sciences Center, Denver, Colorado

Alejandro Arroliga, MD, FCCP
Department of Pulmonary, Allergy, and Critical Care Medicine, The Cleveland Clinic Foundation, Cleveland, Ohio

Ronald Balkissoon, MD
Associate Professor, Department of Medicine, Pulmonary Division, National Jewish Medical and Research Center; Associate Professor, Department of Medicine, Division of Pulmonary Sciences and Critical Care Medicine, Department of Preventive Medicine and Biometrics, University of Colorado Health Sciences Center, Denver, Colorado

Robert D. Ballard, MD
Professor of Medicine, National Jewish Medical and Research Center, University of Colorado Health Sciences Center, Denver, Colorado

Rajesh Bhagat, MD
Assistant Professor and Staff Physician, Division of Pulmonary, Critical Care, and Sleep Medicine, University of Mississippi Medical Center, Jackson, Mississippi

Roy Brower, MD
Pulmonary and Critical Care Medicine, Johns Hopkins University School of Medicine, Baltimore, Maryland

Kevin K. Brown, MD
Director, Interstitial Lung Disease Program, National Jewish Medical and Research Center; Division of Pulmonary Sciences and Critical Care Medicine, University of Colorado Health Sciences Center, Denver, Colorado

Lee K. Brown, MD
Vice Chair, Department of Internal Medicine; Associate Chief, Division of Pulmonary and Critical Care Medicine; Professor of Medicine and Pediatrics, University of New Mexico School of Medicine; Program in Sleep Medicine, University of New Mexico Health Sciences Center, Albuquerque, New Mexico

Marie M. Budev, DO, MPH
Department of Allergy, Pulmonary, and Critical Care Medicine, Lung Transplantation Program, The Cleveland Clinic Foundation, Cleveland, Ohio

Todd M. Bull, MD
Assistant Professor of Medicine, Division of Pulmonary Sciences and Critical Care Medicine, University of Colorado Health Sciences Center, Denver, Colorado

Ellen L. Burnham, MD
Assistant Professor of Medicine, Division of Pulmonary, Allergy, and Critical Care Medicine, Grady Memorial Hospital, Atlanta, Georgia

G. Douglas Campbell, Jr., MD
Division of Pulmonary, Critical Care, and Sleep Medicine, University of Mississippi Medical Center, Jackson, Mississippi

Bartolome R. Celli, MD
Chief, Division of Pulmonary/Critical Care Medicine and Sleep Medicine, Caritas St. Elizabeth's Medical Center; Assistant Professor, Tufts University School of Medicine, Boston, Massachusetts

Richard N. Channick, MD
Associate Professor of Medicine, Pulmonary and Critical Care Division, University of California at San Diego Medical Center, La Jolla, California

Thomas Corbridge, MD
Associate Professor of Medicine, Director of Medical Critical Care, Northwestern University Feinberg School of Medicine, Chicago, Illinois

Anthony M. Cosentino, MD, FACP, FACCP
Chief of Academic Medicine, St. Mary's Medical Center; Clinical Professor of Medicine, University of California at San Francisco School of Medicine, San Francisco, California; Associate Clinical Professor of Medicine, Creighton University School of Medicine, Omaha, Nebraska

Kala Davis, MD
Division of Pulmonary and Critical Care Medicine, Stanford University Medical Center, Stanford, California

Gregory Diette, MD
Pulmonary and Critical Care Medicine, Johns Hopkins University School of Medicine, Baltimore, Maryland

Anne E. Dixon, MD
Assistant Professor, Division of Pulmonary and Critical Care Medicine, University of Vermont College of Medicine, Burlington, Vermont

Karen A. Fagan, MD
LAC + USC Medical Center, Los Angeles, California

Bonnie F. Fahy, RN, MN
Pulmonary Clinical Nurse Specialist, Pulmonary Rehabilitation Coordinator, St. Joseph's Hospital and Medical Center, Phoenix, Arizona

Enrique Fernandez, MD
Professor of Medicine, University of Colorado Health Science Center; National Jewish Medical and Research Center, Denver, Colorado

Stephen K. Frankel, MD
Assistant Professor, Interstitial Lung Disease Program, National Jewish Medical and Research Center; Division of Pulmonary Sciences and Critical Care Medicine, University of Colorado Health Sciences Center, Denver, Colorado

Mark W. Geraci, MD
Professor of Medicine, Head of Division of Pulmonary Sciences and Critical Care Medicine, University of Colorado Health Sciences Center, Denver, Colorado

Mary Gilmartin, BSN, RRT, AE-C
Nurse Specialist, Coordinator of the Chronic Obstructive Pulmonary Disease Clinical Research and NETT, National Jewish Medical and Research Center, Denver, Colorado

Carlos E. Girod, MD
Associate Professor, Division of Pulmonary and Critical Care Medicine, University of Texas Southwestern Medical Center, Dallas, Texas

Philip L. Goodman, MS, RRT
Department of Medicine, Denver Health Medical Center, Denver, Colorado

Marc V. Gosselin, MD
Assistant Professor, Diagnostic Radiology Department, Director of Thoracic Imaging, Oregon Health and Science University, Portland, Oregon

E. Brigitte Gottschall, MD, MSPH
Assistant Professor, Division of Environmental and Occupational Health Sciences, National Jewish Medical and Research Center, Denver, Colorado

Michael P. Gruber, MD
Fellow, Division of Pulmonary Sciences and Critical Care Medicine, University of Colorado Health Sciences Center, Denver, Colorado

Katherine Habeeb, MD, FCCP
Clinical Assistant Professor, Division of Pulmonary and Critical Care Medicine, University of Vermont College of Medicine; Fletcher Allen Health Care, Burlington, Vermont

Mark P. Hamlin, MD, MS
Assistant Professor, Department of Anesthesiology, University of Vermont College of Medicine; Director of Anesthesia Critical Care, Fletcher Allen Health Care, Burlington, Vermont

Michael E. Hanley, MD
Professor of Medicine, University of Colorado School of Medicine, Denver, Colorado

John E. Heffner, MD
Professor of Medicine, Executive Medical Director, Medical University of South Carolina, Charleston, South Carolina

Richard A. Helmers, MD
Consultant in Pulmonary and Critical Care Medicine; Vice-Chair, Department of Internal Medicine, Mayo Clinic Scottsdale, Scottsdale, Arizona

Dean Hess, PhD, RRT
Department of Anesthesiology, Harvard Medical School; Assistant Director of Respiratory Care, Massachusetts General Hospital, Boston, Massachusetts

Nicholas S. Hill, MD
Division of Pulmonary, Critical Care, and Sleep Medicine, Tufts-New England Medical Center, Boston, Massachusetts

R. Hal Hughes, MD
East Tennessee Pulmonary Associates, Oak Ridge, Tennessee

Michael C. Iannuzzi, MD
Chief, Division of Pulmonary, Critical Care, and Sleep Medicine, Florette and Ernst Rosenfeld and Joseph Soloman Professor of Medicine, The Mount Sinai School of Medicine, New York, New York

David H. Ingbar, MD
Professor of Medicine, Physiology, and Pediatrics; Director, Pulmonary Allergy and Critical Care Division, University of Minnesota School of Medicine, Minneapolis, Minnesota

James R. Jett, MD
Professor of Medicine, Consultant in the Division of Pulmonary and Critical Care Medicine, Mayo Clinic College of Medicine, Rochester, Minnesota

Marc A. Judson, MD
Professor of Medicine, Division of Pulmonary and Critical Care Medicine, Medical University of South Carolina, Charleston, South Carolina

David A. Kaminsky, MD
Associate Professor of Medicine, Pulmonary Disease and Critical Care Medicine, University of Vermont College of Medicine, Burlington, Vermont

Robert J. Karman, MD
Private Practice, Pulmonary and Critical Care Medicine, Louisville, Kentucky

Carol A. Kauffman, MD
Section of Infectious Diseases, Department of Internal Medicine, Veterans Affairs Medical Center, Ann Arbor, Michigan

Hyun Joo Kim, MD
Assistant Professor of Medicine, Pulmonary, Allergy, and Critical Care Division, University of Minnesota School of Medicine, Minneapolis, Minnesota

Talmadge E. King, Jr., MD
Chief, Medical Services, San Francisco General Hospital; The Constance B. Wofsy Distinguished Professor and Vice-Chairman, Department of Medicine, University of California at San Francisco School of Medicine, San Francisco, California

Jeffrey S. Klein, MD
Professor, Department of Radiology, University of Vermont College of Medicine; Fletcher Allen Health Care, Burlington, Vermont

James L. Knepler, Jr., MD
Department of Pulmonary and Critical Care Medicine, University of Cincinnati School of Medicine, Cincinnati, Ohio

Steven J. Kolpak, MD
Assistant Professor of Medicine, University of Colorado Health Sciences Center; Resident Clinic Director, Denver Health Ambulatory Care Center, Denver, Colorado

Jonathan Kullnat, MD
Oregon Health and Science University, Portland, Oregon

Y.C. Gary Lee, MBChB, PhD, FCCP, FRACP
Centre for Respiratory Research, University College, London, United Kingdom; Osler Chest Unit, Oxford Centre of Respiratory Medicine, Oxford, United Kingdom; Asthma and Allergy Research Institute, University of Western Australia, Perth, Australia

Teofilo L. Lee-Chiong, Jr., MD
Associate Professor, Department of Medicine, University of Colorado Health Sciences Center; National Jewish Medical and Research Center, Denver, Colorado

David L. Levin, MD, PhD
Department of Radiology, University of California at San Diego School of Medicine, La Jolla, California; University of California at San Diego Medical Center, San Diego, California

Stephanie M. Levine, MD
Professor, Department of Medicine, Pulmonary and Critical Care, University of Texas Health Science Center, San Antonio, Texas

Andrew H. Limper, MD
Professor of Medicine, Mayo Clinic College of Medicine, Mayo Clinic, Rochester, Minnesota

David A. Lynch, MD
Professor of Radiology and Medicine, Department of Radiology, University of Colorado Health Sciences Center; University of Colorado Hospital; National Jewish Center for Immunology and Respiratory Medicine, Denver, Colorado

Joseph P. Lynch III, MD
Division of Pulmonary, Critical Care Medicine, and Hospitalist, Department of Internal Medicine, The David Geffen School of Medicine, University of California at Los Angeles, Los Angeles, California

Thomas D. MacKenzie, MD, MSPH
Associate Professor of Medicine, University of Colorado Health Sciences Center; Director of General Internal Medicine, Denver Health Ambulatory Care Center, Denver, Colorado

Lisa A. Maier, MD, MSPH
Assistant Professor, Division of Environmental and Occupational Health Sciences, National Jewish Medical and Research Center; Assistant Professor, Division of Pulmonary Sciences and Critical Care Medicine, University of Colorado Health Sciences Center, Denver, Colorado

Kamel Marzouk, MD, MS
Division of Pulmonary and Critical Care Medicine, Keck School of Medicine, University of Southern California, Los Angeles, California

Richard A. Matthay, MD
Boehringer Ingleheim Professor of Medicine, Pulmonary and Critical Care Section, Department of Medicine, Yale University School of Medicine, New Haven, Connecticut

Praveen N. Mathur, MBBS
Professor of Clinical Medicine, Indiana University School of Medicine, Indianapolis, Indiana

Janet R. Maurer, MD, MBA
CIGNA HealthCare, Lifesource/CRU, Cleveland, Ohio

Peter Mazzone, MD, MPH, FRCPC, FCCP
Department of Pulmonary, Allergy, and Critical Care Medicine, The Cleveland Clinic Foundation, Cleveland, Ohio

C. Hewitt McCuller, Jr., MD
Louisiana State University Health Science Center, New Orleans, Louisiana

Rebecca L. Meredith, BS, RRT
Department of Emergency Services, The Cleveland Clinic Foundation, Cleveland, Ohio

Albert Miller, MD
Chief, Division of Pulmonary and Critical Care Medicine, Catholic Medical Center of Brooklyn and Queens, Jamaica, New York; Professor of Clinical Medicine, New York Medical College, Valhalla, New York

Melvin Morganroth, MD
Clinical Associate Professor, Department of Internal Medicine, Division of Pulmonary and Critical Care Medicine, Oregon Health and Sciences University; Chief of Critical Care, Providence Portland Medical Center, Portland, Oregon

Marc Moss, MD
Associate Professor of Medicine, Division of Pulmonary, Allergy, and Critical Care, Department of Medicine, Emory University School of Medicine, Atlanta, Georgia

Septimiu D. Murgu, MD
Fellow, Pulmonary and Critical Care Medicine, Department of Medicine, University of California School of Medicine, Irvine, California

Mangala Narasimhan, DO
Fellow, Division of Pulmonary and Critical Care Medicine, Beth Israel Medical Center, New York, New York

Steve Nelson, MD
John H. Seabury Professor of Medicine, Louisiana State University Health Services Center, New Orleans, Louisiana

Francis C. Nichols, MD
Assistant Professor of Surgery, Consultant in the Division of General Thoracic Surgery, Mayo Clinic College of Medicine, Rochester, Minnesota

Michael S. Niederman, MD
Professor of Medicine, State University of New York at Stony Brook Health Sciences Center; Chairman, Department of Medicine, Winthrop University Hospital, Mineola, New York

Alexander S. Niven, MD
Director, Respiratory Care Services, Department of Medicine, Pulmonary/CCM Service, Madigan Army Medical Center, Tacoma, Washington; Clinical Assistant Professor, Department of Medicine, University of Washington School of Medicine, Seattle, Washington

David Ost, MD
Assistant Professor of Medicine, Department of Pulmonary Medicine, New York University School of Medicine, New York, New York; North Shore-Long Island Jewish Health System, Manhasset, New York

Harold I. Palevsky, MD
Professor of Medicine, University of Pennsylvania School of Medicine; Chief, Pulmonary, Allergy and Critical Care, University of Pennsylvania Medical Center–Presbyterian; Director, Pulmonary Vascular Disease Program, Presbyterian Medical Center, Philadelphia, Pennsylvania

Polly E. Parsons, MD
Professor, Department of Medicine, University of Vermont College of Medicine; Chief, Critical Care Services, Fletcher Allen Health Care, Burlington, Vermont

Victor Pinto-Plata, MD
Division of Pulmonary/Critical Care Medicine and Sleep Medicine, Caritas St. Elizabeth's Medical Center, Boston, Massachusetts

Udaya B. S. Prakash, MD
Scripps Professor of Medicine, Mayo Clinic College of Medicine; Consultant, Pulmonary and Critical Care Medicine, Mayo Medical Center and Mayo Clinic, Rochester, Minnesota

Ganesh Raghu, MD, FACP, FCCP
Professor of Medicine and Laboratory Medicine, Division of Pulmonary and Critical Care Medicine, Departments of Medicine and Laboratory Medicine; Chief, Chest Clinic; Director, Lung Transplant Program, University of Washington Medical Center, Seattle, Washington

Carrie A. Redlich, MD, MPH
Professor of Medicine, Occupational and Environmental Medicine Program and Pulmonary and Critical Care Medicine, Department of Medicine, Yale University School of Medicine, New Haven, Connecticut

Cecile Rose, MD, MPH
National Jewish Medical and Research Center, Denver, Colorado

Mark J. Rosen, MD
Chief, Division of Pulmonary and Critical Care Medicine, Beth Israel Medical Center; Professor of Medicine, Albert Einstein College of Medicine, New York, New York

Edward C. Rosenow III, MD, MS
Emeritus Professor of Medicine, Mayo Clinic College of Medicine, Mayo Clinic, Rochester, Minnesota

Deborah Z. Rubin, MD
Division of Radiation Oncology, University of Vermont College of Medicine; Fletcher Allen Health Care, Burlington, Vermont

Steven A. Sahn, MD
Professor of Medicine; Director of the Division of Pulmonary/Critical Care Medicine, Allergy, and Clinical Immunology, Medical University of South Carolina, Charleston, South Carolina

Samer Saleh, MD
Division of Pulmonary and Critical Care Medicine, Keck School of Medicine, University of Southern California, Los Angeles, California

Catherine S.H. Sassoon, MD
Pulmonary and Critical Care Section, Veterans Affairs Long Beach Healthcare System, Long Beach, California; Professor of Medicine, University of California School of Medicine, Irvine, California

Milene T. Saavedra, MD
Assistant Professor of Medicine, University of Colorado Health Sciences Center, Denver, Colorado

Neil W. Schluger, MD
Division of Pulmonary, Allergy, and Critical Care Medicine, Columbia University College of Physicians and Surgeons, New York, New York

Marvin I. Schwarz, MD
Department of Pulmonary Sciences and Critical Care Medicine, University of Colorado Health Sciences Center, Denver, Colorado

Lori Shah, MD
Associate Medical Director, Lung Transplantation Program, Division of Pulmonary, Critical Care, and Sleep Medicine, The Mount Sinai School of Medicine, New York, New York

Om P. Sharma, MD, FRCP
Professor of Medicine, Division of Pulmonary and Critical Care Medicine, Keck School of Medicine, University of Southern California, Los Angeles, California

Akshay Sood, MD, MPH
Assistant Professor of Medicine, Division of Pulmonary and Critical Care Medicine, Southern Illinois University School of Medicine, Springfield, Illinois

James K. Stoller, MD, MS
Associate Chief of Staff; Vice President of the Division of Medicine, Department of Pulmonary, Allergy, and Critical Care Medicine, The Cleveland Clinic Foundation, Cleveland, Ohio

Oyebode A. Taiwo, MD, MPH
Assistant Professor of Medicine, Occupational and Environmental Medicine, Department of Medicine, Yale University School of Medicine, New Haven, Connecticut

Gregory B. Tardie, PhD
Director, Human Performance Laboratory, Pulmonary Medicine Service, William Beaumont Army Medical Center, El Paso, Texas

John M. Taylor, MD
Clinical Fellow, Critical Care Medicine, Department of Anesthesia and Perioperative Care, University of California at San Francisco School of Medicine, San Francisco, California

Mitchell H. Tsai, MD, MS
Clinical Instructor, Department of Anesthesiology, University of Vermont College of Medicine, Burlington, Vermont

Yuan-Po Tu, MD
Staff Physician, The Everett Clinic, Everett, Washington

Marc A. Voelkel, MD
Pulmonary and Critical Care Section, Department of Medicine, University of Colorado Health Sciences Center, Denver, Colorado

Ann Weinacker, MD
Assistant Professor of Medicine, Division of Pulmonary and Critical Care Medicine, Stanford University Medical Center, Stanford, California

Idelle M. Weisman, MD
Associate Professor of Medicine and Anesthesiology, Texas Tech University Health Sciences Center; Chief, Department of Clinical Investigations; Director, Human Performance Laboratory and Pulmonary/Critical Care Services, William Beaumont Army Medical Center, El Paso, Texas

Karen Wesenberg, MD
Pulmonary and Critical Care Medicine, The Oregon Clinic, Portland, Oregon

Jeanine P. Wiener-Kronish, MD
Professor, Departments of Anesthesia and Medicine, Vice-Chairman, Department of Anesthesia, Cardiovascular Research Institute Investigator, University of California at San Francisco School of Medicine, San Francisco, California

Robert F. Wolken, BS, RRT
Critical Care Respiratory Specialist, Denver Health Medical Center, Denver, Colorado

Marie E. Wood, MD
Associate Professor of Medicine, Division of Medical Oncology, University of Vermont College of Medicine; Fletcher Allen Health Care, Burlington, Vermont

Richard G. Wunderink, MD
Professor of Medicine, Division of Pulmonary and Critical Care, Northwestern University Feinberg School of Medicine, Chicago, Illinois

Steve Yang, MBBS, MRCP, FAMS
Associate Consultant, Department of Respiratory and Critical Care Medicine, Singapore General Hospital, Singapore; Division of Pulmonary and Critical Care Medicine, University of Washington Medical Center, Seattle, Washington

PREFACE

In this third edition, we have continued our focus on the concept that pulmonary clinicians and respiratory therapists must first pose proper questions before they can formulate effective solutions to their patients' respiratory problems. Perhaps in no field of medicine is this twin challenge of identifying essential questions and deriving appropriate answers more fundamentally important than in the management of pulmonary disorders. The broad-based nature of pulmonary medicine requires a masterly understanding of diverse immunologic, infectious, traumatic, neoplastic, and inflammatory conditions. Some respiratory conditions arise primarily in the lungs, whereas others pose as "lung diseases" but actually represent pulmonary manifestations of underlying "occult" systemic disorders. Moreover, effective application of respiratory therapeutics requires proficiency in diverse pharmacologic and surgical interventions in addition to a mechanic's (or in some cases an engineer's) grasp of ventilator tubes, principles of gas and fluid flow, and electronic circuitry of ventilatory and monitoring devices. It is no wonder that this complex field presents clinicians with major challenges in identifying the appropriate questions, let alone providing corrects answers to patients' clinical problems.

We have been delighted with the response to the first two editions of *Pulmonary/Respiratory Therapy Secrets*. In this third edition, we have again been fortunate to have many leaders in pulmonary medicine and respiratory therapy contribute chapters in their areas of expertise. These experts have expanded the *Secrets* format to include Top Secrets and Key Points. These new features allow readers to note quickly what experienced clinicians consider the most important concepts presented in their chapters. We believe the authors have succeeded in preserving the "cutting edge" nature of their content while presenting information in a readable and retainable manner that will benefit a broad readership. We hope that this book will continue to be a valuable resource to medical students, residents, fellows, and experienced clinicians alike in their efforts to ask the right questions and discover the best answers.

Polly E. Parsons, MD
John E. Heffner, MD

TOP 100 SECRETS

These secrets are 100 of the top board alerts. They summarize the concepts, principles, and most salient details of pulmonary and respiratory therapy.

1. When evaluating complaints of cough or dyspnea, it is important to include onset, precipitants, exposures, and other associated symptoms in the history of present illness.

2. When evaluating an abnormal chest radiograph, the most important first step is to obtain previous films for comparison.

3. Gynecomastia in a man with cigarette stains on his fingers is a telltale sign of lung cancer. In a middle-aged man with bibasilar inspiratory rales and clubbing, idiopathic pulmonary fibrosis should always be suspected.

4. All patients wishing to stop smoking should be offered nicotine replacement, bupropion sustained-release (SR) therapy, or both. Active physician involvement in attempts at smoking cessation is vital. Even a discussion about smoking as short as 3 minutes can double a patient's chances of quitting successfully.

5. Results from pulmonary function testing should not be used as the sole criterion for referral to pulmonary rehabilitation. Symptoms and functional limitations direct the need for pulmonary rehabilitation.

6. Mortality from chronic obstructive pulmonary disease (COPD) often results from secondary conditions. Pulmonary rehabilitation can change the course of cardiac deconditioning, peripheral muscle dysfunction, decreases in total and lean body mass, anxiety, and poor coping skills.

7. Impairment means loss of physical or physiologic function, whereas disability refers to the impact of the impairment on the person's life. Physicians assess impairment, whereas disability is determined by administrators based on the information provided by physicians and criteria for eligibility. The commonly accepted legal standard of certainty that a respiratory disease was caused by an occupational exposure is one of "more probable than not," or a level of certainty greater than 50%.

8. The presence of chronic lung disease is the most important patient-related risk factor for the development of postoperative pulmonary complications and should prompt careful evaluation and follow-up. A surgical site involving the thorax or upper abdomen carries the highest risk for the development of postoperative pulmonary complications.

9. Acute respiratory distress syndrome (ARDS) can develop over hours or days. Predisposing factors include sepsis, pneumonia, trauma, the aspiration of gastric contents, and transfusion-related acute lung injury. Patients with increasing FiO_2 requirements, decreased pulmonary compliance, and chest radiograph findings consistent with pulmonary edema (in the absence of congestive heart failure) should be ventilated in accordance with the ARDSnet protocol.

10. Atelectasis is the most common cause of postoperative hypoxemia. Profound hypoxemia can be seen in patients with small regions of atelectasis. Predisposing factors include shallow tidal

volumes, mechanical compression, mucous plugging, and secretions. The most effective treatment for atelectasis is coughing. Other treatments include incentive spirometry, positive pressure breathing, and tracheal suctioning.

11. When an anterior mediastinal mass is detected in an adult, the most common cause is a thymic neoplasm or enlarged lymph nodes due to lymphoma.

12. The radiologic features that allow a confident diagnosis of a benign solitary pulmonary nodule include a smooth margin, a central or complete calcification, and an absence of growth over 2 years.

13. On computed tomography (CT) scanning, intravenous contrast is indicated for the evaluation of the pulmonary vasculature, the mediastinal veins and arteries, the heart, the pulmonary hila, suspected lung cancer, and inflammatory pleural disease. High-resolution CT is helpful for the evaluation of known or suspected interstitial lung disease, bronchiectasis, and lung nodules.

14. Although pulmonary angiography does have some risks, the overall complication rate remains very low (<3%).

15. The main causes of hypoxemia are decreased inspired oxygen (caused by high altitude), hypoventilation (caused by respiratory center depression, neuromuscular disease, or respiratory failure), pulmonary or cardiac shunt, ventilation–perfusion (V/Q) mismatch (caused by airway secretions or bronchospasm), and diffusion defect (caused by pulmonary fibrosis, emphysema, or pulmonary resection).

16. The main types of hypoxia are hypoxemic hypoxia, anemic hypoxia, circulatory hypoxia, affinity hypoxia (i.e., a decreased release of oxygen from hemoglobin to the tissues), and histotoxic hypoxia (e.g., cyanide poisoning).

17. Warming cool extremities by placing a glove filled with warm water on the patient's hand may improve the ability of the pulse oximeter to detect an adequate signal.

18. Pulmonary function testing can identify *patterns* of disease such as obstructive impairment with or without reversibility, restrictive lung disease, restrictive chest wall disease, restrictive neuromuscular disease, and pulmonary vascular disease. Additional information from the patient's history, a physical examination, imaging, or a tissue biopsy will usually be required to make a specific diagnosis.

19. Spirometry is the easiest pulmonary function test to obtain but is often difficult to interpret without information from other pulmonary function studies. Do not hesitate to order tests for static lung volumes, the single-breath carbon monoxide diffusing capacity of the lungs (DL_{CO}^{SB}), the maximum inspiratory pressure at residual volume (PI_{max}), and the maximum expiratory pressure (PE_{max}) when clarification is necessary.

20. Exercise testing is a better estimate of functional capacity and quality of life than resting cardiac and pulmonary measurements. If you cannot figure out why a patient is short of breath, cardiopulmonary exercise testing can help you determine the primary and contributing diagnoses and initiate a more timely therapeutic intervention.

21. If the chest x-ray looks weird, think pleural disease.

22. Bronchoalveolar lavage can be safely done in patients with significant bleeding disorders including thrombocytopenia, elevated prothrombin time, and other coagulopathies. Mechanical ventilation is not a contraindication for bronchoscopy.

23. Fluoroscopic guidance is essential for the biopsy of a solitary lung nodule. Universal infection prevention precautions are indicated for all patients, regardless of the indication for bronchoscopy.

24. Endobronchial lesions are treated by endobronchial ablation (such as laser therapy, argon plasma coagulation, or cryotherapy). Extrinsic compression is best treated by stent placement or brachytherapy. Consider an endobronchial lesion whenever the patient has localized wheezing or recurrent pneumonia in the same lobe, especially in patients with risk factors such as known malignancy.

25. Chest tubes are central to the recovery of patients with a sizable pneumothorax, a hemothorax, complicated parapneumonic effusion, or empyema and also to the palliation of selected patients with malignant or paramalignant effusions.

26. Complications from chest tubes, including infection, malposition, bleeding, nerve damage, perforation of adjacent structures, and reexpansion pulmonary edema, are minimized by proper insertion; the regular assessment of function, patency, and location; and timely removal.

27. Only mediastinoscopy allows biopsies of right and left mediastinal lymph nodes through one small neck incision.

28. Positron emission tomography (PET) scanning does not provide histopathologic confirmation of metastatic mediastinal disease; therefore, mediastinoscopy remains essential in the evaluation of patients with lung cancer.

29. Medical thoracoscopy performed with local anesthesia can provide a diagnosis in 90% of cases of exudative pleural effusion.

30. Beware of the talc particle size before using it for pleurodesis. Small particle size can cause ARDS.

31. Inspiratory stridor in a patient with asthma suggests vocal cord dysfunction, which can be diagnosed by a flow-volume loop followed by fiberoptic laryngoscopy.

32. Frequent use of a rescue inhaler, nocturnal awakenings, and high peak-flow variability suggest poorly controlled asthma and a need for increased therapy.

33. Consider cystic fibrosis in a patient with chronic cough and sputum production, persistent infection with characteristic organisms, airflow obstruction, chronic chest radiographic abnormalities, or characteristic extrapulmonary manifestations. Pulmonary disease in cystic fibrosis is characterized by a process of ongoing inflammation, infection, and obstruction. This cycle may be hindered by a combination of antibiotics, mucolytic agents, bronchodilators, anti-inflammatory agents, and airway clearance devices.

34. All patients with community-acquired pneumonia (CAP) need empirical therapy directed against pneumococci, atypical pathogens (often as coinfecting pathogens), and other organisms, as dictated by risk factors. Most patients with CAP show clinical improvement within 3 days of therapy, and those not responding need a careful evaluation for unusual pathogens, drug-resistant organisms, pneumonia complications (i.e., empyema, drug-induced colitis, or pulmonary embolus), and alternate (noninfectious) diagnoses.

35. To avoid inappropriate initial empirical antibiotic therapy for ventilator-associated pneumonia (VAP), always use a different class of antibiotic from that which the patient received earlier in the hospitalization. A negative tracheal aspirate Gram stain has a very high negative predictive value

for VAP. Look for nonpulmonary sources of infection rather than assuming that pneumonia is the cause. Recurrent pneumonia in the same segment should raise suspicion of foreign body aspiration.

36. Microaspiration is seen in up to 45% of the normal population in deep sleep. Thus, oropharyngeal colonization will affect the spectrum of pathogens causing community-acquired pneumonia.

37. Self-limited pulmonary fungal infection does not require antifungal therapy. The treatment for mild to moderate disease is itraconazole. Fluconazole is as effective for coccidioidomycosis but not for histoplasmosis and blastomycosis. The treatment for severe disease is amphotericin B (or a liposomal form).

38. The diagnosis of pleuropulmonary amebiasis should always be considered in an individual with an unexplained right lower lobe pneumonia, mass, or empyema. Tropical pulmonary eosinophilia should be considered in a nonimmune individual who develops refractory asthma after a visit to an endemic area.

39. If a patient with HIV infection has a sustained (i.e., >3 months) increase in HIV helper cell (CD4+) lymphocyte count to > 200 cells/μL after using highly active antiretroviral therapy (HAART), antipneumocystis prophylaxis can be discontinued.

40. New vaccination guidelines have lowered the recommended age for influenza vaccination in healthy adults from $\geq$ 65 years old to $\geq$ 50 years old. During a vaccine shortage, use $\geq$ 65 years of age as the cutoff. All people at high risk for influenza complications should be vaccinated.

41. Gastric acid suppression therapy has been associated with an increased risk for community-acquired pneumonia. Patients hospitalized with or at risk for invasive *Streptococcus pneumoniae* should receive the pneumococcal vaccine prior to hospital discharge.

42. Removing all pleural fluid at the time of thoracentesis in a patient with a parapneumonic effusion may avoid the need for a chest catheter. Patients can then be monitored for fluid reaccumulation.

43. Perform testing for latent tuberculosis infection only in patients at high risk for reactivation. Do not test persons you would not treat, even if they have a positive result.

44. The incidence of infections by atypical mycobacteria has increased dramatically in recent decades. It is often difficult to differentiate true pulmonary infection by atypical mycobacteria from simple colonization.

45. If a patient with human immunodeficiency virus (HIV) infection has intrathoracic lymphadenopathy on routine radiographs or computed tomography, think strongly about tuberculosis or fungal infection.

46. Unlike most HIV-associated disorders, the occurrence of pulmonary hypertension in HIV-infected persons is unrelated to the CD4+ lymphocyte count, and it usually does not improve with antiretroviral therapy.

47. Considering the diagnosis of immune reconstitution inflammatory syndrome usually allows the clinician to avoid unnecessary and invasive diagnostic tests.

48. A negative (i.e., <500 mg/mL) D-dimer assay combined with a low pretest probability of thromboembolic disease can be used in outpatients to exclude thromboembolic disease with a 99% negative predictive value.

49. The classic triad of the fat embolism syndrome includes respiratory insufficiency, neurologic abnormalities, and petechial rash.

50. If a patient develops acute respiratory distress and hemodynamic compromise during central line insertion or removal, consider venous air embolism. Immediately place the patient left side down in Trendelenburg's position and administer 100% FiO_2.

51. The most common tumors associated with tumor emboli are adenocarcinomas of the breast, stomach, and lung.

52. In a patient with unexplained dyspnea, order an echocardiogram looking for signs of pulmonary hypertension. Request specifics including right-sided chamber size, a pulmonary artery (PA) systolic pressure estimate, and right ventricular function. Always perform a complete diagnostic evaluation with echocardiography, V/Q scanning, pulmonary function testing, a sleep study (if indicated), and a right heart catheterization before initiating therapy for pulmonary arterial hypertension.

53. The absence of inspiratory crackles on chest examination in a patient with diffuse interstitial lung disease on chest imaging studies should suggest granulomatous lung diseases, especially sarcoidosis. An obstructive pattern of lung impairment in a patient with diffuse interstitial lung disease (ILD) should suggest a diagnosis of sarcoidosis, lymphangioleiomyomatosis, hypersensitivity pneumonitis, tuberous sclerosis, or COPD with superimposed ILD.

54. Because cardiac sarcoidosis may be sudden and lethal, all patients with sarcoidosis should have a baseline electrocardiogram. All patients with sarcoidosis and an abnormal baseline electrocardiogram or symptoms of palpitations or congestive heart failure should have an aggressive work-up for cardiac sarcoidosis that should include, at a minimum, a Holter monitor and an electrocardiogram.

55. Sarcoidosis may predominantly involve the airways, resulting in an obstructive lung disease that may mimic asthma.

56. No single histopathologic feature in patients with idiopathic pulmonary fibrosis (IPF) and biopsy-confirmed unusual interstitial pneumonia (UIP) predicts the subsequent clinical course or likelihood of responding to therapy. One recent study, however, suggests that patients with more evidence of fibroblast foci have shorter survival times.

57. Thoracic disease may precede the more typical manifestations of collagen vascular disease. Depending on the specific collagen vascular disease, all the elements of the thorax can be involved, including the pleura, causing pleuritis and elusions; the lung parenchyma, resulting in various forms of diffuse parenchymal or interstitial lung disease; the airways, resulting in bronchiolitis; and the pulmonary arteries, resulting in pulmonary hypertension.

58. A newly described, aggressive form of small airways disease—bronchiolocentric interstitial pneumonia—is characterized by a distinctive pattern of interstitial fibrosis extending around the bronchioles. Chart radiographs demonstrate diffuse reticulonodular infiltrates.

59. Approximately 50% of patients with small vessel vasculitis will have one or more recurrences of their disease, and these disease flares may manifest with either familiar or novel signs and symptoms compared with the initial presentation. Cytotoxic or immunosuppressive medications have serious complications and side effects that can mimic a disease flare.

60. Patients with vasculitis are immunocompromised as a result of both their disease and their therapy; thus, infections may present with atypical features. Infections, especially unrecognized infections, represent a major cause of morbidity and mortality in vasculitis patients.

61. If a patient presents with sudden dyspnea, cough, hemoptysis, and diffuse alveolar infiltrates with air space filling on chest radiography, the differential diagnosis must include diffuse alveolar hemorrhage.

62. If you suspect diffuse alveolar hemorrhage, obtain the blood urea nitrogen (BUN) level, the creatinine level, a urinalysis for microscopic hematuria, serologic testing (for autoantibodies and antineutrophil cytoplasm antibodies [ANCAs]), and, in addition to assessing the coagulopathy status (i.e., platelet count, prothrombin time [PT], and activated partial thromboplastin time [APTT]) and the severity of anemia by a complete blood count, consider a bronchoscopy with lavage.

63. Keep a high index of suspicion for obstructive sleep apnea. One study demonstrated that it is present in 9% of adult women and 24% of adult men. Continuous positive airway pressure (CPAP) is a very effective treatment for obstructive sleep apnea, but careful and expert follow-up is crucial.

64. If you start a patient with obesity hypoventilation syndrome on nocturnal nasal continuous positive airway pressure (n-CPAP) for sleep apnea, recheck awake arterial blood gas after 3–4 weeks. The patient may still be hypercapnic and will benefit from a change to nocturnal bilevel positive airway pressure therapy.

65. Silica and coal dust exposure can result in fibrotic or pneumoconiotic lung disease along with airway disease (including chronic bronchitis), airway obstruction, and emphysema.

66. The beryllium lymphocyte proliferation test (BeLPT) is used in the diagnosis of beryllium sensitization and chronic beryllium disease (CBD) and can differentiate CBD from other granulomatous lung disease.

67. Recognize the importance of a complete occupational and environmental history in any patient with an interstitial lung disease.

68. As with other granulomatous lung diseases, hypersensitivity pneumonitis (HP) is more common in nonsmokers than in smokers. However, smokers with HP tend to have more insidious symptoms and a poorer 10-year survival rate. The prognosis for recovery from HP depends on effective antigen exposure removal; permanent fibrosis, emphysema, and airway reactivity are potential sequelae of HP.

69. Occupational asthma is a syndrome of variable airflow limitation and hyperresponsiveness due to exposures in an occupational setting. It may account for up to 20% of cases of adult-onset asthma. Occupational asthma may be triggered by an immune response to a high-molecular-weight (of animal or vegetable origin) or low-molecular-weight compound, or it may be triggered as a nonimmune response to exposure to a high dose of irritant.

70. The physician must know every drug that the patient is taking, including over-the-counter (OTC) drugs and eye drops. The only way this can be accomplished is for the patient or family to bring in *all* medications in their original bottles.

71. The differential diagnosis of diffuse pulmonary infiltrates in the immunocompromised host includes (1) opportunistic infection; (2) recurrence of the underlying disease; (3) drug-induced

lung disease; (4) unrelated disorders such as pulmonary emboli (PE), congestive heart failure (CHF), and CAP; and (5) a combination of two or more of the above.

72. Three-dimensional conformal planning can limit exposure of normal lung tissue to radiation and can decrease the risk of pneumonitis. The mainstay of treatment for radiation pneumonitis and fibrosis is a combination of steroids and pulmonary rehabilitation.

73. If there is a discrepancy between oxygen saturation measured by pulse oximetry and that measured directly by co-oximetry, consider carbon monoxide poisoning.

74. Do not forget the few key antidotes available for toxic inhalational exposures: sodium nitrite and sodium thiosulfate for cyanide toxicity; sodium nitrite for hydrogen sulfide toxicity; calcium gluconate for hydrofluoric acid toxicity; and atropine, pralidoxime, and diazepam for nerve gas poisoning.

75. Tumor growth doubling time refers to the rate at which a lung mass doubles in size over time. A tumor doubles in size when it reaches 1.3 times its last linear dimension. Doubling times of malignant lesions range from 21–400 days. Benign processes have doubling times that are usually either faster or slower.

76. A patient with a large pleural effusion and an absence of contralateral mediastinal shift on a chest radiograph is most likely to have lung cancer obstructing the ipsilateral main-stem bronchus.

77. Paraneoplastic endocrine syndromes are not uncommon. The most effective therapy is treatment of the underlying tumor. Other treatments can effectively relieve symptoms and correct biochemical abnormalities while one awaits therapy for the cancer to take effect.

78. Paraneoplastic neurologic syndromes occur in a minority of patients with lung cancer, most commonly those with small-cell carcinoma. The syndromes often develop before the tumor is evident. The course of the syndrome may be independent of the clinical course of the tumor or its treatment.

79. Hamartomas are the most common benign lung tumor.

80. Lymphangitic carcinoma is a cause of Kerley's B lines on chest radiograph.

81. When initiating mechanical ventilation in a patient with ARDS or acute lung injury (ALI), use a low tidal volume strategy (i.e., 6 cc/kg ideal body weight) with plateau pressures of ≤ 30–35 cmH_2O to limit barotrauma and to improve outcomes.

82. When considering pulmonary artery (PA) catheter placement in a patient with ARDS, have a therapy in mind that you will or will not use, depending on the results of your PA catheter readings. If no therapy modification is being considered, do not place the catheter.

83. Neck flexion and extension affect the position of an endotracheal tube. Remember, the hose follows the nose. Neck flexion may result in endobronchial intubation and neck extension, leading to accidental extubation.

84. A difficult airway can be avoided by anticipating the needs of the patient and the limitations of one's airway management skills. A patient with a known difficult intubation requiring advanced techniques, with physical characteristics predicting difficult airway manipulation, or with injuries preventing cervical movement or oral/nasal instrumentation should prompt a call for assistance from both an anesthesiologist and a surgeon.

85. For ventilator-dependent patients, no duration of translaryngeal intubation is inherently unsafe. The decision to perform a tracheostomy, therefore, does not require calendar watching, but it benefits from an anticipatory approach, wherein tracheostomy is performed when prolonged ventilation appears probable and the patient will likely experience benefits from the procedure. A tracheostomy allows ventilated patients to communicate by articulated speech, which counters feelings of isolation and lack of control.

86. The best predictor of noninvasive positive pressure ventilation (NPPV) failure in acute respiratory failure is the failure of mental status, vital signs, or gas exchange to improve within 1–2 hours. Other predictors of failure include low pH, advanced age, a Glasgow Coma score < 11, severe hypercapnia (i.e., $PaCO_2 > 92$ mmHg), an Acute Physiology and Chronic Health Evaluation (APACHE) II score > 29, lack of dentition, and air leaks around the mask.

87. High airway pressure alarms on mechanical ventilation may signify a medical emergency such as a tension pneumothorax, a kinked or clogged endotracheal tube, or severe bronchospasm.

88. Positive-end expiratory pressure (PEEP) is useful for reducing intrapulmonary shunt and improving arterial oxygenation in patients with pulmonary edema, acute lung injury, and ARDS.

89. In patients with ARDS, in the absence of contraindications, permissive hypercapnia is warranted as part of a lung-protective ventilation strategy.

90. Closed-loop mechanical ventilation improves patient–ventilator interaction and patient comfort.

91. The intensive care unit neuromuscular syndrome may contribute to chronic ventilator dependency; minimize the use of neuromuscular blocking agents and corticosteroids; and utilize insulin and blood glucose protocols.

92. When considering sending a patient home on mechanical ventilation, the patient's and family's willingness and ability to provide care are two of the most important factors to consider. A patient who requires high inspired oxygen concentrations is not a candidate for home ventilation. The goals of home ventilatory care should be consistent with the needs of the patient, not with what the hospital care team thinks is the best option.

93. Use of continuous supplemental oxygen has been shown to prolong life in patients with stable chronic hypoxemia due to COPD. During commercial air travel, ambient cabin pressure may be as high as 8000 feet. Supplemental oxygen is recommended when the patient's in-flight PaO_2 is predicted to be ≤ 50 mmHg.

94. A large disparity exists between the number of potential recipients and the number of available donor organs. Many patients die while on the waiting list. Early referral is key.

95. Factors indicating which patients with a nonpurulent parapneumonic effusion will most likely require pleural space drainage for adequate resolution include prolonged symptoms of pneumonia prior to admission, alcoholism or other risk factors of aspiration, an effusion larger than 50% of the hemithorax, loculation, and pleural fluid pH < 7.20.

96. A pleural fluid analysis diagnostic of spontaneous esophageal rupture includes increased salivary amylase, pleural fluid pH < 7.00, and cytology with squamous epithelial cells and food particles.

97. Hemodynamic instability and contralateral shift of the trachea in the setting of a pneumothorax suggest tension physiology (i.e., tension pneumothorax) and warrant immediate intervention. Virtually all patients with pneumothorax associated with positive-pressure ventilation should have a tube thoracostomy placed due to the risk of subsequent tension pneumothorax.

98. Malignant pleural mesothelioma is an incurable cancer currently reaching pandemic proportion worldwide, and the majority of cases are induced by asbestos exposure. The mainstay of treatment should consist of best supportive care, consideration of pemetrexed-based chemotherapy, and prophylactic radiotherapy to pleural puncture sites. No quality data indicate that radical surgery for mesothelioma actually improves survival or quality of life.

99. Always suspect multiple myelomas in a patient with recurrent pneumonia, bone pains, and increased serum proteins.

100. Transudative pleural effusions occur early in almost all patients after liver transplantation.

I. BEDSIDE EVALUATION

TAKING THE PULMONARY HISTORY

Karen A. Fagan, MD

1. **What is dyspnea and what causes it?**
   Dyspnea is the subjective sensation of uncomfortable or difficult breathing. Most patients report dyspnea as "shortness of breath." Patients report dyspnea when their breathing is excessive for the activity that they are doing. The sensation of dyspnea is produced by stimulation of both central and peripheral receptors that monitor respiratory muscle activity, hypoxia, hypercapnia, acid-base status, airway irritation, and changes in the pressure volume characteristics of the lung (i.e., j receptors in lung fibrosis or emphysema).

   There are many systems and conditions that contribute to dyspnea, including cardiopulmonary, hematologic, psychosocial, and environmental (e.g., high altitude) factors; body habitus (i.e., obesity); fever; and level of exercise. Any situation that increases the work of breathing (i.e., airway obstruction or decreased lung compliance) also contributes to the sensation of dyspnea.

2. **Give the features of dyspnea that are important to distinguish in the pulmonary and respiratory history.**
   Onset: Acute dyspnea is readily recognized by both patient and physician. **Subacute/chronic** and **progressive** dyspnea, however, may be more difficult to characterize. Exercise tolerance or limitation over time may be the most useful way to establish the duration of symptoms in these situations. The patient's report of changes in exercise capacity over time (from months to years) may identify the onset of symptoms. Dyspnea at rest is a late finding in respiratory disease.

   Positional complaints: Platypnea, shortness of breath experienced upon assuming the upright position, is most commonly seen in patients with hepatic disease and intrapulmonary shunts.

   Orthopnea, dyspnea occurring in the supine position, is most commonly a symptom of cardiac dysfunction. **Paroxysmal nocturnal dyspnea** is also a feature of many cardiac diseases. Occasionally, patients with upper airway lesions may present with complaints of dyspnea or cough while recumbent.

   Precipitants: Reliable precipitating factors leading to dyspnea include environmental or occupational exposures, exposure to animals, and exposure to inhalational agents (industrial or recreational).

   Karnani NG, Reisfield GM, Wilson GR: Evaluation of chronic dyspnea. Am Fam Physician 71(8):1529–1537, 2005.

3. **What questions should be asked about a patient's smoking history?**
   Smoking-related lung disease is common; thus, a complete, reliable smoking history, including the following information, is important in the initial assessment of any patient, especially a patient with pulmonary disease:
   - Age at which smoking began
   - Type of tobacco used
   - Breaks in smoking history
   - Amount of smoking (i.e., pack-years, or packs per day multiplied by the number of years smoked)

A physician caring for a smoking patient should assess previous attempts at smoking cessation and should determine ways to improve the patient's success. Information should be sought about the presence of other smokers in the patient's environment, the use of support groups, the use of pharmacologic treatments (i.e., nicotine replacement), and prior input from medical personnel.

4. **Which features of the family history are important when assessing a patient with respiratory complaints?**
There may be a hereditary component in several diseases. All patients should be asked about any respiratory diseases or symptoms in first-degree relatives (i.e., those immediately related to the patient). Early age at onset of emphysema may suggest a deficiency in alpha$_1$ antitrypsin. Cough with purulent sputum production and recurrent infections may suggest a familial form of bronchiectasis (e.g., cystic fibrosis or Williams-Campbell syndrome). Some patients with pulmonary fibrosis may also have familial forms. Approximately 20% of patients with idiopathic pulmonary arterial hypertension have an affected family member.

5. **What information should be obtained from a patient who complains of cough?**
Coughing is a common complaint of patients. Although cough can be a nonspecific symptom of many diseases, a good history should begin to limit the differential diagnosis. The history includes descriptions of the onset, quality, duration, associated expectoration, presence of other respiratory symptoms, and changes in voice. Cough may be caused by inflammatory, chemical, mechanical, or psychosocial mechanisms.
   Sputum production is a key feature of cough. Healthy adults generally do not expectorate any sputum during the course of the day; thus, sputum production may be considered abnormal. The consistency and color of the sputum may help identify the source because purulent sputum usually correlates with infectious causes. The presence and quantity of blood are also important. Fetid-smelling, purulent sputum may indicate the presence of an anaerobic infection or a lung abscess. Large quantities of sputum (bronchorrhea) can be seen in some malignancies, bronchiectases, and inflammatory airway diseases. Thick, tenacious sputum associated with mucous plugs can be seen in patients with cystic fibrosis and asthma (especially allergic bronchopulmonary aspergillosis). Rarely, patients report expectoration of a chalky or stone-like object, a broncholith, which can be associated with tuberculosis and some fungal infections.
   The **time of day** during which the cough is worst may help identify a cause. Sinusitis or sinus drainage may cause a nocturnal or morning cough. Similarly, gastroesophageal reflux may cause symptoms that are worse at night or when the patient is supine. Upper airway obstruction has the same pattern. Cough after exercise may indicate reactive airway disease. Nocturnal coughing may indicate the presence of cardiac disease, especially when associated with paroxysmal nocturnal dyspnea. Cough that occurs during eating may indicate the presence of a tracheoesophageal fistula.

KEY POINTS: ESSENTIALS FOR EVALUATING COMPLAINTS OF DYSPNEA AND COUGH

1. Onset (i.e., acute, chronic, or progressive)

2. Precipitants of symptoms (e.g., environmental exposures or allergens)

3. Positional component (e.g., lying down, sitting up, or eating)

4. Sputum production (including color, consistency, and presence of blood)

A careful list of **past and present medication use** is important in evaluating a cough. Chronic dry coughing is seen with the use of angiotensin-converting enzyme inhibitors in as many as 20% of patients treated with these antihypertensive agents. Fortunately, the coughing resolves with cessation of the drug. However, chronic dry coughing with dyspnea may also be a feature of the pulmonary fibrosing diseases; thus, the medication history may be important in distinguishing the diagnosis.

Aspiration of foreign bodies may also produce both acute and chronic coughing; this possibility should be considered in children with cough and in adults with a history of impaired consciousness. Hoarseness may be associated with laryngeal sources of cough. An often-overlooked cause of chronic cough is hair or wax in the external auditory canal causing stimulation of the vagus nerve.

Holmes RL, Fadden CT: Evaluation of the patient with chronic cough. Am Fam Physician 69(9):2159–2166, 2004.

6. **Which features of an asthmatic patient's history suggest severe disease that may require more aggressive treatment?**
If a patient answers yes to any of the following questions, he or she is at increased risk of developing respiratory failure as a result of an asthma exacerbation:

- Have you required mechanical ventilation for an exacerbation in the past?
- Have you needed to be seen in the emergency department (ED) or to be hospitalized for asthma in the past year?
- Have you been treated with oral corticosteroids for asthma in the past?
- Have you had an increase in the use of rescue medications (i.e., inhalers) in the past week?
- Do you frequently wake at night due to your asthma symptoms?

  http://www.nhlbi.nih.gov/health/prof/lung/asthma/practgde.htm

7. **Define hemoptysis. How are the cause and severity assessed?**
Hemoptysis is the expectoration of blood with coughing. It is a manifestation of a number of different processes. It is a frightening, occasionally life-threatening complaint that brings patients to medical attention promptly. Most important in the patient interview is assessment of the quantity and quality of blood and the presence of any associated symptoms. Massive hemoptysis is usually easily assessed. It is generally greater than 600 cc in a 24-hour period and can be quite dramatic. More commonly, patients complain of lesser quantities such as streaks, specks, or clots. It may be difficult to estimate the amount of blood based on such reports. Use of collection containers may be the best way to establish the amount of blood produced. Other associated symptoms, such as fullness in one side of the chest or a tickle in the airway, can occasionally localize the side from which the bleeding is originating.

There are numerous causes of hemoptysis. The presence of associated symptoms may help form a differential diagnosis of the cause. Sputum production, especially when purulent, may point to an infectious cause of the hemoptysis. Weight loss and chronic cough in a patient with hemoptysis who smokes may be an indication of malignancy. Tuberculosis may present with similar symptoms in a patient exposed to the mycobacterium. Hemoptysis in a patient with heart disease and dyspnea while recumbent may be caused by pulmonary edema. The presence of chest pain and acute dyspnea may suggest pulmonary embolism.

Corder R: Hemoptysis. Emerg Med Clin North Am, 1(2):421–435, 2003.

8. **Can the causes of chest pain be reliably differentiated from one another?**
No. Chest pain arises from several sites in the thorax and surrounding organs. Although there are features that suggest a particular cause of chest pain, it can be frustrating to accurately establish and treat the cause of the chest pain. History alone can rarely identify the cause of chest pain, but attention to the quality, onset, duration, related symptoms, and precipitating and alleviating factors may help the observant historian more carefully evaluate this serious complaint. Chest pain is usually described as pleuritic or nonpleuritic.

Pleuritic chest pain, or pain arising from the parietal surface of the pleura, usually can be distinguished easily from other chest pain syndromes by history. It is usually sharp and relates to respiratory muscle movements such as inspiration or coughs. It is frequently sudden in onset and may be episodic. Causes of pleuritic chest pain include pneumonia, pleural effusion, pulmonary infarction, chest wall muscle inflammation, rib fractures, pneumothorax, and inflammation of the pleura in systemic diseases such as systemic lupus erythematosus and rheumatoid arthritis.

Nonpleuritic chest pain can be more difficult to characterize than pleuritic chest pain because both pulmonary and cardiac disease may present in similar ways. Classic anginal chest pain with pressure-like pain, radiation to the arm and jaw with associated shortness of breath, nausea, and diaphoresis may be difficult to distinguish from similar symptoms seen in pulmonary hypertension. Careful attention to medical history of other conditions and risk factors for coronary artery disease may distinguish the cause of this type of pain. Other important causes of nonpleuritic chest pain include musculoskeletal, gastroesophageal, pericardial, and aortic disorders. Subdiaphragmatic processes can also present with referred pain to the chest through irritation of the diaphragm and its surfaces.

9. **What information should be obtained about potential environmental exposures and occupational history?**

Two distinct environments may be important in evaluating a pulmonary patient: the home and the workplace. Before a detailed history of either of these locations is undertaken, it is important to have a clear understanding from the patient of the primary symptoms and whether they relate to a particular location or activity.

A detailed history of potential exposures in the home encompasses the construction, the site, the furnishings, the heating and cooling systems, any damage to the home (e.g., water damage), the presence of carpeting, the type of linens used, and any pets. This information is of particular interest in patients with hypersensitivity syndromes and asthma or other allergic syndromes. The presence of pets and other animals, currently or previously, may contribute to allergic and asthmatic symptoms. Pet birds are frequently overlooked in reporting animals in the home, so it is important to ask about these specifically.

A detailed occupational history includes all past and current jobs, specific responsibilities at each location, and information regarding chemicals and other hazardous materials at the workplace. It is especially important to ascertain whether respiratory protection was worn and, if so, what type. Documented exposures should be thoroughly reviewed. If necessary, the patient or physician may request job descriptions and material safety data sheets from the work site. This is especially important in patients with concern for particulate-induced lung disease or for workers with exacerbations of their respiratory symptoms in the work environment.

10. **What is the most important information to obtain when a patient is being evaluated for an abnormal chest radiograph?**

The most important questions to be addressed when a patient has been referred for evaluation of an abnormal chest radiograph are the following:

KEY POINTS: ESSENTIALS FOR EVALUATING AN ABNORMAL CHEST RADIOGRAPH

1. Obtain previous chest radiographs for comparison.

2. Evaluate for associated symptoms such as cough, weight loss, chest pain, or fever.

3. Obtain a smoking and occupational history (e.g., exposures that may increase the possibility of cancer, fibrosis).

■ Does the patient have any previous chest radiographs?
■ Are they available for comparison with the current films?
■ Can they be obtained?

Direct comparison of prior radiographs may establish a lesion as benign or may suggest that further evaluation is necessary.

11. **A patient's wife complains that he snores and stops breathing at night and that he falls asleep at embarrassing times during the day. What else do you want to know about the patient?**

■ Does he stop snoring for brief intervals in the night? If so, how does he resume snoring?
■ Does he ever have quick, jerky limb movements while asleep?
■ Does he complain of not sleeping well or of feeling very sleepy during the day?
■ Does he frequently take naps?
■ Does he have headaches in the morning?
■ Has he experienced sexual dysfunction?

These questions may help characterize several sleep disorders, especially obstructive sleep apnea, which can affect as many as 20% of adults in the United States. Although the patient can frequently provide adequate information to the interviewer, it is always important to obtain additional data from family and sleep partners because the patient may have frequent awakenings that do not fully arouse him but that significantly disturb his sleep.

CHAPTER 2

PHYSICAL EXAMINATION

Samer Saleh, MD, and Om P. Sharma, MD, FRCP

1. **Describe the general principles underlying a successful physical examination.**
   The physical examination of the chest should be pursued in an orderly manner through inspection, palpation, percussion, and auscultation. The physical examination is not a routine exercise, but rather a systemic intellectual activity that should be pursued logically and diligently.

2. **Which clinical signs best indicate respiratory distress?**
   Rapid respiratory rate and the use of accessory muscles of respiration denote the presence of respiratory discomfort. The rate of normal quiet respiration varies from 12–18 breaths per minute. The diaphragm and the intercostal muscles perform respiration. Accessory muscles of respiration include the scalene muscles and the pectorals. During their use, the nostrils flair, the alae nasi contract, and the sternomastoids elevate the clavicles and the sternum. Large changes in intrathoracic pressure during inspiration and expiration produce retraction of the intercostal muscles during inspiration, particularly if tracheal obstruction exists. Patients with advanced emphysema breathe through pursed lips, a maneuver that helps to increase expiratory flow time.

3. **What is the significance of paradoxical respiration?**
   Normal respiration is of two types, thoracic and abdominal. Thoracic respiration, performed by the upper part of the chest, is seen in normal women, anxious subjects, patients with ascites, and patients with diaphragmatic paralysis. In men and young children, respiration is abdominal. During normal respiration, the diaphragm moves down in inspiration (seen as outward movement of the abdominal viscera) and upward in expiration. In paradoxical respiration, the diaphragm moves down in expiration and is sucked in during inspiration. This finding represents diaphragmatic fatigue or paralysis and indicates impending respiratory arrest. In ventilated patients, it reflects ventilator–patient dysynchrony and requires either adjustment of the ventilator or sedation of the patient.

4. **How can inspection be useful in a patient with a chest disease?**
   The patient with a barrel-shaped chest whose supraclavicular spaces are retracted on inspiration clearly has emphysema. Retraction of the lower lateral chest wall during inspiration in the same patient is a characteristic called Hoover's sign. A tripod sign is present in patients with respiratory distress when they lean forward on both upper extremities to help stabilize the clavicle for the action of the accessory respiratory muscles. The presence of dilated veins on the chest wall is pathognomonic of superior vena cava syndrome. Impaired movement of part or all of the hemithorax may result from pleural effusion, pneumothorax, pleural tumor, or fibrosis. Gynecomastia in a man with cigarette stains on the fingers is a telltale sign of lung cancer.

   Sharma O: Symptoms and signs in pulmonary medicine. Dis Mon 41:577–640, 1995.

5. **Define subcutaneous emphysema.**
   Subcutaneous emphysema is the presence of air in the subcutaneous tissues. It may be caused by the following: air leaking from within the pleura, for example, from a pneumothorax; mediastinal air, for example, from a ruptured esophagus; or gas-forming organisms. Subcutaneous emphysema also may be caused iatrogenically from insertion of chest tubes and central lines.

6. **What is Tietze's syndrome?**

   Careful palpation of the chest sometimes reveals costochondral tenderness, often with swelling, which may be the source of unexplained pain in the chest. The condition, also called costochondritis, may be caused by stress or trauma to rib structures at one or more costochondral junctions.

   Gilliland B: Relapsing polychondritis and other arthritides. In Braunwald E, Fauci AS, Kasper DL, et al (eds): Harrison's Principles of Internal Medicine, 15th ed. New York, McGraw-Hill, 2001, p 2013.

7. **How is consolidation distinguished from pleural effusion on pulmonary examination?**

   A combination of percussion and auscultatory findings distinguishes consolidation from effusion (Table 2-1).

TABLE 2-1.   PHYSICAL FINDINGS IN PULMONARY CONSOLIDATION AND PLEURAL EFFUSION

Condition	Inspection	Palpation	Percussion	Auscultation
Consolidation	Respiratory rate increased; movements decreased on affected side	No mediastinal shift; tactile (vocal) fremitus increased	Dull	Bronchial breathing; bronchophony; whispering pectoriloquy; fine crepitations
Pleural effusion	Movements diminished	If large, mediastinum shifted to opposite side; tactile (i.e., vocal) fremitus absent	Flat or stony dull	Breath sounds absent; sometimes bronchial and egophonic above level of fluid

8. **Describe egobronchophony.**

   Egobronchophony or egophony is a nasal character imparted to the spoken word because of the presence of overtones. It is easily recognized: when a patient says "E," it sounds like "A." Egobronchophony is best heard over an effusion. It represents the area of consolidated or collapsed lung above the effusion.

9. **What are rales, crackles, or crepitations?**

   Crepitations sound like bursting air bubbles and indicate that secretions are present. Table 2-2 summarizes the differences between fine and coarse crackles.

10. **How is airway obstruction identified?**

   The presence of wheezes or rhonchi is suggestive of airway obstruction. Both are produced by the rapid flow of air through narrowed bronchi. The walls and secretions of the bronchi vibrate between the closed and barely open positions, similar to the way a reed vibrates in a musical instrument. Wheezes tend to be of a higher pitch and a greater intensity than rhonchi, which have a snoring or moaning quality (Table 2-3).

TABLE 2-2. DIFFERENCES BETWEEN FINE AND COARSE CRACKLES

Features	Fine Crackles	Coarse Crackles
Sound	Explosive interrupted sounds (<250 msec); higher in pitch, simulated by rubbing a lock of hair between the fingers	Explosive interrupted sounds (<250 msec); lower in pitch, simulated by bubbling liquid
Cause	Sudden opening up of previously collapsed alveoli and small airways	Sudden opening up of previously collapsed bronchi and large airways; air bubbling through secretions
Phase of respiratory cycle	End inspiration	Early inspiration or, often, expiration
Effect of cough	Does not clear	May clear
Settings	Pulmonary fibrosis, pneumonia, and heart failure	Acute bronchitis, severe pulmonary edema, and chronic bronchitis

TABLE 2-3. DIFFERENCES BETWEEN WHEEZES AND RHONCHI

Features	Wheezes	Rhonchi
Sound	Continuous (>250 msec), high-pitched musical sound; usually polyphonic	Continuous (>250 msec), low-pitched moaning sound; frequently monophonic
Cause	Vibration of small airways at point of closure	Vibration of larger airways at point of closure
Phase of respiratory cycle	Almost always inspiratory; occasionally expiratory	Almost always inspiratory; occasionally expiratory
Effect of cough	May change with cough	Clears, at least temporarily
Diseases	Asthma or extrinsic compression of airway by foreign body, tumor, or secretion	Acute bronchitis; chronic obstructive pulmonary disease; extrinsic compression of airway; or obstruction of the airway by foreign body, tumor, or secretions

11. **Which findings in a patient with bronchospasm are most ominous?**
A silent chest in a tired and lethargic patient with airway obstruction signifies exhaustion and impending respiratory arrest. Previously heard wheezes disappear because airflow velocity is decreased in obstructed airways and no sounds are produced. Such a situation requires prompt intubation and mechanical ventilation.

12. **How is the severity of bronchospasm assessed?**
Although respiratory rate and pulsus paradoxus are useful indicators, they are neither sensitive nor specific enough for assessing the severity of airway obstruction. The only way to reliably measure airway obstruction is by measuring flow rate either by spirometry or by peak-flow meters.

13. **Describe clubbing and name the five most common pulmonary causes of clubbing.**
Clubbing is a bilateral, symmetric fingernail deformity, originally described by Hippocrates. When associated with periostitis and arthritis, this syndrome is called hypertrophic pulmonary osteoarthropathy. Pulmonary causes of clubbing include bronchiectasis, lung abscesses, pulmonary malignancy, cystic fibrosis, and idiopathic pulmonary fibrosis. Clubbing is not a feature of chronic bronchitis, emphysema, or bronchial asthma.

KEY POINTS: COMMON PULMONARY CAUSES OF CLUBBING

1. Lung cancer

2. Bronchiectasis

3. Lung abscesses

4. Cystic fibrosis

5. Idiopathic pulmonary fibrosis

14. **What is the significance of hypertrophic pulmonary osteoarthropathy (HOA)?**
Finger clubbing and HOA are different manifestations of the same disease process. HOA includes clubbing, periosteal inflammation, and synovial effusions. The most frequent cause of HOA is lung cancer. Removal of the cancer may result in disappearance of HOA.

Martinez-Lavin M: Hypertrophic osteoarthropathy. In Klippel JH, Dieppe PA (eds): Rheumatology. London, Mosby, 1998, p 8.

15. **What are the usual clinical signs in emphysema?**
Patients with emphysema present with a relatively quiet chest that is often barrel-shaped and is diffusely hyperresonant. Breath sounds are vesicular but significantly reduced in intensity. Adventitious sounds are unusual unless there is concomitant bronchitis or asthma. The expiratory phase of respiration is usually prolonged.

Badgett RG, Tanaka DJ, Hung DK, et al: Can moderate chronic obstructive pulmonary disease be diagnosed by historical and physical findings alone? Am J Med 94:188–196, 1993.

16. **Which eye disorders are seen in patients with pulmonary diseases?**
Episcleritis and uveitis may be seen in patients with systemic lupus erythematosus and rheumatoid arthritis. Patients with ankylosing spondylitis and up to 25% of patients with sarcoidosis have uveitis. Optic nerve involvement with gradual progressive visual loss is also seen in sarcoidosis. Bilateral episodic anterior uveitis is a feature of Behçet's syndrome. It is often associated with retinal vasculitis.

Keratoconjunctivitis sicca is a feature of Sjögren's syndrome. Choroid tubercles may be seen in patients with tuberculosis. Wegener's granulomatoses may produce lid edema, nasolacrimal duct obstruction, proptosis, and conjunctival chemosis.

James DG, Graham E: Oculo-pulmonary syndromes. Semin Respir Med 9:380–384, 1988.

17. **Describe the skin findings associated with pulmonary disease.**
See Table 2-4.

Sharma O: Selected pulmonary cutaneous syndromes. Semin Respir Med 9:239–246, 1988.

TABLE 2-4.	SKIN FINDINGS IN PULMONARY DISEASE	
Skin Finding	Description	Pulmonary Disease
Cyanosis	Bluish discoloration of extremities, usually the tips of fingers or lips	Any disease causing hypoxemia, including cardiac disease; seen with peripheral vascular disease.
Lupus pernio	Chronic bluish granulomatous infiltration of the nose, cheeks, ears, and, sometimes, the lips and chin	Sarcoidosis
Erythema nodosum	Painful red nodules occurring mainly on the shins	Primary tuberculosis, cocci-dioidomycosis, sarcoidosis, brucellosis, Behçet's disease
Lupus vulgaris	Reddish-brown, flat plaques with yellowish-brown nodules on the head, face, neck, arms, and legs (in descending order of frequency); ulceration and scarring are characteristic	Tuberculosis
Splinter hemorrhages		Psittacosis pneumonia
Horder's spots	Faint pink spots on the trunk	Psittacosis pneumonia
Vesicles	Clear lesions 2–5 mm in diameter	Varicella pneumonia
Cutaneous ulcers		Tularemia pneumonia
Stevens-Johnson syndrome		Mycoplasma pneumonia

KEY POINTS: FINDINGS ON FUNDUS EXAMINATION OF THE PULMONARY PATIENT

1. Choroid tubercles in tuberculosis

2. Papilledema in sarcoidosis

3. Retinal vasculitis in collagen vascular disease and Behçet's disease

4. Papilledema and retinal hemorrhages in hypercapneic respiratory failure

18. **What are the pulmonary changes in hepatic cirrhosis?**
Pleural effusions, namely hepatic hydrothorax, can occur in up to 10% of patients with liver cirrhosis. They are more common on the right side than on the left side and can occur in the absence of ascites. Spontaneous bacterial empyema can complicate these effusions. Hepatopulmonary syndrome is characterized by hypoxemia, platypnea (worsening dyspnea in the upright position), and orthodeoxia (worsening hypoxemia in the upright position). It

results from right-to-left intrapulmonary shunts. Portopulmonary hypertension is pulmonary arterial hypertension in patients with portal venous hypertension.

deCampos J, Filho L, Werebe E, et al: Hepatic hydrothorax. Semin Resp Critical Care Med 22:665–673, 2001.

19. **What is the BODE index?**
The BODE index is a grading system that consists of four variables. The B stands for body mass index. The O stands for the degree of airflow obstruction, measured by the forced expiratory volume in 1 second (FEV_1) after a dose of albuterol. The D stands for dyspnea, which is measured by the modified medical research council (MMRC) dyspnea scale. The E stands for exercise capacity, measured by the 6-minute walk test. The BODE index has a score of 0–10; the higher the score, the higher the mortality. It is better than the FEV_1 at predicting the risk of death from any cause and from respiratory causes among patients with COPD.

Celli BR, Cote CG, Marin JM, et al: The body-mass index, air flow obstruction, dyspnea and exercise capacity index in chronic obstructive pulmonary disease. N Eng J Med 350:1005–1012, 2004.

20. **What are the neurologic signs of worsening hypercapnia in a patient with COPD?**
Hypoxia and acute on top of chronic hypercapnia cause many manifestations in patients with decompensated chronic respiratory failure. Headaches, drowsiness, confusion, and coma (in late stages) can occur. Muscle twitching, tremors, and asterixis are some of the motor signs. Papilledema can occur in up to 10% of patients with respiratory insufficiency and reflects the raised intracranial pressure from hypercapnia-induced cerebral vasodilation. Flame-shaped retinal hemorrhages and distended retinal veins can also be seen on examination of the fundus.

Jozefowicz RF: Neurologic manifestations of pulmonary disease. Neurol Clin 7:605–617, 1989.

CHAPTER 3

SMOKING CESSATION

Steven J. Kolpak, MD, and Thomas D. MacKenzie, MD, MSPH

1. **Describe the prevalence of cigarette smoking in the United States in this century.**

   Cigarette smoking became the most popular form of tobacco consumption in the 1920s. Per-capita cigarette consumption rose sharply during World War II and eventually peaked in the late 1960s at over 4000 cigarettes per capita per year. The prevalence of cigarette smoking (i.e., the percentage of the adult population who smoke regularly) peaked at 41% and declined annually until 1990 when the prevalence reached 25%. Since then, the decline has been much less rapid, reaching 23% in 2002. The good news is that the prevalence of smoking among high school students has fallen to a new 12-year low after rising steadily in the 1990s. Currently, 22% of high school students have smoked on at least 1 of the last 30 days, down from a high of 36% in 1997.

   Centers for Disease Control and Prevention (CDC): Cigarette Smoking Among Adults—United States, 2002. Morb Mortal Wkly Rep 53(20):427–431, 2004.
   Centers for Disease Control and Prevention (CDC): Cigarette Smoking Among High School Students—United States, 1991–2003. Morb Mortal Wkly Rep 53:499–501, 2004.

2. **What two questions best assess a patient's level of nicotine dependence?**
   1. How soon after awakening do you smoke your first cigarette? (Less than 30 minutes after awakening indicates more severe dependence.)
   2. How many cigarettes do you smoke per day? (More than 25 indicates severe dependence.)

3. **How do you quantify a person's smoking history?**

   Multiply the average number of packs smoked per day by the number of years of smoking to get the number of pack-years of smoking. For example, a 55-year-old woman who began smoking at age 15 and thinks she smoked an average of 1.5 packs (30 cigarettes) per day has a 60 pack-year smoking history (1.5 packs/day × 40 years).

4. **Is smoking cessation counseling effective?**

   With intervention, smoking abstinence rates can be significantly increased. There is a strong dose-response relationship between the intensity (i.e., time spent) of counseling and its effectiveness. Brief advice (<3 minutes) increases quit rates by 30%, low-intensity counseling (3–10 minutes) increases rates by 60%, and high-intensity counseling (>10 minutes) increases rates by over 100%. Likewise, the number of sessions included in the intervention shows a positive association with cessation rates.

5. **Describe strategies used to promote smoking cessation in a clinical setting.**

   Programs that use several modes of repeated counseling and intervention are the most effective for initial and long-term cessation. Interventions include clinician (physician and nonphysician) individualized counseling, telephone counseling, and group counseling. Self-help materials such as pamphlets, cassettes, and videos work best as an adjunct to clinician advice. The use of carbon monoxide testing and pulmonary function testing to give feedback on parameters related to smoking can double quit rates in primary care settings.

6. **List the five A's of smoking cessation counseling.**
   The U.S. Public Health Service lists five steps in the provision of office-based interventions (Fig. 3-1).
   1. **Ask** about smoking at every opportunity: Tobacco exposure should be assessed at every office visit as the fifth vital sign. It raises the awareness of smokers, nonsmokers, and office staff to the importance of cessation.
   2. **Advise** all smokers to stop: Physician advice is a powerful and inexpensive tool for smoking cessation, especially when given in a "teachable moment" such as an office visit for bronchitis or a tobacco-related hospitalization.
   3. **Assess** the patient's willingness to quit: To tailor counseling to the individual patient, determine his or her readiness to quit and interest in doing so. If the patient is not interested in quitting, provide a motivational intervention (see question 7). Patients interested in quitting should be offered assistance or referred for intensive treatment.
   4. **Assist** patients in the cessation effort: Any health care provider can assist the patient in setting a quit date, which should be scheduled as soon after the initial counseling session as possible. Offer recommended pharmacotherapies (first-line therapies, such as nicotine replacement systems and sustained-release bupropion [bupropion SR], or second-line therapies, such as clonidine and nortriptyline) to all patients unless these are specifically contraindicated.
   5. **Arrange** follow-up: A follow-up visit or telephone call should occur shortly after the quit date, preferably within the first week. A second follow-up is recommended within the first month, with further contact as needed.

7. **List the five R's of motivational interventions.**
   The following components of clinical interventions are designed to enhance motivation to quit smoking in patients who are not ready to make an attempt at quitting.
   1. **Relevance:** Information should be provided that is relevant to the patient's sociodemographic characteristics, disease status, health concerns, and social situation.
   2. **Risks:** Acute, long-term, and environmental risks should be discussed with the patient.
   3. **Rewards:** The clinician should highlight potential rewards of stopping that seem relevant to the patient.
   4. **Roadblocks:** Barriers to quitting should be elicited. Discuss characteristics of the different treatments that could eliminate these barriers.
   5. **Repetition:** The motivational intervention should be repeated every time an unmotivated smoker visits the clinic.

8. **Name the typical nicotine withdrawal symptoms.**

Craving for nicotine	Irritability	Frustration
Anger	Anxiety	Difficulty concentrating
Restlessness	Increased appetite	

9. **In the absence of treatment, how long can the symptoms of nicotine withdrawal be expected to last?**
   Nicotine withdrawal symptoms begin quickly, as soon as several hours after the last cigarette. They generally peak within the first few days and are usually minimal by 30 days. Some smokers, however, complain of tobacco cravings for months or even years after quitting.

10. **What happens to pulmonary function tests with smoking? Upon cessation?**
    The forced expiratory volume in 1 second (FEV_1) has been used as the primary measure of pulmonary function in several studies. Among all persons over the age of 45 years, the FEV_1 declines at a rate of approximately 20 mL/yr as a natural consequence of aging. In the Lung Health Study, patients with chronic obstructive pulmonary disease (COPD) who continued to

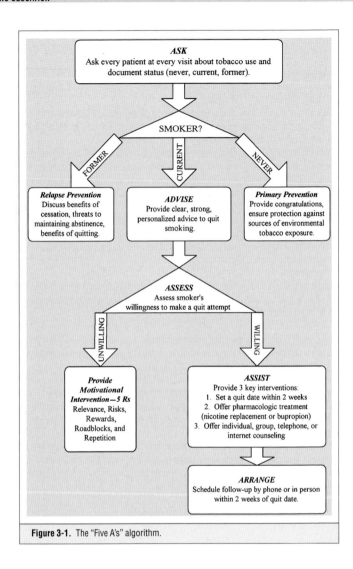

Figure 3-1. The "Five A's" algorithm.

smoke showed a steeper rate of decline in FEV_1 of about 62 mL/yr. Patients who were able to quit successfully reduced their rate of decline to that of nonsmokers.

Scanlon PD, Connett JE, Waller LA, et al: Smoking cessation and lung function in mild-to-moderate chronic obstructive pulmonary disease—The Lung Health Study. Am J Respir Crit Care Med 161:381–390, 2000.

11. **What are some short-term health benefits of smoking cessation?**
    1. The excess risk of premature coronary heart disease falls by one-half within 1 year of abstinence.
    2. Some of the toxic effects of cigarette smoking that may lead to cardiac events, such as increased platelet activation, elevated carbon monoxide levels, and coronary artery spasm, are immediately reversible with cessation.

3. Pregnant women who stop during the first 3–4 months of pregnancy eliminate their excess risk of having a low-birth-weight baby.

12. **What are some long-term benefits of smoking cessation?**
    Data from 50 years of follow-up on male British physicians suggest that
    1. Men who stop smoking before age 50 cut their age-specific mortality rate in half and extend their life by 6 years compared to continuing smokers.
    2. Men who quit smoking by age 30 have a similar life expectancy to those who never smoked, which is 10 years longer than that of continuing smokers.

    Doll R, Peto R, Boreham J, Sutherland I: Mortality in relation to smoking: 50 years' observations on male British doctors. BMJ 328:1519, 2004.

KEY POINTS: FIVE CANCERS CAUSALLY RELATED TO CIGARETTE SMOKING

1. Lung (all types)

2. Oral cavity (lip, tongue, mouth floor, and pharynx)

3. Laryngeal

4. Esophageal

5. Pancreatic

---

13. **How much weight do people gain after they quit smoking?**
    Several studies on the effects of smoking on weight have shown that ex-smokers gain more weight over time than nonsmokers or active smokers. The typical weight gain associated with smoking cessation ranges from 2.5–4.5 kg (5–10 lb). Women tend to gain slightly more weight than men. Genetic predisposition, younger age, and reduced physical activity may increase the risk for weight gain.

    Rigotti N: Treatment of tobacco use and dependence. N Engl J Med 346: 506–512, 2002.

14. **Who should receive nicotine replacement therapy (NRT) when trying to quit smoking?**
    The U.S. Public Health Service recommends that all persons who are ready to make a quit attempt, in the absence of contraindications, should be offered NRT when trying to quit smoking.

    Fiore MC, Bailey WC, Cohen SJ, et al: Treating Tobacco Use and Dependence: A Clinical Practice Guideline. Rockville, MD, U.S. Department of Health and Human Services, 2000, pp 71–75.

15. **How do different types of nicotine replacement therapy work?**
    Nicotine gum contains nicotine bound in a gum base, which allows the nicotine to be released slowly. Once released, the nicotine is absorbed through the buccal mucosa.
    The nicotine inhalation system consists of a mouthpiece and a cartridge that contains 10 mg of nicotine. Nicotine is released when air is inhaled through the assembled device. Each puff delivers 13 μg of nicotine, so 80 puffs are needed to obtain the amount of nicotine found in a typical cigarette.
    The nicotine nasal spray is an aqueous solution of nicotine. One spray is delivered to each nostril, and the nicotine is rapidly absorbed through the mucous membranes. Because of its rapid absorption, the nasal spray has been found to have more dependence potential than other forms of nicotine replacement.

The nicotine transdermal patch is composed of an adhesive base with a thin film of nicotine. The nicotine is absorbed across the skin, giving relatively steady serum nicotine concentrations.

Nicotine lozenges, the most recently approved replacement formulation, contain nicotine in a hard base. The slowly dissolving base allows nicotine to be absorbed through the mucous membranes of the mouth.

16. How should smokers use nicotine gum and lozenges?

Nicotine gum and lozenges are both available over the counter in 2- and 4-mg strengths. Patients should be instructed to chew the gum on a fixed schedule, at least one piece every 1–2 hours, and to continue for at least 1–3 months. The patient should chew it slowly until a tingling sensation is felt and then should hold it between the cheek and teeth for maximal buccal absorption. Heavy smokers (i.e., those who used more than 25 cigarettes per day) should use the 4-mg dose of gum.

For the lozenges, users should be instructed to use 1–2 lozenges every hour for 6 weeks and then to taper the dose over the next 6 weeks. Patients should not chew or swallow the lozenge or eat or drink anything while using it because these activities will decrease buccal absorption of nicotine.

17. How do you decide which form of NRT to use?

All forms of NRT have similar efficacy, resulting in quit rates nearly double those of placebo. Choice of NRT is largely dictated by patient preference. Patches appear to be the easiest to use and are generally preferred by patients. Smokers who struggle with the habitual nature of smoking behavior may prefer an inhaler, lozenges, or gum.

18. What are the contraindications to NRT?

Although package inserts recommend caution in using nicotine products in patients with cardiovascular disease, studies of patch use show no association between NRT and acute cardiovascular events, even in patients who smoke intermittently while using the patch. The nicotine nasal spray should not be used in persons with severe reactive airway disease. Pregnant and breast-feeding smokers should be urged to quit first without any pharmacologic therapy. NRT should be offered only if the potential benefits of the increased chance of abstinence afforded by these products outweigh their risks.

19. What is the role of bupropion SR (Zyban) in smoking cessation?

Bupropion SR is a dopamine and norepinephrine reuptake inhibitor. It is the only antidepressant approved in the United States for smoking cessation. The Cochrane Review reports that initial quit rates with bupropion SR are double those of placebo. Bupropion may be more effective in heavier smokers and may also assist in preventing relapse in successful quitters.

Hays JT, Hurt RD, Rigotti NA, et al: Sustained-release bupropion for pharmacologic relapse prevention after smoking cessation: A randomized, controlled trial. Ann Intern Med 135(6):423–433, 2001.

Hughes J, Stead L, Lancaster T: Antidepressants for smoking cessation. Cochrane Database Syst Rev (4): CD000031, 2004.

20. How is bupropion SR prescribed?

Patients should be instructed to begin bupropion therapy 1 week before their target smoking quit date. The recommended dosage is 150 mg per day for 3 days and then 150 mg twice daily for the duration of treatment. There is, however, evidence that success rates are just as high in patients using just 150 mg per day and that adverse effects may be more common with the higher dose. While smokers are encouraged to continue bupropion for 7–12 weeks after their quit date, use for several months may improve long-term quit rates.

21. What are the contraindications to bupropion SR therapy?

Bupropion SR should not be prescribed to patients who have a seizure disorder, who have a current or former diagnosis of bulimia or anorexia nervosa, or who have used a monoamine oxidase (MAO) inhibitor within the previous 2 weeks. Bupropion SR is a Food and Drug

KEY POINTS: FDA-APPROVED PHARMACOLOGIC THERAPIES FOR SMOKING CESSATION

1. Bupropion SR (Zyban)

2. Nicotine gum

3. Nicotine inhalers

4. Nicotine nasal sprays

5. Nicotine patches

6. Nicotine lozenges

Administration (FDA) Class B drug in pregnancy. As with use of nicotine replacement therapy, bupropion SR should be used only after a pregnant woman has failed to quit without pharmacotherapy and the benefits of an increased chance of smoking cessation outweigh the risks of using it.

22. **Can combination therapies be used effectively?**
    1. **Nicotine patch with nicotine gum or nasal spray:** A meta-analysis of three studies found that combination nicotine therapy is almost twice as effective as monotherapy. While the patient is receiving a relatively constant amount of nicotine through the patch, he or she can adjust the dose on an acute basis using a second agent. Combination therapy is recommended only when monotherapy has failed.
    2. **Nicotine patch and bupropion SR:** One randomized, controlled trial comparing the nicotine patch alone, bupropion SR alone, and a combination of bupropion SR and the patch found that the combination is safe and significantly increases quit rates compared to the patch alone but not compared to bupropion SR alone.

23. **Are there other effective pharmacologic therapies for smoking cessation?**
    Two other drugs, nortriptyline and clonidine, are considered second-line therapies for tobacco dependence. Neither is FDA approved for this indication. Patients failing first-line treatments may be candidates for either drug.
    1. **Nortriptyline:** Dosing ranges from 25–150 mg per day, with treatment periods from 12 weeks to 1 year. Side effects of nortriptyline, such as dry mouth and sedation, often limit its usefulness.
    2. **Clonidine:** An alpha$_2$ receptor agonist, it has been shown to nearly double the rate of successful quitting. It is initially started at 0.1 mg twice daily, and therapy generally lasts from 1–3 months. Side effects similar to nortriptyline can be problematic.

24. **Which societal interventions have been instituted to help curb smoking?**
    1. Increased tobacco taxes
    2. Mass-media tobacco education and counteradvertising campaigns
    3. Business and workplace indoor smoking bans
    4. Restricted youth access to tobacco
    5. Phone "quitlines" and internet-based counseling resources for patients and healthcare providers

    http://www.quitnet.com
    http://www.surgeongeneral.gov/tobacco

CHAPTER 4

PULMONARY REHABILITATION

Bonnie F. Fahy, RN, MN

1. **What is the definition of pulmonary rehabilitation?**
   Pulmonary rehabilitation was defined in 1999 by the American Thoracic Society (ATS) as "a multidisciplinary program of care for patients with chronic respiratory impairment that is individually tailored and designed to optimize physical and social performance and autonomy."

   American Thoracic Society: ATS statement: Pulmonary rehabilitation—1999. Am J Respir Crit Care Med 159:1666–1682, 1999.

2. **Who is a candidate for pulmonary rehabilitation?**
   Pulmonary rehabilitation should be considered for every patient with chronic lung disease, both obstructive and restrictive, who, despite optimal medical management, has dyspnea or other respiratory symptoms, reduced exercise tolerance, any restriction in activities because of lung disease, or impaired health status.

   Global Initiative for Chronic Obstructive Lung Disease (GOLD) 2005 Guidelines for the care of the patient with chronic obstructive pulmonary disease (COPD) recommends that all patients with GOLD Stage II (moderate), GOLD Stage III (severe), or GOLD Stage IV (very severe) lung disease have pulmonary rehabilitation added to their therapeutic regime.

   http://www.goldcopd.com

3. **Who is *not* a candidate for pulmonary rehabilitation?**
   Patients who are unable to participate (e.g., because of severe arthritis or a psychiatric disorder) or who have an unstable concomitant condition (e.g., unstable angina) that may place them at risk are usually not candidates for pulmonary rehabilitation.

4. **Patients with pulmonary hypertension (PH) were once thought not to be candidates for pulmonary rehabilitation. Has this thinking changed?**
   Yes. Since the inclusion of patients with PH in pulmonary rehabilitation programs as part of pre-transplant care has been shown to result in improved physical conditioning, patients with PH are now receiving pulmonary rehabilitation at specialty centers with staff who have experience caring for PH patients.

   American Association of Cardiovascular and Pulmonary Rehabilitation: AACVPR Guidelines for Pulmonary Rehabilitation Programs, 3rd ed. Champaign, IL, Human Kinetics, 2004, pp 77–79.

5. **What are the goals of pulmonary rehabilitation?**
   The goals of pulmonary rehabilitation are:
   - Relief of symptoms
   - Improvement in exercise tolerance
   - Improvement in health status
   - Prevention of disease progression by avoidance of complications and exacerbations
   - Reduction in mortality

   Pulmonary rehabilitation does not change lung function except for a minimal change that can be attributed to instruction in the effective use of bronchodilators.

6. **Why is it important to refer a patient to a comprehensive pulmonary rehabilitation program rather than sending the patient to a program that provides only exercise training?**
If the patient is going to invest time and energy in rehabilitation, he or she will appreciate receiving the most comprehensive services available. Additionally, some insurance providers reimburse for pulmonary rehabilitation only once in a lifetime, and it is unfortunate when a patient has utilized this one-time benefit on a suboptimal program.

7. **How will I know if I am referring my patient to a comprehensive pulmonary rehabilitation program?**
Question the program coordinator regarding program content or locate a program that has been nationally certified by the American Association of Cardiovascular and Pulmonary Rehabilitation (AACVPR). An AACVPR-certified program has been evaluated and found to have the essential standards of care for pulmonary rehabilitation. A listing of AACVPR-certified programs is available at http://www.aacvpr.org/certification/

8. **What is meant by self-management education?**
Traditional patient education, which simply provides the patient with information related to the condition and its therapy, is being enhanced in pulmonary rehabilitation programs by emphasis being given to self-management education. Self-management education teaches specific skills to manage chronic disease and to guide health behavior modification. These skills increase self-efficacy with the goal of improving clinical outcomes including adherence to therapies. An example of a self-management skill is early identification of an exacerbation.

KEY POINTS: ESSENTIAL COMPONENTS OF COMPREHENSIVE PULMONARY REHABILITATION

1. Exercise training

2. Self-management education

3. Psychosocial and behavioral intervention

4. Nutritional therapy

5. Outcome assessment

6. Promotion of long-term adherence

9. **What specific topics should be taught during the education sessions?**
The curriculum presented must be individualized to the patient's needs, with the needs being identified during the initial assessment. Educational topics include:
- Breathing strategies
- Normal lung function and pathophysiology of lung disease
- Proper use of medications, including oxygen
- Bronchial hygiene techniques
- Benefits of exercise and maintaining physical activities
- Energy conservation and work-simplification techniques
- Eating right

- Irritant avoidance, including smoking cessation
- Prevention and early treatment of respiratory exacerbations
- Indications for calling the health care provider
- Leisure, travel, and sexuality
- Coping with chronic lung disease and end-of-life planning
- Anxiety and panic control, including relaxation techniques and stress management

10. **Which breathing strategies should be taught in pulmonary rehabilitation?**
Traditionally, the breathing strategies that are taught in pulmonary rehabilitation are pursed lip breathing and diaphragmatic breathing. Pursed lip breathing is known to help prevent airway collapse and to reduce respiratory rate and dyspnea while improving tidal volume and oxygen saturation. Results from the use of diaphragmatic breathing have not been as convincing; no data from controlled studies support this breathing strategy. Despite these findings, patients find that diaphragmatic breathing, in combination with pursed lip breathing, allows them to remain in control of their breathing instead of having their breathing control them.

11. **How do you exercise a dyspneic, frightened patient?**
Start slowly and offer much reassurance. The patient's baseline exercise ability is assessed by a simple exercise tolerance test (e.g., a walk distance test). From these data, an individualized exercise prescription is devised, emphasizing endurance rather than speed or strength. Although treadmills are the most common exercise mode in pulmonary rehabilitation, treadmills may be intimidating to the severely limited patient. Pushing a rollator (a walker with four large wheels) will build confidence, and transference to the treadmill will follow. Upper extremity exercises are equally important and follow the same tenet of first building endurance and then building strength.

12. **What are the benefits of adding strength training to endurance training in pulmonary rehabilitation?**
Strength training has greater potential for increasing muscle mass and strength than endurance training. Strength training may result in less dyspnea, thereby making this type of exercise easier to tolerate than aerobic training in some patients. For improvements in muscle strength and endurance, a combination of strength and endurance exercise is optimal.

> Ortega F, Toral J, Cejudo P, et al: Comparison of effects of strength and endurance training in patients with chronic obstructive pulmonary disease. Am J Respir Crit Care Med 166:669–674, 2002.

13. **Is a group setting preferred over one-to-one instruction in pulmonary rehabilitation?**
Yes. The major advantage of a group setting is that it brings patients with similar problems together. "Misery loves company" rings true. Patients who exhibit what is thought to be situa-

---

KEY POINTS: SIGNIFICANT AND CLINICALLY MEANINGFUL IMPROVEMENTS FROM PULMONARY REHABILITATION

1. Decrease in dyspnea

2. Increase in exercise ability and functional capacity

3. Improved health status

4. Decreased healthcare utilization

tional depression may improve markedly when they find they are not the only ones with dyspnea or the need for supplemental oxygen. An occasional patient requires referral for in-depth psychological counseling, which should be available in rehabilitation programs. Many rehabilitation programs have ongoing maintenance exercise that serves as a support group. Space should be available for family members to meet while patients are exercising so that they, too, have a support system.

14. **What professional disciplines are included in the pulmonary rehabilitation team?**

The core pulmonary rehabilitation team includes the referring physician, the program medical director, and the program coordinator, who will be an experienced healthcare provider such as a registered nurse, physical therapist, or respiratory therapist. Other team members may include:

- Exercise physiologists
- Dietitians
- Occupational therapists
- Social workers
- Psychologists

http://www.thoracic.org/COPD

15. **Describe the cost and duration of a pulmonary rehabilitation program.**

The cost and duration of pulmonary rehabilitation programs vary regionally because of different policies established by Medicare fiscal intermediaries and other insurance providers. There is no national coverage policy for pulmonary rehabilitation, resulting in each fiscal intermediary establishing a local coverage determination (LCD) for pulmonary rehabilitation. Generally, the cost of a program is far less than one hospital admission. GOLD guidelines state that the optimal length of a program has not been determined, but that the longer the program continues, the more effective the results.

http://www.goldcopd.com

CHAPTER 5

PULMONARY DISABILITY EVALUATION

Oyebode A. Taiwo, MD, MPH, Carrie A. Redlich, MD, MPH, and Akshay Sood, MD, MPH

1. **Explain the difference between impairment and disability.**

   Impairment means a loss of physical or physiologic function. **Disability** refers to the impact of the impairment on the person's life. Impairment may occur without disability. For example, a patient with moderate emphysema working on a word processor may have measurable impairment and little resultant disability. Conversely, disability may occur without impairment. For example, an autobody painter with isocyanate asthma may be disabled from work but may have no measurable impairment if removed from work when the disease process is at an early stage. Two people with the same impairment may have different resultant disabilities.

KEY POINTS: DIFFERENCES BETWEEN DISABILITY AND IMPAIRMENT EVALUATION

1. Impairment means loss of physical or physiologic function.

2. Disability refers to the impact of the impairment on the person's life.

3. Impairment assessment is a medical evaluation performed by physicians.

4. Disability determination is made by administrators based on the information provided by physicians and on criteria for eligibility.

2. **What guides exist for the evaluation of pulmonary impairment and disability?**

   There are several guides with varying standards that often result in different ratings of pulmonary impairment and disability. Social Security, the Department of Veterans' Affairs, and the State Workers' Compensation Boards use different criteria. Other commonly used documents are the American Medical Association (AMA) *Guides to the Evaluation of Permanent Impairment* and the American Thoracic Society (ATS) official statements. Physicians are encouraged to read through the latest editions of these documents before evaluating patients under different compensation systems. Many, but not all, states use the AMA *Guides* for determining workers' compensation. Some pulmonary diseases such as coal workers' pneumoconiosis have their own specific criteria for impairment and disability (see question 17).

   American Medical Association: Guides to the Evaluation of Permanent Impairment, 5th ed. Chicago, American Medical Association, 2001, pp 87–115.

   American Thoracic Society: Evaluation of impairment/disability secondary to respiratory disorders. Am Rev Respir Dis 133(6):1205–1209, 1986.

   Social Security Administration: Disability Evaluation under Social Security. Washington, DC, U.S. Department of Health and Human Services, 2005, pp 24–35. Available at http://www.ssa.gov/disability/professionals/bluebook/Entire-Publication1-2005.pdf.

   Electronic Code of Federal Regulations (e-CFR) Title 38: Pensions, Bonuses, and Veterans' Relief, Volume 1 (Part 4). Schedule for Rating Disabilities: The Respiratory System 4:96–97. Available at http://ecfr.gpoaccess.gov.

3. **Explain the differences between permanent and temporary disability and between partial and total disability.**

A disability may be characterized as either permanent or temporary. A permanent disability is not expected to improve with time and treatment. On the other hand, a temporary disability is likely to be short-term and the patient can be expected to improve to a higher level of function. In addition, a disability may be characterized as partial or total. Total disability usually implies that an individual is unable to do any work, whereas partial disability allows for some level of functioning in the workplace.

4. **Describe the role of a physician in respiratory impairment and disability assessment.**

Physicians determine the presence and severity of a respiratory impairment using objective criteria. Disability determination is made by administrators (often nonclinicians) based on the information provided by physicians on impairment.

5. **What is the Americans with Disabilities Act (ADA)?**

The ADA of 1990 is the federal law that protects individuals who have a disability as defined in the ADA but are qualified to perform the essential functions of a job, with or without reasonable accommodations. A disability is defined by the ADA as a physical or mental impairment that *substantially* limits one or more of the major life activities of such an individual. The ADA prohibits pre-employment medical examinations. An employer is also prohibited from making inquiries of a job applicant as to whether he or she is an individual with a disability or as to the nature or severity of any such disability.

Department of Justice: Americans with Disability Act, Public Law, 1990, pp 101–336. Available at http://www.usdoj.gov/crt/ada/publicat.htm#Anchor-14210.

Matson CC, Holleman WL, Nosek M, Wilkinson W: Impact of the Americans with Disabilities Act on family physicians. J Fam Pract 36(2):201–206, 1993.

6. **What is the role of a physician under the ADA?**

After a conditional offer of employment, an employer may require an employment entrance examination. The purpose of this examination is to determine if an individual can perform the essential functions of a job in a safe manner. These examinations must be given to all individuals offered the job conditionally, regardless of health status. The clinician performs the employment entrance examination keeping all the medical information obtained confidential and advises the employer and nonmedical personnel on issues regarding restrictions on the work or duties of the employee and necessary accommodations.

Matson CC, Holleman WL, Nosek M, Wilkinson W: Impact of the Americans with Disabilities Act on family physicians. J Fam Pract 36(2):201–206, 1993.

7. **What is accommodation?**

Accommodation is the process of making workplace adjustments to permit a person with impairment to continue to work. Even when impairment cannot be eliminated by medical treatment following an illness, a physician may serve as a member of an interdisciplinary team to significantly diminish the consequent disability. For example, modification of chemical exposures may be possible or a worker may be transferred to another department that does not deal with a specific chemical agent or process.

8. **What is workers' compensation?**

Workers' compensation is a no-fault system of insurance in which insurers or employers pay benefits to an employee with an injury or illness caused by a workplace exposure or accident. In return, the worker gives up his or her rights to sue the employer for the injury. Workers' compensation laws vary from state to state. Physicians play an important role in workers' compensation. They are obligated to diagnose and treat work-related illness and to assist the patient with the documentation to file claim for benefits. Some states require that all work-related diseases be reported to the State Department of Health.

9. **How does one determine whether a respiratory disease is work related?**
A detailed occupational exposure history is required to establish the diagnosis of an occupational lung disease. This includes all employments. Exposures to specific respiratory agents in the workplace, such as dusts, fumes, vapors, and allergens, should be noted, clarifying the timing, duration, and dose of exposure when possible, as well as the use of a personal respiratory protective device. Temporal associations between exposures and symptoms should be carefully documented, including onset and changes in relationship to work. Presence of similar complaints or diseases in coworkers is also helpful in establishing an occupational etiology.

10. **Define a preexisting respiratory condition.**
This refers to any impairment or disease that existed prior to the onset of another disease. For example, an individual may have a history of preexisting childhood asthma which was made worse by workplace exposure to respiratory irritants. A preexisting condition can be *exacerbated* if the individual temporarily became worse and then returned to his or her baseline, or the preexisting condition can be *aggravated* if the individual became worse but never returned to baseline (i.e., the individual now has persistence of symptoms and requires more asthma medications). In practice, both new-onset respiratory disorders and preexisting respiratory disorders made worse by workplace exposures are considered work-related lung diseases; thus, both are compensable.

11. **How certain do I need to be that an impairment is due to an occupational exposure when dealing with workers' compensation cases?**
The level of certainty required in determining causation for workers' compensation is different from the usual standard of 95% certainty used in medical research. The commonly accepted standard of certainty that an illness was caused by an occupational exposure is one of "more probable than not," or a level of certainty greater than 50%.

12. **What is the role of pulmonary function tests in evaluating lung impairment?**
The most commonly used test of pulmonary function is spirometry. In obstructive airway disease, the spirometry should be done after the administration of inhaled bronchodilators. In Crapo et al, test results are expressed as percentage of predicted normal values, which are based on the individual's height, age, and gender, and need to be race-corrected for African Americans. In addition, the lower limit of normal is calculated as lying at the 5th percentile of the reference population. The AMA classification of respiratory impairment is outlined below (Table 5-1). At least one of these measures of ventilatory function should be abnormal to the degree described in that class if the impairment is to be rated in that class.

American Medical Association: Guides to the Evaluation of Permanent Impairment, 5th ed. Chicago, American Medical Association, 2001, pp 87–115.
Crapo RO, Morris AH: Standardized single breath normal values for carbon monoxide diffusing capacity. Am Rev Respir Dis 123(2):185–189, 1981.
Crapo RO, Morris AH, Gardner RM: Reference spirometric values using techniques and equipment that meet ATS recommendations. Am Rev Respir Dis 123(6):659–664, 1981.

13. **Should arterial blood gas levels be measured routinely in evaluating lung impairment?**
Blood-gas determination is considered invasive, difficult to standardize, and poorly correlated with exercise capacity. For most persons with obstructive lung diseases, the forced expiratory volume in 1 second (FEV_1) correlates better with exercise capacity than does PaO_2. However, if hypoxemia is suspected, blood-gas measurement is recommended. According to the AMA guide, resting hypoxia indicates severe impairment; it is defined as PaO_2 of 55 mmHg on room

TABLE 5-1.   AMERICAN MEDICAL ASSOCIATION CLASSIFICATION OF RESPIRATORY IMPAIRMENT

Test Parameter	Class 1:	Class 2:	Class 3:	Class 4:
(As Percentage of Predicted Normal Value)	0–9% Impairment of the Whole Person	10–25% Impairment of the Whole Person	26–50% Impairment of the Whole Person	51–100% Impairment of the Whole Person
FVC	≥Lower limit of normal	≥60 and <lower limit of normal	51–59%	≤50%
FEV$_1$	≥Lower limit of normal	≥60 and <lower limit of normal	41–59%	≤40%
D$_L$CO	≥Lower limit of normal	≥60 and <lower limit of normal	41–59%	≤40%
VO$_2$max (mL/kg-min)	≥25	≥20 and <25	≥15 and <20	<15 (or <1.05 L/min)
METs	≥7.1	5.7–7.1	4.5–5.6	<4.5

D$_L$CO = diffusing capacity of carbon monoxide; FEV$_1$ = forced expiratory volume in 1 second; FVC = forced vital capacity; METs = multiple of basal oxygen consumption, approximately 3.5 mL/min/kg; VO$_2$max = maximal oxygen uptake, a measure of maximum exercise capacity.
Adapted from American Medical Association: Guides to the Evaluation of Permanent Impairment, 5th ed, Chicago, American Medical Association, 2001.

air at sea level or PaO$_2$ of less than 60 mmHg in the presence of pulmonary hypertension, cor pulmonale, erythrocytosis, or increasingly severe hypoxia during exercise. Hypoxemia should be documented on two occasions that are at least 4 weeks apart.

American Medical Association: Guides to the Evaluation of Permanent Impairment, 5th ed. Chicago, American Medical Association, 2001, pp 87–115.

14. **When should a cardiopulmonary exercise test be ordered?**
In patients in whom subjective dyspnea is disproportionate to the pulmonary function test result or for those in whom the latter is difficult to interpret because of submaximal performance, a cardiopulmonary exercise test may be considered. Although some have suggested that this test may also be used to determine if a patient can perform a job with a known energy requirement, this is rarely needed. Determination of work capacity can usually be predicted based on the severity of the respiratory disorder and the job description.

American Thoracic Society: Evaluation of impairment/disability secondary to respiratory disorders. Am Rev Respir Dis133(6):1205–1209, 1986.
American Thoracic Society, American College of Chest Physicians: ATS/ACCP Statement on cardiopulmonary exercise testing. Am J Respir Crit Care Med, 2003. 167(2):211–277. Available at http://www.thoracic.org/adobe/statements/cardioexercise.pdf.

15. **List some conditions in which the subjective symptoms may exceed the measured pulmonary impairment.**
- Reversible and episodic pulmonary diseases such as asthma and vocal cord dysfunction
- Nonpulmonary diseases such as myocardial ischemia, pulmonary vascular diseases, and anemia

- Psychogenic causes such as panic attacks
- Multiple chemical sensitivity syndrome
- Malingering
- Deconditioning

16. **Does any test identify malingering?**
Fortunately, frank malingering is uncommon. Unfortunately, there is no perfect test to identify a malingerer. However, the following steps can be taken to evaluate a patient when malingering is suspected:
   - Make sure the patient understands the purpose and the performance of the pulmonary function test.
   - Review test results to ensure that the patient has given a good and reproducible effort.
   - Cardiopulmonary exercise testing may be helpful when a disparity exists between subjective symptoms and objective findings.

17. **Are there any pulmonary diseases that have their own specific criteria for impairment and disability?**
Several pulmonary diseases, such as asthma and certain pneumoconiosis, have their own specific criteria for impairment and disability. For example, miners with coal workers' pneumoconiosis can apply for compensation under a specific federal legislation popularly known as the "Black Lung Act." According to the AMA guide, lung cancers are a cause of severe impairment at the time of diagnosis. If, at reevaluation 1 year later, no evidence of tumor is found, then impairment is calculated on the basis of the degree of physiologic impairment present at that time.

   American Medical Association: Guides to the Evaluation of Permanent Impairment. 5th ed. Chicago, American Medical Association, 2001, pp 87–115.
   http://www.oalj.dol.gov/public/blalung/refrnc/30_cont.htm.

18. **Since airflow obstruction in asthmatics varies at different times, how is their impairment rated?**
Under the ATS and AMA guides, an asthmatic's impairment is scored on the following three parameters:
   - Post-bronchodilator FEV_1
   - Percentage of change in FEV_1 after bronchodilator use or degree of airway hyper-responsiveness as defined by the concentration of a test agent, commonly methacholine, that provokes a fall in FEV_1 of 20% from baseline PC_{20}
   - The need for bronchodilators and steroids to control symptoms
   The sum of the above scores is used to calculate the degree of impairment. Before an asthmatic is permitted to return to work, the workplace should be assessed to ensure that no triggers for asthma are present.

   American Medical Association: Guides to the Evaluation of Permanent Impairment, 5th ed. Chicago, American Medical Association, 2001, pp 87–115.
   American Thoracic Society, Medical Section of the American Lung Association: Guidelines for the evaluation of impairment/disability in patients with asthma. Am Rev Respir Dis 147(4):1056–1061, 1993.

19. **How are impairment and disability determined in patients with occupational asthma?**
The ATS and AMA guides place patients with asthma induced by sensitizers such as isocyanates in a unique category. The recommended treatment for this condition is to completely remove the worker from further exposure. In some individuals, in the absence of exposure to the specific agent, physiologic tests may be normal and symptoms may be absent. Such patients are considered 100% disabled (even though they may not have measurable impairment) for any job that exposes them to the causative agent. A respirator may not be able to protect such a patient from low levels of the sensitizing agent that might trigger an attack. Relocation to a new job and vocational

training should be considered. Assessment for long-term disability should be done approximately 2 years after removal from exposure when improvement has been shown to plateau. The evaluation should then be done using the guide for nonoccupational asthma.

American Medical Association: Guides to the Evaluation of Permanent Impairment, 5th ed. Chicago, American Medical Association, 2001, pp 87–115.

American Thoracic Society, Medical Section of the American Lung Association: Guidelines for the evaluation of impairment/disability in patients with asthma. Am Rev Respir Dis 147(4):1056–1061, 1993.

20. **When several factors are responsible for causing lung disease, how does a physician apportion the different factors to the resultant disease?**
Apportionment describes the relative contribution of multiple factors to the disease. For example, cigarette smoking may be a contributory factor in certain occupational diseases, such as lung cancer, in asbestos-exposed workers. Often it is difficult, if not impossible, to determine the relative roles of different factors in disease causation. In these conditions, physicians are asked to state their opinion, taking into consideration the body of available knowledge in that area. The usual standard for workers' compensation is whether the occupational exposure has been a substantial contributing factor in causing or increasing the impairment.

KEY POINTS: STEPS FOR IMPAIRMENT AND DISABILITY EVALUATION

1. Establish a diagnosis of respiratory disorder.

2. Determine the severity of the respiratory disorder using objective criteria (e.g., pulmonary function tests, cardiopulmonary exercise tests, and imaging studies).

3. Assess impairment using appropriate criteria (e.g., AMA, ATS, and Social Security criteria).

4. Answer any other questions asked (e.g., apportionment, restrictions, causality, or work-relatedness).

5. Generate a report for use by administrators to determine disability or eligibility for benefits.

21. **What should a physician write in an impairment evaluation report?**
All is lost if an appropriate evaluation report is not written. The following suggestions are helpful:
- The diagnosis and severity of the respiratory disorder should be stated clearly.
- The specific questions asked should be answered in clear lay terminology.
- The specific compensation system guidelines should be followed to evaluate the presence and severity of impairment. Furthermore, the impairment should be rated as temporary or permanent.
- In occupational cases, the work relationship to disease causation should be stated and, if asked, apportionment should be addressed.
- It is also appropriate to describe work that a patient can and cannot perform and to make recommendations for vocational rehabilitation, if necessary.

CHAPTER 6

PREOPERATIVE ASSESSMENT OF THE PULMONARY PATIENT

Katherine Habeeb, MD, FCCP

1. **What is the definition of postoperative pulmonary complications (PPCs)?**

   PPCs can be defined as pulmonary abnormalities that result in identifiable disease or dysfunction and adversely impact the patient's clinical course. They include atelectasis, acute infection such as tracheobronchitis or pneumonia, exacerbation of underlying chronic lung disease, bronchospasm, respiratory failure with prolonged mechanical ventilation, and thromboembolic disease. These conditions are a significant cause of morbidity and mortality. Approximately one-fourth of deaths occurring within 6 days of surgery are attributed to postoperative pulmonary complications.

   Arozullah A, Conde M, Lawrence V: Preoperative evaluation for postoperative pulmonary complications. Med Clin North Am 87:153–173, 2003.
   Smetana G: Preoperative pulmonary evaluation. N Engl J Med 340:937–944, 1999.

2. **Which patients are at increased risk of developing PPCs?**

   Several patient-related factors are known to be associated with an increased risk of PPCs. These include the presence of chronic obstructive pulmonary disease (COPD), asthma, active smoking, current respiratory infection, and poor general health status as classified by the American Society of Anesthesiologists (ASA); in other words, ASA Class II or greater. The most important patient-related factor is chronic lung disease, which has an odds ratio of development of a PPC as high as 5.8. Advanced age and morbid obesity, while once thought to relate to increased risk, have not consistently been shown to be independent predictors.

   McAlister FA, Kahn NA, Straus SE, et al: Accuracy of the preoperative assessment in predicting pulmonary risk after nonthoracic surgery. Am J Respir Crit Care Med 167:741–744, 2003.
   Smetana G: Preoperative pulmonary evaluation. N Engl J Med 340:937–944, 1999.

3. **Does smoking cessation prior to surgery lower the risk of postoperative pulmonary complications?**

   Prospective studies have found that in patients undergoing elective noncardiac surgery, smoking is associated with more than a fivefold risk of PPCs. The risk is increased even in the absence of chronic lung disease, especially for those patients with a more than 20 pack-year history. Data inferred from cohort studies on cardiac bypass patients suggests that smokers can reduce their rate of PPCs by refraining from smoking for at least 8 weeks prior to elective surgery. Short-term abstinence has not been shown to lower the rate of PPCs, and some evidence suggests that it may actually lead to increased risk, possibly due to decreased sputum clearance.

   Regardless of the time frame, smoking cessation is always encouraged, and the clinician should use the preoperative evaluation as an opportunity to counsel patients on the benefits of lifelong smoking cessation.

   Arozullah A, Conde M, Lawrence V: Preoperative evaluation for postoperative pulmonary complications. Med Clin North Am 87:153–173, 2003.
   Rock P, Passannante A: Preoperative assessment: Pulmonary. Anesthesiol Clin North Am 22: 77–91, 2004.

4. **What surgical factors can affect the risk of developing postoperative pulmonary complications?**

Surgical factors that may affect pulmonary risk include the surgical site, the duration of the surgery, the type of anesthesia, and the type of neuromuscular blockade. Complication rates are significantly greater with thoracic or upper abdominal surgery. Surgical procedures of greater than 4 hours in duration have been shown to increase the risk for postoperative pneumonia. Although it is somewhat controversial, a recent review of 141 trials comparing outcomes from neuraxial blockade versus general anesthesia concluded that there is a risk reduction with the use of either epidural or spinal anesthesia. Lastly, long-acting neuromuscular blockers such as pancuronium lead to residual neuromuscular blockade and should be avoided in patients who are at a higher risk of developing pulmonary complications.

Arozullah A, Conde M, Lawrence V: Preoperative evaluation for postoperative pulmonary complications. Med Clin North Am 87:153–173, 2003.

Pedersen T, Eliasen K, Henriksen E: A prospective study of risk factors and cardiopulmonary complications associated with anaesthesia and surgery: Risk indicators of cardiopulmonary morbidity. Acta Anaesthesiol Scand 34: 144–155, 1990.

Rodgers A, Walker N, Schug S, et al: Reduction of postoperative mortality and morbidity with epidural or spinal anesthesia: Results from overview of randomized trials. BMJ 321:1493, 2000.

5. **Why is the surgical site so important?**

The surgical site is the most important factor when it comes to predicting overall risk for the development of PPCs. In fact, the incidence of PPCs is inversely related to the surgical site's distance from the diaphragm. The highest rates are seen with thoracic and upper abdominal surgeries and are due to diaphragmatic dysfunction, splinting, and the inability to take deep breaths. Perioperative alterations in lung volumes and ventilation patterns may result in hypoxemia and atelectasis. Complication rates range from 19–59% for thoracic surgery and 17–76% for upper abdominal surgery, as compared to 0–5% for lower abdominal surgery. Abdominal aortic aneurysm repair carries among the highest risk rates for PPC. Randomized trials have shown that some laparoscopic procedures can significantly reduce the risk of respiratory complications.

Arozullah A, Conde M, Lawrence V: Preoperative evaluation for postoperative pulmonary complications. Med Clin North Am 87:153–173, 2003.

Arozullah A, Khuri S, Henderson W, et al: Development and validation of a multifactorial risk index for predicting postoperative pneumonia after major noncardiac surgery. Ann Intern Med 135:847–857, 2001.

Smetana G: Preoperative pulmonary evaluation. N Engl J Med 340:937–944, 1999.

6. **Describe the expected postoperative changes in pulmonary function tests.**

After cardiac or upper abdominal surgery there is a reduction in vital capacity (VC), tidal volume, and functional residual capacity (FRC), which can lead to ventilation/perfusion (V/Q) mismatch and hypoxemia. VC can temporarily be reduced to 50–60% of the preoperative measurement. The respiratory rate is generally increased so that overall minute ventilation does not change. The FRC is reduced to 50% of baseline but generally returns toward normal by the fifth postoperative day. In comparison, lower abdominal surgery can be associated with a 35% loss in VC, but this is usually clinically insignificant and resolves within 24 hours. Laparoscopic surgery can also be associated with a transient 30% reduction in VC as well as diaphragmatic dysfunction. Compared to open procedures, however, there is less impairment of the forced expiratory volume in 1 second (FEV_1), the forced vital capacity (FVC), arterial oxygenation, and ventilation with the laparoscopic approach.

Olsen G: Preoperative assessment of the pulmonary patient. In Parsons P, Heffner J (eds): Pulmonary/Respiratory Therapy Secrets, 2nd ed. Philadelphia, Hanley & Belfus, 2002, p 494.

Putensen-Himmer G, Putensen C, et al: Comparison of postoperative respiratory function after laparoscopy or open laparotomy for cholecystectomy. Anesthesiology 77:675–80, 1992.

KEY POINTS: POSTOPERATIVE PULMONARY COMPLICATIONS

1. The most important *patient-related* risk factor for the development of postoperative pulmonary complications is the presence of chronic lung disease.

2. The incidence of postoperative pulmonary complications is inversely related to the distance of the surgical site from the diaphragm.

3. Active smokers are at increased risk of developing pulmonary complications; smoking cessation at least 8 weeks prior to surgery can reduce this risk.

4. Management of chronic pulmonary diseases such as COPD, asthma, or obstructive sleep apnea (OSA) should be maximized prior to surgery.

7. **How is diaphragmatic function altered after surgery?**
Diaphragmatic dysfunction occurs following thoracic or upper abdominal surgery and contributes significantly to PPCs. This dysfunction is not necessarily related to residual neuromuscular block-ade or to suboptimal pain relief. Physiologic studies have shown that the inherent contractility of the diaphragm itself does not appear to be impaired and the phrenic nerves respond normally when maximally stimulated. The important etiologic factor for diaphragmatic dysfunction appears to be inhibitory reflexes from sympathetic, vagal, or splanchnic receptors. This reduced function can persist for up to 7 days postoperatively.

   Olsen G: Preoperative assessment of the pulmonary patient. In Parsons P, Heffner J (eds): Pulmonary/Respiratory Therapy Secrets, 2nd ed. Philadelphia, Hanley & Belfus, 2002, p 494.
   Rock P, Passannante A: Preoperative assessment: pulmonary. Anesthesiol Clin North Am 22:77–91, 2004.

8. **When is it appropriate to obtain preoperative pulmonary function tests (PFTs)?**
The role of preoperative PFTs prior to noncardiothoracic surgery is unclear. Many studies have concluded that individual PFT abnormalities do not accurately predict PPC risk. Often, PFTs only confirm the clinical impression of severe lung disease, which should also be obtained during a complete preoperative history and physical. In 1990, the American College of Physicians (ACP) issued guidelines that recommend preoperative PFTs on the following groups of patients:
   - All lung resection patients
   - Those undergoing coronary bypass surgery or upper abdominal surgery with a history of tobacco use or dyspnea
   - Those with unexplained pulmonary symptoms who are undergoing prolonged or extensive lower abdominal surgery
   - Those with unexplained pulmonary disease who are undergoing head and neck or orthopedic surgery

   American College of Physicians: Preoperative pulmonary function testing. Ann Intern Med 112:793–794, 1990.

9. **Are routine preoperative arterial blood gases (ABGs) useful?**
Routine ABG analysis does not appear to significantly contribute to preoperative pulmonary risk assessment. Several small case series previously identified a higher risk of PPCs for patients with hypercarbia (PaCO$_2$ >45) likely reflecting more severe chronic lung disease. These patients should be identified from other aspects of the preoperative evaluation, however, and there is no level of hypercarbia that is necessarily prohibitive for surgery, even in respect to lung resection. The American College of Physicians recommends preoperative ABG analysis on the following patients:
   - Those undergoing coronary bypass or upper abdominal surgery with a history of tobacco use or dyspnea
   - All patients undergoing lung resection

Hypoxemia has been associated with an increased risk for PPCs in lung resection patients but is otherwise not considered to be an independent risk factor.

American College of Physicians: Preoperative pulmonary function testing. Ann Intern Med 112:793–794, 1990.

Smetana G: Preoperative pulmonary evaluation. N Engl J Med 340:937–944, 1999.

10. **Which patients should have preoperative chest radiographs?**
Routine chest radiographs are of little benefit in risk stratification of healthy patients. A meta-analysis of studies involving 14,390 preoperative chest radiographs found only 14 cases in which the chest radiograph was unexpectedly abnormal and management was influenced. It is well known, however, that chest radiograph abnormalities are seen more frequently with increased age. There are no evidence-based guidelines regarding which patients may benefit from preoperative chest radiographs. One reasonable approach is to consider obtaining a film for all patients over the age of 60 and also for those patients whose clinical findings suggest cardiopulmonary disease and who have not had a film within the last 6 months.

Archer C, Levy AR, McGregor M: Value of routine preoperative chest x-rays: A meta-analysis. Can J Anaesth 40:1022–1027, 1993.

Smetana G: Preoperative pulmonary evaluation. N Engl J Med 340:937–944, 1999.

11. **True or false: The patient with obstructive sleep apnea (OSA) is at increased risk for development of postoperative pulmonary complications.**
True. Sleep-disordered breathing can occur in any patient following major surgery, even without prior OSA diagnosis. A recent retrospective study concluded that patients with OSA undergoing hip and knee replacement had a higher rate of postoperative complications compared with case-matched controls. Patients with OSA are at risk for developing increased episodes of apnea and more severe hypoxemia. Sedatives, anesthetics, and analgesic agents can lead to decreased pharyngeal tone and decreased ventilatory and arousal responses to hypoxia, hypercarbia, and airway obstruction. Supine positioning can also aggravate symptoms of OSA, and airway management is often challenging. Preoperative diagnosis and treatment of OSA is very important from a risk-stratification standpoint. Proper treatment of OSA preoperatively can improve heart function, reduce pulmonary artery hypertension, and normalize blood pressure.

Grupta R, Parvizi J, Hanssen A, Gay P: Postoperative complications in patients with obstructive sleep apnea syndrome undergoing hip of knee replacement: A case-control study. Mayo Clin Proc 76:897–905, 2001.

Rock P, Passannante A: Preoperative assessment: Pulmonary. Anesthesiol Clin North Am 22:77–91, 2004.

12. **Which patients with OSA should be considered for postoperative intensive care unit (ICU) admission?**
Not all patients with OSA will need to be monitored in an ICU setting after surgery. Guidelines for consideration of postoperative ICU admission include:
- Severe OSA, as revealed by preoperative assessment
- Difficult airway management in the operating room
- Morbid obesity (body mass index [BMI] > 30)
- Patient's inability to manage continuous positive airway pressure (CPAP) alone
- Patient very sedated postoperatively and requires opioids for pain control

Rock P, Passannante A: Preoperative assessment: Pulmonary. Anesthesiol Clin North Am 22:77–91, 2004.

Ulnick K, Debo R: Postoperative management of the patient with obstructive sleep apnea. Otolaryngol Head Neck Surg 122:233–236, 2000.

13. **How is the patient with asthma managed?**
Although complication rates for asthmatics undergoing surgery are much lower today than years ago, bronchospasm is one of the most significant complications that can occur during surgery. Risk factors for the development of PPCs in the asthmatic patient include:

- Recent increased asthma symptoms or home rescue beta agonist use
- Recent emergency room visit or requirement of asthma therapy at a medical facility
- Prior history of tracheal intubation for asthma exacerbation

Oral or intravenous steroids in the perioperative period should be considered for all asthmatics at risk for PPCs. Ideally, the steroids should be started 24–48 hours prior to surgery and can be stopped without taper during the postoperative period if there is no evidence of bronchospasm. Higher-dose inhaled steroids may be a reasonable alternative. If wheezing appreciates prior to surgery, inhaled beta agonist, in addition to steroids, should be given. If the wheezing persists, elective surgery should be postponed.

Rock P, Passannante A: Preoperative assessment: pulmonary. Anesthesiol Clin North Am 22:77–91, 2004.

14. **What can be done to reduce the risk for postoperative pulmonary complications in the patient with COPD?**
Patients with COPD should be optimized with routine pulmonary medications including beta-agonists, anticholinergics, and steroids, if appropriate. Preoperative examination should assess and treat for unrecognized cor pulmonale. Additionally, patients with COPD may have chronically fatigued respiratory muscles, which can be exacerbated by poor nutritional status as well as electrolyte and endocrine disorders. These should all be corrected prior to surgery, if possible. Other considerations include antibiotics if there is evidence of lower respiratory tract infection and instruction on lung expansion maneuvers to be used postoperatively. A preoperative finding of hypoxemia warrants further investigation and treatment. Elective surgeries should be postponed until adequate oxygen therapy has been instituted.

Rock P, Passannante A: Preoperative assessment: Pulmonary. Anesthesiol Clin North Am 22:77–91, 2004.
Smetana G: Preoperative pulmonary assessment of the older adult. Clin Geriatr Med 10:35–55, 2003.

KEY POINTS: PREOPERATIVE PULMONARY ASSESSMENT

1. Routine PFTs are not useful in predicting the risk for pulmonary complications and are recommended only in certain groups of patients.

2. ABG analysis does not contribute significantly to the postoperative pulmonary risk assessment in most patients and therefore should not be routinely ordered.

3. Hypercarbia ($PaCO_2 > 45$) is not an absolute contraindication to surgery.

4. Preoperative chest radiographs should be considered in all patients over the age of 60 and in those patients who have not had a recent film and whose clinical assessment reveals cardiopulmonary disease.

5. In evaluating patients for lung resection, a FEV_1 or diffusing capacity for carbon monoxide (DLCO) < 80% of predicted necessitates additional testing to predict postoperative lung function.

15. **What preoperative testing should be done prior to lung resection for cancer?**
The goal of preoperative physiologic testing prior to lung resection is to identify patients who are at high risk for perioperative complications as well as those who will be chronically disabled from the projected loss of lung function. These goals should be achieved using the least invasive testing available. A preoperative cardiovascular risk assessment is essential in all patients given their general advanced age and higher risk of atherosclerosis from cigarette smoking. Spirometry and DLCO are complementary tests that are most commonly used to predict a patient's ability to withstand surgery for lung cancer. $FEV_1 > 2$ liters or $\geq 80\%$ predicted for

pneumonectomy and >1.5 liters for lobectomy are generally levels held to be safe. DLCO can have an even higher correlation with PPC and death. DLCO should be > 80% predicted for consideration of pneumonectomy. The most recent evidence-based recommendations are that if either the FEV_1 or DLCO is <80% predicted, additional testing to predict postoperative lung function should be performed.

Beckles M, Spiro S, Colice G, Rudd R: The physiologic evaluation of patients with lung cancer being considered for resectional surgery. Chest 123:105S–114S, 2003.

16. **How is the predicted postoperative (ppo) lung function calculated?**
Methods to predict postoperative lung function include ventilation scans, perfusion scans, quantitative computed tomography (CT), and simply counting the number of segments removed. The most popular method is to measure the relative function of each lung with a split perfusion scan using tetracycline-labeled macroaggregates of albumen. This technique is easy to perform and allows quantification of the contribution of the parenchyma to be resected. The values are usually reported as a percentage of ppo lung function (%ppo) in order to take into account patient variables such as age, gender, and weight. The %ppo from this method has been shown to correlate well with $ppoFEV_1$ and $ppoD_{LCO}$. The formula for pneumonectomy is:

$$ppoFEV_1 = preoperative\ FEV_1 \times (1 - fraction\ of\ total\ perfusion\ for\ the\ resected\ lung)$$

There is a similar calculation for $ppoFEV_1$ following lobectomy. These formulas can also be used for $ppoD_{LCO}$ calculations. A value of < 40% for $ppoFEV_1$ or $ppoD_{LCO}$ predicts a high risk of cardiopulmonary complications and perioperative mortality. These patients should undergo exercise testing.

Beckles M, Spiro S, Colice G, Rudd R: The physiologic evaluation of patients with lung cancer being considered for resectional surgery. Chest 123:105S–114S, 2003.

Schuurmans M, Diacon A, Bolliger C: Functional evaluation before lung resection. Clin Chest Med 23:159–172, 2002.

17. **How is exercise testing used to evaluate patients for lung resection?**
Oxygen delivery to the entire body, including the heart, the lungs, and the pulmonary and systemic vasculature, can be evaluated through exercise testing. Maximal oxygen consumption (VO_2 max) can estimate a patient's fitness and has been shown to correlate well with postoperative outcome. The VO_2 max can therefore be used as a guide to stratify risk for perioperative complications in lung-resection candidates:
- Patients with a preoperative VO_2 max > 20 mL/kg/min are at no increased risk of complications or death.
- Patients with a VO_2 max < 15 mL/kg/min are at increased risk of complications.
- Patients with a VO_2 max < 10 mL/kg/min are at very high risk of complications and death.

Not all clinicians agree that complication rates can be clearly divided by the above. In general, however, patients with both low %ppo FEV_1 and DLCO values (< 40% predicted) and a VO_2 max of <15 mL/kg/min are at very high surgical risk. These patients should be counseled about nonoperative treatment choices.

Beckles M, Spiro S, Colice G, Rudd R: The physiologic evaluation of patients with lung cancer being considered for resectional surgery. Chest 123:105S-114S, 2003.

CHAPTER 7

POSTOPERATIVE PULMONARY CARE

Jeanine P. Wiener-Kronish, MD, and John M. Taylor, MD

1. **How does general anesthesia affect pulmonary function?**
   Exposure to general anesthetic agents may impair pulmonary gas exchange and result in intraoperative and postoperative hypoxemia. The supine position has been shown to cause a 20% decrease in
   functional residual capacity (FRC). Obesity further worsens FRC as the increased intraabdominal
   pressure results in additional cephalad displacement of the diaphragm. With the induction of general
   anesthesia and muscle relaxation, FRC is reduced. Patients with elevated closing capacities are more
   predisposed to the development of atelectasis. Residual effects of both intravenous and inhalation
   anesthetics blunt the ventilatory responses to hypercapnia and hypoxia. Anesthetic agents also atten-
   uate the protective hypoxic pulmonary vasoconstriction reflex. These effects persist for several hours
   and may contribute to the intrapulmonary shunting and hypoxia seen in the recovery room.
   Prolonged pulmonary dysfunction (longer than 24 hours) is usually not caused by anesthesia.

   Benumof JL: Respiratory physiology and respiratory function during anesthesia. In Miller RD (ed):
   Anesthesia, 5th ed. New York, Churchill Livingstone, 2000, pp 602–614.

2. **How does surgery affect pulmonary function?**
   The location of the surgery determines whether postoperative pulmonary dysfunction occurs.
   Immediately after upper abdominal surgery, vital capacity (VC) is reduced to 40% of preoperative values. FRC is reduced to 70% of preoperative values. These pulmonary abnormalities are
   slow to resolve; the vital capacity and FRC gradually return to normal over 7–14 days following
   a nadir at postoperative day 2. Lower abdominal surgery also decreases ventilation variables
   to 60–80% of preoperative values over a similar time frame. A thoracotomy decreases vital
   capacity by almost 4 liters. Superficial and extremity surgery results in little, if any, change in
   postoperative FRC. Mechanisms thought to be important in causing the decreases in FRC and
   VC include an increase in negative signaling along the phrenic nerve, resulting from stimulation
   of the abdominal splanchnic nerves. Laparoscopic surgical approaches are associated with
   significantly less impairment of respiratory function than comparable open procedures, perhaps
   because of the decrease in splanchnic nerve stimulation.

   McKeague H, Cunningham AJ: Postoperative respiratory dysfunction: Is the site of surgery crucial?
   Br J Anaesth 79(4):415–416, 1997.
   Joris J, Kaba A, Lamy M: Postoperative spirometry after laparoscopy for lower abdominal or upper abdom-
   inal surgical procedures. Br J Anaesth 79(4):422–426, 1997.
   Nguyen NT, Lee SL, Goldman C, et al: Comparison of pulmonary function and postoperative pain after
   laparoscopic versus open gastric bypass: A randomized trial. J Am Coll Surg 192(4):469–476, 2001.

3. **What are the general principles of immediate postoperative pulmonary care?**
   Postoperative pulmonary dysfunction can be caused by mechanical, hemodynamic, and
   pharmacodynamic factors related to the surgery and to the anesthesia. The postanesthesia
   care unit (PACU) is the area designed for monitoring and care of patients recovering from the
   immediate effects of these derangements. The drugs and equipment available to provide
   routine care include supplemental oxygen, suction, vital sign monitors, pulse oximeters, and
   electrocardiographs. Advanced support equipment (i.e., ventilators, intravascular pressure
   monitors, and defibrillators) must also be available. Airway patency and protection are continuously monitored. Supplemental oxygen therapy is always provided to help ensure that

systemic oxygenation is adequate, and oximetry has become the standard of care to document the presence of adequate oxygenation. Prophylactic measures employed to prevent potential pulmonary complications such as atelectasis include the following:

- Patient positioning with the head of the bed elevated 30 degrees to minimize the incidence of aspiration
- Early ambulation
- Coughing
- Incentive spirometry

For those patients who will remain intubated, confirming proper endotracheal tube placement and endotracheal tube cuff inflation pressure can prevent airway trauma and complications related to mainstem intubation or excessive air leak around the endotracheal cuff. Lastly, hand cleansing with alcohol-based gel before and after contact with each patient can greatly reduce transmission of nosocomial infection.

Feeley TW, Macario A: The postanesthetic care unit. In Miller RD (ed): Anesthesia, 5th ed. New York, Churchill Livingstone, 2000, pp 2308–2311.

4. **Describe some maneuvers for treatment of postoperative airway obstruction.**
The tongue and pharyngeal soft tissues falling backward and occluding the airway most commonly cause airway obstruction. Airway obstruction is often the result of over-sedation. Signs of airway obstruction include a lack of air movement, retractions of the accessory muscles, and a lack of chest wall movement.

The following maneuvers are used to reestablish airway patency:
- Neck extension (if not contraindicated) accompanied by a jaw thrust
- Moving the patient into a lateral position
- Insertion of an oral or nasal airway (with caution because this may cause vomiting or gagging)
- Examination of the oropharynx for obstructing material
- Mask ventilation, endotracheal intubation, or cricothyrotomy (to be used if conservative measures fail)

If the patient has undergone a procedure on the neck and intubation has failed, consideration should be given to opening the wound, relieving airway compression, and reattempting intubation. Laryngospasm is an infrequent cause of airflow obstruction that usually responds to the positive pressure generated by mask ventilation. Patients with known or suspected obstructive sleep apnea (OSA) may benefit from continuous positive airway pressure (CPAP) or bilevel positive airway pressure (bilevel-PAP), providing the patient is able to protect the airway.

Stoelting RK, Miller RD: Basics of Anesthesia, 4th ed. New York, Churchill Livingstone, 2000, pp 411–414.

5. **What criteria are used to determine when a patient may be extubated after an anesthetic?**
Think of the mnemonic "When you think, the patient will **SOAR**."
- **S = S**ecretions. Lower respiratory tract **secretions** are not more excessive than the patient's ability to clear them.
- **O = O**xygenation is adequate. Usually a PaO_2 of 80 mmHg with an FiO_2 of 0.4 provides for some margin of safety because the maximum FiO_2 that can be dependably delivered to nonintubated patients is approximately 0.5.
- **A = A**irway. The patient is able to protect his or her airway. This is easily determined by testing a gag reflex.
- **R = R**espiratory effort is adequate. This is assessed by clinical examination or quantified with variables such as a maximum inspiratory pressure (MIP) or a vital capacity (VC). The patient must be able to generate a MIP more negative than -30 cmH_2O or have a VC greater than 10 cc/kg.

Additionally, one must consider the type of surgery, especially those involving head and neck or positioning that may lead to airway edema. If airway edema is suspected, maneuvers to assess airway edema (either qualitative or quantitative) must be employed. Qualitative measures include the cuff-leak test and the tube occlusion test. Quantitative measures include the difference in delivered and returned tidal volumes while using the ventilator assist-control mode.

Jaber S, Chanques G, Matecki S, et al: Post-extubation stridor in intensive care unit patients. Intensive Care Med 29(1):69–74, 2003.

6. **What is the differential diagnosis of hypoxemia in the recovery room?**
   More-common causes:
   - Pain-causing splinting
   - Anesthesia or surgery resulting in atelectasis or shunting
   - Sedation (i.e., narcotics or benzodiazepines) resulting in hypoventilation
   - Shivering or hyperthermia resulting in increased O_2 consumption
   - Decreased alveolar ventilation resulting in decreased alveolar O_2 concentration

   Less-common causes:
   - Bronchospasm from intubation
   - Pneumothoraces
   - Pulmonary edema from volume overload or cardiac failure
   - Pulmonary emboli
   - Aspiration of gastric contents
   - Sepsis
   - Hemorrhage

   Medication-related causes:
   - Attenuation of hypoxic vasoconstriction, seen with nitrates, nitroprusside, dopamine, and epidural local anesthetics
   - Methemoglobinemia from benzocaine, bupivacaine, lidocaine, amyl nitrate, or inhaled nitric oxide

   Ajayi T, Grapper MA: Methemoglobinemia. Plum Pers 18:1–7, 2001.

7. **What clinical scenarios are associated with acute lung injury (ALI) and acute respiratory distress syndrome (ARDS)?**
   Common causes of ALI and ARDS are pneumonia, sepsis, and aspiration of gastric contents. Other causes include fat emboli, transfusion-related acute lung injury, inhalation injury, near-drowning, pulmonary contusion, and lung reperfusion injury.

8. **How are ARDS and ALI diagnosed and treated?**
   The 1994 North American–European Consensus Committee (NAECC) consensus definition of ALI and ARDS describes an acute or persistent pulmonary process. The underlying process has chest radiograph findings of bilateral infiltrates consistent with pulmonary edema in the absence of left atrial hypertension. ALI is diagnosed by $PaO_2/FiO_2 < 300$, and ARDS is diagnosed by $PaO_2/FiO_2 < 200$. Treatment guidelines are outlined in the ARDSnet protocol. Briefly, the ARDSnet protocol calls for lung-protective ventilation using higher positive end-expiratory pressure (PEEP) and lower FiO_2. To achieve this, the assist-control ventilation mode is chosen, with tidal volumes of 6–8 cc/kg, based on ideal body weight. Tidal volumes and PEEP are adjusted to maintain inspiratory plateau pressures <30 cmH_2O. A pH of 7.3–7.45 is targeted by adjusting the respiratory rate up to 35 breaths per minute.

   Brower RG, Ware LB, Berthiaume Y, Matthay MA: Treatment of ARDS. Chest 120(4):1347–1367, 2001.

9. **What causes inaccurate pulse oximetry readings?**
   Pulse oximeters use the oxyhemoglobin absorption of infrared light transmitted across a pulsatile peripheral vascular bed (i.e., a finger or earlobe) to determine the degree of arterial oxygen saturation. Decreases in oxygen saturation are detected only when the arterial oxygen tension falls below the level of full hemoglobin oxygen saturation. Certain situations are associated with inaccurate pulse oximetry readings. Pulse oximetry readings often cannot be obtained from patients who are hypothermic or vasoconstricted because of vasopressor therapy or hypoten-

sion due to lack of pulsatile flow. Pulse oximetry is accurate between 50% and 100% saturation. Pulse oximetry probes placed directly over large pulsing vascular structures may give erroneous low saturation (SpO_2) readings. Spurious pulse oximetry readings may be caused by fluorescent or infrared lights (such as those used to warm small infants) or by movement of the extremity on which the probe is located. Other causes of inaccurate readings include severe anemia, intravascular dyes (e.g., methylene blue), fingernail polish, and the presence of other hemoglobin species such as methemoglobin or carboxyhemoglobin. Ambient light, skin color, and venous blood do not cause inaccurate readings because they are not pulsatile.

Tremper KK, Barker SJ: Pulse oximetry. Anesthesiology 70:98–108, 1989.

10. **What is the differential diagnosis of hypercapnia in the recovery room?**
Hypercapnia is the result of either decreased clearance or increased production of carbon dioxide. Decreased central respiratory drive may result from a neurologic defect or, more commonly, from residual anesthetic effects. Narcotic-induced depression may be reversed by naloxone, whereas benzodiazepines may be counteracted by flumazenil. Impairment of the chest bellows mechanism may occur if residual neuromuscular blockade, chest pain, or abdominal distention is present. Patients with intrinsic lung disease may have greater sensitivity to postoperative stresses, which may cause an exacerbation of hypercapnia. The increased carbon dioxide production associated with shivering or hyperthermia is usually not problematic unless ventilation cannot be appropriately increased. An uncommon, yet the most serious, cause of hypercapnia may be malignant hyperthermia.

Feeley TW, Macario A: The postanesthetic care unit. In Miller RD (ed): Anesthesia, 5th ed. New York, Churchill Livingstone, 2000, pp 2308–2311.

KEY POINTS: THE MOST COMMON POSTOPERATIVE AIRWAY COMPLICATIONS

1. Atelectasis

2. Airway obstruction

3. Alveolar hypoventilation

4. Bronchospasm

11. **Describe the differential diagnosis of postoperative wheezing.**
Wheezing may occur secondary to bronchospastic asthma, exacerbation of COPD or bronchitis, airway edema, pneumothorax, pulmonary embolus, or congestive heart failure. In the intubated patient, obstruction of the endotracheal tube by mucus, cuff overinflation, a kinked endotracheal tube, an endobronchial intubation, or nasogastric tube misplacement should also be considered. Less-common causes are medication reactions and transfusion reactions.

Stoelting EA, Dierdorf SF: Anesthesia and Co-Existing Disease, 4th ed. New York, Churchill-Livingstone, 2002.

12. **Which patients are at risk for OSA and complications associated with OSA?**
Patients who smoke, postmenopausal women, patients with nasal congestion due to allergies. OSA has an association with several comorbid conditions. Patients with diabetes in association with metabolic syndrome, hypertension, coronary artery disease, congestive heart failure, and previous strokes are at an increased risk for OSA and associated complications.

Young T, Skatrud J, Peppard P: Risk factors for obstructive sleep apnea in adults. JAMA 291:2013–2016, 2004.

13. **Should smokers stop smoking before an operation?**

    Cigarette smoking is a risk factor for postoperative complications. Depending on several factors, smokers may present to the operating room with significant levels of carboxyhemoglobin (i.e., >3%). An elevated carboxyhemoglobin will reduce the amount of hemoglobin available to bind oxygen and will also shift the oxygen–hemoglobin saturation curve to the left. Nicotine has significant vasoconstrictive effects and will increase pulse rates. Decreases in heart rate, blood pressure, and catecholamine levels can be seen within 20 minutes of discontinuing smoking. The maximal benefit from discontinuing smoking does not occur for 4–6 weeks; however, all smokers should be encouraged to stop at least 12–24 hours prior to surgery. Although recent studies have shown an increase in sputum production in patients who stopped smoking <2 months prior to surgery, this increase was not associated with an increase in perioperative pulmonary complications.

    Moller A, Villebro N, Pedersen T: Interventions for preoperative smoking cessation. Cochrane Database Syst Rev (4):CD002294, 2001.

    Moller AM, Villebro N, Pedersen T, Tonnesen H: Effect of preoperative smoking intervention on postoperative complications: A randomized clinical trial. Lancet 359:114–117, 2002.

14. **Can you predict which patients with chronic obstructive lung disease will require prolonged mechanical ventilation?**

    The postoperative complications associated with chronic obstructive lung disease (COLD) include atelectasis, pneumonia, and exacerbation of bronchitis. Identification of patients who will require prolonged postoperative mechanical ventilation has been difficult. In a study of 51 smokers with COLD who were to have elective abdominal vascular procedures, 25% required mechanical ventilation for more than 1 day. These ventilated patients also had longer hospital stays and a higher mortality rate than the patients who did not require mechanical ventilation. Preoperative data that were predictive of the requirement for prolonged ventilation included an extensive history of smoking (72 pack-years, versus 44 pack-years in the nonventilated group) and a low preoperative arterial oxygen tension (68 mmHg, versus 77 mmHg in the nonventilated group). Preoperative spirometry was not helpful in predicting postoperative respiratory failure.

    COLD has been shown to be a risk factor associated with increased likelihood of postoperative respiratory failure requiring prolonged mechanical ventilation, increased risk of pneumonia, and increased mortality.

    Arozullah AM, Daley J, Henderson WG, Khuri SF: Multifactorial risk index for predicting postoperative respiratory failure in men after major noncardiac surgery. The National Veterans Administration Surgical Quality Improvement Program. Ann Surg 232(2):242–253, 2000.

    Arozullah AM, Khuri SF, Henderson WG, et al: Development and validation of a multifactorial risk index for predicting postoperative pneumonia after major noncardiac surgery. Ann Intern Med 135(10):847–857, 2001.

15. **What is the role of pulmonary function testing (PFT) in preoperative risk assessment?**

    PFT should be viewed as a management tool to optimize preoperative pulmonary function as well as to provide an individual's baseline performance so that more accurate comparative assessments may be made in the postoperative phase of care. For example, spirometry or peak flows may be useful monitors of the status of the asthmatic patient. Preoperative assessment of vital capacity in the patient with myasthenia gravis gives clinicians a realistic benchmark to determine optimal recovery of ventilation mechanics after the dysfunction caused by anesthesia and a surgical procedure.

    Patients scheduled for pneumonectomy may benefit from PFTs to assess the ratio of the forced expiratory volume in 1 second (FEV_1) to the forced vital capacity (FVC). More importantly, patients scheduled for pneumonectomy may benefit from perfusion scan to assess the ventilation/perfusion (V/Q) relationship in the lung to be removed.

The BODE index demonstrated that a multivariate grading system (including body mass index [BMI], FEV_1, the degree of dyspnea, and exercise tolerance) was more valuable than FEV_1 alone in predicting death from respiratory causes in patients with COPD.

Celli BR, Cote CG, Marin JM, et al: The body-mass index, airflow obstruction, dyspnea, and exercise capacity index in chronic obstructive pulmonary disease. N Engl J Med 350:1005–1012, 2004.

16. **Describe the postoperative problems of patients with restrictive lung disease.**
There are few recent studies on postoperative problems of patients who have restrictive lung disease from lung fibrosis, interstitial lung disease, or spinal deformities. In contrast, many studies have suggested that irreversible pulmonary failure occurs in patients with scoliosis who have upper thoracic curves exceeding 70 degrees. Pulmonary function is improved in adolescents and children whose scoliosis is surgically corrected. It is unclear whether pulmonary function improves in adults with severe scoliosis after surgical repair of their spinal deformities. Patients with restrictive lung disease have high minute ventilations and may not meet the standard criteria for extubation because of their high respiratory frequencies. Patients with restrictive lung disease have noncompliant lungs that may require positive pressure ventilation through either mechanical ventilation or intermittent positive pressure breathing (IPPB).

17. **How should patients be evaluated for thoracotomy prior to surgery?**
Preoperative evaluation of patients for lung resection should include exercise studies because several investigators have shown that oxygen consumption levels during exercise are helpful in predicting whether a patient can undergo lung resection and have an uneventful postoperative course. In a recent study, if a patient had a VO_2 max >75% of predicted, the patient had a 90% chance of not having complications, even after a pneumonectomy. The ability to achieve a high VO_2 max during exercise suggests that the patient has ample pulmonary and cardiac function and that he or she is capable of moderate exercise (i.e., not debilitated). Static pulmonary function studies are not as helpful in predicting postoperative complications in this patient population. Patients having pneumonectomy may benefit from a nuclear medicine perfusion scan to determine the differential flow to the lungs.

Reilly JJ Jr: Evidence-based preoperative evaluation of candidates for thoracotomy. Chest 116(6 Suppl):474S–476S, 1999.

18. **What complications occur after thoracotomy?**
Thoracotomy is associated with the most serious postoperative pulmonary dysfunction because the lungs are affected as well as the rib cage (Table 7-1). Furthermore, thoracotomies are often performed on patients who already have severe underlying lung disease. Preoperative evaluation of patients with bronchogenic carcinoma who are candidates for pulmonary resection or pneumonectomy has therefore been extensively investigated. Surgery is the only possible cure for lung cancer, but the rate of complications is high (10–15% in patients who have had pneumectomy); the complications seen after thoracotomy include respiratory failure, myocardial infarction, pneumonia, atelectasis, and death. Preoperative evaluation of candidates for lung resection should include exercise studies because several investigators have shown that oxygen consumption levels during exercise are helpful in predicting whether a patient can undergo lung resection and have an uneventful postoperative course. In a recent study, if a patient had a VO_2 max of more than 75% of predicted, the patient had a 90% chance of not having complications, even after a pneumonectomy. The ability to achieve a high VO_2 max during exercise suggests that the patient has good pulmonary and cardiac function and is capable of moderate exercise (i.e., not debilitated). Static pulmonary function studies are not as helpful in predicting postoperative complications in this patient population.

TABLE 7-1. DEFINITION OF POST-THORACOTOMY COMPLICATIONS (WITHIN 30 DAYS OF SURGERY)

Acute carbon dioxide retention (partial pressure of arterial carbon dioxide >45 mmHg)	Pneumonia (temperature >38°C, purulent sputum, infiltrate seen on chest radiograph)
Prolonged mechanical ventilation (≥48 hours)	Pulmonary embolism
Symptomatic cardiac arrhythmias requiring treatment	Lobar atelectasis (necessitating bronchoscopy)
Myocardial infarction	Death

Adapted from Bolliger CT, Jordan P, Soler M, et al: Exercise capacity as a predictor of postoperative complications in lung resection candidates. Am J Respir Crit Care Med 151:1472–1480, 1995.

19. **Identify the most common postoperative pulmonary complication and describe sequelae of that complication.**
Atelectasis is the most common postoperative pulmonary complication. Thoracic and upper abdominal surgery can result in pain, splinting, and a shallow monotonous breathing pattern resulting in atelectasis. Consequences of atelectasis include hypoxemia, myocardial ischemia, infection, and delayed ambulation. Atelectasis can be treated with either positive pressure (IPPB) or negative pressure treatment (incentive spirometry). Studies have shown positive and negative pressure treatments to be equally efficacious, although negative pressure treatments are far more cost effective. Administration of epidural narcotics appears to reduce atelectasis, pulmonary infections, and the overall pulmonary complication rate.

Savel R, Wiener-Kronish JP, Gropper MA: Postoperative care. In Wachter RM, Goldman L, Hollander H (eds): Hospital Medicine. Philadelphia, Lippincott Williams & Wilkins, 2004, pp 261–269.

20. **What causes atelectasis?**
Atelectasis usually occurs in the basal lobes of the lung (with 100% incidence after thoracotomies) and is secondary to trauma to the lung, reduced respiratory effort caused by an increase in negative nervous signals along the phrenic nerve, splinting, obesity, intrathoracic fluid, pulmonary edema, and decreased compliance. Intra-abdominal surgery, intra-abdominal

KEY POINTS: TREATMENTS OF POSTOPERATIVE AIRWAY OBSTRUCTION

1. Jaw thrust or chin lift

2. Oral or nasal airway

3. CPAP or bilevel-PAP

4. Intubation

5. Cricothyrotomy or tracheotomy

masses, ascites, bowel obstruction, and viscus dilation all decrease diaphragmatic excursion. These factors and a rapid, shallow respiratory pattern predispose the patient to small airway closure and alveolar collapse. Mucous plugging, inspissated secretions, and a poor cough contribute to persistent atelectasis. The diagnosis is made by clinical examination, chest radiograph, and arterial blood gas analysis.

21. How should atelectasis be treated?

The most effective therapy for atelectasis is the use of a respiratory maneuver that increases inspiration and has the patient hold his or her inspiratory breath, allowing the inspired gas to enter collapsed alveoli through the pores of Kohn. No study has shown a benefit of one maneuver over another; IPPB, blow gloves, and incentive spirometers are all equivalent in their ability to treat atelectasis, to decrease hospital stays, and to decrease respiratory failure. Other therapeutic interventions used for atelectasis include extended mechanical ventilation, chest percussion, coughing, bronchodilators, enhanced analgesia, and nasotracheal suction-ing. Patient positioning is also important. The sitting position places the diaphragm at a better mechanical advantage and increases FRC. The lateral decubitus position, with the expanded lung in the dependent position, improves V/Q matching and facilitates mucus clearance from the atelectatic nondependent lung. Application of PEEP in the form of CPAP or bilevel-PAP has generally been shown to be an effective adjunct. Bronchoscopy has proven to be a controversial therapy.

Care must be taken when treating atelectasis: hemodynamic changes may occur with large tidal volumes and inspiratory holds. There are experimental models demonstrating profound reduction in cardiac output associated with lung recruitment maneuvers in the setting of lung injury.

Lim SC, Adams AB, Simonson DA, et al: Transient hemodynamic effects of recruitment maneuvers in three experimental models of acute lung injury. Crit Care Med 32(12):2378–2384, 2004.

22. What methods may be used to mobilize and remove secretions in postoperative patients?

Manual lung hyperinflation has been shown to improve lung static compliance and to promote mobilization of secretions; however, these effects have not been linked to reduction in morbidity or mortality. Inspiratory gases may be humidified. This decreases mucus viscosity and supports ciliary function. Adequate intravascular hydration helps to maintain the humidification capacity of the nasopharynx and the tracheal mucosa. Mucolytic agents such as N-acetylcysteine have been suggested as a way of decreasing the viscosity of secretions, but their potential for causing bronchospasm limits their utility. Blind nasal suctioning with a soft catheter is an effective way of generating a cough, especially in the uncooperative patient. During the suctioning procedure, electrocardiographic monitoring is used to detect reflex arrhythmias and bradycardias. Bronchoscopy is reserved for the most refractory cases of thickened, retained secretions.

Berney S, Denehy L: A comparison of the effects of manual and ventilator hyperinflation on static lung compliance and sputum production in intubated and ventilated intensive care patients. Physiother Res Int 7(2):100–108, 2002.

23. Describe the various measures for delivery of oxygen therapy in nonintubated patients.

The major considerations in the selection of a supplemental oxygen device are patient comfort and compliance as well as the level of FiO_2 required. Nasal cannulas are well tolerated, but the delivered FiO_2 decreases with increased minute ventilation. Because of poor humidification, flow rates greater than 6 L/min may dry nasal mucosa. A venturi mask entrains a controlled amount of room air into a high flow of oxygen, which provides a more constant FiO_2 independent of minute ventilation and inspiratory flow rate. This device is less comfortable and has limited humidification ability. An open face mask, when tightly fitted, can deliver up to 50% FiO_2 and higher levels of humidity because of larger bore tubing. Face tents are more comfortable but vary in the amount of oxygen delivered. Masks with reservoir bags (i.e., nonrebreathing masks) have enhanced oxygen delivery capacity (60–80% FiO_2). Combinations of nasal cannulas and face masks are sometimes used. They are able to deliver enriched oxygen concentrations, but the high flows necessary are seldom tolerated for prolonged periods. Patients may receive very high FiO_2 delivery from face masks with large volume tubing and reservoir tubing or nasal high-flow gas therapy. High-flow warmed and humidified oxygen therapy can provide 10–40 L/min of variable FiO_2.

Waugh JB, Granger WM: An evaluation of 2 new devices for nasal high-flow gas therapy. Resp Care 49(8):902–906, 2004.

24. **How can stridor and bronchospasm be reversed?**
Stridor (suggested by a wheezing during inspiration) is indicative of partial upper airway obstruction, which is often caused by swelling or paralysis of the laryngeal or supraglottic soft tissues. Therapy should be aimed at reduction of swelling. Nebulized racemic epinephrine is useful if the side effects of tachycardia and hypertension can be tolerated. Dexamethasone is an effective anti-inflammatory but requires several hours for effect. If epiglottitis is likely, the patient's airway (especially that of a small child) should be evaluated in the operating room because the airway may become totally obstructed after being manipulated. In all patients with stridor, equipment should be readily available for intubation or tracheotomy in case clinical deterioration makes one or both of these measures necessary.

Bronchospasm initially should be treated, if possible, by removal of any precipitating agents (e.g., beta-blockers). The cornerstones of inhalation therapy are $beta_2$ agonists. Albuterol has the fewest $beta_2$ effects and may be administered through a metered dose inhaler or continuously as an aerosol. The aerosol form of the anticholinergic ipratropium may also facilitate bronchodilatation. Steroid therapy has become the primary treatment for bronchospasm caused by asthma. In severe asthma, steroids need to be given early and in large amounts because deaths in asthmatics tend to occur in patients who received too little steroid treatment or who were given steroids too late in the attack. In asthmatic patients who have a history of intubation for their disease, preoperative administration of steroids should be considered. Asthmatic patients on steroids, either long-term or acutely, are at high risk for prolonged paralysis if they receive more than one dose of nondepolarizing paralytic agents.

Although a combination of helium and oxygen (heliox) will not reverse bronchospasm, it may reduce the turbulent flow encountered during bronchospasm and allow for more effective gas exchange in distal airways by providing laminar flow. More studies are needed to evaluate the efficacy of heliox for the treatment of acute bronchospasm. Bronchospasm is not reversed, but resultant hypoxemia can be attenuated.

Rodrigo G, Pollack C, Rodrigo C, Rowe BH: Heliox for nonintubated acute asthma patients. Cochrane Database Syst Rev (4):CD002884, 2003.

25. **Describe the commonly used modalities of mechanical ventilation.**
Volume ventilation: In assist control (A/C) ventilation, when the patient initiates an inspiration, the ventilator delivers a preset tidal volume. If the patient's respiratory rate falls below a preset level, the machine delivers breaths automatically at a backup rate. With intermittent mandatory ventilation (IMV), the ventilator delivers a preset tidal volume at a preset rate, but the patients may breathe spontaneously between cycles and assume a greater portion of their ventilatory needs. Synchronization is possible between the expiratory phase of the patient's breath and a mandatory ventilation cycle through synchronized intermittent mandatory ventilation (SIMV). With volume-regulated ventilation, variables such as mode of ventilation, tidal volume, respiratory rate, inspiratory rate, and flow rate must be set.

Pressure ventilation: With pressure-regulated ventilation, inspiratory pressure, inspiratory time, and respiratory rate need to be set. In pressure-regulated ventilation, the tidal volume varies if the patient has an unexpected increase or decrease in lung compliance. For example, a patient with severe bronchospasm whose initial inspiratory pressure was set at 50 cmH_2O to deliver a 500-mL tidal volume would receive a much larger tidal volume when the bronchospasm resolved and compliance increased. All modes of ventilation also require the clinician to dictate the FiO_2 and the level of desired PEEP.

Continuous positive airway pressure can be used in both intubated and nonintubated patients; the patient breathes spontaneously through a high-flow system that does not allow the patient's inspiratory pressure to go to zero at any time during the respiratory cycle. If the patient is intubated, preset levels of pressure support may be added during the patient's inspiratory effort. This is intended to overcome the excess work of breathing through demand valves and ventilator tubing as well as that caused by the patient's underlying pathology.

Pressure support with PEEP will prevent airway pressure from going to zero during end-expiration (allowing a patient to initiate the next breath from a more favorable point on the compliance curve) and also will provide assistance in maintaining adequate tidal volumes with positive pressure delivered during inspiration.

New modes of ventilation, termed dual-mode ventilation, try to combine the advantages of volume and pressure-cycled ventilation modes by limiting inspiratory pressure while controlling minute ventilation. A theoretical advantage is improved patient comfort since the ventilator can respond instantaneously to increased flow demand.

26. **What are the variables commonly used in postoperative ventilation?**
See Table 7-2.

TABLE 7-2. COMMON VENTILATOR SETTINGS IN THE POSTOPERATIVE PERIOD		
	Volume Control	**Pressure Control**
Tidal volume or inspiratory pressure	10 cc/kg*	Titrate to maintain 10 cc/kg (10–30 cmH$_2$O)
Respiratory rate	10–12 BPM	10–12 BPM
Inspiration-to-expiration ratio	—	1:2 to 1:3
FiO$_2$	100% with titration to 50% based on PaO$_2$ or SaO$_2$	100% with titration to 50% based on PaO$_2$ or SaO$_2$
PEEP	5 cmH$_2$O	5 cmH$_2$O

* Provided there is no evidence of lung injury.
BPM = breaths per minute; PEEP = positive end-expiratory pressure.

27. **Are there potential hazards to oxygen therapy?**
Pulmonary oxygen toxicity manifests as thickening and edema of the lung interstitium. It is a function of the oxygen dose and the duration of therapy. Even with 100% oxygen supplementation, days may be required before microscopic damage may be detected. Toxicity is unlikely to develop at levels of up to 60% oxygen, even for prolonged periods of exposure. Thus, the benefits of oxygen therapy greatly outweigh the risks in the postoperative period.

Because oxygen diffuses into pulmonary capillary blood much faster than nitrogen, periods of 100% oxygen supplementation in smaller alveoli may actually promote their collapse. The resulting atelectasis may cause increased intrapulmonary shunting and hypoxia despite the enhanced oxygen support. Retrolental fibroplasia is a hazard of oxygen therapy that occurs in neonates of low birth weight or less than 34 weeks of gestational age.

Davis WB, Rennard SI, Bitterman PB, Crystal RG: Pulmonary oxygen toxicity. Early reversible changes in human alveolar structures induced by hyperoxia. N Engl J Med 309(15):878–883, 1983.

28. **What is the difference between a humidifier and a nebulizer?**

    Nebulizers are devices that generate aerosolized suspensions of particles in a carrier gas. They are categorized as jet (pneumatic) and ultrasonic. The jet nebulizer utilizes the Bernoulli effect of a directed high-velocity gas stream drawing surface liquids into the stream as aerosolized particles. They are frequently used to humidify gases and to deliver bronchodilator drugs.

    Humidifiers are used to provide dry medical gases with a water content similar to that normally present in room air. Passover humidifiers depend on evaporation to add water vapor to gases that pass over a water surface. In bubble-through humidifiers, gas passes as bubbles through a reservoir of heated water. This increases the capacity of the gas to hold water vapor. Humidifiers of this type are frequently used when the humidification function of the upper airway is bypassed, such as during mechanical ventilation.

29. **Which postoperative volume recruitment therapy is best to prevent postoperative pulmonary complications?**

    Several techniques have been studied, including IPPB, deep-breathing exercises, incentive spirometry, and chest physiotherapy. Critical review, as well as a meta-analysis, demonstrates that all are equally efficacious in reducing the rate of pulmonary complications by a factor of two compared with no therapy after abdominal surgery. Currently, incentive spirometry is popular as a simple, inexpensive modality that provides objective goals for monitoring efficacy. Although there is little evidence, preoperative education may improve patient compliance and performance in the postoperative period. The most cost-effective maneuver to reduce postoperative pulmonary complications is patient positioning. Provided there are no absolute contraindications, raising the head of the patient's bed to a minimum of 30 degrees decreases the likelihood of aspiration and ventilator-associated pneumonia. Early ambulation is another inexpensive and effective method to recruit atelectatic lung segments and to increase functional residual capacity.

    Overend TJ, Anderson CM, Lucy SD, et al: The effect of incentive spirometry on postoperative pulmonary complications: A systematic review. Chest 120(3):971–978, 2001.

CONTROVERSIES

30. **Does epidural analgesia improve pulmonary function?**

    Although many studies have demonstrated improved radiologic markers in patients receiving epidural analgesia compared with those receiving general anesthesia and systemic opioids, the effects of epidural therapy on serious pulmonary complications (e.g., pneumonia and respiratory failure) remain unclear. The studies that observed a benefit from epidural analgesia examined high-risk patients, used intraoperative epidural anesthesia, and continued epidural analgesia (local or opioid) into the postoperative period. On the other hand, those studies that did not observe a difference used healthy patients, did not study high-risk procedures, or did not control postoperative analgesia. There are data, however, showing that complete pain relief achieved by epidural narcotics will not improve VC or FRC. In contrast, local anesthetics appear to improve pulmonary function after upper abdominal surgery. Thus, epidural analgesia that includes local anesthesia may offer additional benefit to patients at high risk for pulmonary complications. Epidural analgesia should be considered for patients with COPD undergoing thoracic surgery.

    Rock P, Passannante A: Preoperative assessment: Pulmonary. Anesthesiol Clin North Am 22(1):77–91, 2004.

    Fotiadis RJ, Badvie S, Weston MD, Allen-Mersh TG: Epidural analgesia in gastrointestinal surgery. Br J Surg 91(7):828–841, 2004.

KEY POINTS: ARDSNET SUMMARY

1. Diagnosis: PaO_2-to-FiO_2 ratio <300 for ALI and <200 for ARDS

2. Chest radiograph: bilateral patchy infiltrates consistent with pulmonary edema

3. Ventilation: low tidal volumes (6–8 cc/kg) based on ideal body weight

4. Oxygenation: facilitated by use of PEEP

5. Weaning: daily spontaneous breathing trials with minimal ventilatory support

---

31. Which is most effective for bronchodilator therapy: jet nebulization, continuous nebulization, or metered-dose inhalers?

Many studies have shown little difference between these three modalities in both intubated and nonintubated patients. However, several studies show (by filter collection and radio-labeled techniques) that in intubated patients, administration of bronchodilators with a metered-dose inhaler attached to a spacing device or delivered by catheter to the distal end of the endotracheal tube results in improvement of deposition by 5–30%. Metered-dose inhalers with spacing devices have also been shown to improve delivery in the nonintubated patient. It is not clear, however, whether this technique is more effective than nebulized therapy because it is difficult to show dosage equivalency, and there are problems with patient cooperation in the acute setting. Metered-dose therapy, used appropriately, can substantially decrease the cost of respiratory care services. Additionally, there is no clear evidence demonstrating a benefit of continuous neb-ulized bronchodilator therapy over intermittent treatment in severe bronchospastic disease.

32. Is bronchoscopy effective for the treatment of atelectasis?

Fiberoptic bronchoscopy has been used as a therapeutic modality for selected cases of atelecta-sis. Atelectasis usually can be managed with vigorous respiratory therapy alone. Many anecdotal reports of the use of bronchoscopy to resolve lobar atelectasis exist in the literature, but prospective studies demonstrate no advantage of bronchoscopy over vigorous pulmonary toilet for these cases. Although not proven prospectively, consideration for bronchoscopy may be given to patients in whom lobar or more widespread atelectasis has not responded to vigorous respiratory care (i.e., suctioning, postural drainage, and chest percussion) or those with life-threatening acute whole-lung atelectasis. One study suggests that bronchoscopy is useful only when the lung is not totally consolidated, as suggested by the radiologic presence of air bronchograms.

Kreider ME, Lipson DA: Bronchoscopy for atelectasis in the ICU: A case report and review of the literature. Chest 124(1):344–350, 2003.

33. How often should ventilation circuits and humidification reservoirs be changed?

The Centers for Disease Control recommendations from 1981 urged ventilator circuit changes every 24–48 hours. However, these recommendations were established before bacteriostatic innovations such as heat moisture exchangers, nonaerosolizing humidifiers, and heated wire circuits. Several studies have shown that highly contaminated condensate from the patient in the ventilator circuit may be a significant risk factor in the development of nosocomial pneumonia, but studies have failed to reveal an increased incidence of pneumonia even when the interval between circuit changes is as long as 1 week. Based on the apparent lack of significant adverse sequelae, the American Association for Respiratory Care in a practice guideline statement recommends establishment of circuit change intervals based on local surveillance programs.

Circuits employing the aforementioned innovations may, in the absence of soilage, require change only every 5–7 days. Humidification systems should be changed every 48 hours. These recommendations have significant implications in terms of reducing use of intensive care unit (ICU) resources.

American Association for Respiratory Care: AARC Guidelines. Resp Care 48(9):869–880, 2003.

34. **Explain the rationale behind weaning ventilatory support.**
Patients with no significant pulmonary pathology who remain intubated in the PACU warrant extubation after they meet criteria discussed in Question 5. Patients who remain intubated for reasons pertaining to significant pulmonary pathology or weakness may require weaning from the ventilator. A common scenario finds a patient with likely aspiration oversedated and left intubated on assist-control. When the patient is appropriately responsive, current recommendations for ventilator liberation call for a spontaneous breathing trial on minimal ventilator support or T-piece oxygen supply. There is no evidence that supports one mode of weaning over another.

35. **What is the evidence for use of CPAP or bilevel-PAP in the treatment of congestive heart failure, acute myocardial infarction, or subacute myocardial infarction?**
Both CPAP and bilevel-PAP have been shown to be superior to supplemental oxygen alone. Initial studies showed that bilevel-PAP was associated with an increase in morbidity and mortality compared to CPAP and supplemental oxygen therapy. New evidence suggests CPAP and bilevel-PAP to be superior to O_2 therapy alone, with an increase in morbidity and mortality in the O_2-therapy group.

Park M, Sangean MC, Volpe Mde S, et al: Randomized, prospective trial of oxygen, continuous positive airway pressure, and bilevel positive airway pressure by face mask in acute cardiogenic pulmonary edema. Crit Care Med 32(12):2407–2415, 2004.

36. **Are lung protective ventilation strategies applicable to the operating room?**
Evidence from a retrospective study demonstrates that >20% of incidence of acute lung injury following surgery requires mechanical ventilation in patients without lung injury prior to initiation of mechanical ventilation. The study also found that women received larger tidal volumes based on ideal body weight and had higher incidence of lung injury than the men in the study. The same study also suggested an association between blood product transfusion and acute lung injury.

Care must be taken to ventilate patients with appropriate tidal volumes based on ideal body weight. It is clear that patients with known acute lung injury should be ventilated according to the ARDSnet protocol. Prospective studies are indicated to evaluate whether smaller tidal volumes should be utilized in patients who are transfused.

Gajic O, Dara SI, Mendez JL, et al: Ventilator-associated lung injury in patients without acute lung injury at the onset of mechanical ventilation. Crit Care Med 32(9):1817–1824, 2004.

37. **What are the pros and cons of lung recruitment maneuvers?**
Experimental evidence suggests that utilization of typical lung recruitment maneuvers may result in severe hemodynamic compromise in the presence of acute lung injury. Atelectasis is often treated with lung hyperinflation and PEEP. To achieve recruitment in the presence of pneumonia, it is common to use large tidal volumes (>10 cc/kg) and a sustained peak inspiratory pressure (PIP) of 35–35 cmH_2O. This model does produce dramatic reduction in cardiac output in experimental models.

Lim SC, Adams AB, Simonson DA, et al: Transient hemodynamic effects of recruitment maneuvers in three experimental models of acute lung injury. Crit Care Med 32(12):2378–2384, 2004.

38. **Which postoperative complications are most prevalent in morbidly obese patients?**

The morbidly obese patient is more prone to have asthma, thromboembolism, hyperglycemia, airway obstruction, hypoventilation, an increased incidence of ICU admission, and an increased incidence of death in ICU. Morbid obesity is an independent risk factor for death in the ICU.

Bercault N, Boulain T, Kuteifan K, et al: Obesity-related excess mortality rate in an adult intensive care unit: A risk-adjusted matched cohort study. Crit Care Med 2:998–1003, 2004.

CHEST RADIOGRAPHS

David L. Levin, MD, PhD, and Jeffrey S. Klein, MD

CHAPTER 8

ORDERING

1. When should a portable chest radiograph be ordered?

Portable chest radiographs are inferior to films obtained in the radiology department because of technical limitations. Portable radiographic equipment uses lower energy (measured in kVp), which requires a longer exposure time to adequately penetrate the patient and results in greater motion artifact. The focal length (i.e., the distance between the x-ray source and the film) is reduced in portable radiography, which leads to magnification of the heart and the anterior thoracic structures, making assessment of cardiac size difficult. Poor contact between the patient and the film cassette produces further magnification and causes indistinctness of margins. Portable chest radiography is often performed with the patient in the supine or semierect position, which limits the degree of inspiration.

Given these limitations, portable radiographs should be obtained only when it is impossible for the patient to be brought to the radiology department. This occurs most commonly in the intensive care and postoperative settings.

Dietrich P, Klein JS: Methods of examination and normal anatomy. In Brant WE, Helms CA (eds): Fundamentals of Diagnostic Radiology. Baltimore, Williams & Wilkins, 1997, pp 291–292.

2. What are the indications for an expiratory chest radiograph?

An expiratory radiograph may be obtained to evaluate for a possible pneumothorax. In full expiration, the density of the lung is increased while the amount of pleural air is unchanged. Therefore, the greater contrast between the lung and the air in the pleural space should enhance detection of pneumothorax. Additionally, the greater volume of pleural air relative to the lung at end-expiration displaces the visceral pleural reflection away from the inner ribs and should enhance its visibility. Despite these theoretical advantages, clinical studies have shown no improvement in the rate of pneumothorax detection using expiratory radiographs.

Expiratory radiographs can assess for unilateral air trapping, as might be seen with an aspirated foreign body. In this situation, a normal lung increases in density and decreases in volume on the expiratory film, whereas an obstructing foreign body produces a lucent lung that remains unchanged in volume.

Seow A, Kazerooni EA, Pernicano PG, Neary M: Comparison of upright inspiratory and expiratory chest radiographs for detecting pneumothoraces. Am J Roentgenol 166:313–316, 1996.

3. When should a lateral decubitus film be ordered?

For a lateral decubitus film, the patient lies on his or her side and the x-ray beam is directed horizontally toward the body. This study is usually obtained to determine the presence and size of a pleural effusion. A free-flowing effusion will layer between the inner cortex of the ribs and the lung, producing a sharply defined homogeneous opacity traversing the length of the chest. A loculated pleural effusion is immobile and will not layer dependently.

An additional indication for a decubitus chest radiograph is the evaluation of possible pneumothorax. Although an upright chest film is usually obtained for this purpose, a decubitus radiograph made with the affected side up may detect a pneumothorax in a patient who cannot sit or stand. On decubitus radiographs, the pleural air is seen as a lucency in the nondependent thorax that outlines the visceral pleura medially and the inner surface of the ribs laterally.

McLoud TC: The pleura. In McLoud TC (ed): Thoracic Radiology: The Requisites. St. Louis, Mosby, 1998, pp 483–490.

4. **Should the radiology requisition include a clinical history?**
   The request for a radiologic study is a request for consultation with a radiologist. Although some physicians believe that providing clinical information on the radiograph requisition will bias the radiologist, studies show that awareness of the clinical data aids the radiologist in accurate interpretation of the study. The clinical history also may suggest alternative imaging modalities that may prove more useful.

5. **What is the difference between conventional radiography and digital radiography?**
   For a **conventional radiograph**, x-ray beams pass from the source through the patient and strike a radiographic cassette. The cassette contains photographic film and a screen that emits photons when activated by x-rays. The film is developed to provide an image. In this setting, the film serves three separate functions: it detects the incoming x-ray energy, it displays the image, and it acts as a permanent record of the examination.

   The term **digital radiography** can be applied to any system that uses an array of numbers to represent the x-ray signal. In most cases, the information is captured from the phosphor and can be transferred to film or displayed on a high-resolution monitor. The image data can be routed through a **picture archiving and communications system** (PACS). The advantage of digital radiography within a PACS environment is the ability to provide images to anyone connected to the system. For example, a patient's study might be viewed simultaneously and at different locations by radiologists, emergency room physicians, and primary care physicians. An additional advantage of digital radiography is that the contrast and brightness of the image can be adjusted to improve visualization of specific regions of the patient such as the mediastinum or osseous structures.

Freedman MT: Digital chest radiography. In Boiselle PM, White CS (eds): New Techniques in Thoracic Imaging. New York, Marcel Dekker, 2001, pp 315–348.

INTERPRETATION

6. **What should be examined first on a chest radiograph?**
   The most important initial observation to make on any radiographic study is the demographic data provided on the film: the patient's name, gender, and date of birth, and the date of the study. The metallic marker indicating the right or left side of the patient should be identified to guide proper film display (the patient's right should correspond to the viewer's left) and to detect congenital abnormalities of organ migration that may be associated with disease. Use of this routine before the radiograph is interpreted prevents mistakes and provides useful information that may aid in image interpretation.

7. **How should a chest radiograph be evaluated?**
   After the patient's data are verified, the films should be examined in a systematic manner. Any pattern that examines all regions of the film is acceptable. A reasonable method would begin with evaluation of the soft tissues of the neck, shoulders, breasts, axillae, diaphragms, and upper abdomen. The skeletal structures are examined next. The pleural surfaces are evaluated for the presence of effusion, pneumothorax, focal or diffuse thickening, and calcification. The mediastinal, hilar, and cardiac interfaces are assessed for contour abnormalities. The trachea

and main bronchi are studied for displacement, narrowing, or intraluminal masses. Finally, the lung parenchyma is examined for abnormally increased or decreased density, either localized or diffuse. A comparison with the opposite lung is helpful to detect subtle localized parenchymal disease. Both frontal and lateral radiographs should be evaluated in this fashion.

8. **How are the anterior, middle, and posterior mediastinal compartments defined?**
The mediastinum is often divided into anterior, middle, and posterior compartments to aid in the differential diagnosis of masses. The division used by radiologists is based on the lateral radiograph. The anterior mediastinum includes the region posterior to the sternum and anterior to the heart and great vessels. The posterior mediastinum extends posteriorly from the posterior margins of the trachea and heart; this compartment includes the descending aorta and the esophagus. The middle mediastinum includes the heart, great vessels, pericardium, pericardial spaces, trachea, and main bronchi.

9. **What are the most common causes of mediastinal masses?**
See Table 8-1.

TABLE 8-1. COMMON MEDIASTINAL MASSES		
Anterior Mediastinum	**Middle Mediastinum**	**Posterior Mediastinum**
Lymphoma	Lymphadenopathy	Neurofibroma (schwannoma)
Thymoma	Tracheobronchial duplication cyst	Vertebral tumors (metastases, myeloma)
Thyroid goiter	Vascular lesions (e.g., aneurysm)	Paraspinal abscess or hematoma
Germ cell tumor (teratoma)	Tracheobronchial tumors	Descending aortic aneurysm Esophageal neoplasms

Strollo DC, Rosado de Christenson M, Jett JR: Primary mediastinal tumors. Part 1: Tumors of the anterior mediastinum. Chest 112:511–522, 1997.
http://www.amershamhealth.com/medcyclopaedia/medical/volume%20V%201/mediastinal%20mass.asp

10. **What lung diseases are associated with increased radiographic density?**
Lung disease can produce increased radiographic density (in which the lungs are too white or opaque) or decreased radiographic density (in which the lungs become too black or lucent). Increased radiographic density due to air space filling reflects replacement of alveolar air with water (in edema), pus (in pneumonia), or blood (in the presence of hemorrhage). Uncommon causes of air space disease include alveolar filling with malignant cells (bronchoalveolar cell carcinoma or lymphoma) or proteinaceous material (pulmonary alveolar proteinosis or acute silicosis). Air space disease is confluent and ill-defined at its margins. It obscures pulmonary vessels and tends toward lobar or segmental distribution as the process extends from involved to uninvolved lung through interalveolar channels (the pores of Kohn). Branching tubular lucencies coursing through regions of confluent opacity represent patent, air-filled bronchi surrounded by consolidated lung and are termed "air bronchograms."

Increased radiographic density also may be caused by interstitial disease. In contrast to air space disease, which usually reflects an acute process, interstitial disease may reflect either acute or chronic infiltration of the supporting structures of the lung. The most common cause of acute interstitial disease is pulmonary edema, although viral or atypical pneumonias can produce similar findings. Chronic interstitial disease most often results from noninfectious interstitial inflammation and fibrosis or metastatic tumor infiltration. The conditions most often associated with chronic interstitial inflammation are collagen vascular diseases (such as scleroderma or rheumatoid arthritis), asbestos exposure, sarcoidosis, and drug reactions. Interstitial edema or inflammation appears radiographically as curvilinear (reticular) or linear opacities, whereas granulomatous processes and metastatic neoplasms can cause diffuse small (miliary) nodules.

11.   What lung diseases are associated with decreased radiographic density?
Decreased radiographic lung density is difficult to detect. When generalized, it is most often associated with chronic obstructive pulmonary disease (e.g., emphysema). Generalized decreased density (hyperlucency) is usually associated with findings of hyperinflation such as flattening or inversion of the diaphragms and an increased anteroposterior diameter of the chest.

12.   What should be examined on the lateral chest radiograph?
The lateral film is useful in evaluating regions of the chest not well displayed on the frontal projection. Such regions include the retrosternal clear space (i.e., the lucent region behind the sternum and anterior to the heart and great vessels) and the posterior lung bases. On the lateral film, these regions are roughly triangular in shape and are radiolucent (i.e., black). An opacity in either region is abnormal and should prompt further evaluation. The lateral film helps confirm the intrathoracic location of focal lesions and aids in accurate compartmentalization of mediastinal masses detected on the frontal radiograph.

Proto AV, Speckman JM: The left lateral radiograph of the chest. Part I. Med Radiog Photogr 55:30–74, 1979.

Proto AV, Speckman JM: The left lateral radiograph of the chest. Part II. Med Radiog Photogr 56:38–64, 1980.

13.   How is the size of a pneumothorax determined?
A pneumothorax is usually estimated from the frontal radiograph as small, moderate, or large. If a more precise determination is needed, three measurements are obtained from an upright film: the vertical height of the pneumothorax at the lung apex and the lateral width of the pneumothorax at 25% and 75% of the height of the thorax. The average of the three measurements, expressed in millimeters, corresponds to the percentage of pneumothorax present. An average of 10 mm indicates a 15% pneumothorax, 15 mm indicates a 20% pneumothorax, and 40 mm corresponds to a 40% pneumothorax.

Collins CD, Lopez A, Mathie A, et al: Quantification of pneumothorax size on chest radiographs using interpleural distances: Regression analysis based on volume measurements from helical CT. Am J Roentgenol 165:1127–1130, 1995.

14.   How is the size of a pleural effusion estimated?
A 50-mL pleural fluid collection will produce blunting of the posterior costophrenic sulcus on the lateral film. A pleural effusion of 200 mL will blunt the lateral costophrenic angle on the frontal radiograph. A pleural collection of 500 mL is necessary to obscure the diaphragmatic contour. On a lateral decubitus view, pleural collection 1 cm thick represents approximately 200 mL of fluid.

Blackmore CC, Black WC, Dallas RV, et al: Pleural fluid volume estimation: A chest radiograph prediction rule. Acad Radiol 3:103–109, 1996.

KEY POINTS: SIZING OF PLEURAL EFFUSIONS ON UPRIGHT CHEST RADIOGRAPHS

1. Blunted posterior costophrenic sulcus = 50 mL pleural fluid

2. Blunted lateral costophrenic sulcus = 200 mL pleural fluid

3. Obscured diaphragm = 500 mL pleural fluid

CLINICAL USES

15. **Describe the radiologic evaluation of a solitary pulmonary nodule.**

    A solitary pulmonary nodule is detected on approximately 0.2% of chest radiographs. The majority of solitary pulmonary nodules are one of four entities: granuloma, bronchogenic carcinoma, hamartoma (a benign pulmonary neoplasm), or solitary metastasis. The radiographic evaluation should result in classifying the nodule as benign (not requiring further evaluation) or possibly malignant (requiring further evaluation).

    The initial step in the evaluation of a nodule is a comparison with the patient's prior chest films. A complete lack of growth for at least 2 years is an accurate indication of benignancy. If old films are unavailable, the nodule should be studied for its size, margins, and the presence of calcification or fat. This is most frequently performed using computed tomography (CT). Nodules exceeding 3 cm in diameter have a high likelihood of malignancy regardless of their density and usually require biopsy. Similarly, a lobulated or spiculated margin is highly suggestive of malignancy. Benign patterns of calcification in a smoothly marginated nodule include complete, central, laminated, and popcorn calcification. Although a benign pattern of calcification is occasionally recognized on plain radiographs, CT is usually necessary for definitive evaluation. The detection of fat in a smooth nodule is indicative of a hamartoma.

    Despite evaluation with CT, many of these nodules will remain radiographically indeterminate—that is, they could be either benign or malignant. In this case, there are many possible options. In some patients, the most appropriate step is to obtain a pathological diagnosis immediately, either through surgical resection or percutaneous biopsy. For nodules greater than 7 mm in size, positron emission tomography (PET) may be used to determine whether a nodule is metabolically active. Unfortunately, this can be seen with malignancy and some infections. Additionally, not all malignancies are "hot" on PET scanning. Lastly, indeterminate nodules may be followed over time to evaluate for interval growth. A nodule that increases in size is highly suspicious.

    Webb WR: Radiologic evaluation of the solitary pulmonary nodule. Am J Roentgenol 154:701–708, 1990. http://www.chestx-ray.com/Lectures/SPNtalk/SPNFlash.html

KEY POINTS: FEATURES OF A SOLITARY PULMONARY NODULE SUGGESTING MALIGNANCY

1. Greater than 3 cm in diameter

2. Lobulated or spiculated margin

3. Growth as determined by prior radiographs

16. **What is the best method for detection of a fractured rib?**

   In patients sustaining blunt chest trauma, rib fractures are common and simply indicate significant trauma. A rib series can be performed to detect rib fractures, but the results rarely alter the patient's management. It is more appropriate to obtain frontal and lateral chest radiographs to detect complications of blunt trauma that require emergency intervention such as pneumothorax, hemothorax, and hemomediastinum.

17. **What is the proper radiographic position for indwelling tubes, lines, and catheters?**

   The tip of an **endotracheal tube** should lie between 3 and 6 cm above the tracheal carina when the patient's head is in a neutral position (with the mandible overlying C6 or C7). This position allows the tube to move 2 cm superiorly (with full neck extension) or inferiorly (with full neck flexion) while remaining safely within the trachea.

   A **central venous catheter** is optimally placed with its tip in the superior vena cava, although a position within a brachiocephalic, central internal jugular, or subclavian vein is acceptable. Positioning of the catheter tip within the right atrium increases the incidence of cardiac perforation and arrhythmia. The tip of a Swan–Ganz catheter should be located within the right or left main pulmonary artery. A tip positioned more than 1.5 cm from the lateral margin of the hilum may lead to vessel injury or occlusion.

   An **intra-aortic balloon pump** is ideally placed with its radiopaque tip just inferior to the aortic knob, which ensures that the catheter tip will not occlude the origin of the left subclavian artery. Placement of the pump too far distally in the aorta may lead to obstruction of the origins of the celiac, mesenteric, or renal arteries during balloon insufflation.

   A **nasogastric tube** should extend into the stomach. Both the distal end of the tube and the proximal port, marked by a break in the radiographic stripe, should lie within the stomach. Any tube that does not course straight past the carina should be removed because it is likely within the airway.

   Klein JS: Intensive and coronary care radiology. In Higgins CB (ed): Essentials of Cardiac Radiology and Imaging. Philadelphia, J.B. Lippincott, 1992, pp 92–103.

COMPUTED TOMOGRAPHY SCANS AND ULTRASOUND

David A. Lynch, MD

1. **Is it ever safe to give intravenous iodinated contrast to a patient with an elevated serum creatinine?**

   The decision to administer IV contrast to a patient with an elevated creatinine always requires careful consideration by the radiologist and the responsible clinician. Administration of IV contrast to such patients may result in further impairment of renal function, sometimes requiring dialysis. The risk of renal failure is increased by the presence of concomitant disease such as diabetes, treatment with nephrotoxic drugs, or hypotension. Performance of noncontrast computed tomography (CT), an alternative test (such as ultrasound or ventilation-perfusion (V/Q) lung scanning), or magnetic resonance (MR) angiography should be considered.

   If contrast-enhanced CT is thought to be critical for management of the patient, adequate hydration and use of N-acetylcysteine (600 mg twice daily on the day before and on the day of the examination) may decrease the risk of renal failure in those with modest renal impairment. However, some studies do not support the use of this agent. If a patient already has irreversible dialysis-dependent renal failure, the administration of IV contrast is unlikely to result in further harm.

   Maeder M, Klein M, Fehr T, Rickli H: Contrast nephropathy: Review focusing on prevention. J Am Coll Cardiol 44:1763–1771, 2004.

2. **Does contrast allergy preclude administration of IV contrast?**

   Again, the decision to administer IV contrast to a patient with previous contrast reaction requires careful consideration, and alternative tests should be considered. Factors to consider include the severity of the prior reaction. If contrast administration is deemed essential, the risk of severe reaction may be reduced by the use of low-osmolar contrast agents and by premedication with corticosteroids and antihistamines.

3. **What are the indications for CT scanning of the chest in the intensive care unit (ICU) setting?**

   The most common indications in critically ill patients are evaluation for pulmonary thromboembolism and evaluation of complex pleural effusion or pneumothorax. The benefits of CT in these patients must be weighed against the risk of transporting the patients.

4. **What is the radiation dose from a routine chest CT? How does it compare with the dose from a chest radiograph?**

   The radiation dose from a routine chest CT is about 5–8 mSv. For comparison, the radiation dose from a frontal and lateral chest radiograph is about 0.06 mSv, and the average annual background radiation is 3.6 mSv.

   Leswick DA, Webster ST, Wilcox BA, Fladeland DA: Radiation cost of helical high-resolution chest CT. Am J Roentgenol 184:742–745, 2005.

5. **What general problems may be encountered in CT scanning of the chest?**

   The most commonly encountered problem in chest CT scanning is the presence of an absolute or relative contraindication to the administration of intravenous contrast, usually either a history of contrast allergy or elevated creatinine. Patients who are morbidly obese may exceed the maximal weight allowed on the table portion of the scanner (usually 300–400 lbs) or may be too large to fit in the scan aperture, particularly with their arms elevated. Even if these patients can fit in the scanner, their scans are often suboptimal because of image noise and motion artifact. Patients with restricted shoulder-girdle movements (e.g., frozen shoulder) may be unable to place or maintain their arms in the optimal position. Metallic orthopedic devices, such as Harrington rods or metallic shoulder replacements, may cause significant artifact. Rarely, patients who are claustrophobic may be unable to tolerate CT scanning; this may usually be handled by appropriate sedation. Respiratory motion artifact is common in those unable to comply with breathing instructions.

6. **Are all CT scans of the thorax performed in the supine position?**
   The **supine** position, with arms elevated above the head, is the standard position for a CT examination of the thorax. **Prone** imaging is often included in high-resolution scan protocols to negate gravitational effects on the dependent portions of the lungs, particularly in interstitial lung diseases that have a predilection for the posterior lungs (e.g., asbestosis). The **lateral decubitus** position is particularly useful in the evaluation of pleural fluid collections, notably when there is associated consolidation.

7. **Are all CT scans of the chest performed in the same phase of respiration?**
   Routine scanning of the thorax is performed at end-inspiration. If the patient cannot suspend respiration for the required length of time, the scan may be performed during gentle mouth-breathing to minimize motion artifact. In dyspneic patients, breath-holding may be facilitated by encouraging prior gentle hyperventilation or by administration of oxygen. End-expiratory scanning is important in patients being evaluated with a high-resolution protocol for diffuse lung disease and in patients being evaluated for tracheobronchomalacia (abnormal tracheal or bronchial collapsibility). In some cases of suspected tracheomalacia, dynamic CT may be performed at one or two levels, with images obtained during a forced expiration; this technique is probably more sensitive than end-expiratory scanning for detection of large or small airway obstruction.

8. **What is meant by spiral CT?**
   Spiral, or helical, CT is a technique whereby image data are acquired continuously. The x-ray tube and detector rotate around the patient, who is moving continuously through the scan plane. This generates a spiral pattern of motion of the patient relative to the image receptor. Advantages of this technique include faster scan acquisition times, more efficient vascular imaging with reduced volumes of intravenous contrast, and improved ability to reconstruct images in

KEY POINTS: COMPUTED TOMOGRAPHY TECHNIQUE

1. Administration of intravenous contrast is indicated for evaluation of the pulmonary vasculature, mediastinal veins and arteries, the heart, the pulmonary hila, suspected lung cancer, and inflammatory pleural disease.

2. High-resolution CT is indicated for evaluation of known or suspected interstitial lung disease, bronchiectasis, and lung nodules.

3. Spiral CT with coronal and sagittal reconstructions may be helpful for evaluation of suspected airway stenosis.

4. Positron emission tomography (PET) scanning can be complementary to CT in diagnosis and staging of lung cancer.

the sagittal, coronal, and oblique planes. Scan slices may be reconstructed at variable thicknesses. Advanced image processing techniques can be used to produce three-dimensional or virtual bronchoscopic images. With progressive technologic improvements and increasing numbers of CT detector rows (currently up to 64 rows), excellent contiguous images of the entire thorax can now be obtained in 10–30 seconds.

9. **What is meant by high-resolution CT (HRCT)?**
The HRCT technique is designed for detailed evaluation of the interstitial structures of the lung. It requires the use of narrow slice thickness (1–2 mm, compared with 5–10 mm for routine scans) with high-resolution, edge-enhancing reconstruction algorithms to maximize depiction of lung detail. Additional prone and expiratory images are typically obtained. Contiguous thicker slices may or may not be acquired in conjunction with the noncontiguous thinner sections.

10. **How safe is CT-guided transthoracic needle biopsy (TNB)?**
Mortality from CT-guided TNB is reported to be 0.02%. Pneumothorax is the most common morbidity (typically 5–30%), but less than half of all patients who develop a pneumothorax require treatment with chest tube drainage. Postprocedure surveillance is critical in the first hour because >90% of pneumothoraces requiring intervention will be evident within that time. This is one of the reasons TNB can be safely performed on an outpatient basis.

Hemorrhage, with or without hemoptysis, occurs in 1–10% of cases and, in the absence of a bleeding diathesis, is usually self limiting. Other complications are uncommon and include vasovagal reactions, subcutaneous emphysema, malignant seeding of the biopsy track, and air embolism (which may be fatal).

Westcott JL: Percutaneous transthoracic needle biopsy. Radiology 169:593–601, 1988.

11. **Can one predict who will get a pneumothorax after TNB?**
Several prospective and retrospective studies have identified factors associated with *increased* risk of pneumothorax. These can be divided into three general categories, but many of these are interrelated.
- **Patient:** Increasing age, increased total lung capacity, PaO_2 <59 mmHg, ratio of forced expiratory volume in 1 second (FEV_1) to forced vital capacity (FVC) <70% predicted, intractable cough, and mechanical ventilation.
- **Target (lesion):** Deeper lesions, smaller lesions, cavitary lesions, and lymphangitic carcinoma.
- **Technique:** Number of pleural passes, increasing external diameter of biopsy needles, use of core-cutting needles rather than aspiration needles, increased duration of the procedure, and inexperience of the operator.

12. **Are there any contraindications to CT-guided TNB?**
- Absence of informed consent from the patient or his or her representative
- Biopsy by an inexperienced person without direct supervision
- Lack of adequate personnel and equipment to effectively manage all potential complications, including cardiopulmonary arrest
- Situations in which biopsy results, whether positive or negative, would have no effect on the patient's management or prognosis
- Severe obstructive lung disease (FEV_1 < 1.0 liter)
- A patient who is uncooperative or unable to maintain a constant position
- Intractable cough
- Bullae in the needle path
- Patients on a positive end-expiration pressure (PEEP) ventilation
- Possible echinococcal cyst
- Possible pulmonary arteriovenous malformation or other vascular lesion

- Severe pulmonary hypertension
- Uncorrectable bleeding diathesis or thrombocytopenia
- Recent myocardial infarction, unstable angina, cardiac decompensation, or uncontrolled cardiac arrhythmia
- Uremia
- Superior vena cava obstruction

The risk-to-benefit ratio should be assessed in each individual in whom there are relative contraindications to TNB.

KEY POINTS: COMPUTED TOMOGRAPHY DIAGNOSIS

1. The characteristic CT finding in pulmonary embolism is an intraluminal filling defect (Fig. 9-1).

2. The typical CT features of usual interstitial pneumonia are peripheral-predominant, basal-predominant, reticular abnormalities with honeycombing (Fig. 9-2).

3. Emphysema is readily recognized on CT by areas of decreased lung attenuation, often surrounding small vessels (Fig. 9-3).

4. Cavities on CT should suggest neoplasm, infection, infarction, or vasculitis (Fig 9-4).

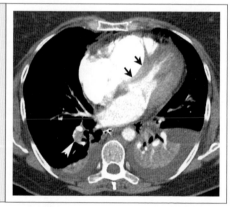

Figure 9-1. A 35-year-old woman with an acute pulmonary embolism. CT angiogram shows a filling defect partially outlined by contrast in the right lower lobe pulmonary artery *(arrowhead)*. Note the marked dilation of the right ventricle, with leftward shift of the septum *(arrows)*.

13. **When is ultrasound needed in thoracentesis?**
    Experienced clinicians can aspirate most pleural collections without image guidance. Small pleural effusions and those in which blind aspiration may be associated with increased risk are best aspirated with the help of ultrasound. In these situations, ultrasound can be used to identify the precise location of pleural fluid in an upright patient and may also determine the presence of loculations or abnormal echogenicity. In addition, ultrasound may identify local pleural abnormalities (e.g., metastases) when present.

14. **When can biopsy procedures be performed under ultrasound guidance?**
    Ultrasound cannot "see" through bone or aerated lung parenchyma, and, therefore, lesions accessible to ultrasound are usually apical, juxtadiaphragmatic, involving the chest wall, in the anterior mediastinum, or having a broad area of contact with the pleura. As a general rule, with ultrasound, "If it can be seen, it can be biopsied."

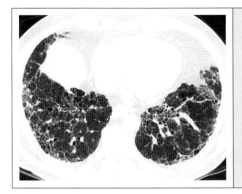

Figure 9-2. A 64-year-old man with idiopathic pulmonary fibrosis. High-resolution chest CT through the lower lungs shows a peripheral predominant, basal predominant, reticular abnormality with subpleural honeycombing, highly predictive of the histologic pattern of usual interstitial pneumonia.

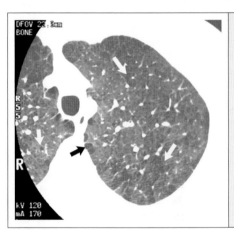

Figure 9-3. A 65-year-old man with emphysema. High-resolution CT shows small, poorly defined areas of decreased lung attenuation *(white arrows)* due to centrilobular emphysema. There is also subpleural (paraseptal) emphysema *(black arrow)*.

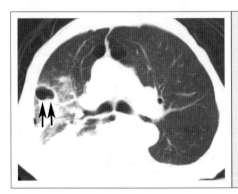

Figure 9-4. A 52-year-old man with staphylococcal pneumonia. Chest CT shows right upper lobe consolidation with a cavity, which contains an air-fluid level *(arrows)*.

15. **What is the role of ultrasound in the diagnosis of pulmonary thromboembolic disease?**

Ultrasound is very accurate in the diagnosis of above-calf deep vein thrombosis (DVT). The sensitivity of compression scanning is >90% with a specificity >98%, and sensitivity can be increased by the addition of Doppler and color-flow imaging. These additional techniques are essential in evaluating pelvic veins. However, the yield from evaluation of asymptomatic limbs is low. The calf veins are more difficult to image but are well visualized in 50–90% of cases, with a sensitivity for DVT diagnosis of approximately 80%, at the expense of an additional 15–30 minutes of scanning time. If pulmonary CT angiography is being performed for evaluation of pulmonary thromboembolism, CT venography, performed as an adjunct to the same study, can effectively evaluate pelvic, femoral, and popliteal veins for thrombus.

Stevens SM, Elliott CG, Chan KJ, et al: Withholding anticoagulation after a negative result on duplex ultra-sonography for suspected symptomatic deep venous thrombosis. Ann Intern Med 140:985–991, 2004.

16. **Is CT superior to fiberoptic bronchoscopy in the investigation of patients with hemoptysis?**
The most commonly identified causes of hemoptysis are bronchogenic carcinoma and bronchiectasis. Most patients with carcinoma can be diagnosed with either CT or bronchoscopy, but bronchoscopy has the advantage of detecting early mucosal abnormalities, inflammation, and squamous metaplasia and may identify blood in an airway when an actual bleeding point is not identified. If a lesion is identified at bronchoscopy, it may be biopsied directly. CT has the advantage of being noninvasive, less operator-dependent, and better at diagnosing peripheral tumors and bronchiectases, which are usually beyond the reach of the endoscopist. Ideally, CT should be performed and reviewed before bronchoscopy to optimize procedure planning.

Set PA, Flower CD, Smith IE, et al: Hemoptysis: Comparative study of the role of CT and fiberoptic bron-choscopy. Radiology 189:677–680, 1993.

17. **What is the role of CT in the staging of lung cancer?**
CT has an important role in distinguishing between resectable and unresectable lung cancer. Lung cancer is generally considered unresectable if there is involvement of the main bronchus within 2 cm of the carina; invasion of a vital mediastinal structure (e.g., the heart, esophagus, aorta, or superior vena cava), a malignant pleural effusion; metastases to the contralateral hilar, contralat-eral mediastinal, or extrathoracic lymph nodes; or metastases to the lung or distal organs.

However, patients usually should not be denied surgery solely on the basis of CT evidence; unresectability should, in general, be proven histologically or at surgery. In particular, since CT identifies lymph node metastases solely on the basis of nodal size (usually >1 cm in short axis), it cannot distinguish reactive from neoplastic enlargement, and it cannot identify metastases in normal-sized lymph nodes. Positron emission tomography (PET) scanning, using 18-fluorodeoxyglucose as an index of metabolic activity, has recently emerged as an important complementary technique to CT for lung cancer staging. Integration of CT with PET imaging may be useful in increasing the sensitivity and specificity of CT for identifying nodal and distant metastases, but it does not eliminate the need for tissue confirmation of suspected metastases.

Erasmus JJ, Truong MT, Munden RF: CT, MR, and PET imaging in staging of non-small-cell lung cancer. Semin Roentgenol 40:126–142, 2005.

18. **Is CT pulmonary arteriography as accurate as conventional pulmonary angiography in detecting pulmonary emboli (PE)?**
Contrast-enhanced spiral CT scanning can reliably detect PE in central pulmonary arteries. With single-detector CT scanners, reported sensitivity and specificity for CT diagnosis of PE in the main, lobar, and segmental vessels are both greater than 90%. For subsegmental PE, the angio-graphic gold standard is flawed, but sensitivity for subsegmental PE appears to have increased with the use of multi-detector CT scans (*see* Fig. 9-1).

Untreated patients without evidence of PE on a good-quality CT pulmonary arteriogram are unlikely to develop PE on follow-up over 3–6 months. The 1% incidence of subsequent fatal or nonfatal PE in this group is similar to that found following normal V/Q scans or pulmonary arteriography.

Goldhaber SZ: Multislice computed tomography for pulmonary embolism—A technological marvel. N Engl J Med 352:1812–1814, 2005.

19. **What is the role of chest CT in screening for lung cancer?**

    In high-risk patients, use of annual low-dose screening CT results in detection of lung cancer in 1–2% of cases at the first screen and in about 0.5% of cases per year at subsequent annual visits. Most screen-detected lung cancers appear to be early stage and ostensibly curable. However, uncontrolled cohort studies of screening are difficult to evaluate because of potential biases (i.e., over-diagnosis, lead-time bias, and length-time bias), and there is no proof that screening decreases mortality from lung cancer. Moreover, the false-positive rate from detection of incidental benign nodules ranges from 25–75%. The results of an ongoing randomized controlled trial (the National Lung Screening Trial) in the United States are awaited to determine whether CT screening is effective in reducing mortality.

    Swensen SJ, Jett JR, Hartman TE, et al: CT screening for lung cancer: Five-year prospective experience. Radiology 235:259–265, 2005.

20. **How accurate is high-resolution CT for diagnosis of usual interstitial pneumonia (UIP)?**

    In the classification of idiopathic interstitial pneumonias, UIP is the morphologic pattern associated with the clinical diagnosis of idiopathic pulmonary fibrosis. HRCT has an important role in identifying this morphologic pattern and in distinguishing it from other conditions. The characteristic CT features of this condition are basal-predominant, peripheral-predominant, reticular abnormalities associated with honeycombing (*see* Fig. 9-2). Features that suggest another condition include nodules, consolidation, discrete cysts, abundant ground-glass abnormalities, and evidence of air trapping. When the typical features of UIP are present and atypical clinical or imaging features are absent, the diagnosis may be correctly made in over 90% of cases.

    Hunninghake GW, Lynch DA, Galvin JR, et al: Radiologic findings are strongly associated with a pathologic diagnosis of usual interstitial pneumonia. Chest 124:1215–1223, 2003.

CHAPTER 10

PULMONARY ANGIOGRAPHY AND MAGNETIC RESONANCE IMAGING OF THE CHEST

Jonathan Kullnat, MD, and Marc V. Gosselin, MD

PULMONARY ANGIOGRAPHY

1. **What are the indications for pulmonary angiography?**

   Historically, the most common indication for pulmonary angiography was the detection of pulmonary embolism when lung ventilation/perfusion (V/Q) scanning was nondiagnostic. However, with the advent and increasing availability of multi-detector spiral computed tomography (CT) scanners, at many institutions, pulmonary angiography is diagnostically reserved for use in conjunction with interventional procedures; these include embolization of pulmonary arteriovenous malformations, aneurysms, and congenital vascular anomalies; embolectomy; and thrombolysis. The Prospective Investigation of Pulmonary Embolism Diagnosis (PIOPED) II database has formally begun evaluating the sensitivity, specificity, positive predictive value, and negative predictive value of contrast-enhanced spiral CT for pulmonary emboli (PE).

2. **List the contraindications to pulmonary angiography.**

   Contraindications to pulmonary angiography relate to one of the following three factors:

   1. **Iodinated contrast:** A previous severe contrast reaction warrants pretreatment with oral corticosteroids (32 mg of methylprednisolone 12 and 2 hours before the procedure) and the use of nonionic contrast. This regimen limits the overall incidence of contrast reactions to less than 2%. Pulmonary angiography is also contraindicated in patients with renal insufficiency (i.e., serum creatinine levels >2.0 mg/dL).
   2. **Cardiac disease:** Patients with a left bundle-branch block are at risk for complete heart block if the angiographic catheter induces a right bundle-branch block as it courses through the heart. In such patients, prophylactic placement of a transvenous pacemaker is necessary before the procedure. Patients susceptible to frequent ventricular tachyarrhythmias may require intravenous lidocaine (or, increasingly, amiodarone) treatment to suppress ventricular ectopy induced by the tip of the catheter as it traverses the right ventricle.
   3. **Pulmonary arterial hypertension and cor pulmonale:** Pulmonary artery systolic pressure exceeding 80 mmHg or right ventricle end-diastolic pressure exceeding 20 mmHg is associated with an increased risk of death from pulmonary angiography. (Indeed, this subgroup of patients accounts for nearly all of the procedure-related mortality). The vasoconstrictive effects of hypertonic contrast on the pulmonary arteries produce a sudden elevation in pulmonary pressures and can result in right heart failure.

   Kaufman JA, Lee CV: Vascular and Interventional Radiology. St. Louis, Mosby, 2003.

3. **How is a pulmonary angiogram performed?**

   This procedure is usually performed under fluoroscopic guidance in the angiography suite of the radiology department. It entails puncturing the femoral vein and placing a pigtail or balloon-tipped catheter into the inferior vena cava (IVC). The catheter is advanced into the right atrium, through the tricuspid valve, and into the right ventricle as the electrocardiogram (ECG) is monitored closely for ventricular arrhythmias. The catheter is then advanced into the pulmonary artery, and the pressure is measured. Routinely, direct anteroposterior and ipsilateral posterior oblique projections are obtained, each using an injection of 40–50 cc at a rate of 25 cc/sec. The study has traditionally been performed with conventional cut-film techniques, which have superior resolution and are less susceptible to motion artifact compared with digital subtraction angiography (DSA). However, DSA is being increasingly utilized because of its decreased associated costs, shorter procedure and hospital times, and increased contrast resolution. The evaluation is complete when an embolus is detected or all pulmonary arteries in question have been visualized. Thus, the angiogram may be complete after a single injection or may require six to eight injections to evaluate the entire arterial system.

If pulmonary embolism is diagnosed in a patient with a contraindication to anticoagulant therapy, an IVC filter can be placed immediately following the angiogram. This requires an additional 30 minutes and is performed through the same venotomy site. A properly positioned IVC filter limits the rate of recurrent pulmonary embolism to 2–5%. Long-term patency rates range between 65% and 98%.

Kaufman JA, Lee CV: Vascular and Interventional Radiology. St. Louis, Mosby, 2003.

4. **What monitoring is recommended during a pulmonary angiogram?**
Cardiac monitoring is necessary during pulmonary angiography, particularly since catheter manipulation through the right ventricle often induces ventricular ectopy. Blood pressure and oxygen saturation are monitored continuously during the procedure. Once the catheter has been placed into the pulmonary artery, a transducer is used to measure the pulmonary artery pressure. If pulmonary hypertension (defined as systolic pressure exceeding 40 mmHg) is present, the rate and volume of contrast injected are reduced to prevent sudden right ventricular overload.

5. **Describe the angiographic findings of acute and chronic thromboembolism.**
Two direct angiographic findings are considered specific for acute pulmonary embolus: a central intraluminal filling defect, which is the most common appearance (94%), and an abrupt contrast cut-off outlining the proximal convex margin of the embolus. In 65% of patients, multiple emboli are found; bilateral emboli are seen in 42%, most commonly in the lower lobes (due to their relatively greater perfusion). Secondary findings include diminished peripheral perfusion, delayed or absent venous filling, and the presence of tortuous arterial collaterals. Unfortunately, these findings are nonspecific; they can be seen in several other disease processes including vasculitis and chronic obstructive pulmonary disease (COPD).

Chronic pulmonary thromboembolism exists when intraluminal organization of the thrombus is incomplete. This can produce several angiographic findings including proximal arterial dilation and distal occlusion with a tapered or rounded edge, stenosis, webs, or eccentric plaques.

Grainger RG, Allison DJ, Adam A, et al (eds): Diagnostic Radiology: A Textbook of Medical Imaging, 4th ed. New York, Churchill Livingstone, 2001.

6. **How accurate is pulmonary angiography?**
Although pulmonary angiography is considered the gold standard for the diagnosis of pulmonary embolism, no studies have compared the accuracy of pulmonary angiography with autopsy findings. It should also at least be recognized that although DSA is being utilized increasingly, much of the literature is based on traditional angiographic techniques. Nevertheless, retrospective and small prospective studies comparing traditional pulmonary angiography with DSA have found no differences with respect to diagnostic accuracy.

Studies comparing interobserver variability in pulmonary angiographic interpretation show a 98% agreement rate for lobar emboli, 90% for segmental emboli, and 66% agreement for subsegmental emboli. These data suggest that the sensitivity of pulmonary angiography is limited when only subsegmental emboli are present. The significance of small subsegmental emboli is controversial. It is likely that they are occasionally missed; yet, follow-up of untreated patients with subsegmental emboli shows a recurrence rate of symptomatic embolism of only 0.6%; the overall rate of thromboembolic events was < 3%. For this reason, a negative pulmonary angiogram is associated with a good prognosis.

Baile EM, King GG, Muller NL, et al: Spiral computed tomography is comparable to angiography for the diagnosis of pulmonary embolism. Am J Respir Crit Care Med 161(3 Pt 1):1010–1015, 2000.

KEY POINTS: COMPLICATIONS OF PULMONARY ANGIOGRAPHY

1. Mild, moderate, or severe contrast reaction

2. Serious cardiac arrhythmias or cardiac arrest (1%)

3. Death (0.2–0.05%), almost exclusively in patients with severe pulmonary arterial hypertension and right ventricular failure

4. Papillary muscle or tricuspid valve injury may occur if the pigtail catheter is not carefully withdrawn upon completion of the angiogram

5. Hematoma

7. **What are the risk factors for a contrast reaction? How is it treated?**
   There are two forms of contrast reactions: nonidiosyncratic and idiosyncratic.
   Nonidiosyncratic reactions are related to the chemical properties of contrast agents and include nausea, vomiting, arrhythmias, congestive heart failure, angina, renal failure, and seizures. Patients at greater risk for contrast-induced nephrotoxicity and renal failure include those with diabetes, congestive heart failure (or other causes of decreased intravascular volume), nephrotic syndrome, and multiple myeloma. The use of a smaller volume of nonionic contrast reduces the incidence of nephrotoxicity. Hydrating with HCO_3^-, as well as pretreatment with N-acetylcysteine (NAC), appears to further reduce the incidence of contrast-related nephrotoxicity relative to preprocedural hydration with NaCl alone. Although the literature is somewhat conflicting and the studies are not without flaws, because of the low cost involved and minimal associated side effects, the use of NAC and HCO_3^- should be considered, as follows:
   - **NAC:** 600 mg twice a day on the day prior and the day of the procedure.
   - **HCO_3^-:** 750 mL of 0.154 mol/L $NaHCO_3$.
   Finally, it has been increasingly recognized that intraprocedural and postprocedural hydration are perhaps the most helpful preventive measures available.
   Symptoms of a mild **idiosyncratic** reaction occur in 5–10% of patients and include pruritus, urticaria, and flushing. Antihistamines may be administered to symptomatic patients. Moderate reactions, including bronchospasm or angioedema, are treated with supplemental oxygen, parenteral bronchodilators, and antihistamines.
   Major reactions included arrhythmias, myocardial infarction, hypotension, anaphylactoid shock, and death. The fatality rate from intravascular contrast injection is less than 1 in 10,000 patients. Patients at increased risk for severe idiosyncratic contrast reaction include those with a history of prior contrast reaction (who are elevenfold more likely than the general population), asthma (who face a fivefold increase), and multiple food or medication allergies (with a fourfold increase). If a patient is considered to be at high risk for a contrast reaction, pretreatment with corticosteroids 12 and 2 hours before the procedure and the use of nonionic contrast decrease the incidence and severity of reactions.
   Hypotension due to a vasovagal reaction is not uncommon; the presence of bradycardia helps distinguish this form of hypotensive reaction from anaphylactoid shock. In the former case, the bradycardia contributes to the hypotension, whereas in the latter, the relative tachycardia observed occurs as a compensatory response. As such, severe hypotension from anaphylaxis is treated with vasopressors (epinephrine, 1–3 mg of 1:10,000 IV or 0.1–0.3 mg of

1:1000 SQ); vasovagal hypotension is effectively managed with atropine (0.5–1.0 mg IV to a total of 2 mg).

Severe respiratory complications are managed by airway maintenance and may require intubation and mechanical ventilation in severe cases.

Merten GJ, Burgess WP, Gray LV, et al: Prevention of contrast-induced nephropathy with sodium bicarbonate: A randomized control trial. JAMA 291(19):2328–2334, 2004.

MAGNETIC RESONANCE IMAGING

8. **How does magnetic resonance imaging (MRI) work?**
    MRI uses the properties of nuclear magnetic resonance (NMR) to produce images. Nuclei with unpaired protons, neutrons, or both have a net spin and angular momentum, or magnetic moment, and can be used to produce an NMR signal. Normally, only hydrogen atoms are sufficiently abundant to be useful in imaging applications. When referring to MRI, unless it is otherwise specified, hydrogen is implied.

    Whereas individual nuclear magnetic moments are miniscule, the powerful magnetic field employed in an MRI (1 tesla is approximately equal to 20,000 times the strength of the earth's magnetic field) aligns the many spinning hydrogen protons and produces a measurable net electromagnetic vector. This proton alignment is then disrupted with different carefully selected sequences of radiofrequency pulses over milliseconds. As the protons return to their original configuration within the large magnetic field, they induce an electromagnetic signal in the unit's receiving coils. After several repetitions over a preset region, the total information is processed mathematically (using variations of a Fourier transformation) and is converted to a cross-sectional image. Unlike CT and other ionizing modalities, tissue differentiation is based not on density but on several other factors, including the relative number of protons, the local heterogeneities within the magnetic field, the relation of excited protons inherent within various tissues (known as T1 and T2 relaxation times), as well as the type of pulse sequence employed. Because there are numerous sequences available to depict different information, the radiologist requires an adequate history to tailor the MRI examination to the clinical situation.

    Mirowitz SA, White CS (eds): MRI Images of the Thorax. MRI Clin North Am 8(1), 2000.

9. **What are the advantages of thoracic MRI versus CT?**
    Although CT is the most widely used cross-sectional imaging modality for depicting chest disease, there are situations in which MRI can be helpful. The ability of MRI to perform direct coronal and sagittal imaging is particularly useful in the evaluation of brachial plexus involvement by a superior sulcus (i.e., Pancoast's tumor), posterior mediastinal masses, and diaphragmatic and juxtacardiac lesions. Because of its excellent depiction of vascular anatomy and direct multiplanar imaging capabilities, MRI has traditionally been the primary modality in the evaluation of congenital cardiovascular disease, aortic dissections, and aneurysms in stable patients and in examining the relationship of a mediastinal or hilar mass to central vascular structures. However, with the increasing availability of multidetector spiral CTs with image reformations and its superior visualization of the pulmonary vasculature, MRI's relative advantage in the diagnosis of these disease processes is lessened.

    MRI does provide superior tissue contrast (although with decreased spatial resolution) that can be useful in the detection of mediastinal or chest wall invasion by lung cancer. In addition, residual or recurrent mediastinal lymphoma can be potentially differentiated from post-treatment fibrosis. Another advantage of MRI is its ability to demonstrate blood flow without the use of intravenous contrast, which is particularly useful in patients with renal insufficiency or a severe contrast allergy. Although contrast may still be given, it is noniodinated, does not cause renal nephropathy, and is associated with a very low risk of allergic reaction. The lack of ionizing radiation and the increasing ability to evaluate physiologic parameters are further advantages of this imaging modality.

10. **What are the disadvantages of thoracic MRI?**
    The thorax is the most difficult region of the body to image with MRI. Since only 10–20% of the lung parenchyma is composed of tissue and blood vessels, there are few protons available to generate a signal. Also, the innumerable tissue–air interfaces give the local magnetic field tremendous heterogeneity, which limits the utility of the T2-weighted spin-echo pulse sequence. Another limitation is motion artifact from the heart, great vessels, and respiration, which, without gated sequences, results in poor spatial resolution. Respiratory and cardiac gating, as well as the development of rapid sequence techniques, have greatly improved the quality of the (non-lung parenchymal) images obtained. Finally, relative to CT, MRI typically requires greater scan times, has greater cost, and does not demonstrate calcification, which would be useful in differentiating benign from malignant processes. Certain patients may find the required breath holding problematic.

11. **What role does MRI have in diagnosing pulmonary embolus?**
    MRI has the ability to diagnose PE through multiple methods: magnetic resonance angiography (MRA), V/Q MRI, and direct clot imaging (which takes advantage of characteristic signal changes from hemoglobin). MRI is unable to reliably visualize pulmonary vessels beyond the segmental level. Because of its increased relative costs, technical requirements, and lesser availability, it is doubtful that MRI/MRA will be used routinely in the evaluation of PE. Nevertheless, when available, in patients with contraindications to IV iodinated contrast, it offers an alternative means of diagnosis.

12. **Discuss some more investigational applications in which thoracic MRI may eventually become useful.**
    In addition to its numerous current applications, cardiac MRI is a rapidly evolving field. Applications under current investigation include contrast-enhanced coronary MRA, infarct sizing, assessment of valvular disease and arthroscopic plaques, myocardial perfusion imaging, and phosphorus-31 cardiac stress tests.

KEY POINTS: POTENTIAL CLINICAL SITUATIONS FOR THORACIC MRI

1. Assessment of neurovascular involvement by superior sulcus tumor

2. Differentiation between recurrent lymphoma and post-therapeutic fibrosis

3. Chest wall, hilar, and mediastinal invasion by tumor

4. Diagnosis of constrictive pericarditis, tumor invasion of the pericardium, and differentiation between hemorrhagic and nonhemorrhagic effusions

5. Aortic dissection or aneurysm (in stable patients)

6. Evaluation of congenital heart disease and cardiac masses

7. Evaluation of myocardial viability and contractile function

8. Differentiation of various cardiomyopathies

9. Estimation of the degree of cardiac shunt

10. Diaphragmatic evaluations

Although MRI has traditionally been extremely limited in its ability to evaluate the lungs, current research and trials employing inhaled He-3, Xe-129, or oxygen (because of its paramagnetic properties) have been promising. Because of the unique properties of MRI, physiologic as well as anatomic information can be obtained. These techniques can differentiate between normal and emphysematous lung tissue and can aid in the planning and follow-up of lung volume reduction surgeries. He-3, in particular, is also able to demonstrate changes associated with graft versus host disease following lung transplantation earlier and more extensively than HRCT. Finally, these techniques have also shown promise in the response to therapy evaluation of asthmatics and those with cystic fibrosis, groups in which repeated imaging with ionizing modalities may be undesirable.

13. **What are the absolute and relative contraindications to MRI?**
   - **Absolute:** Pacemakers and even inactive pacing leads act like an antenna to induce arrhythmias from the strong electromagnetic field. Any ferromagnetic metal within or adjacent to vital structures can shift in the strong magnetic field and cause tissue damage. Before the MRI examination, the patient should be questioned about the presence of such devices, which may include older aneurysm clips, metallic foreign bodies in the orbit, cochlear implants, and older Starr–Edwards cardiac valve prostheses.
   - **Relative:** Since the MRI tunnel is confining, a claustrophobic patient must be sedated before entering the MRI area; otherwise, an alternative imaging modality should be selected. Similarly, uncooperative patients and children need to be sedated to reduce motion artifacts. As a result of the rapidly changing magnetic fields, the MRI machine generates a repetitive loud banging noise that can agitate a disoriented patient or child. Although there is no evidence of any harmful effects on the fetus, elective MRI examinations on pregnant patients should be postponed until the postpartum period unless absolutely necessary. In the case of neurostimulators, bone stimulators, hearing aids, and certain dental implants, the relative benefits and risks should be considered.

14. **What techniques are used to reduce motion artifacts?**
   Cardiac motion is reduced with the use of ECG cardiac gating. The electromagnetic pulses are synchronized to set points in the cardiac cycle, usually the R-wave of the QRS complex. This allows imaging to occur at the same phase of the cardiac cycle, which substantially diminishes motion artifact and only minimally increases the length of the examination. Cardiac gating can only be implemented in patients with a regular cardiac rate and rhythm; it cannot be used in patients with frequent ectopy or atrial arrhythmias such as atrial fibrillation.

   Respiratory compensation is usually accomplished with a sensor device on the chest wall that matches chest wall motion with the acquisition of images, thereby allowing the computer to compensate for significant respiratory motion. This technique, however, increases the total length of the study by 200–300% unless the number of sequence repetitions is decreased (sacrificing the signal-to-noise ratio). Alternatively, fast sequences that enable the study to be completed within a single breath hold, as well as other nongated methods of minimizing artifact, have been developed that further improve image quality.

CHAPTER 11

ARTERIAL BLOOD GASES

Dean Hess, PhD, RRT

1. **What are arterial blood gases (ABGs)?**

   The term *arterial blood gases* (ABGs) refers to measurements of hydrogen ion concentration (pH), partial pressure of carbon dioxide (PCO_2), and partial pressure of oxygen (PO_2) in arterial blood. Measured values for hemoglobin saturation with oxygen (O_2Hb), carboxyhemoglobin (COHb), and methemoglobin (metHb) may be included. Many laboratories also report calculated values of oxygen saturation, bicarbonate concentration, and base excess. These measurements assess oxygenation, ventilation, and acid–base status.

2. **How can the complications of arterial puncture be avoided?**

   The rare risk of complications is decreased with the radial artery because there is collateral blood flow to the hand (commonly assessed using the modified Allen's test), the radial artery (unlike the brachial artery) is far enough away from nerves (e.g., the medial nerve) that damage to the nerve is unlikely, the radial site is generally more aseptic than the femoral site, the radial artery is often near the surface so it is easy to palpate, and pain from the puncture is lessened. The risk of bleeding complications is increased with anticoagulant or thrombolytic therapy; in these cases, pressure must be manually applied to the puncture site until all signs of bleeding are absent (a minimum of 5–10 minutes). The risk of pain is decreased by use of a 22- or 23-gauge needle, and a local anesthetic (e.g., lidocaine) can be used to lessen the pain associated with arterial puncture.

   Giner J, Casan P, Belda J, et al: Pain during arterial puncture. Chest 110:1443–1445, 1996.

3. **Describe the complications associated with arterial catheters.**

   An arterial catheter is indicated for continuous blood pressure monitoring and the need for frequent ABG samples or other laboratory assessments. Routine insertion of arterial catheters is unwarranted because this practice increases the number of unnecessary laboratory tests obtained. Serious complications of arterial catheters, although rare, include hemorrhage, vascular occlusion, and infection. Thrombus formation is avoided by use of a continuous irrigation system, although the presence of heparin in the irrigation may not be necessary. When blood is collected from arterial catheters, the irrigation solution must be cleared from the connected tubing, which can cause considerable blood loss if samples are collected frequently and blood conservation procedures are not used.

4. **Why are blood gas samples transported on ice?**

   Metabolism by blood cells continues in the syringe until the sample is analyzed, causing a decrease in PO_2, an increase in PCO_2, and a decrease in pH. This can be diminished by transport of the sample in an ice-water slush unless the sample is analyzed within 10 minutes. The metabolic effects on the blood sample are caused primarily by the activity of leukocytes. In patients with leukocytosis > 100,000 cells/μL, the PaO_2 of the blood sample may decrease very quickly, which is called **leukocyte larceny**. It may be impossible to accurately determine the PaO_2 of patients in extreme leukocytosis, and *in vivo* methods (e.g., pulse oximetry) may be more reliable.

5. **Why is heparin used in blood gas syringes?**
Coagulation of the blood sample must be avoided because clots interfere with the function of the blood gas analyzer. Dry lyophilized lithium heparin is used so that electrolyte measurements can be performed using the blood gas sample. Moreover, dry heparin reduces the risk of preanalytic errors caused by dilution of the sample with the volume of the liquid form of heparin. The PO_2 and PCO_2 of liquid heparin are virtually the same as the PO_2 and PCO_2 of ambient air (about 150 mm Hg and 0 mm Hg, respectively, at sea level). Heparin dilution causes the measured PCO_2 of the sample to decrease and the PO_2 of the sample to move toward 150 mm Hg (the measured PO_2 increases if the true value is less than 150 mm Hg and decreases if the true value is more than 150 mm Hg). High concentrations of heparin are acidic (pH less than 7) and lower the pH of the sample. If liquid heparin is used, its effects can be minimized by using only enough to fill the dead volume of the needle and syringe.

6. **Why must arterial blood gas samples be obtained anaerobically?**
A common preanalytic error related to blood gases is contamination of the sample with room air. At sea level, air has a PO_2 of about 150 mm Hg and a PCO_2 of about 0 mm Hg. Thus, if the sample is contaminated with air, the measured PO_2 of the sample increases if the true value is less than 150 mm Hg and decreases if the true value is more than 150 mm Hg. Contamination of the sample with air lowers the PCO_2 of the sample with a resultant increase in pH.

7. **Are blood gas levels stable or are they variable in apparently stable patients?**
ABG levels may vary considerably over brief 5- to 10-minute intervals in critically ill mechanically ventilated patients who otherwise appear stable. Different measured values may reflect physiologic alterations such as subtle changes in cardiopulmonary function or patient repositionings that alter distribution of blood flow to the lungs, or they may result from preanalytic error. Variability is greatest for PO_2 and less for PCO_2 and pH. It is important not to react too strongly to a single blood gas result that differs from previous results in an otherwise clinically stable patient.

Sasse SA, Chem PA, Mahutte CK: Variability of arterial blood gas values over time in stable medical ICU patients. Chest 106:187–193, 1994.

8. **Why can't venous blood gases be used instead of ABGs?**
Arterial blood gases reflect lung function. Venous blood gases reflect the adequacy of tissue oxygenation and tissue carbon dioxide clearance. A low mixed venous PO_2 (<35 mm Hg) reflects tissue hypoxia and may be the result of decreased oxygen delivery or increased tissue oxygen uptake. Venous PO_2 is typically much lower than arterial PO_2, and there is often little relationship between the two. For example, the mixed venous PO_2 may be low and the arterial PO_2 may be high if cardiac output is reduced, lung function is normal, and FiO_2 is high. Normally, the mixed venous PCO_2 is only slightly greater than the arterial PCO_2. However, venous PCO_2 depends on blood flow and, in cases of low blood flow (e.g., cardiac arrest), the mixed venous PCO_2 may be high even though the arterial PCO_2 is normal or decreased.

9. **Can the PaO_2 normally be less than 75 mm Hg or more than 100 mm Hg?**
The PaO_2 can never be greater than the partial pressure of oxygen that exists in the alveolar space (PAO_2). The modified alveolar gas equation is used to calculate the PAO_2:

$$PAO_2 = (EBP \times FiO_2) - (1.25 \times PaCO_2)$$

where effective barometric pressure (EBP) is the effective barometric pressure. EBP is the difference between barometric pressure and water vapor pressure at body temperature (47 mm Hg at 37°C). For an individual breathing room air (FiO_2 0.21) at sea level (barometric pressure = 760 mm Hg) with a normal $PaCO_2$ (40 mm Hg), the PAO_2 is ≈ 100 mm Hg. Considering the alveolar-to-arterial (A-a) gradient of 5–10 mm Hg, the measured PaO_2 would be 90–95 mm Hg. The alveolar gas equation predicts that the PAO_2 will be <100 mm Hg if the barometric pressure is <760 mm Hg.

Thus, the normal PaO_2 is lower at higher altitudes. For example, the PaO_2 is ≈ 75 mm Hg at an altitude at which ambient barometric pressure is 650 mm Hg. On the other hand, PaO_2 will be > 100 mm Hg with hyperbaric conditions (e.g., patients treated with hyperbaric oxygen). PaO_2 also increases with an increase in FiO_2. The alveolar gas equation predicts that the PAO_2 will be ≈ 675 mm Hg when 100% oxygen is breathed at sea level; thus, the PaO_2 is normally > 600 mm Hg when FiO_2 is 1.0.

10. **What is the highest possible PaO_2 for a normal person breathing 50% oxygen at sea level, and what is the highest possible PaO_2 for a normal person breathing room air at an ambient pressure of 500 mm Hg?**
The highest possible PaO_2 for a normal person breathing 50% oxygen at sea level is:

$$PAO_2 = (713 \times 0.50) - (1.25 \times 40) = 300 \text{ mm Hg}$$

Because the A-a gradient increases with FiO_2, the measured PaO_2 in a person breathing 50% oxygen at sea level would be less than the PAO_2 of 300 mm Hg. The highest possible PaO_2 for a normal person breathing room air at an ambient pressure of 500 mm Hg (EBP = 453 mm Hg) is:

$$PAO_2 = (453 \times 0.21) - (1.25 \times 40) = 45 \text{ mm Hg}$$

11. **How does hypoxia differ from hypoxemia?**
Hypoxemia refers to decreased delivery of oxygen from the atmosphere to the blood. Hypoxemia is defined by a PaO_2 of less than 80 mm Hg in a person breathing room air at sea level. **Hypoxia** refers to decreased delivery of oxygen to the tissues. It is important to recognize that hypoxemia may occur without hypoxia, and vice versa.

KEY POINTS: CAUSES OF HYPOXEMIA

1. **Decreased inspired oxygen**: Altitude

2. **Hypoventilation**: Respiratory center depression, neuromuscular disease, or respiratory failure

3. **Shunt**: Pulmonary (e.g., atelectasis, pneumonia, pulmonary edema, or acute respiratory distress syndrome) or cardiac (i.e., patent foramen ovale)

4. **V/Q mismatch**: Airway secretions or bronchospasm

5. **Diffusion defect**: Pulmonary fibrosis, emphysema, or pulmonary resection

KEY POINTS: CAUSES OF HYPOXIA

1. **Hypoxemic hypoxia**: Lower-than-normal PaO_2 (hypoxemia)

2. **Anemic hypoxia**: Decreased red blood cell count, carboxyhemoglobin, methemoglobin, or hemoglobinopathy

3. **Circulatory hypoxia**: Decreased cardiac output or decreased local perfusion

4. **Affinity hypoxia**: Decreased release of oxygen from hemoglobin to the tissues

5. **Histotoxic hypoxia**: Cyanide poisoning

12. **What determines hemoglobin oxygen saturation?**
    The saturation of hemoglobin is determined by the oxyhemoglobin dissociation curve
    (Fig. 11-1), for which oxygen saturation is a function of PO_2. The affinity of hemoglobin for
    oxygen is high at high saturations and less at lower saturations. This effect facilitates oxygen
    loading in the lungs (where the PO_2 is high) and oxygen unloading to the tissues (where the PO_2
    is low). The position of the oxyhemoglobin dissociation curve is not fixed. Factors that shift the
    curve to the left increase the affinity of hemoglobin for oxygen, and factors that shift the curve to
    the right decrease the affinity of hemoglobin for oxygen. Saturation of hemoglobin is also
    affected by conditions such as COHb and metHb. Carbon monoxide attaches to oxygen binding
    sites of hemoglobin with a high affinity and decreases the ability of hemoglobin to carry oxygen.
    Thus, the hemoglobin oxygen saturation cannot be greater than 70% if the COHb level is 30%.
    Methemoglobin is produced when the iron in the hemoglobin molecule is converted from its
    reduced state (Fe^{2+}) to its oxidized state (Fe^{3+}). Hemoglobin can carry oxygen only if the iron is
    in the reduced state. Thus, metHb decreases the ability of hemoglobin to transport oxygen.

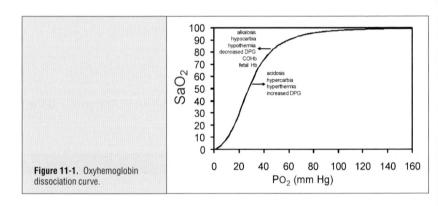

Figure 11-1. Oxyhemoglobin dissociation curve.

13. **How is oxygen saturation of arterial blood measured?**
    Oxygen saturation is measured by CO-oximetry. The CO-oximeter measures oxygen saturation
    by light absorption. Multiple wavelength CO-oximetry can measure COHb and metHb in addition
    to oxyhemoglobin. Oxygen saturation (SaO_2) can be calculated from PaO_2 and pH. However, the
    calculated SaO_2 may differ considerably from the measured SaO_2. The calculated SaO_2 consid-
    ers only the effects of PaO_2 and pH and disregards other physiologic effects on the oxyhemoglo-
    bin dissociation curve. The calculated SaO_2 also does not consider the effects of COHb and
    metHb, resulting in an overestimation of SaO_2 when these are present.

14. **Why might a patient have a high PaO_2 but a low measured oxygen saturation?**
    From the oxyhemoglobin dissociation curve, one would predict an oxygen saturation of nearly
    100% when the PaO_2 is 150 mm Hg. A low saturation with a high PaO_2 means that something
    has decreased the ability of hemoglobin to bind oxygen. One explanation is the presence of
    COHb or metHb. Pulse oximetry is not appropriate for this evaluation because it uses only two
    wavelengths of light and is unable to differentiate among oxyhemoglobin, COHb, and metHb.

15. **What determines the $PaCO_2$?**
    $PaCO_2$ is determined by carbon dioxide production ($\dot{V}CO_2$) and alveolar ventilation. Alveolar ven-
    tilation is determined by minute ventilation ($\dot{V}_E$) and the ratio of dead space to total ventilation
    (V_D/V_T). Thus,

    $$PaCO_2 = \dot{V}CO_2/[\dot{V}_E \times (1 - V_D/V_T)]$$

As seen in Figure 11-2, $PaCO_2$ will increase with an increase in V_D/V_T, an increase in $\dot{V}CO_2$, and a decrease in $\dot{V}_E$.

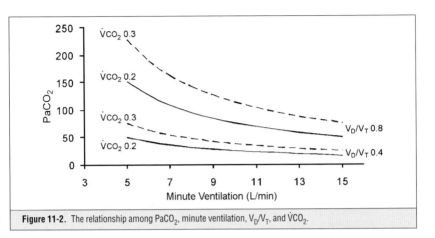

Figure 11-2. The relationship among $PaCO_2$, minute ventilation, V_D/V_T, and $\dot{V}CO_2$.

KEY POINTS: CAUSES OF INCREASED PaCO₂

1. **Increased $\dot{V}CO_2$:** Fever, sepsis, high calorie intake, high carbohydrate intake, or exercise

2. **Increased V_D/V_T:** Pulmonary embolism, pulmonary hypoperfusion, positive pressure ventilation or high rate–low tidal volume ventilation

---

16. **What is the Henderson-Hasselbalch equation?**
    The Henderson-Hasselbalch equation describes the relationship among pH, HCO_3^-, and PCO_2:

$$pH = 6.1 + \log \frac{[HCO_3^-]}{(0.03 \times PCO_2)}$$

17. **What is the difference between a respiratory and a metabolic acid–base disturbance?**
    Changes in pH resulting from changes in HCO_3^- are called *metabolic* acid–base disorders, and changes in pH resulting from changes in PCO_2 are called *respiratory* acid–base disorders (Table 11-1). An increase in pH caused by an increase in HCO_3^- is a metabolic alkalosis, and an increase in pH caused by a decrease in PCO_2 is a respiratory alkalosis. A decrease in pH caused by a decrease in HCO_3^- is a metabolic acidosis, and a decrease in pH caused by an increase in PCO_2 is a respiratory acidosis.

18. **What is a compensated acid–base disturbance?**
    Whenever the ratio of HCO_3^- to $(0.03 \times PCO_2)$ is 20:1, the pH is normal (7.40). A compensated respiratory acid-base disorder occurs when a physiologic change in HCO_3^- occurs secondary to a PCO_2 change so that the ratio of HCO_3^- to $(0.03 \times PCO_2)$ is 20:1 and, thus, the pH is normal. Likewise, a physiologic change in PCO_2 may occur secondary to a HCO_3^- disorder so that the ratio of HCO_3^- to $(0.03 \times PCO_2)$ is 20:1 and, thus, the pH is normal (respiratory compensation for a metabolic disturbance). The expected compensation is given in Table 11-2.

TABLE 11-1. COMMON ACID–BASE DISTURBANCES

Disorder	pH	PaCO$_2$	HCO$_3^-$
Respiratory acidosis			
Uncompensated	↓↓	↑↑	nl
Partially compensated	↓	↑↑	↑
Fully compensated	nl	↑↑	↑↑
Respiratory alkalosis			
Uncompensated	↑↑	↓↓	nl
Partially compensated	↑	↓↓	↓
Fully compensated	nl	↓↓	↓↓
Metabolic acidosis			
Uncompensated	↓↓	nl	↓↓
Partially compensated	↓	↓	↓↓
Fully compensated	nl	↓↓	↓↓
Metabolic alkalosis			
Uncompensated	↑↑	nl	↑↑
Partially compensated	↑	↑	↑↑
Fully compensated	nl	↑↑	↑↑

↓↓ = very decreased; ↑↑ = very increased; ↓ = decreased; ↑ = increased; nl = normal.

TABLE 11-2. EXPECTED COMPENSATION FOR ACID–BASE DISTURBANCES*

Respiratory acidosis:	$\Delta HCO_3^- = 0.10 \times \Delta PaCO_2$ (acute)
	$\Delta HCO_3^- = 0.35 \times \Delta PaCO_2$ (chronic)
Respiratory alkalosis:	$\Delta HCO_3^- = 0.2 \times \Delta PaCO_2$ (acute)
	$\Delta HCO_3^- = 0.5 \times \Delta PaCO_2$ (chronic)
Metabolic acidosis:	$\Delta PaCO_2 = 1.2 \times \Delta HCO_3^-$
Metabolic alkalosis:	$\Delta PaCO_2 = 0.9 \times \Delta HCO_3^-$

*If the acid–base status exceeds the expected level of compensation, a mixed acid–base disturbance is present.

19. **Describe the acid–base disorder associated with pH = 7.54, PaCO$_2$ = 55 mm Hg, and HCO$_3^-$ = 15 mmol/L.**
It is impossible for the pH to be greater than 7.40 if the PaCO$_2$ is greater than than 40 mm Hg and the HCO$_3^-$ is less than 24 mmol/L. Therefore, there must be a laboratory or transcription error, because either the pH, the PaCO$_2$, or the HCO$_3^-$ is incorrect. It is impossible to know which is wrong without examining the patient or repeating the blood gas analysis.

KEY POINTS: CAUSES OF ACID–BASE DISTURBANCES

1. Respiratory acidosis (i.e., hypoventilation)
   - Respiratory center depression: Pathologic or iatrogenic
   - Disruption of neural pathways affecting respiratory muscles: Neuropathy or trauma
   - Neuromuscular blockade: Disease or paralyzing agents
   - Respiratory muscle weakness: Fatigue or disease

2. Respiratory alkalosis (i.e., hyperventilation)
   - Respiratory center stimulation: Hypoxia, anxiety, or central nervous system pathology
   - Iatrogenesis: Excessive mechanical ventilation

3. Metabolic acidosis
   - Lactic acidosis (e.g., hypoxia)
   - Ketoacidosis (e.g., uncontrolled diabetes)
   - Uremic acidosis (e.g., renal failure)
   - Loss of base from lower gastrointestinal tract (e.g., diarrhea)
   - Loss of base from kidneys (e.g., acetazolamide or renal tubular acidosis)
   - Poisons (e.g., methanol, ethylene glycol, or aspirin)

4. Metabolic alkalosis
   - Hypokalemia
   - Loss of acid from upper gastrointestinal tract (e.g., vomiting or gastric suction)
   - Bicarbonate administration

20. **How is the anion gap useful in explaining acid–base disturbances?**
    The anion gap is useful to differentiate causes of metabolic acidosis. Metabolic acidosis can be associated with a normal anion gap (i.e., hyperchloremic acidosis) or with an increased anion gap (i.e., normochloremic acidosis). The anion gap is calculated as:

    $$\text{anion gap} = Na^+ - (Cl^- + HCO_3^-)$$

    A normal anion gap is 8–12 mmol/L. Causes of metabolic acidosis with an increased anion gap include lactic acidosis, diabetic ketoacidosis, and azotemic (i.e., renal) acidosis. Causes of metabolic acidosis with a normal anion gap include loss of bicarbonate from the gastrointestinal tract (e.g., diarrhea), acetazolamide therapy, renal tubular acidosis, or excessive chloride administration (e.g., volume expansion with normal saline, HCl, and NH_4Cl).

21. **What is the strong ion difference?**
    The strong ion difference (SID) is a method of evaluating acid–base disturbances based on the Stewart physiochemical approach to acid–base chemistry. Using this approach, the only variables that affect pH are PCO_2, SID, and the concentration of unmeasured strong ions. The normal value for SID is 40 mmol/L and is calculated as:

    $$SID = HCO_3^- + 0.28 \times [\text{albumin (gm/L)}] + [\text{inorganic phosphate (mmol/L)}]$$

    Metabolic acidosis is associated with a decreased SID, and metabolic alkalosis is associated with an increased SID (*see* Table 11-3).

    Fencl V, Jabor A, Kazda A, Figge J: Diagnosis of metabolic acid-base disturbances in critically ill patients. Am J Respir Crit Care Med 162:2246–2251, 2000.

TABLE 11-3. CLASSIFICATION OF ACID–BASE DISTURBANCES USING STEWART'S APPROACH

	Acidosis	Alkalosis
Respiratory	$\uparrow PCO_2$	$\downarrow PCO_2$
Metabolic		
Water excess or deficit	$\downarrow SID, \downarrow Na^+$	$\uparrow SID, \uparrow Na^+$
Chloride excess or deficit	$\downarrow SID, \uparrow Cl^-$	$\uparrow SID, \downarrow Cl^-$
Unmeasured strong ion excess	$\downarrow SID, \uparrow$ unmeasured anions	

22. **Should arterial blood gas results be corrected to the patient's temperature?**
Blood gases and pH are measured at 37°C. If the patient's temperature is abnormal, the *in vivo* blood gas and pH values will differ from those measured and reported by the blood gas laboratory. Using empirical equations, the blood gas analyzer can adjust the measured values to the patient's body temperature. Two ventilation strategies for hypothermic acid-base management have been suggested. During alpha-stat management, $PaCO_2$ is maintained at 40 mm Hg when measured at 37°C. The dissociation fraction of the imidazole moiety of histidine is thereby constant, whereas pH changes parallel to the neutral point of water. During pH-stat management, $PaCO_2$ is corrected to the patient's actual body temperature. Due to the increased gas solubility during hypothermia, the alpha-stat strategy results in relative hyperventilation and a decrease in cerebral blood flow. This issue is becoming increasingly important with the use of induced hypothermia after cardiac arrest and in the treatment of focal cerebral ischemia. Animal studies suggest that pH-stat management, compared with alpha-stat management, results in improved cerebral blood flow and neurological outcomes. The pH-stat approach allows differentiation of temperature-related changes from physiologic changes. Temperature-adjusted values should be used to compare blood gas levels with exhaled gas values (e.g., end-tidal PCO_2) and to calculate oxygen content indices (e.g., shunt arterial) or tension indices (e.g., $P(A-a)O_2$).

Kollmar R, Frietsch T, Georgiadis D, et al: Early effects of acid-base management during hypothermia on cerebral infarct volume, edema, and cerebral blood flow in acute focal cerebral ischemia in rats. Anesthesiology 97:868–874, 2002.

Ye J, Li Z, Yang Y, et al: Use of a pH-stat strategy during retrograde cerebral perfusion improves cerebral perfusion and tissue oxygenation. Ann Thorac Surg 77:1664–1670, 2004.

CHAPTER 12

PULSE OXIMETRY

Philip L. Goodman, MS, RRT, and Robert F. Wolken, BS, RRT

1. **What is pulse oximetry?**
   Pulse oximetry is a noninvasive method of determining oxygen saturation of hemoglobin in pulsating arterial blood vessels.

2. **How does pulse oximetry work?**
   The pulse oximeter compares the amount of red light absorbed to the amount of infrared light absorbed by both deoxygenated hemoglobin (Hb) and oxyhemoglobin (HbO_2). The result is displayed as SpO_2 (saturation obtained by pulse oximetry).

   http://www.nda.ox.ac.uk/wfsa/html/u11/u1104_01.htm

3. **On which physical principles is pulse oximetry based?**
   Pulse oximeters rely on a combination of the principles of spectrophotometry and photoplethysmography. Spectrophotometry is based on the Beer–Lambert law, which relates the amount of light transmitted through a solution with the concentration of a solvent. Photoplethysmography measures changes in tissue properties during the cardiac cycle, allowing the pulse oximeter to differentiate between arterial blood and venous blood.

   Jubran A: Pulse oximetry. Intens Care Med 30:2017–2020, 2004.

4. **How accurate are pulse oximeters? Are there differences among various models?**
   Most manufacturers report an accuracy of ±2% for saturations that are greater than 70%. The reported accuracy drops to ±3% for saturations between 50% and 70%. These claims can be somewhat misleading as studies have shown that SpO_2 values fall within ±4–5% of CO-oximetry values (SaO_2) 95% of the time.

   Van de Louw A, Cracco C, Cerf C, et al: Accuracy of pulse oximetry in the intensive care unit. Intens Care Med 27:1606–1613, 2001.

5. **Does nail polish affect pulse oximetry?**
   Polish that absorbs light at the oximeter's transmission wavelengths (660 nm and 940 nm) will alter the SpO_2. Green and blue polish have increased absorbency at 660 nm, which will produce a lower SpO_2 reading. Black nail polish has increased absorbency at both 660 and 940 nm and will also cause a lower SpO_2 reading, but to a lesser extent than green and blue. Although red nail polish does not exhibit absorbency in the oximeter's range and should not affect SpO_2 readings, it is usually recommended to remove any nail polish prior to the use of finger probes.

   If signal interference caused by nail polish is suspected, try placing the finger probe in a side-to-side position rather than the traditional top-to-bottom position.

   Chan MM, Chan MM, Chan ED: What is the effect of fingernail polish on pulse oximetry? Chest 123: 2163–2164, 2003.

   Cote CJ, Golstein EA, Fuchsman WH, Hoaglin DC: The effect of nail polish on pulse oximetry. Anesth Analg 67(7):683–686, 1988.

6. **If the pulse oximeter reads 90% or greater, does it mean that the patient has an acceptable PaO_2?**
Not necessarily. It is important to remember those factors that can shift the position of the oxyhemoglobin dissociation curve and alter the relationship of a given PaO_2 and the corresponding level of hemoglobin saturation. These factors include temperature, pH, $PaCO_2$, and 2,3-diphosphoglycerate (2,3-DPG).

7. **How does dyshemoglobinemia affect pulse oximetry?**
Carboxyhemoglobin (COHb) and methemoglobin (metHb) can account for variances between SpO_2 and SaO_2. Given that COHb and metHb absorb red and infrared light at the same wavelengths as Hb and HbO_2, their presence affects the SpO_2 measurements, but they cannot be differentiated. COHb is read as HbO_2, and any amount will falsely elevate the value of the SpO_2 reading. In the presence of high levels of metHb, SpO_2 is erroneously low when the SaO_2 is greater than 85%. Increased metHb levels therefore can result in either overestimation or underestimation of SpO_2, depending on the actual SaO_2.

   Barker SJ, Tremper KK, Hyatt J, et al: Effects of methemoglobinemia on pulse oximetry and mixed venous oximetry. Anesthesiology 67:A171, 1987.

8. **What is the difference between functional and fractional saturation?**
Although not entirely correct, saturation measurements by pulse oximetry are commonly referred to as *functional saturation*, whereas saturation measurements made by CO-oximeters are referred to as *fractional saturation*. The following equations point out the differences between these two types of saturation measurements and help to explain why SpO_2 readings can differ from SaO_2 measurement:

$$\text{Functional } SaO_2 = \frac{HbO_2}{HbO_2 + Hb} \times 100$$

$$\text{Functional } SaO_2 = \frac{HbO_2}{HbO_2 + Hb + COHb + metHb} \times 100$$

9. **What are some other limitations of pulse oximetry?**
Most errors in pulse oximetry measurement are the result of poor signal quality (i.e., low perfusion) or excessive noise (i.e., motion artifact). Methylene blue has been reported to cause falsely low SpO_2 values. Severe anemia may affect accuracy since oximetry is dependent on light absorption by hemoglobin. Hyperbilirubinemia does not appear to affect SpO_2. Although conflicting data exist, skin pigmentation and the presence of sickle cell disease may yield less accurate values due to various technical problems such as poor signal strength.

   Chellar L, Snyder JV, et al: Accuracy of pulse oximetry in patients with hyperbilirubinemia. Respir Care 36:1383–1386, 1991.

KEY POINTS: LIMITATIONS OF PULSE OXIMETRY

1. Not an indicator of acid–base status

2. Not a reliable indicator of ventilatory status (e.g., hypoventilation)

3. Less reliable in low perfusion states

4. Motion artifact is a significant source of error and false alarms

5. Dyshemoglobinemias may cause inaccurate values

10. **What is the penumbra effect?**

Penumbra (from Latin *paene*, meaning *almost*, and *umbra*, meaning *shade*) refers to the partially lighted area surrounding the complete shadow of a body, as in an eclipse. Incorrectly positioned pulse oximetry probes may still provide a pulsatile signal yet prevent adequate illumination of the photodetector by the light-emitting diode (LED). Light shunted from the LED to the photodetector can theoretically cause a falsely low SpO_2 if the SaO_2 is more than 85% and a falsely high SpO_2 if the SaO_2 is less than 85%.

Kelleher JF, Ruff RH: The penumbra effect: Vasomotion-dependent pulse oximeter artifact due to probe malposition. Anesthesiology 7:787–791, 1988.

11. **In addition to its effect on the oxyhemoglobin dissociation curve, how will body temperature affect pulse oximeter readings?**

Body temperature above or below normal will cause the sensor LEDs to shift their spectral outputs 0.2 nm/°C, which can result in an overestimation or underestimation of SpO_2. Correcting for this temperature-induced wavelength shift is not clinically relevant in most instances.

12. **Is there any advantage to using a particular sensor type or monitoring site?**

Sensors are available in a variety of sizes and configurations. Fingers, toes, and earlobes are the most common locations for probe placement. Selection of a sensor site should be based on where the most stable and strongest signal can be obtained. Nondisposable clothespin probes are best used for spot checks or for patients who are not too active. Adhesive-backed sensors are probably better suited for neonatal and pediatric patients, measurements during transport, and in patients who are restless and therefore more likely to cause displacement of the clothespin probe.

13. **What about the risk of cross-contamination when a nondisposable sensor is used?**

Similarly to other clinical devices such as blood pressure cuffs and stethoscopes implicated in the spread of nosocomial infections, pulse oximetry probes should be suspected as potential reservoirs of infection. A report on residual bacterial contamination of nondisposable sensors found that 66% of the sensors that were identified as ready for patient use were contaminated with bacteria. The development of more effective cleaning protocols and single-patient-use sensors will decrease the risk of the spread of infection.

Wilkin MC: Residual bacterial contamination on reusable pulse oximetry sensors. Respir Care 38:1155–1160, 1993.

14. **Are there any potential complications to pulse oximetry use?**

Since the probes contain electronic circuitry, there is potential for malfunction causing thermal burns. Pressure sores and tissue necrosis can be caused by improper probe placement or failure to monitor and to change probe placement. Pressure injuries are more common when using spring-loaded sensors and in those patients who have impaired peripheral perfusion, are receiving vasoconstrictors, or have other conditions that make them susceptible to cutaneous tissue breakdown. False results for normoxemia or hyperoxemia may lead to inappropriate treatment.

Murphy KG, Secunda JA, Rockoff MA: Severe burns from a pulse oximeter. Anesthesiology 73:350–352,1990.

15. **What are some other uses for pulse oximetry?**

Other less proven uses include:

- Assessing collateral circulation prior to arterial cannulation
- Monitoring of vascular blood flow of transplanted digits
- Screening for desaturation while eating

- Feedback device for patients with chronic obstructive pulmonary disease (COPD) during breathing retraining
- Noninvasive detection and estimation of the degree of pulsus paradoxus

16. **When should pulse oximetry be used?**
   Pulse oximetry has become the standard of care in many clinical settings and is frequently referred to as the fifth vital sign. Continuous pulse oximetry monitoring is recommended for patients requiring mechanical ventilatory support; during patient transport; and during procedures such as bronchoscopy, endoscopy, cardiac catheterization, and sleep apnea screening. Intrapartum fetal pulse oximetry is available for monitoring fetal oxygenation status but has yet to be accepted into widespread clinical practice.

   Neff T: Routine oximetry. A fifth vital sign? Chest 94:227, 1988.

17. **Are there any significant technological advances in pulse oximetry on the horizon?**
   Pulse oximeter manufacturers offer technological advances that generally deal with issues related to sensor probes, portability, and battery life. Advances that have a more significant clinical impact address limitations inherent in oximeters, specifically, motion artifact and low perfusion states.

KEY POINTS: CLINICAL APPLICATIONS OF PULSE OXIMETRY

1. Detection of hypoxemia

2. Titration of fractional inspired oxygen concentration

3. Screening for cardiopulmonary disease

4. Assessment of oxygenation status during patient transport

18. **Describe a clinical example that highlights the limitations of pulse oximetry.**
   Arterial blood gases (ABGs) were drawn from a patient breathing room air. The pH was 7.40, $PaCO_2 = 36$ mmHg, and $PaO_2 = 61$ mmHg. SpO_2 was 90%. The patient was breathing at a respiratory rate of 20 breaths per minute (BPM). Later, the patient became tachypneic with a respiratory rate of 44 BPM. The SpO_2 was 90%, and the results of subsequent ABGs were pH = 7.50, $PaCO_2 = 24$ mmHg, and $PaO_2 = 50$ mmHg.

19. **What is the explanation of the SpO_2 values seen in the clinical example described above?**
   This patient had clearly become hypoxemic even though the pulse oximeter was showing an acceptable SpO_2. Hyperventilation caused an acute respiratory alkalosis, shifting the oxyhemoglobin dissociation curve to the left. The left shift resulted in the same hemoglobin saturation at a significantly lower PaO_2. This situation exemplifies that it is important to remember those factors that can cause a shift in the oxyhemoglobin dissociation curve. Other factors include temperature and abnormal levels of 2,3-DPG.

CHAPTER 13

PULMONARY FUNCTION TESTING

Lee K. Brown, MD, and Albert Miller, MD

1. What is spirometry?

Spirometry is the measurement of the volume of air that can be inhaled or exhaled. The various lung volumes and capacities (a capacity is defined as the sum of two or more volumes) are depicted graphically in Figure 13-1. Since residual volume (RV) is defined as the volume of air that remains in the lungs after maximal exhalation, spirometry can never measure RV itself or any capacity that includes RV. Modern spirometers may measure respired volume directly or, more commonly, measure instantaneous flow and compute volume by mathematic integration.

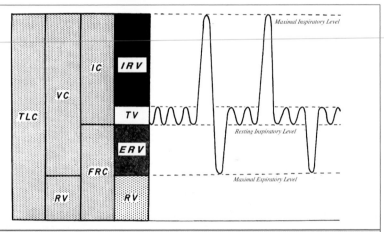

Figure 13-1. Spirogram depicting the various subdivisions of total lung capacity (TLC). Vital capacity (VC), inspiratory capacity (IC), tidal volume (TV), and expiratory reserve volume (ERV) are measurable by spirometry. Residual volume (RV), functional residual capacity (FRC), and TLC can only be measured by special techniques since their RV component, by definition, cannot be exhaled. (From Comroe JH, Forster RE, DuBois AB, et al: The Lung. Chicago, Year Book, 1962, p 8.)

2. What maneuvers are used in the performance of spirometry?

- **Slow vital capacity (SVC):** The patient breathes tidally and then inhales slowly to total lung capacity (TLC), followed by a slow exhalation to RV, much as depicted in Figure 13-1.
- **Forced vital capacity (FVC):** The patient breathes tidally, inhales slowly to TLC, and then exhales, as hard and as fast as possible, to RV. In most cases, the patient is then instructed to inhale once more, also as hard and as fast as possible, back to TLC.
- **Maximal voluntary ventilation (MVV):** The patient breathes in and out through the spirometer, as rapidly and deeply as possible, for either 12 or 15 seconds. The total volume of air exhaled or inhaled during that period of maximal breathing is measured, expressed in terms of liters per minute, and reported as the MVV.

3. **What measurements are made using the SVC maneuver?**
    Not surprisingly, the SVC maneuver is used to measure slow vital capacity. The SVC maneuver is also an essential element in the determination of static lung volumes, which are the lung volumes and capacities that include RV: functional residual capacity (FRC), TLC, and, of course, RV itself. Rather than measure each of these volumes individually, common practice is to measure FRC and then to perform an SVC maneuver to obtain the expiratory reserve volume (ERV) and inspiratory capacity (IC). A quick look at Figure 13-1 demonstrates that TLC can easily be obtained by adding IC to FRC, and RV is obtained by subtracting ERV from FRC.

4. **What measurements are made using the FVC maneuver?**
    When spirometrically measured volume is plotted against time during the expiratory portion of an FVC maneuver, a curve termed the forced expiratory spirogram results (Fig. 13-2). Volumes, timed volumes, and average flows are easily derived from this curve; the four most commonly used parameters thus obtained are FVC, ERV, forced expiratory volume in 1 second (FEV_1), and the forced expiratory flow at 25–75% of forced vital capacity (FEF_{25-75}).

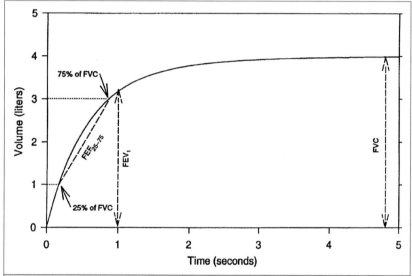

Figure 13-2. Spirogram of a forced expiratory effort from TLC to RV, depicting forced vital capacity (FVC) and the forced expiratory volume after 1 second of exhalation (FEV_1). The average flow between 25% and 75% of vital capacity (FEF_{25-75}) is obtained from the slope of the line connecting these two points on the spirogram, as shown.

5. **Does reduced FVC indicate a restrictive disorder?**
    Figure 13-1 demonstrates graphically that FVC is dependent on the values of both TLC and RV: FVC will decline if TLC falls or if RV rises. The dependence of FVC on TLC led to its use as an indicator of restrictive impairment, as a result of either lung disease or chest wall disease. Lung disorders that fill or obliterate alveoli (e.g., consolidation or interstitial fibrosis) or remove alveolar volume (e.g., lung resection) will reduce TLC and, thus, FVC. Chest wall disorders that interfere with the expansion of the lungs within the thorax (e.g., kyphoscoliosis) or weaken the inspiratory muscles (e.g., amyotrophic lateral sclerosis, myasthenia gravis, or other causes of diaphragmatic paresis) will also reduce TLC and, thus, FVC.

6. **Can airflow obstruction reduce FVC?**
Yes. FVC will also decline if RV is elevated from air trapping, a phenomenon that frequently occurs in obstructive lung disease when dynamic collapse of small airways prevents complete emptying of alveoli in the time available for expiration. Elevated RV can also be related to weakness of the expiratory muscles (primarily the abdominal wall muscles: *rectus abdominis* and *transversus abdominis*) due to neuromuscular disorders.

Gilbert R, Auchincloss JH: What is a "restrictive" defect? Arch Intern Med 146:1779–1781, 1986.

7. **Why is ERV measured?**
ERV is highly dependent on the mobility of the diaphragm and is reduced in neuromuscular disorders. Abdominal processes that interfere with diaphragmatic movement, such as obesity, ascites, or pregnancy, also reduce ERV. ERV also falls immediately after abdominal surgery. Studies indicate that this is likely due to inhibition of diaphragmatic motion from mechanical or irritative factors rather than incisional pain.

Simonneau G, Vivien A, Sartene R, et al: Diaphragm dysfunction induced by upper abdominal surgery. Role of postoperative pain. Am Rev Respir Dis 128:899–903, 1983.

8. **Why are timed volumes such as FEV_1 measured?**
Timed volumes are defined as the volume of air exhaled during an FVC maneuver during the first 0.5, 1.0, 2.0, or 3.0 seconds after the start of exhalation. Thus, FEV_1 is the volume exhaled during the first 1 second of the maneuver. Timed volumes are actually average flow rates during the specified period of time, and, therefore, they decline when airway obstruction is present. Timed volumes are relatively insensitive to obstruction limited to the small airways (i.e., those <2 mm in diameter) but are useful in disorders that affect larger airways or the upper airway.

9. **What is different about exhaled flow measured at low lung volumes compared to high volumes?**
At lung volumes less than approximately 70% of FVC, flow will not increase with additional expiratory force once a minimum threshold of effort is achieved (Fig. 13-3). During a forced exhalation, airway pressure progressively declines, traveling from the alveolus (i.e., upstream) to the mouth (i.e., downstream). This pressure drop is attributable to airway resistance and exists only when airflow is present. At some downstream point in the conducting airways (i.e., the equal pressure point), intraluminal pressure falls below the pressure compressing the airway (which is equivalent to pleural pressure + lung elastic recoil pressure), and the airway will collapse. Since this interrupts airflow, intraluminal pressure will rise and reopen the airway. In reality, these bronchi probably do not open and close, but rather they reach equilibrium in diameter such that increases in expiratory force (above a minimum threshold) will not increase airflow.

Robinson DR, Chaudhary BA, Speir WA Jr: Expiratory flow limitation in large and small airways. Arch Intern Med 144:1457–1460, 1984.

10. **What is FEF_{25-75}?**
FEF_{25-75} is the average flow during the middle half of the FVC maneuver, starting when 25% of the FVC has been exhaled and ending when 75% of the FVC has been collected in the spirometer. (Figure 13-2 demonstrates that FEF_{25-75} is actually the slope of the line connecting these two points on the spirogram.) FEF_{25-75} is reduced when resistance to airflow increases due to airway obstruction, and it often correlates with FEV_1. However, FEF_{25-75} and other flows measured at low lung volumes may more closely reflect the status of the small airways, although this is controversial.

11. **Why might flows at low lung volumes reflect disease in these small airways?**
At low lung volumes, airflow becomes proportional to lung elastic recoil divided by the resistance of the airways between the alveoli and the equal pressure point, which are mainly those

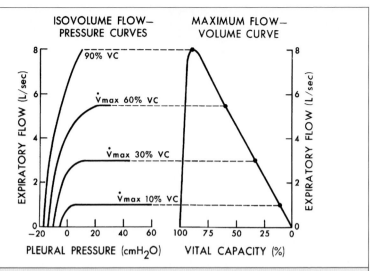

Figure 13-3. Effort-independence of flow during forced expiration at lower lung volumes. The left panel depicts the flow versus pleural pressure curves at four different lung volumes (expressed as percent of vital capacity [VC]). Note that at 90% of VC, increased pleural pressure (i.e., effort) results in increased flow, whereas at the lower lung volumes, flow does not increase once a minimum pleural pressure is exceeded. A forced expiratory flow-volume loop from a single maximal effort is depicted in the right panel. (From Murray JF: The Normal Lung: The Basis for Diagnosis and Treatment of Pulmonary Disease, 2nd ed. Philadelphia, WB Saunders, 1986, p 100.)

<2 mm in diameter. If it can be assumed that lung elastic recoil is normal, a reduction in FEF_{25-75} or any of the other flows at low lung volume would represent an increase in the resistance of these small airways. There exist more accurate tests of small airway function that depend on measuring the degree of inhomogeneous ventilation between lung units (e.g., multiple-breath nitrogen washout curves or frequency dependence of lung compliance), but these are usually only available in research laboratories.

12. **Is reduced FEV_1 or FEF_{25-75} always diagnostic of airway obstruction?**
No. These indices of obstruction will frequently decline to some extent in restrictive disorders as well. Consider a patient with severe kyphoscoliosis, such that measured FVC is 2.0 liters despite a predicted FVC of 5.0 liters. Predicted FEV_1 for this patient might be 3.5 liters, but there is obviously no chance that the patient will achieve this since only 2.0 liters can be exhaled for the entire breath. Thus, spirometric flows will often decline, as will volumes, in the presence of restrictive impairment.

13. **How then can restrictive impairment be distinguished from obstructive?**
The parameters FEV_1/FVC and forced expiratory time (FET_{25-75}) can help. FEV_1/FVC defines obstruction in terms of the fraction of FVC that can be exhaled in 1 second, rather than its absolute value; if FEV_1 falls to a greater degree than FVC, FEV_1/FVC will decline and obstruction is present. FEV_1/FVC is somewhat age dependent, and the following guidelines are helpful: for adults less than 40 years old, at least 75% of FVC should be exhaled in 1 second; between the ages of 40 and 60 years, this value should be 70% or greater; and for subjects aged 60 years or older, it should be greater than 65%. FET_{25-75} represents the time it takes for the "middle half" of

KEY POINTS: INTERPRETING THE FORCED EXPIRATORY SPIROGRAM

1. If FVC is normal, restrictive ventilatory impairment (as defined by reduced TLC) is only rarely present.

2. Reduced FVC may be due to restrictive ventilatory impairment or air trapping from obstructive lung disease. If there is spirometric evidence of obstruction, measure TLC to determine if restrictive impairment is also present.

3. FEV_1 and FEF_{25-75} may be low in either restrictive or obstructive impairment. Look at FEV_1/FVC and FET_{25-75} to make the distinction.

4. Recommended criteria for a positive bronchodilator response only apply to FVC and FEV_1. Using FEF_{25-75} or other flows at low lung volumes to assess reversibility is complicated and not recommended in clinical situations.

5. When ordered to assess upper airway obstruction, the forced flow-volume loop must include inspiratory and expiratory phases.

FVC to be exhaled (i.e., the time during which FEF_{25-75} is computed) and is another relatively volume-independent marker of obstruction.

Allen GW, Sabin S: Comparison of direct and indirect measurement of airway resistance. Am Rev Respir Dis 104:61–71,1971.

Crapo RO: Pulmonary-function testing. N Eng J Med 331:25–30, 1994.

14. What is a flow-volume loop?
The flow-volume loop is simply another way of displaying the same information collected during the forced spirogram. Instead of showing volume versus time, the flow-volume loop displays instantaneous flow versus volume (Fig. 13-4).

15. List the advantages of the flow-volume loop.
- Instantaneous flows are easily read off the curve. This includes peak flow (i.e., the maximum flow achieved, characteristically inscribed early in the effort) as well as the various flows at low lung volumes.
- The overall shape of the curve can yield important information.
- All of the spirometric indices available from the forced expiratory spirogram (see Fig. 13-2) can still be obtained from the flow-volume loop as long as a timing mark is generated by the apparatus to indicate the 1-second point so that FEV_1 can be measured.

16. What information is derived from the shape of the flow-volume loop?
- Inadequate expiratory effort may result in a delayed upstroke to peak flow; early termination of effort is evidenced by flow that drops abruptly to zero rather than gradually declining as the curve meets the volume axis at the end of the breath; coughing and extra breaths are also readily apparent.
- Small airway obstruction: An expiratory effort with a long, upwardly concave tail (see Fig.13-4) indicates that much of the FVC at low lung volumes is exhaled at low flow rates, consistent with small airway obstruction.
- Upper airway obstruction: Obstruction cephalad to the mainstem bronchi characteristically affects peak flow the most, resulting in flattening of the flow-volume loop (Fig. 13-5).

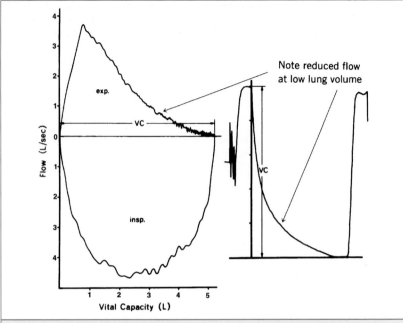

Figure 13-4. Maximal expiratory and inspiratory flow-volume loop and the spirogram from the same effort. The expiratory limb demonstrates the upwardly concave tail associated with small airway obstruction. (From Petty TL, Lakshminarayan S: Practical pulmonary function tests. In Petty TL [ed]: Pulmonary Diagnostic Techniques. Philadelphia, Lea & Febiger, 1975, p 23, with permission.)

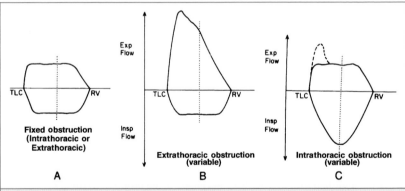

Figure 13-5. Flow-volume loops in upper airway obstruction. **A,** Fixed obstruction, intrathoracic or extrathoracic. **B,** Variable extrathoracic obstruction. **C,** Variable intrathoracic obstruction. Incomplete flattening of the expiratory limb (dashed line) is occasionally observed.

17. **Can the flow-volume loop distinguish different patterns of upper airway obstruction?**

This is possible when both the expiratory and inspiratory limbs of the flow-volume loop are collected. Flattening of both the expiratory and inspiratory limbs of the loop occurs when upper airway obstruction is fixed (e.g., tracheal stenosis). Nonfixed (i.e., variable) lesions in the extrathoracic airway (e.g., bilateral vocal cord paralysis) will primarily affect the inspiratory limb when the vocal cords are drawn more closely together by suction; the cords will be pushed apart during exhalation so that the expiratory limb will look relatively normal. Variable lesions in the intrathoracic airway (e.g., tracheomalacia) will be relieved during inhalation because negative intrathoracic pressure pulls open intrathoracic airways, causing the inspiratory limb to appear normal while the expiratory limb flattens.

Guntupalli KK, Bandi V, Sirgi C, et al: Usefulness of flow volume loops in emergency center and ICU settings. Chest 111:481–488, 1997.

18. **Is there any other reason to measure peak expiratory flow?**
Peak expiratory flow is inscribed early in the forced exhalation, at a high lung volume. Consequently, it reflects obstruction in the larger airways and varies greatly with effort. Peak flow is most often used as an index of the degree of obstruction of airways during exacerbations of bronchial asthma since it is easily measured in the emergency department with simple equipment. In fact, the equipment is simple enough that patients can be supplied with a peak flow meter to use in the home; this leads to a second use, that of anticipating an exacerbation of asthma before significant symptomatic deterioration. Patients with brittle asthma, who frequently require trips to the emergency department or hospital admission for treatment, can measure their own peak flow at home on a regular (e.g., daily) basis and call their medical practitioner for instructions if peak flow declines.

Li JTC: Home peak expiratory flow rate monitoring in patients with asthma. Mayo Clin Proc 70:649–656, 1995.

19. **What is the significance of an improvement in FVC or FEV_1 following a bronchodilator aerosol treatment?**
Such a procedure is known as an assessment of reversibility. Patients with obstructive ventilatory impairment on initial spirometry are given a bronchodilator aerosol (most frequently, a beta-adrenergic agonist such as albuterol), and spirometry is repeated. An increase in either parameter beyond what might be expected from the normal variability of the measurement itself indicates a response to the bronchodilator. One commonly used guideline defines reversibility as a 12% or greater improvement in FVC or FEV_1. (The value must also increase by more than 200 mL.) Reversibility is consistent with bronchial asthma or at least supports the use of bronchodilator therapy in that patient.

American Thoracic Society: Lung function testing: Selection of reference values and interpretive strategies. Am Rev Respir Dis 144:1202–1218, 1991.

20. **What is bronchial challenge testing?**
Bronchial challenge testing is most frequently used to diagnose occult bronchial asthma. The cholinergic drug methacholine chloride is used, prepared as a solution in buffered normal saline and administered as an aerosol. Baseline spirometry is performed following inhalation of the diluent alone and then after inhalation of increasing concentrations of the drug. The procedure is stopped if and when FEV_1 declines by 20% or more below baseline or after a maximum concentration of methacholine is administered. Patients with bronchial asthma or other conditions leading to airway hyperreactivity will demonstrate this 20%-or-greater decrease in FEV_1 at lower concentrations of methacholine than normal subjects.

21. **What does measurement of MVV reflect?**
The MVV maneuver integrates the activity of many different parts of the ventilatory apparatus: respiratory muscles, chest wall, pulmonary parenchyma, and airways. However, derangement in some components of the ventilatory apparatus affects MVV more than derangement in others. MVV is typically reduced when obstructive impairment is present, but it is usually preserved in

restrictive disease (with the exception of neuromuscular disease) until the disorder is quite severe since patients with most restrictive conditions are able to compensate for reduced tidal volume simply by increasing respiratory frequency. In contrast, any attempt to increase MVV in obstructive disease necessarily requires an increase in flow, which is the limiting factor in obstruction. MVV can be helpful in distinguishing obstructive from restrictive lung disease, and it is also a sensitive indicator of neuromuscular disorders that impair the strength and endurance of the ventilatory muscles.

22. **Is it useful to compare SVC and FVC?**

SVC is usually quite similar to FVC except in obstructive airway disease and pulmonary emphysema. In these disorders, a forced expiration will often cause dynamic collapse of the airways, either because they are narrowed from disease or because reduced elastic recoil of the destroyed lung parenchyma fails to hold the airways open to the usual extent. The result is trapped air behind the obstruction, elevated RV, and reduced FVC. Thus, a significant disparity between SVC and FVC (with FVC smaller than SVC) suggests obstructive disease or pulmonary emphysema.

Chan ED, Irvin CG: The detection of collapsible airways contributing to airflow limitation. Chest 107:856–859, 1995.

23. **How are static lung volumes measured?**

There are currently three common methods used to determine FRC. Two of the methods, helium wash-in and nitrogen wash-out, are so-called "gas dilution" techniques that depend upon a marker gas that is distributed throughout the lungs at FRC. The other technique, body plethysmography, encloses the patient in a sealed booth; FRC is calculated by applying Boyle's law to the changes in mouth pressure and box volume that occur when the patient pants against an occluded mouthpiece.

24. **List the advantages and disadvantages of each technique.**

The gas dilution methods are somewhat easier for patients to perform since they only need to breathe normally on a mouthpiece. However, this measurement takes longer than using the body plethysmograph since time is required either for helium to equilibrate throughout the lungs in the wash-in technique or for nitrogen to be flushed out of the lungs in the wash-out technique. This time interval can be quite prolonged in the patient with obstructive airway disease. Body plethysmography requires a cooperative patient who does not mind being locked within the small booth and who can perform an adequate panting maneuver. The measurement itself takes only a few seconds, especially using modern computerized equipment.

25. **Is there any utility in measuring FRC both ways?**

Body plethysmography measures the volume of *any* gas-containing space in the thorax, including bullae. In some patients with chronic obstructive lung disease, it is sometimes useful to both perform a determination of FRC plethysmographically and use a gas dilution technique. The difference between the two measurements (plethysmographic FRC will be larger) is then a reflection of the volume of gas contained in bullae.

26. **When is it important to measure static lung volumes?**

These volumes are frequently useful when spirometry alone presents a confusing or mixed picture. The most common situation occurs when spirometry indicates that restriction (i.e., reduced FVC) and obstruction (i.e., reduced FEV_1-to-FVC ratio) coexist. The question is then raised as to whether FVC is reduced simply because RV is elevated due to air trapping or whether true restriction is also present. If the determination of static lung volumes demonstrates that RV is elevated and TLC normal, pure obstructive impairment is diagnosed; if TLC is reduced, both obstruction and restriction are present.

27. **Is there a standardized noninvasive test for assessment of gas exchange across the lung?**

Such a test does exist and is called the diffusing capacity of the lung (D_L) in the United States and transfer factor (T_L) in Great Britain and Europe. The test gas contains carbon monoxide, and the standard method involves a 10-second breath hold ("single breath" in pulmonary function jargon) at full inspiration, so the full abbreviation is $DL_{CO}SB$. Carbon monoxide, like oxygen, has a special affinity for hemoglobin, so its uptake during the breath hold is not limited by the receiving reservoir, the pulmonary blood flow, but by the surface area and nature of the air–blood interface, the tissues and fluid that make up the alveolar–capillary membrane. Other assessments of gas exchange require arterial blood gases and are therefore invasive (*see* below).

28. **In what types of disease does the $DL_{CO}SB$ provide information?**

Decreases in $DL_{CO}SB$ reflect loss of or damage to the gas-exchanging surface of the lung, as occurs in emphysema, interstitial lung disease, and pulmonary vascular diseases. In chronic obstructive pulmonary disease (COPD), decrease in $DL_{CO}SB$ helps distinguish emphysema from obstructive chronic bronchitis or chronic asthma, in which $DL_{CO}SB$ remains normal. In interstitial lung disease, including sarcoidosis, decrease in $DL_{CO}SB$ often precedes abnormality in other measurements of lung function. In pulmonary vascular disease, decrease in $DL_{CO}SB$ may be the only abnormality in standard pulmonary function tests.

Miller A: Physiologic pulmonary diagnosis: The spectrum of impairments. Allergy Proceedings 14:401–407, 1993.

29. **Is there a relationship between $DL_{CO}SB$ and invasive measurements of gas exchange?**

The $DL_{CO}SB$ is frequently reduced in interstitial lung disease even when invasive measurements such as resting arterial pO_2 or the alveolar–arterial difference in pO_2 [$(A-a)D_{O2}$] are normal. These invasive tests of gas exchange may be made more sensitive by performing them during exercise; for instance, widening of the $(A-a)D_{O2}$ during exercise generally correlates with substantial reduction in the $DL_{CO}SB$.

Miller A, Brown LK, Sloane MF, et al: Cardiorespiratory responses to incremental exercise in sarcoidosis patients with normal spirometry. Chest 107:323–329, 1995.

KEY POINTS: STATIC LUNG VOLUMES, DIFFUSING CAPACITY, AND RESPIRATORY MUSCLE STRENGTH

1. Be familiar with the method used in your laboratory to measure static lung volumes because there are advantages and disadvantages to each possible method.

2. In patients with smoking-related obstructive lung disease, use $DL_{CO}SB$ to determine the presence of pulmonary emphysema.

3. Consider pulmonary vascular disease or early interstitial lung disease in the patient with normal TLC but reduced $DL_{CO}SB$.

4. Reduction in both TLC and $DL_{CO}SB$ most often indicates interstitial lung disease but can also be seen in alveolar filling processes and after pulmonary resection.

5. Reduced TLC with normal $DL_{CO}SB$ suggests chest wall or neuromuscular disease. Physical examination can help clarify the situation; radiologic studies can confirm the former, and measurement of PI_{max} and PE_{max} can identify the latter.

30. **Does cigarette smoking affect the $DL_{CO}SB$?**
    Yes. By increasing venous CO-hemoglobin, cigarette smoking limits transfer of this gas across the alveolar capillary membrane. This effect is minimized by having patients undergoing the test refrain from smoking for 24 hours.

    Smokers have values for $DL_{CO}SB$ that are about 20% lower than nonsmokers. All of this difference cannot be explained by CO-hemoglobin. Since ex-smokers have values intermediate between continuing smokers and lifetime nonsmokers, some of this difference is likely due to effects on the alveolar–capillary membrane that are not clinically detectable.

    Miller A, Thornton JC, Warshaw R, et al: Single breath diffusing capacity in a representative sample of the population of Michigan, a large industrial state: Predicted values, lower limits of normal and frequencies of abnormality by smoking history. Am Rev Resp Dis 127:270–277, 1983.

31. **What else affects the $DL_{CO}SB$?**
    $DL_{CO}SB$ decreases with age and increases with height; therefore, predicted values are computed using age and height as variables. $DL_{CO}SB$ varies directly with pulmonary capillary blood volume, and the value of $DL_{CO}SB$ must be corrected for erythrocytosis or anemia. The presence of extravasated blood (i.e., due to pulmonary hemorrhage) can also raise $DL_{CO}SB$. Exercise causes pulmonary capillary recruitment and will increase $DL_{CO}SB$; this may also happen during the first trimester of pregnancy, when expansion of blood volume occurs.

    Marrades RM, Diaz O, Roca J, et al: Adjustment of DLCO for hemoglobin concentration. Am J Respir Crit Care Med 155:236–241, 1997.

32. **What clinical tests of pulmonary function assess respiratory muscle strength?**
    Many ways to evaluate respiratory muscle strength are used in research studies but are not clinical tests (e.g., diaphragmatic electromyography and transdiaphragmatic pressure). A simple measurement of respiratory muscle strength is the maximal inspiratory pressure (PI_{max}) or maximal expiratory pressure (PE_{max}), measured by a pressure transducer at the mouth when a subject makes a maximal inspiratory effort from RV or a maximal expiratory effort from TLC.

    Black LF, Hyatt RE: Maximal respiratory pressures: Normal values and relationship to age and sex. Am Rev Resp Dis 99:696–702, 1969.

33. **What is the relationship between PI_{max} or PE_{max} and the standard tests of pulmonary function?**
    PI_{max} and PE_{max} reflect respiratory muscle weakness: PI, of the inspiratory muscles (primarily the diaphragm), and PE, of the expiratory muscles, including abdominal muscles. Depending on the type and level of muscle involvement, reduction in PI_{max} or PE_{max} is frequently seen in neuromuscular respiratory disease even when spirometric tests and lung volumes are normal. ($DL_{CO}SB$ is not directly affected by respiratory muscle disease). Therefore, reduction in PI_{max} or PE_{max} is a sensitive indicator of disorders characterized by respiratory muscle involvement, such as motor neuron disease (e.g., amyotrophic lateral sclerosis) and Guillain–Barré syndrome. As the disease progresses, the inspiratory capacity, vital capacity, FEV_1, and flow rates will progressively fall and will predict the advent of respiratory failure.

    American Thoracic Society/European Respiratory Society: ATS/ERS Statement on respiratory muscle testing. Am J Respir Crit Care Med 166:518–624, 2002.

CHAPTER 14

CLINICAL EXERCISE TESTING

Alexander S. Niven, MD, Gregory B. Tardie, PhD, and Idelle M. Weisman, MD

1. Why do exercise testing?

Clinical exercise testing is an important tool in the assessment and management of patients with known or suspected cardiac and pulmonary disease. There is increasing awareness that resting cardiac and pulmonary tests cannot reliably predict functional capacity. Exercise testing provides a reproducible objective measurement of exercise tolerance, which has been shown to correlate better than resting measurements with available health status and quality-of-life assessments.

Johnson BD, Weisman IM: Clinical exercise testing. In Crapo J, Hassroth J, Karlinsky J, King TE (eds): Baum's Textbook of Pulmonary Diseases, 7th ed. Philadelphia, Lippincott Williams & Wilkins, 2004, pp 55–78.

2. What are the most popular types of clinical exercise testing?

Exercise testing can be performed in a variety of ways. Some methods are low-tech and simple, whereas others require more complex technology but provide a more complete assessment. In order of increasing complexity, the most popular clinical exercise tests are (1) the 6-minute walk test (6MWT), (2) the shuttle walk test, (3) exercise challenge testing, (4) the cardiac stress test, and (5) the cardiopulmonary exercise test (CPET). The clinical question, functional capacity of the patient, and available facilities are the major factors that determine which method to use.

American Thoracic Society: ATS/ACCP statement on cardiopulmonary exercise testing. Am J Respir Crit Care Med 167:211–277, 2003.

3. What is a 6MWT?

The 6MWT measures the maximum distance that a patient can walk at his or her own pace in a 6-minute interval. This self-paced test is performed in an indoor corridor 30 meters long. The 6MWT provides a global assessment of functional capacity and is generally used for patients with relatively severe functional impairment. It does not provide specific information about each of the organ systems involved in exercise or the mechanism of exercise limitation. The 6MWT therefore has limited diagnostic capability, especially in patients with cardiac ischemia and combined heart–lung disease. This test has been used (1) for preoperative and postoperative evaluation of patients undergoing lung resection, lung transplantation, or lung volume reduction surgery; (2) to monitor response to therapeutic interventions and pulmonary rehabilitation; and (3) to predict morbidity and mortality in patients with cardiac and pulmonary vascular disease. Reference values are now for normal aduts.

American Thoracic Society: Guidelines for the six minute walk test. Am J Respir Crit Care Med 166:111–117, 2002.

Enright PL, Sherril DL: Reference equations for the six-minute walk in healthy adults. Am J Respir Crit Care Med 158:1384–1387, 1998.

4. What is a shuttle walk test?

The shuttle walk test measures the maximal distance a patient can walk on a 10-meter course at a pace set by audio signals from a cassette tape. Minute-by-minute walking speed is increased until the patient achieves exhaustion. This is a maximal symptom-limited test comparable in intensity to maximal tests performed on the treadmill. The test can also be modified for submaximal exercise testing. The shuttle walk test correlates better with maximal oxygen consumption ($\dot{V}O_2$ max) than the 6MWT, but it is probably less reflective of functional capacity during daily activities. Lack of cardiac monitoring during shuttle walk testing may place patients at higher risk of medical complications compared to more complex exercise testing.

Singh SJ, Morgan MD., Scott S, et al: Development of a shuttle walking test of disability in patients with chronic airway obstruction. Thorax 47:1019–1024, 1992.

5. What is exercise challenge testing?

Exercise challenge testing (also known as exercise-induced bronchoconstriction [EIB] testing) is used to identify airway hyperreactivity in suspected or known asthmatics with exercise-induced bronchospasm. The test involves constant work exercise on a treadmill or cycle ergometer for 6–8 minutes at an intensity that keeps the heart rate at approximately 80% of the predicted maximum. The resulting increase in minute ventilation generally triggers airway hyperreactivity if present. Spirometry (the forced vital capacity [FVC] and the forced expiratory volume in 1 second [FEV_1]) is measured before and at 5, 15, and 30 minutes postexercise. A drop of 10–15% in FEV1 or FVC after exercise is considered a positive test. Exercise-induced bronchoconstriction is observed in 70–80% of patients with asthma, but EIB is less sensitive and less specific than methacholine bronchoprovocation testing.

American Thoracic Society: Guidelines for methacholine and exercise challenge testing—1999. Am J Respir Crit Care Med 161:309–329, 2000.

Eliasson AH, Phillips YY, Rajagopal KR, et al: Sensitivity and specificity of bronchial provocation testing. An evaluation of four techniques in exercise-induced bronchospasm. Chest 102:347–355, 1992.

6. What is a cardiac stress test?

A cardiac stress test is an incremental treadmill exercise test used primarily to diagnose myocardial ischemia and to assess therapeutic interventions (i.e., medications, percutaneous interventions, and surgery). It is the most widely used clinical exercise testing modality in the United States. The test consists of serial electrocardiogram (ECG) and blood pressure monitoring while a subject exercises with progressively increasing intensity to exhaustion. The Bruce protocol is the most popular and consists of five progressive stages, each lasting for 3 minutes (Stage I, 1.7 mph and 10% grade; Stage II, 2.5 mph and 12% grade; Stage III, 3.4 mph and 14% grade; Stage IV, 4.2 mph and 16% grade; Stage V, 5.0 mph and 18% grade). The single most reliable indicator of exercise-induced ischemia is ST-segment depression, although other ECG abnormalities are also used as supplementary indicators.

American College of Cardiology/American Heart Association: ACC/AHA 2002 guidelines update for exercise testing: A report of the American College of Cardiology/American Heart Association Task Force on practice guidelines (Committee on Exercise Testing). Circulation 106:1883–1892, 2002.

Bruce RA, McDonough JR: Stress testing in screening for cardiovascular disease. Bull N Y Acad Med 45:1288–1305, 1969.

7. What is a CPET?

CPET improves upon standard exercise testing methods by adding concurrent measurements of respiratory gas exchange. It is a test that measures oxygen consumption ($\dot{V}O_2$), carbon dioxide production ($\dot{V}CO_2$), and minute ventilation ($\dot{V}_E$), during a symptom-limited incremental exercise test on a cycle ergometer or treadmill. Patient symptoms, ECG, blood pressure, and pulse oximetry are also monitored, and arterial blood gas (ABG) measurements can be added to provide more accurate information on pulmonary gas exchange. CPET provides a more complete picture of functional capacity, the integrated responses of major organ systems to exercise, and the mechanisms of exercise limitation.

American Thoracic Society: ATS/ACCP statement on cardiopulmonary exercise testing. Am J Respir Crit Care Med 167:211–277, 2003.

Zeballos RJ, Weisman IM: Modalities of clinical exercise testing. In Weisman IM, Zeballos RJ (eds): Clinical Exercise Testing. Basel, Karger, 2002, pp 30–42.

KEY POINTS: INDICATIONS FOR CARDIOPULMONARY EXERCISE TESTING

1. Evaluation of exercise intolerance

2. Evaluation of unexplained dyspnea

3. Functional evaluation of cardiovascular, respiratory, and metabolic diseases

4. Preoperative evaluation and risk stratification

5. Measurement of therapeutic response to treatment

6. Determination of functional impairment for disability evaluation

7. Evaluation of mechanisms of exercise limitation

8. Exercise prescription

8. **Why do a cardiopulmonary exercise test?**
Dyspnea on exertion and exercise intolerance are common problems in many conditions and diseases. CPET is increasingly used in the diagnostic evaluation of these disorders. Cardiac stress tests primarily focus on ischemia and generally cannot define other underlying pathophysiology that results in exercise intolerance. CPET can diagnose the cause of exertional symptoms, identify the principal factor limiting exercise in patients with multiple contributing clinical conditions, and prioritize treatment. Exercise tolerance can also be used to manage clinical outcomes of therapy, and it provides prognostic information in many populations. Common contraindications to CPET testing are listed in Table 14-1.

TABLE 14-1. CONTRAINDICATIONS TO CARDIOPULMONARY EXERCISE TESTING

Absolute

- Acute coronary syndrome or recent myocardial infarction
- Uncontrolled congestive heart failure or symptomatic arrhythmia
- Symptomatic severe aortic stenosis
- Recent venous thromboembolism
- Uncontrolled severe asthma
- Inability to cooperate with testing

Relative

- Hypertrophic cardiomyopathy
- Uncontrolled hypertension (i.e., systolic blood pressure [BP] > 200 mmHg, diastolic BP > 120 mmHg)
- Severe pulmonary hypertension
- Advanced or complicated pregnancy
- Orthopedic conditions that compromise exercise performance

Adapted from American Thoracic Society: ATS/ACCP statement on cardiopulmonary exercise testing. Am J Respir Crit Care Med 167:211–277, 2003.

9. **What cardiopulmonary variables are measured during a CPET?**
The number of measurements obtained during CPET depends on the individual patient and the indications for testing. The most important measurements are listed in Table 14-2.

   Weisman IM, Zeballos RJ: Clinical exercise testing. Clin Chest Med 22(4):679–701, 2001.

TABLE 14-2. MEASURED CARDIOPULMONARY VARIABLES DURING CARDIOPULMONARY EXERCISE TESTING		
Variables	**Noninvasive**	**Invasive***
Metabolic	Oxygen consumption (VO_2) Cardiac dioxide production (VCO_2)	Lactate
Cardiovascular	Heart rate (HR) Blood pressure (BP) Oxygen pulse (O_2 pulse)	
Ventilatory	Minute ventilation (V_E) Tidal volume (V_T) Respiratory rate (f)	
Pulmonary gas exchange	End tidal PO_2 and PCO_2 Ventilatory efficiency Oxygenation (SpO_2)	V_D/V_T SaO_2, PaO_2 pH, $PaCO_2$
Acid–base symptoms	Dyspnea Leg fatigue Chest pain	

* Requires ABG measurement.
Adapted from Weisman IM, Zeballos RJ: Clinical exercise testing. Clin Chest Med 22(4):679–701, 2001.

10. **How are cardiopulmonary variables measured during CPET?**
During exercise, the patient breathes into a mouthpiece connected to a computerized system that provides breath-by-breath analysis of respiratory gas exchange. Averaging of 30- or 60-second intervals is generally performed to minimize breath-by-breath measurement artifact. The computer processes three primary signals: (1) air flow, (2) oxygen fraction (concentration), and (3) carbon dioxide fraction. When heart rate is added, these four signals form the basis for most of the measured and derived cardiopulmonary variables generated during CPET.

    Beck KC, Weisman IM: Methods for cardiopulmonary exercise testing. In Weisman IM, Zeballos RJ (eds): Clinical Exercise Testing. Basel, Karger, 2002, pp 43–59.
    Zeballos RJ, Weisman IM: Behind the scenes of cardiopulmonary exercise testing. Clin Chest Med 15:193–213, 1994.

11. **Should a bicycle ergometer or treadmill be used for CPET?**
Although both modalities are acceptable for clinical testing, an electronically braked cycle may be preferable because it (1) offers a direct measurement of work rate, (2) minimizes ECG artifact, (3) allows for easier blood sample collection during exercise, and (4) has a better cost and safety profile. Maximum $\dot{V}O_2$ measurements are 5–11% less using a cycle ergometer compared to treadmill testing, possibly due to more local muscle fatigue.

    Beck KC, Weisman IM: Methods for cardiopulmonary exercise testing. In Weisman IM, Zeballos RJ (eds): Clinical Exercise Testing. Basel, Karger, 2002, pp 43–59.

12. **How is a maximal incremental CPET performed?**
    1. The patient is connected and familiarized to the exercise equipment.
    2. Cardiopulmonary measurements are obtained for 3 minutes at rest.
    3. Unloaded cycling is performed (1–3 minutes, optional).
    4. Incremental exercise is performed with steady increases in work rate to volitional exhaustion (5–30 W/min, based on the patient's functional capacity, for 8–12 minutes).
    5. Postexercise recovery and monitoring (10 minutes).

    American Thoracic Society: ATS/ACCP statement on cardiopulmonary exercise testing. Am J Respir Crit Care Med 167:211–277, 2003.

13. **When should a constant work protocol be performed?**
    Constant work exercise should be considered when CPET is used to monitor therapeutic responses to medication, surgery, or pulmonary rehabilitation. A constant work protocol is commonly performed after a maximum CPET and consists of at least 6 minutes of constant exercise at an intensity of 50–80% of the previously measured maximum work rate. Maximal pulmonary gas exchange information can also be approximated using a single arterial blood gas measurement obtained between minutes 5 and 6 of constant exercise at 70% of the maximum work rate.

    Oga T, Nishimura K, Tsukino M, et al: The effects of oxitropium bromide on exercise performance in patients with stable chronic obstructive pulmonary disease. Am J Respir Crit Care Med 161:1897–1901, 2000.
    Zeballos RJ, Weisman IM, Connery SM: Comparison of pulmonary gas exchange measurements between incremental and constant work exercise above the anaerobic threshold. Chest 113:602–611, 1998.

14. **What is the best index of exercise capacity?**
    $\dot{V}O_2$ max is the maximum amount of oxygen utilized per minute during exhaustive exercise; it is modulated by physical activity and remains the best available index for the assessment of exercise capacity and level of fitness. A normal $\dot{V}O_2$ max provides reassurance that no significant functional abnormality exists. A reduced $\dot{V}O_2$ max may reflect abnormalities in oxygen delivery (i.e., heart, lung, and systemic and pulmonary circulation), peripheral utilization (i.e., peripheral circulation or muscle), poor effort, or obesity (Fig. 14-1).

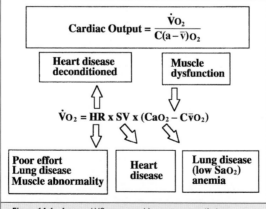

Figure 14-1. A normal VO_2 max provides reassurance that no significant functional abnormality exists. A reduced VO_2 max may reflect abnormalities in oxygen delivery (i.e., heart, lung, or systemic and pulmonary circulation), peripheral utilization (i.e., peripheral circulation or muscle), poor effort, or obesity.

15. **What are the normal physiologic responses to CPET?**

During exercise, there is an increase in oxygen demand to meet the metabolic requirements of the exercising muscles. The increased oxygen demand is met through an integrated response of the cardiopulmonary system, blood redistribution, and oxygen utilization by exercising muscles. At maximal exercise, oxygen consumption can increase up to 18-fold; heart rate, by twofold to threefold; stroke volume, twofold; cardiac output, fivefold; minute ventilation, 20- to 25-fold; and muscles oxygen extraction, twofold to threefold. The anaerobic threshold (AT) occurs at approximately 50% of $\dot{V}O_2$ max in normal adults and can be used both as an indicator of level of fitness and as a supplementary variable in the diagnosis of exercise limitation (Fig. 14-2).

Jones NL, Killian KJ: Exercise limitation in health and disease. N Engl J Med 343:632–641, 2000.

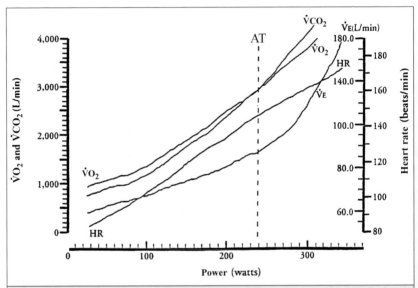

Figure 14-2. The anaerobic threshold (AT) occurs at approximately 50% of $\dot{V}O_2$ max in normal adults and can be used both as an indicator of level of fitness and as a supplementary variable in the diagnosis of exercise limitation. HR = heart rate. (Adapted from Weisman IM, Zaballos RJ: Clinical exercise testing. Clin Chest Med 22[4]:679–701, 2001).

KEY POINTS: NORMAL RESPONSES TO EXERCISE

1. $\dot{V}O_2$ increases linearly with work rate, and $\dot{V}O_2$ max is normal.

2. HR and O_2 pulse approach maximum predicted values at peak exercise.

3. There is ample ventilatory reserve (i.e., >20%) at peak exercise.

4. Oxygenation remains normal, and V_D/V_T decreases with exercise.

16. **What are the normal cardiovascular responses to CPET?**

Measurement of cardiac output is the best index of cardiac function during exercise. CPET uses noninvasive measurements, $\dot{V}O_2$ and heart rate, to estimate changes in the cardiac output during testing. $\dot{V}O_2$ and heart rate both increase linearly with increases in work rate, whereas O_2 pulse (a noninvasive estimator of stroke volume in patients without lung disease) also increases linearly but plateaus late in exercise. Oxygen delivery is the product of cardiac output and arterial oxygen content. As arterial oxygen content is normally maintained even at peak exercise, cardiac output is the limiting factor for $\dot{V}O_2$ max in normal subjects. Heart rate and O_2 pulse therefore generally approximate maximal predicted values at peak exercise.

17. **What are the normal ventilatory responses to CPET?**

In a normal adult, both respiratory rate and tidal volume progressively increase with exercise until tidal volume reaches approximately 50% of vital capacity. Further increases in minute ventilation at higher work rates are primarily due to elevations in respiratory rate. Ventilatory efficiency can be determined by measuring how much minute ventilation is achieved for a given level of metabolic demand ($\dot{V}_E/\dot{V}CO_2$ or $\dot{V}_E/\dot{V}O_2$). Ventilatory inefficiency due to reduced cardiac output and consequent ventilation/perfusion (V/Q) abnormalities is an important prognostic indicator of cardiovascular mortality.

> Chua TP, Ponikowski P, Harrington D, et al: Clinical correlates and prognostic significance of the ventilatory response to exercise in chronic heart failure. J Am Coll Cardiol 29:1585–1590, 1997.

18. **How does exercise affect pulmonary gas exchange?**

Oxygenation during exercise improves or remains the same in normal healthy subjects. Minute ventilation increases proportionally to compensate for the increased production of CO_2, resulting in a relatively stable concentration of exhaled CO_2 (also called end-tidal CO_2 [$ETCO_2$]) until near peak exercise. Better V/Q matching, particularly in the upper lung zones during exercise, results in a decrease in physiologic dead space. This is frequently expressed as a reduction in the ratio of dead space to tidal volume (V_D/V_T). Pulse oximetry is usually adequate to assess trends in oxygenation during exercise in subjects with normal lung function.

19. **When should ABGs be measured during CPET?**

ABGs are recommended when pulmonary gas exchange abnormalities are suspected or when pulse oximetry measurements are unreliable (e.g., because of poor signal, active smoking, or dark skin). ABGs are needed to calculate of the alveolar arterial oxygen gradient [$P(A-a)O_2$] and V_D/V_T. Patients with pulmonary diseases will often have pulmonary gas exchange abnormalities. Abnormal widening of $P(A-a)O_2$ with exercise usually reflects V/Q mismatch, but diffusion abnormalities or anatomical shunt may also contribute. Failure of V_D/V_T to decrease normally with exercise suggests V/Q abnormalities caused by increased physiologic dead space (i.e., wasted ventilation).

20. **What mechanisms are involved in exercise limitation?**

Exercise limitation is defined by a reduced $\dot{V}O_2$ max and can be caused by three broad categories:

1. **Cardiovascular limitation:** Due to problems with the heart, pulmonary or systemic circulation, or blood (i.e., anemia or carboxyhemoglobin)
2. **Respiratory limitation:** Due to ventilatory or gas exchange factors
3. **Peripheral limitation:** Due to a broad spectrum of neuromuscular conditions that affect oxygen utilization and mechanisms of muscle contraction

Other potential factors that can affect exercise include deconditioning, effort, individual perceptions, and environmental conditions. Exercise limitation is commonly multifactorial, with one exercise pattern serving as the predominant limiting factor.

21. **How can CPET differentiate patients with heart and lung diseases?**

    The difference between maximal predicted values and measured values for a variable during exercise is called a reserve. CPET permits the evaluation of both cardiovascular and ventilatory reserves. If $\dot{V}O_2$ max is less than predicted, a cardiovascular limitation to exercise can be suspected if the measured heart rate (HR) is near or equal to the maximal HR (i.e., no heart rate reserve [HRR]) and there is ventilatory reserve (VR). A ventilatory limitation to exercise can be suspected if the ventilatory demand ($\dot{V}_E$max) is near or equal to the patient's maximum ventilatory capacity (i.e., no VR) and there is HRR. Patients can have both cardiac and ventilatory limitation to exercise (i.e., no HRR and no VR). The table below reflects the usual response to exercise of patients with either cardiac or pulmonary disease (Table 14-3).

    Weisman IM, Zeballos RJ: A practical approach to the interpretation of cardiopulmonary exercise testing. In Weisman IM, Zeballos RJ (eds): Clinical Exercise Testing. Basel, Karger, 2002, pp 299–324.

TABLE 14-3.   RESPONSE TO EXERCISE IN HEART DISEASE AND LUNG DISEASE

	Heart Disease	Lung Disease
$\dot{V}O_2$	Decreased	Decreased
Heart rate reserve*	Variable	Increased
Ventilatory reserve†	Normal	Decreased
PaO_2	Normal	Decreased
Exercise ECG	Usually abnormal	Normal

*Heart rate reserve (HRR) = predicted maximal HR – measured maximal HR
†Ventilatory reserve (VR) = (MVV – $\dot{V}_E$max) or ($\dot{V}_E$max)/MVV; MVV is the maximal voluntary ventilation at rest, an estimate of ventilatory capacity. MVV can be measured directly or calculated ($FEV_1 \times 40$).

22. **What are exercise tidal flow-volume loops?**

    Diagnosing ventilatory limitation based on ventilatory reserve alone can be problematic. Plotting exercise tidal flow-volume loops within the resting maximal flow volume envelope is an increasingly popular method to better assess ventilatory impairment and to gain insight into a patient's breathing strategy and operational lung volumes during exercise (Fig. 14-3). Normal subjects increase their tidal volume during exercise by increasing end inspiratory lung volume (EILV) and decreasing end expiratory lung volume (EELV). At peak exercise, there is still substantial room to increase both flow and volume. In contrast, a patient with chronic obstructive lung disease may develop early flow limitation with increasing respiratory rate, leading to dynamic hyperinflation due to air trapping. This is reflected by an increase in operational lung volumes (i.e., EELV). By peak exercise, flow limitation is present throughout expiration, and EILV approaches total lung capacity—with no ventilatory reserve.

    Johnson BD, Weisman IM, Zeballos RJ, et al. Emerging concepts in the evaluation of ventilatory limitation during exercise. Chest 116:488–503, 1999.

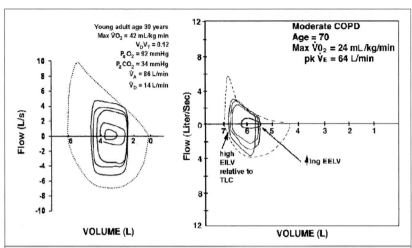

Figure 14-3. CPET in a healthy young adult at age 30 years and in a patient with moderate COPD. (Adapted from Johnson BD, Weisman IM, Zeballos RJ, et al: Emerging concepts in the evaluation of ventilatory limitation during exercise. Chest 116:488–503, 1999.)

THORACENTESIS AND PERCUTANEOUS PLEURAL BIOPSY

CHAPTER 15

Polly E. Parsons, MD, and Yuan-Po Tu, MD

1. **What are the chest x-ray findings in a pleural effusion?**
   Remember the axiom: *If the chest x-ray looks weird, think pleural disease*. The possibility of a pleural effusion should be considered in any abnormal chest x-ray. Increased densities on a chest x-ray are often attributed to parenchymal disease when they actually represent pleural fluid. Classically, intrapleural fluid gives rise to relatively homogeneous opacifications, the appearance of which depends on the volume of fluid, the anatomic location, and the presence or absence of intrapleural air.
   - Massive effusions can cause opacification of all or most of the hemithorax with or without mediastinal shift. The major differential is a drowned lung.
   - Moderate-sized effusions have the classic appearance of a homogeneous shadow occupying the lower portion of the hemithorax, obliterating the margins of the adjacent heart and diaphragm.
   - Minimal or small effusions may cause a haziness of the costophrenic angle or may be completely hidden behind the dome of the diaphragm on the posteroanterior (PA) x-ray projection. Often a lateral x-ray view will be helpful because it will show blunting of the posterior gutter.
   - Subpulmonic effusions collect between the inferior surface of the lung and the superior surface of the diaphragm and mimic the findings of an elevated hemidiaphragm on x-ray.
   - Interlobular effusions have a fusiform homogeneous shadow with well-defined margins lying in the long axis of an interlobar fissure. Effusions in the minor fissures are best seen on the PA projection, and those in the major fissures are best seen on the lateral projection. The x-ray findings of interlobular effusions are classically pseudotumors.
   - Hydropneumothorax gives a picture of a linear air fluid interface when the x-ray is taken with the patient in the upright position. The major differential diagnosis is a juxtapleural intrapulmonary cavity partially filled with fluid.

   Sahn SA: The pleura. Am Rev Respir Dis 138:184–234, 1988.

2. **What additional x-rays are helpful in evaluating a pleural effusion?**
   Lateral decubitus films are often helpful in determining how much fluid is present and whether it is free-flowing or loculated. The lateral decubitus view ordered should correspond to the side of the effusion. Therefore, if the patient has a left-sided pleural effusion, order a left lateral decubitus chest x-ray. The film will then be taken with the patient lying on his or her left side, allowing the pleural fluid to track along the lateral pleural space, where it is easily visualized.

   Levin DL, Klein JS: Imaging techniques for pleural space infections. Semin Respir Infect 14:31–38, 1999.

3. **What is the rule of thumb for estimating the amount of pleural fluid present on a chest x-ray?**
   - **200 cc:** Blunting of the costophrenic angle on the PA radiograph
   - **1–1.5 L:** Effusion occupying half of the hemithorax
   - **2.5–3 L:** Effusion occupying an entire hemithorax

4. **When should a diagnostic thoracentesis be considered?**
   Most patients with more than 10 mm of free-flowing pleural fluid demonstrated on a lateral decubitus x-ray should undergo diagnostic thoracentesis. Small effusions, less than 10 mm, often can be observed, but if thoracentesis is indicated, ultrasound guidance may be necessary.

KEY POINTS: INDICATIONS FOR THORACENTESIS

1. New effusions of uncertain etiology greater than 10 mm on a lateral decubitus x-ray

2. Suspected infection

3. Suspected malignancy

4. Effusion interferes with comfort and the ability to breathe (may require large-volume thoracentesis)

5. **When should ultrasound guidance for thoracentesis be considered?**
   - Patient is undergoing direct ultrasound guidance performed during thoracentesis (to decrease the pneumothorax complication rate).
   - Patient has a small pleural effusion, <10 mm, when clinically indicated.
   - Patient has loculated pleural fluid.
   - Patient has a pleural effusion on the side of an elevated hemidiaphragm.
   - Patient is on mechanical ventilation.
   - Patient has a bleeding diathesis.

   Jones PW, Moyers JP, Rogers JT, et al: Ultrasound-guided thoracentesis: Is it a safer method? Chest 123:418–423, 2003.

6. **What are the relative contraindications to a thoracentesis?**
   - Uncooperative patients (many clinicians consider this an absolute counterindication)
   - Inability to clearly palpate the rib margins
   - Inability to correct a coagulopathy
   - Patients on mechanical ventilation (especially those on positive end-expiratory pressure [PEEP])
   - Patients with severe chronic obstructive pulmonary disease (COPD)
   - Patients with one lung
   - Patients in whom the benefit from the procedure is unlikely to outweigh the risk
   - Operator inexperience

7. **Which alternative procedures are often considered instead of thoracentesis?**
   - Chest tube placement
   - Diagnostic and therapeutic interventional radiologically placed catheters for loculated effusions

8. **What are the common complications of thoracentesis?**
   - **Pneumothorax:** Estimated to occur in 11% of patients, although only 2% will require chest tubes. The incidence varies with the size of the needle used for the procedure. Pneumothorax is more frequent when the thoracentesis is performed blindly and is less frequent when it is performed with ultrasound guidance.
   - **Pain:** Up to 20% of patients may complain of anxiety and pain at the site of the thoracentesis.

9. **What are the uncommon complications of thoracentesis?**
   - Introduction of air into the pleural space
   - Seroma at the procedure site
   - Bleeding
   - Infection
   - Hypotension
   - Hypoxemia or air embolism
   - Splenic and liver laceration
   - Tumor seeding of the tract
   - Catheter fragment left in the pleural space
   - Death (rare)

   Barbers R, Patel P: Thoracentesis made safe and simple. J Respir Dis 15:841–851, 1994.
   Collins TA, Sahn SA: Thoracentesis: Clinical value, complications, technical problems, and patient experience. Chest 91:817–822, 1987.

10. **Is a postprocedure chest x-ray needed after every thoracentesis?**
    No. Several studies have now shown that the incidence of pneumothorax in asymptomatic patients is very low. However, chest x-rays should be performed in symptomatic patients and in any patient in whom a complication is suspected.

    Aleman C, Alegre J, Armadan L, et al: The value of chest roentgenography in the diagnosis of pneumothorax after thoracentesis. Am J Med 107:340–343, 1999.
    Capizzi SA, Prakash UB: Chest roentgenography after outpatient thoracentesis. Mayo Clinic Proc 73:940, 1998.

11. **What do you do if you see bright red blood back while performing a thoracentesis?**
    Although pleural effusions can be hemorrhagic, the appearance of bright red blood in the absence of chest trauma should raise concern that an intercostal artery, the spleen, or the liver has been punctured or lacerated. Although massive hemorrhage from a thoracentesis is rare, it is critical to carefully monitor the patient's hemodynamic status, to follow the patient's hematocrit, and to correct any coagulation abnormalities. If there is evidence of persistent blood loss, a surgeon should be consulted.

12. **Which patients are at increased risk for laceration of an intercostal artery during thoracentesis?**
    Elderly patients. With increasing age, the tortuosity of intercostal blood vessels increases such that the amount of space between two ribs that is safe (i.e., free of blood vessels and nerves) is decreased. Increased intercostal vessel tortuosity may start as early as age 40. Therefore, it is always important when performing a thoracentesis to insert the needle directly over the superior border of the rib to avoid puncturing a vessel. Thoracentesis for removal of fluid is best performed in the posterior gutter since the intercostal arteries are most closely adherent to the posterior rib and the intercostal space is greatest in the posterior chest.

    Carney M, Ravin CE: Intercostal artery laceration during thoracentesis. Chest 75:520–522, 1979.

13. **I am in the middle of drawing off pleural fluid, and I am drawing back air. Does this mean that I punctured the lung?**
    Not necessarily. Sometimes air enters the pleural space during a thoracentesis if the system (i.e., needle, stopcock, or syringe) is open to air inadvertently during the procedure. Take your time and familiarize yourself with the system you are going to use prior to beginning the procedure.

14. **Should I quit if I am not able to get any fluid back?**
    The inability to obtain pleural fluid (i.e., a dry tap) occurs when the thoracentesis has been performed in the wrong location or when the fluid is too viscous to be drawn through the needle. The first step is to reassess your clinical localization of the pleural fluid. If there is any question as to the location of the pleural fluid, ultrasound guidance would be appropriate for the next attempt. If you suspect that the patient has an empyema and, therefore, the fluid is very viscous, an attempt with a larger needle may be indicated. Again, assuring the location of the pleural fluid with ultrasound guidance may be prudent.

15. **What is post-thoracentesis reexpansion pulmonary edema?**
    Unilateral pulmonary edema and hypoxemia may develop following a thoracentesis. This usually occurs when the pleural effusion has been present and compressing underlying lung tissue for more than 7 days and when more than 1–1.5 L of pleural fluid is removed at a time.

16. **How much fluid do you need to obtain for a diagnostic thoracentesis?**
    Usually 35–50 mL are more than adequate for routine diagnostic studies, although more fluid may be helpful if cytology studies are needed.

17. **What routine tests should be ordered on pleural fluid?**
    Cell count and differential, lactate dehydrogenase (LDH), total protein, glucose, and hydrogen ion concentration (pH). Additional studies can be ordered, depending on the differential diagnosis of the pleural effusion in the patient being evaluated. These studies include gram stain, acid-fast bacillus (AFB) stain, cytology, amylase, cholesterol, triglycerides, and special serologies, as well as aerobic, anaerobic, AFB, and fungal cultures.

    Light RW: Clinical practice. Pleural effusions. N Engl J Med 346:1971–1977, 2002.

18. **Are there any gross characteristics of the pleural fluid that help one make the diagnosis even while doing the thoracentesis?**
    1. Grossly bloody effusions with a red blood cell count per cubic millimeter (RBC/mm^3) greater than 100,000:
       - Traumatic tap
       - Malignancy: malignant mesothelioma or metastatic neoplasms
       - Pulmonary embolism and postpericardiotomy syndrome (less common)

KEY POINTS: PLEURAL EFFUSIONS AND CONGESTIVE HEART FAILURE

1. Congestive heart failure is the most common cause of a pleural effusion.

2. Performing a thoracentesis on a patient with congestive heart failure usually does not add any new or helpful clinical information.

3. Approximately 80% of pleural effusions due to congestive heart failure are bilateral.

4. Approximately 75% of pleural effusions due to congestive heart failure respond within 48 hours after initiating diuretics.

5. Classically, the pleural effusions associated with congestive heart failure are transudates; however, diuretic therapy may change the pleural effusion characteristics so that they have exudative features.

6. If a patient with clinical congestive heart failure develops fever, pleuritic chest pain, or a marked discrepancy in the size of bilateral effusions, a diagnostic thoracentesis should be performed.

2. White, milky appearance, suggesting injury to the lymphatic channels
   - Chylothorax
   - Chyliform pleural effusion
   - Lymphoma
   - Surgical trauma
3. Putrid smell
   - Empyema
   - Anaerobic pleural parapneumonic process

   Shinto RA, Light RW: Effects of diuresis on the characteristics of pleural fluid in patients with congestive heart failure. Am J Med 88:230–234, 1990.
   Villena V, Lopes-Encuentra A, Garcia-Lujan R, et al: Clinical implications of appearance of pleural fluid at thoracentesis. Chest 125:156–159, 2004.

19. **Do small effusions associated with pneumonia need to be investigated?**
    - Small parapneumonic effusions (i.e., less than 10 mm) associated with pneumonia will usually resolve with treatment of the pneumonia.
    - Large parapneumonic effusions and effusions that persist after appropriate treatment associated with ongoing fever and pain should be investigated.

      Cohen M, Sahn SA: Resolution of pleural effusions. Chest 119:1547–1562, 2001.

20. **When should a percutaneous pleural biopsy be considered?**
    In patients with an undiagnosed exudative effusion. The majority of these patients have either tuberculosis or a malignancy. Percutaneous pleural biopsy has a diagnostic yield of greater than 75% for tuberculosis. In general, malignant pleural effusions can be diagnosed with cytology studies, so a percutaneous pleural biopsy does not significantly increase the diagnostic yield in these patients. Pleural biopsies are best performed before draining the pleural effusion. A larger pleural effusion provides a larger separation between the pleural and parietal surfaces.

21. **What are the contraindications to a percutaneous pleural biopsy?**
    - **Uncooperative patient:** Ideally, patients need to be able to sit upright, to follow directions, and to hold their breath on command.
    - **Inadequate pleural fluid in the pleural space:** If the pleural space is obliterated, the biopsy needle is likely to enter the lung.
    - **Bleeding diathesis or coagulopathy:** Beware of patients with renal failure who may have a prolonged bleeding time, and do not perform the procedure in patients who are anticoagulated.

22. **What are the risks of a percutaneous pleural biopsy?**
    The risks are similar to those from thoracentesis and include pneumothorax, hypotension, hemorrhage, infection, and air embolism. To minimize the likelihood of biopsying an intercostal vessel, an adage to specifically remember when doing pleural biopsies is "Never biopsy at 12 o'clock," meaning do not biopsy directly above the biopsy needle entry site (i.e., the equivalent of the position of the hands of the clock at 12 o'clock) because you may catch the vessel with the biopsy needle.

23. **How many percutaneous pleural biopsies do I need to take?**
    Usually 4–6 biopsies taken at a single site are adequate for diagnosis. Despite the fact that pleural metastases and tuberculosis lesions are scattered and patchy, the few studies available suggest that performing biopsies at multiple sites at the same time does not improve the diagnostic yield of the procedure.

    Jimenez D, Perez-Rodrigues E, Diaz G, et al: Determining the optimal number of specimens to obtain with needle biopsy of the pleura. Respir Med 96:14–17, 2002.

24. **Is there an advantage to computed tomography (CT) guided needle biopsies of the pleura compared to blind percutaneous biopsies?**
A recent study suggested that CT-guided cutting needle biopsies had a much higher diagnostic yield in patients with suspected malignancy and negative pleural fluid cytology.

Maskell NA, Gleeson FV, Davies RJ: Standard pleural biopsy versus CT-guided cutting needle biopsy for diagnosis of malignant disease in pleural effusions: A randomised controlled trial. Lancet 361:1326–1330, 2003.

WEBSITE

http://www.thoracic.org/assemblies/cc/ccprimer/infosheet11.html

BIBILIOGRAPHY

1. Kennedy L, Sahn SA: Noninvasive evaluation of the patient with a pleural effusion. Chest Surg Clin North Am 4:451–465, 1994.
2. McElvein RB: Procedures in the evaluation of chest disease. Clin Chest Med 13:1–9, 1992.
3. Quigley RL: Thoracentesis and chest tube drainage. Crit Care Clin 11:111–126, 1995.
4. Sokolowski JW, Burgher LW, Jones FL, et al: Guidelines for thoracentesis and needle biopsy of the pleura. Am Rev Respir Dis 140:257–258, 1989.

CHAPTER 16

BRONCHOSCOPY

Udaya B. S. Prakash, MD

1. What is bronchoscopy?

Bronchoscopy is a diagnostic and therapeutic procedure that permits direct visualization of the tracheobronchial lumen with the help of the bronchoscope, a specialized optical device. Bronchoscopy permits collection of respiratory secretions from the tracheobronchial tree and tissue samples from the airway mucosa, lung parenchyma, and lymph nodes and other masses located immediately adjacent to but outside the tracheobronchial lumen. Bronchoscopy is also used to treat the airway luminal obstruction caused by various diseases including cancer, bleeding from respiratory structures, and many pulmonary disorders. Bronchoscopy is the most commonly performed invasive procedure in pulmonology.

Colt HG, Prakash UBS, Offord KP: Bronchoscopy in North America: Survey by the American Association for Bronchology, 1999. J Bronchol 7:8–25, 2000.

Utz JP, Prakash UBS: Indications for Ind contraindications to bronchoscopy. In Prakash UBS (ed): Bronchoscopy. New York, Raven Press, 1994, pp 81–89.

Prakash UBS: Bronchoscopy. In Albert RK, Spiro SG, Jett JR (eds): Clinical Respiratory Medicine, 2nd ed. Philadelphia, Elsevier, 2004, pp 143–160.

Prakash UBS: Bronchoscopy. In Mason RJ, Broaddus VC, Murray JF, Nadel, JA (eds): Murray and Nadel's Textbook of Respiratory Medicine, 4th ed. Philadelphia, Saunders, 2005, pp 1617–1650.

Prakash UBS: Bronchoscopy unit, expertise, and personnel. In Bollinger C, Mathur P (eds): Interventional Bronchoscopy. Prog Respir Res 30:1–13, 2000.

Prakash UBS, Offord KP, Stubbs SE: Bronchoscopy in North America: The ACCP Survey. Chest 100:1668–1675, 1991.

2. What is a bronchoscope?

It is an instrument that permits examination of the tracheobronchial tree (see above). The two main types of bronchoscopes are the flexible (i.e., fiberoptic) and rigid bronchoscopes (Figs. 16-1 and 16-2). The flexible bronchoscopes can be inserted through a nasal passage, mouth, or tracheostomy stoma, whereas the rigid scopes can only be inserted through the mouth or tracheostomy stoma. The flexible bronchoscope is used in over 95% of all bronchoscopy procedures.

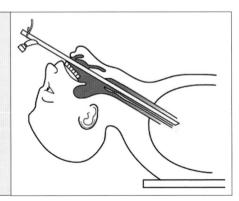

Figure 16-1. Rigid bronchoscopy requires hyperextension of the patient's neck to permit passage of the instrument into the airways. To prevent discomfort, intravenous sedation or general anesthesia is required in most patients. (Elsevier Science, 2005.)

3. **What are the indications for rigid bronchoscopy?**
   In adults, a rigid bronchoscope is preferred by many for laser therapy, placement of tracheobronchial prostheses (i.e., stents), dilatation of tracheobronchial strictures, and mechanical debridement of obstructing tumors in the major airways. Although these procedures can be performed with flexible bronchoscopes, the rigid instrument permits the procedure to be done more quickly and allows for better management of complications. Rigid bronchoscopy is preferred by many for extraction of airway foreign bodies in children.

   Swanson KL, Prakash UBS, McDougall JC, et al: Airway foreign bodies in adults. J Bronchol 10:107–111, 2003.

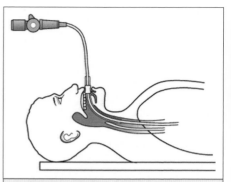

Figure 16-2. Flexible bronchoscopy performed by oral insertion. Most flexible bronchoscopy procedures can be performed by oral or nasal insertion after topical anesthesia is applied to the nasal or oropharyngeal mucosa. (Elsevier Science, 2005.)

KEY POINTS: MOST COMMON INDICATIONS FOR BRONCHOSCOPY

1. Abnormal chest x-ray

2. Hemoptysis

3. Suspected opportunistic lung infections

4. Retained airway secretions and mucous plugs

5. Unexplained cough of >6 weeks in duration

4. **How is bronchoscopy performed?**
   Almost all flexible bronchoscopies can be performed safely under topical anesthesia and intravenous sedation. Lidocaine is the most commonly used topical anesthetic. It is applied by spraying it with a canister or through the working channel of the flexible bronchoscope. Lidocaine is applied as needed to control cough during bronchoscopy. General anesthesia may be required for most rigid bronchoscopies. Pediatric patients frequently require general anesthesia.

5. **Where does one perform bronchoscopy?**
   Most medical centers may assign a physical location (e.g., an operating room, a bronchoscopy laboratory, or a specially equipped room) for bronchoscopy. However, the procedure is frequently performed by the bedside, especially in critical care units and emergency departments. Many medical centers in which invasive or specialized bronchoscopy procedures are routinely provided have a dedicated location with facilities to administer general anesthesia and necessary equipment for both rigid and flexible bronchoscopies.

6. **What are the indications for bronchoscopy?**
   The two broad indications are diagnostic and therapeutic (Tables 16-1 and 16-2). In many patients, both indications are used simultaneously.

TABLE 16-1. COMMON INDICATIONS FOR DIAGNOSTIC BRONCHOSCOPY

Cough

Hemoptysis

Wheezing and stridor

Abnormal chest roentgenogram

Pulmonary infections
  Localized
  Diffuse
  In immunocompromised patients

Diffuse lung disease (noninfectious)
  Interstitial lung diseases
  Drug-induced lung disorders

Intrathoracic lymphadenopathy or mass
  Pulmonary nodules
  Bronchogenic carcinoma
    Positive or suspicious sputum cytology
    Staging of bronchogenic carcinoma
    Follow-up of bronchogenic carcinoma
  Metastatic carcinoma (endobronchial or parenchymal)
  Esophageal and mediastinal tumors
  Foreign body in the airways (suspected)
  Tracheobronchial strictures and stenoses

TABLE 16-2. COMMON INDICATIONS FOR THERAPEUTIC BRONCHOSCOPY

Airway secretions, mucous plugs, clots, and necrotic debris

Atelectasis

Mucoid impaction syndromes
  Plastic bronchitis
  Asthma
  Cystic fibrosis

Foreign body in the tracheobronchial tree

Neoplasms of the tracheobronchial tree
  Bronchoscopic debridement
  Laser therapy
  Argon plasma coagulation
  Electrocautery
  Cryotherapy
  Brachytherapy
  Balloon dilatation
  Placement of a tracheobronchial stent

Strictures and stenoses
  Bronchoscopic dilatation
  Laser, electrocautery, or argon plasma coagulation
  Balloon dilatation
  Stent placement

Respiratory failure
  Endotracheal tube placement
  Endotracheal tube exchang

Harrow EM, Abi-Saleh W, Blum J, et al: The utility of transbronchial needle aspiration in the staging of bronchogenic carcinoma. Am J Respir Crit Care Med 161:601–607, 2000.

Wahidi MM. Ernst A: The role of bronchoscopy in the management of lung transplant recipients. Resp Care Clin N Am 10:549–562, 2004.

7. **List the absolute contraindications to bronchoscopy**
   - Totally uncooperative patient
   - Hemodynamic instability
   - New myocardial infarction
   - Unstable angina
   - Life-threatening arrhythmias
   - Worsening asthma or status asthmaticus
   - Rapidly worsening hypercarbia
   - Lack of appropriate instruments and personnel (including an insufficiently trained bronchoscopist)

KEY POINTS: ABSOLUTE CONTRAINDICATIONS FOR BRONCHOSCOPY

1. Lack of cooperation by the patient

2. Unstable angina pectoris

3. Uncontrolled cardiac arrhythmias

4. Refractory hypoxemia in spite of supplemental oxygen

5. Lack of bronchoscopy expertise

8. **What are the major complications of bronchoscopy?**
   Bronchoscopy is a safe procedure. Low-grade fever is seen in 10–20% of patients, but septicemia is extremely rare. Other complications include mild bronchospasm and dyspnea. Bronchoscopic lung biopsy is complicated by pneumothorax in 1–2% of cases. The incidence of postbiopsy bleeding (i.e., >100 mL) is 1–2%.

   Culver DA, Gordon SM, Mehta AC: Infection control in the bronchoscopy suite: A review of outbreaks and guidelines for prevention. Am J Respir Crit Care Med. 167:1050–1056, 2003.

   Picard E, Schwartz S, Goldberg S, et al: A prospective study of fever and bacteremia after flexible fiberoptic bronchoscopy in children. Chest 117:573–577, 2000.

9. **What precautions are required before bronchoscopy is performed?**
   Unless clinical details indicate the presence of underlying coagulopathy or diseases that predispose to excessive bleeding, routine screening for bleeding diathesis is not indicated. Biopsies are not recommended if the platelet count is <60,000 µL and a serum creatinine is >3.0 mg/dL. Other precautions are listed in Table 16-3.

10. **What special precautions are necessary for the bronchoscopy team?**
    Universal infection prevention precautions are indicated for all patients, regardless of the indication for bronchoscopy. All bronchoscopy personnel must wear eyeglasses, gloves, and face masks to prevent spread of infection. Proper sterilization of the bronchoscope and ancillary equipment is imperative.

TABLE 16-3.   PREBRONCHOSCOPY CHECKLIST

1. Is there an appropriate indication for bronchoscopy?
2. Has there been a previous bronchoscopy?
3. If the answer to (2) is yes, were there any problems or complications?
4. Does the patient (or legal guardian, if patient is unable to communicate) fully understand the goal, risks, and complications of bronchoscopy?
5. Does the patient's past medical history (including allergy to medications or topical anesthesia) or present clinical condition pose special problems or predispose the patient to complications?
6. Are all the appropriate tests completed, with results available?
7. Are the premedications appropriate and the dosages correct?
8. Does the patient require special consideration before bronchoscopy (e.g., corticosteroid for asthma, insulin for diabetes mellitus, or prophylaxis against endocarditis) or during bronchoscopy (e.g., supplemental oxygen, extra sedation, or general anesthesia)?
9. Is the plan for postbronchoscopy care appropriate?
10. Are all the appropriate instruments and personnel available to assist during bronchoscopy and to handle the potential complications?

Adapted from Prakash UBS, Cortese DA, Stubbs SE: Technical solutions to common problems in bronchoscopy. In Prakash UBS (ed): Bronchoscopy. New York, Raven, 1994, pp 111–113.

11. **Which pharmacologic agents are routinely used in most flexible bronchoscopies?**
An antisialagogue (atropine or glycopyrrolate) is used by some bronchoscopists to reduce airway secretions. Sedatives are recommended for most patients to allay anxiety and to induce antegrade amnesia. Almost all patients require a topical anesthetic such as lidocaine. Supplemental oxygen is recommended for all patients. Normal saline is essential for bronchial washings and bronchoalveolar lavage (BAL).

12. **Can bronchoscopy be performed in severely hypoxemic patients?**
Yes. Although severe hypoxemia is a relative contraindication, if intraoperative supplemental oxygen can maintain a satisfactory oxygen saturation (i.e., $SO_2 > 90\%$), often bronchoscopy can be performed. Blood gas analysis and pulmonary function tests are not necessary before bronchoscopy.

13. **Is the presence of a coagulopathy a contraindication?**
No. Bronchoscopy to inspect airways and to obtain BAL can be safely done in patients with significant bleeding disorders, including thrombocytopenia, elevated prothrombin time, and other coagulopathies. However, biopsies and other interventional procedures are contraindicated.

14. **Are biopsies performed in patients with coagulopathies?**
Yes. If the platelet count is <60,000/μL, 4–6 units of platelets are transfused 30–45 minutes before biopsy. In patients taking warfarin (Coumadin), the international normalized ratio (INR) should be reduced to ≤1.5 before biopsy. Aspirin therapy is not a contraindication to biopsies. Antiplatelet agents (e.g., clopidogrel) increase the risk of postbiopsy bleeding.

15. **Is mechanical ventilation a contraindication to bronchoscopy?**
    No. Critically ill patients and patients on mechanical ventilation frequently require flexible bron-choscopy for the removal of retained secretions, the placement or change of endotracheal tubes, diagnostic BAL, bronchoscopic lung biopsy, and assessment of hemoptysis and other pulmonary problems.

16. **What are the indications for bronchoalveolar lavage?**
    BAL is used most commonly to identify pulmonary infections; it is now preferred to protected-specimen brush to identify bacteria in the distal respiratory tract. BAL has a high diagnostic rate (>95%) in lung infection caused by *Pneumocystis carinii* and is also helpful in the diagnosis of noninfectious conditions such as lymphangitic metastasis, lymphangioleiomyomatosis, pulmonary eosinophilic granuloma, and pulmonary alveolar proteinosis. BAL is not helpful to diagnose idiopathic pulmonary fibrosis, sarcoidosis, and other diffuse lung diseases.

    http://www.thoracic.org/criticalcare/bal.asp
    Meyer KC: The role of bronchoalveolar lavage in interstitial lung disease. Clin Chest Med 25:637–49, 2004.

17. **Describe the BAL technique.**
    The tip of the flexible bronchoscope is advanced as far as possible and wedged into the bronchus that leads to the most abnormal segment, as seen on chest x-ray or on chest computed tomography (CT). Normal saline, in five aliquots of 20 mL each, is instilled into the lung segment through the working channel of the bronchoscope. The effluent is then suctioned back through the bronchoscope into a container (Fig. 16-3).

18. **What ancillary instruments can be used with bronchoscopy?**
    Cytology brushes, biopsy forceps, catheter needles, and specialized instruments such as lasers, electrocauters, cryoprobes, brachytherapy catheters (for intraluminal radiation), argon plasma coagulators, ultrasound probes, balloons, stents, and others.

19. **How is the bronchoscopic lung biopsy (BLB) performed?**
    The flexible bronchoscope is introduced into the bronchus that leads to the lung parenchymal abnormality identified by chest x-ray or chest CT. The biopsy forceps are then passed through the bronchoscope, and when they reach the lesion, the forceps are opened and closed after a tissue sample is caught, at which point the forceps with tissue are withdrawn. Usually, 4–6 biopsies are obtained. Once the absence of bleeding is confirmed, the bronchoscope is withdrawn from the bronchus. Although BLB can be obtained without fluoroscopic guidance, fluoroscopic guidance significantly reduces the risk of pneumothorax. If a localized lesion (such as a lung nodule) is to be biopsied, fluoroscopic guidance is essential.

    Prakash UBS, Utz JP: Bronchoscopic lung biopsy. In Wang KP, Mehta AC, Turner KF Jr (eds): Flexible Bronchoscopy. Malden, MA, Blackwell Publishing, 2004, pp 89–102.

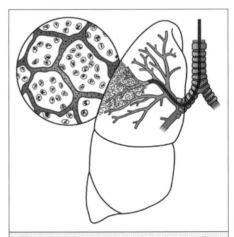

Figure 16-3. Technique of bronchoalveolar lavage. The tip of the flexible bronchoscope is advanced and wedged in the distal-most bronchus leading to the pulmonary parenchymal abnormalities, and aliquots of saline (20 mL, five times) are instilled and suctioned back. (Elsevier Science, 2005.)

20. **Can BLB be performed in patients receiving mechanical ventilation?**
Yes. The risk of pneumothorax, however, is slightly increased, particularly if the patient is receiving positive end-expiratory pressure (PEEP) breathing. Prior to biopsy, PEEP should be discontinued and the patient taken off the ventilator and oxygenated with hand-bagging. Reinstitution of PEEP should be withheld for at least 30 minutes after BLB.

Olopade CO, Prakash UBS: Bronchoscopy in the critical care unit. Mayo Clin Proc 64:1255–1263, 1989.

21. **What are palliative bronchoscopic therapies?**
These are treatments to provide symptomatic relief of dyspnea and hemoptysis in patients with advanced major airway obstruction caused by unresectable or otherwise untreatable tumors. The treatments include bronchoscopic dilatation, laser ablation, cryotherapy, electrocautery, brachytherapy (intraluminal irradiation), phototherapy, and placement of airway prostheses.

KEY POINTS: TYPES OF BRONCHOSCOPIC PALLIATIVE THERAPIES

1. Laser ablation

2. Electrocautery

3. Argon plasma coagulation

4. Cryotherapy

5. Brachytherapy

22. **Name some of the new developments in bronchoscopic techniques that are being tested.**
- Bronchoscopic lung volume reduction by inserting endobronchial valves
- Electromagnetic navigation to sample localized lung lesions
- Different types of airway prostheses (i.e. stents) to keep open obstructed airways
- Ultrasound-guided sampling of thoracic lymph nodes
- Gene therapy of tumors

CHAPTER 17

INTERVENTIONAL PULMONOLOGY

James L. Knepler, Jr., MD, and Praveen N. Mathur, MBBS

1. **What is the definition of interventional pulmonology?**

   We define interventional pulmonology as "the art and science of medicine as related to the performance of diagnostic and invasive therapeutic procedures that require additional training and expertise beyond that required in a standard pulmonary medicine training program." Disease processes encompassed within this discipline include complex airway management problems, benign and malignant central airway obstruction, and pleural diseases.

   > Beamis J, Mathur PN (eds): Interventional Pulmonology. New York, McGraw-Hill, 1999.
   > Bolliger CT, Mathur PN (eds): Interventional Bronchoscopy: Progress in Respiratory Research, Vol. 30. Basel, Karger, 2000.
   > http://www.aabronchology.org

2. **Which pulmonary procedures fall under of the category of interventional?**

   Diagnostic and therapeutic procedures include, but are not limited to, rigid bronchoscopy, laser bronchoscopy, endobronchial electrosurgery, argon plasma coagulation, cryotherapy, airway stent insertion, balloon bronchoplasty and dilatation techniques, endobronchial radiation (i.e., brachytherapy), endobronchial ultrasound, transthoracic needle aspiration and biopsy, percutaneous dilatational tracheotomy, transtracheal oxygen catheter insertion, transbronchial needle aspiration, and medical thoracoscopy.

   > Seijo LM, Sterman DH: Interventional Pulmonology. N Engl J Med 344:740–749, 2001.

3. **What are the common clinical findings in patients with a tracheobronchial lesion?**

   Patients with a tracheobronchial lesion can present with dyspnea, cough, chest discomfort, hemoptysis, stridor, or a localized wheeze. The patient's history may include known cancer, aspiration of a foreign body, prior airway surgery or intubation, recurrent pneumonia, or other underlying illnesses that may involve the airways, such as sarcoidosis or tuberculosis.

   Although a tracheobronchial lesion may be detected on chest radiography or a computed tomography (CT) scan, direct airway visualization with bronchoscopy is often needed to define the extent of the lesion.

   > Sheski FD, Mathur PN: Endoscopic options for tracheo-bronchial obstruction. ACCP Pulmonary and Critical Care Update, Volume 14, pp 21–24.

4. **What is the difference between an endobronchial lesion and extrinsic compression?**

   - Endobronchial lesions are found within the tracheobronchial tree and can be visualized by bronchoscopy.
   - In extrinsic compression, the lesion compresses the tracheobronchial tree from outside the lumen. The actual lesion cannot be visualized; however, its effects can be seen.
   - Frequently, endobronchial and extrinsic lesions coexist.

5. **Are endobronchial lesions and extrinsic compression treated differently?**
   Endobronchial lesions are much more amenable to ablation of the lesion. This may be done with laser therapy (neodymium/yttrium–aluminum–garnet [Nd/YAG]), argon plasma coagulation (APC), cryotherapy, electrocautery, or brachytherapy. These will remove the lesion that was seen with the bronchoscopy and will recanalize the airway. You have to careful to remove only the endobronchial component. Extraluminal lesions causing extrinsic compression are usually treated with bronchoscopic or balloon dilatation, stent placement, and external beam radiation if they are malignant. The mucosa of the endobronchial tree is pushed in and may be normal in appearance. Extrinsic compression is not amenable to endobronchial ablation.

6. **What does "laser" stand for? What are the two types of lasers used in the airway?**
   Laser is an acronym for **l**ight **a**mplified by the **s**timulated **e**mission of **r**adiation. The two lasers most commonly used in removing endobronchial lesions are the carbon dioxide and Nd/YAG lasers. Table 17-1 describes the difference between these two lasers. The Nd/YAG laser is used more often by interventional pulmonologists because it can be used in a rigid or a flexible bronchoscope.

   Cavaliere S, Foccoli P, Farina PL: Nd:YAG laser bronchoscopy: A 5-year experience with 1936 applications in 1000 patients. Chest 94:15–21, 1988.

TABLE 17-1.	THE DIFFERENCES BETWEEN THE CO_2 LASER AND THE ND/YAG LASER	
	CO_2	Nd/YAG
Penetration of tissue	Shallow (0.1–0.5 mm)	Deeper (3–5 mm)
Bronchoscope	Rigid	Rigid or flexible
Hemostasis	Poor	Good
Precision in cutting	Very precise	Less precise
Wavelength	Long	Short
Operator	Otolaryngologist	Pulmonologist
Area of lung	Larynx	Tracheobronchial tree

7. **What are the potential complications of Nd/YAG laser use?**
   Many of the complications are the same as for bronchoscopy, including reaction to anesthesia and hypoxia from obstruction of an airway by the bronchoscope or associated equipment. Debris from the removed lesion can also cause hypoxia. Potentially, the most catastrophic complication is endotracheal fire or even explosion. Patients who require an endotracheal tube or a high concentration of O_2 are at the greatest risk. Lastly, perforation of an underlying or contiguous structure can occur. This can lead to fatal hemorrhage, pneumomediastinum, pneumothorax, or tracheoesophageal fistula. The laser itself can cause retinal damage, which could potentially affect the patient, operator, and other staff; therefore, it must always be in standby mode when it is not directed at its target. In addition, all members in the operating room should wear eye protection.

8. **What is cryotherapy?**
   Cryotherapy is using cold as a treatment. In the 1960s, Gage was the first to use cryotherapy to treat a patient with carcinoma obstructing a bronchus. Today, most endobronchial cryotherapy is performed using a flexible cryoprobe or rigid bronchoscopy. In the United States, it is usually performed with flexible bronchoscopy. The goal of cryotherapy is to destroy diseased tissue

while sparing normal tissue. This does not happen immediately. Cryotherapy effect is a consequence of various cellular mechanisms, including intracellular dehydration, mechanical damage from ice crystals, and vasoconstriction and the formation of microthrombi.

Knepler JL Jr, Mathur PN: Cryotherapy. In Beamis JE, Mathur PN, Mehta AC (eds): Interventional Pulmonary. Marcel Dekker, 2004, pp 157–165.

Mathur PN, Wolf KF, Busk MF, et al: Fiberoptic bronchoscopic cryotherapy in the management of tracheobronchial obstruction. Chest 110:718–723, 1996.

9. **Which tissues are cryosensitve, and which are cryoresistant?**
   Cryosensitve tissues include skin, mucus membranes, nerves, endothelium, and granulation tissue. Cryoresistant tissues include fat, cartilage, nerve sheaths, connective tissue, and fibrosis. There are also some data that suggest that lung cancer may be more cryosensitive than normal lung tissue.

10. **What are the advantages and disadvantages of cryotherapy?**
    Cryotherapy is relatively safe compared to other modalities for removing endobronchial lesions. Side effects are rare, but they can include cardiopulmonary arrest, massive hemoptysis, and tracheoesophageal fistula. Furthermore, beside being used to debulk and removed endobronchial masses, cryotherapy can be used to remove foreign bodies, blood clots, and mucus plugs; the probe will stick to these objects. The biggest disadvantage of cryotherapy is that it may take 2–4 weeks for the full effects to be obtained; therefore, it is not useful to treat lesions causing impending respiratory failure. Stenting, laser photo ablation, or electrocautery may be better in these circumstances.

11. **What are electrocautery and APC?**
    Electrocautery uses an electric current to produce heat and to destroy tissue. Electrocautery uses an alternating current at a high frequency (105–107 Hz) to generate heat that coagulates, vaporizes, or cuts tissue, depending on the power. The indications for electrocautery are similar to those for cryotherapy and Nd/YAG laser. Electrocautery is usually a palliative treatment in patients with malignancy, but it is not useful in removing foreign bodies.

    APC is similar to electrocautery, but no tissue–probe contact occurs; rather, ionized argon gas acts as a conductor between the probe and tissue. APC penetrates tissue only 5 mm; therefore, it may not be as effective at debulking endobronchial masses as laser or normal electrocautery.

    Sheski FD, Mathur PN: Endobronchial electrosurgery: Argon plasma coagulation and electrocautery. Semin Respir Crit Care Med 25:367–374, 2004.

12. **What are the complications of electrocautery?**
    Like Nd/YAG laser, electrocautery can cause endobronchial fire. There are reports of patient and operator burns, but there is little literature on this subject. There is also a chance of airway stenosis or tracheomalacia. Lastly, there is concern in using electrocautery in patients with a pacemaker or an automatic implantable cardiac defibrillator as these may malfunction when exposed to an electric current.

13. **Describe the clinical utility of endobronchial ultrasound.**
    Endobronchial ultrasound is useful in determining the depth of tumor invasion in tracheobronchial lesions, as well as in demonstrating the relationship of such tumors to hilar vascular structures. It is also useful for visualizing paratracheal and peribronchial nodes, which helps in transbronchial needle aspiration. In addition, it has some benefits in localizing peripheral lesions.

14. **What is brachytherapy?**
    Brachytherapy is the delivery of endobronchial radiation therapy. Initially, rigid bronchoscopy was used to place the source of radiation. Today, the flexible bronchoscope is used to place a

thin polyethylene catheter into the area of the tumor. The radiation source can then be delivered remotely to minimize exposure. The goal of brachytherapy is palliation of symptoms caused by airway obstruction of tumor tissue. It can also be used as an adjunct to external beam radiotherapy for treatment in unresectable lung cancer.

15. Who performed the first brachytherapy?
In 1922, Yankauer reported two cases in which he implanted radium into an endobronchial tumor using a bronchoscope. He had the radium in capsules attached to a string that exited through the patients' mouths.

16. What are the contraindications for brachytherapy?
Obviously, brachytherapy is only indicated in patients with malignant lesions. Patients with high-grade obstruction are at risk for complete obstruction secondary to postradiation edema; therefore, they should first undergo debulking by Nd/YAG laser, electrocautery, or cryotherapy. Also, patients with fistulas leading to nonpulmonary areas should not receive brachytherapy.

17. What is the difference between high-dose-rate (HDR) and low-dose-rate (LDR) brachytherapy?
LDR brachytherapy is defined as 2 Gy/hr at the point of reference, whereas a HDR is greater than 10 Gy/hr. Traditionally, LDR brachytherapy was used, but with the availability of iridium 192 and better shielding techniques, HDR brachytherapy has become the procedure of choice. The main advantage of HDR brachytherapy is the shorter therapy time. Most patients are treated once a week as opposed to every day.

Gustafson G, Vicini F, Freedman L, et al: High-dose rate endobronchial brachytherapy in the management of primary and recurrent bronchogenic malignancies. Cancer 75:2345–2350, 1995.

18. What is photodynamic therapy (PDT)?
Certain compounds (e.g., hematoporphyrin derivatives) act as photosensitizing agents. This allows selective damage from monochromatic light. The light is administered through the bronchoscope. Malignant cells uptake more agent and therefore are more susceptible to damage. Endobronchial masses and minimally invasive central airway lesions are most amenable to PDT.

19. What are the indications for a stent?
The major indication is extrinsic compression of a large airway, secondary to malignant neoplasm. Stents are also indicated for patients with malignant endobronchial lesions that have failed cryotherapy or laser resection and those currently undergoing external beam radiation. Stents are also indicated in benign conditions that result in large airway compression. These include benign tumors (e.g., amyloid) and various strictures including postintubation, postinflammatory, postinfectious, and anastomotic strictures, especially post-transplant. Tracheobronchomalacia due to radiation or relapsing polychondritis is also an indication.

Bolliger CT, Mathur PN: Expandable endobronchial stents. Beamis J, Mathur PN (eds): Interventional Pulmonology. New York, McGraw-Hill, 1999, pp 113–127.

20. Where does the word *stent* come from?
The British dentist Charles R. Stent developed a device to promote the healing of gingival grafts. It has now come to mean any device that maintains the lumen of a hollow structure. Anecdotal reports of stents in the airway date back to 1915; however, the first really useful airway stent was the Montgomery T-tube in the 1960s.

KEY POINTS: CHARACTERISTICS OF AN IDEAL STENT

1. Ease of insertion and removal

2. Availability in different sizes, to match the obstruction

3. Ability to maintain its position without migration

4. Resistance to compressive forces, yet sufficiently elastic to conform to the airway contours

5. Construction of inert material that will not irritate the airway, precipitate infection, or promote granulation tissue

6. Possession of the same characteristics of the normal airway so that mobilization of secretions is not impaired

Of note, these have never all been obtained in clinical practice.

21. **What are the different kinds of stents used in airways?**
    Tracheobronchial stents consist of silicon, metal, or a hybrid of the two. Table 17-2 summarizes the major differences. Metal stents, inherently inert, can be made from stainless steel, tantalum, or alloys incorporating cobalt, chromium, and molybdenum (e.g., Vitallium and nobelium). Some metal stents need to be placed with a dilating balloon, whereas others are self expanding. They should not be placed for benign conditions because they cannot be removed after several months in place. Hybrid stents are made of metal covered with silicon. They combine the advantages of metal stents and silicon stents. The silicon does not allow tumor to grow between the struts.

    Bolliger CT, Mathur PN: Expandable endobronchial stents. Beamis J, Mathur PN (eds): Interventional Pulmonology. New York, McGraw-Hill, 1999, pp 113–127.
    Saito Y: Endobronchial stents: Past, present, and future. Semin Respir Crit Care Med 25:375–380, 2004.

TABLE 17-2. THE DIFFERENCES BETWEEN METAL STENTS AND SILICON STENTS		
	Metal	**Silicon**
Bronchoscope	Flexible or rigid	Rigid
Price	Expensive	Relatively inexpensive
Removable	No	Yes
Problems with migration	Less (1%)	Yes (30%)
Granulation tissue or tumor growth	Between the struts	At the edges

CHAPTER 18

CHEST TUBES

Thomas Corbridge, MD, and David Ost, MD

1. **What are the indications for chest tube placement?**
   The main indications for chest tube placement are pneumothorax, hemothorax, symptomatic pleural effusion, empyema, complicated parapneumonic effusion, pleurodesis of a recurrent malignant effusion, and chylothorax. The decision to place a chest tube depends on the particulars of the case and a risk–benefit analysis.

   Miller KS, Sahn SA: Chest tubes: Indications, technique, management, and complications. Chest 91:258, 1987.

2. **What are the contraindications to chest tube placement?**
   There are no absolute contraindications to chest tube placement in a life-threatening situation. However, extreme caution is warranted in patients with coagulopathy, and correction of clotting abnormalities is recommended before insertion whenever possible. A bleeding diathesis is a relative contraindication to semi-elective tube placement (as in drainage and pleurodesis of a malignant effusion) that should be considered during the risk–benefit analysis. Cellulitis at the puncture site is a contraindication to an elective procedure. A complicated pleural space with multiple loculations is a relative contraindication to blind tube placement. Image-guided placement of one or more tubes is preferable in this situation.

3. **Is a chest tube always required for pneumothorax?**
   No. If the pneumothorax is less than 15% of lung volume on a chest radiograph and the patient is stable, watchful waiting may be appropriate, provided that there is close follow-up, serial radiographs can be performed, and a chest tube can be placed quickly if necessary. If the patient is hospitalized, supplemental oxygen can be administered to facilitate resorption of pleural air. If a pneumothorax is large or if the patient is unstable, is receiving mechanical ventilation, or is scheduled for general anesthesia, a chest tube should be placed. Similarly, if a patient cannot be followed closely or has severe underlying lung disease or life-threatening comorbidities, chest tube placement should be considered.

   Sahn SA, Heffner JE: Spontaneous pneumothorax. N Engl J Med 342:868, 2000.

KEY POINTS: CHEST TUBES AND EFFUSIONS

1. Chest tubes are indicated for complicated parapneumonic effusions characterized by pH < 7.20 and glucose < 60 mg/dL.

2. Empyemas require one or more chest tubes, depending on loculations, for adequate drainage; a 32- to 26-Fr tube is preferred for viscous fluids, but 10- to 14-Fr catheters may be required for image-guided drainage of loculations. Instillation of a fibrinolytic agent helps dislodge loculations.

3. Pleurodesis of a malignant pleural effusion should be considered when the lung is fully inflated, there is symptomatic improvement after large-volume drainage, and short-term prognosis is good.

4. **Under what circumstances should a patient with pleural effusion have a chest tube?**
Many pleural effusions can be managed with thoracentesis and treatment of the underlying problem. Chest tubes are required when effusions cause respiratory or hemodynamic compromise or when drainage of infected fluid is critical for recovery. Clinical conditions include hemothorax (particularly when there is penetrating chest trauma), complicated parapneumonic effusion, and empyema. A chest tube is also required for pleurodesis of symptomatic malignant or paramalignant effusions.

5. **How is a patient positioned and prepared for chest tube placement?**
Hemodynamically stable patients should be premedicated with narcotics and a sedative hypnotic. The patient is placed in the supine position with the involved side elevated, supported by pillows or towels, and the arm is flexed overhead. The entry site is sterilely prepared and draped. The skin and subcutaneous tissue are infiltrated with 1–2% lidocaine, followed by infiltration of the periosteum, subcutaneous tissue, and parietal pleura. As much as 30–40 mL of 1% lidocaine may be necessary for adequate anesthesia. Aspiration of pleural fluid or air confirms entry into the pleural space.

6. **Where should the incision be made for chest tube placement?**
Chest tubes are generally placed in the fourth or fifth intercostal space along the anterior axillary line, anterior to the superior iliac crest and the latissimus dorsi muscle. In cases of pneumothorax, the tube can be inserted in the second intercostal space at the midclavicular line, but penetration of breast tissue and muscle makes this approach more difficult, and care must be taken to avoid the internal mammary artery, which lies just medial to the proper insertion site.

7. **How is a chest tube inserted?**
An incision of 2–3 cm is made with a scalpel over the rib, extending into the subcutaneous tissues. Subcutaneous tissue over the superior aspect of the rib is bluntly dissected with a large clamp using an opening and spreading maneuver, taking care to avoid the neurovascular bundle of the adjacent rib. Considerable force may be required to pop through the parietal pleura into the pleural space. The index finger is used to explore the pleural space, to ensure proper position, and to identify adhesions. Thin adhesions can be disrupted manually, but care must be taken not to injure the patient or cause bleeding. A medium-sized clamp is used to direct the tube into proper position. For drainage of pleural fluid, the tube is placed inferiorly and posteriorly. For pneumothorax, the catheter is directed apically.

Symbas PN: Chest drainage tubes. Surg Clin North Am 69:41, 1989.

8. **What size chest tube should be used?**
The choice of size is determined by the indication for chest tube placement: for drainage of pleural fluid of low viscosity, a 28-Fr tube is adequate; for higher viscosity fluids such as those found in empyema, a 32- to 36-Fr tube is preferred. Chest tubes for patients who have sustained trauma with hemothorax or hemopneumothorax should be even larger (36–40 Fr). Smaller tubes, in the range of 12–22 Fr, are adequate for treatment of spontaneous pneumothorax. For image-guided drainage of a pleural loculation, a 10- to 14-Fr catheter may be used.

Klein JS, Schultz S, Heffner JE: Interventional radiology of the chest: Image-guided percutaneous drainage of pleural effusions, lung abscess, and pneumothorax. Am J Roentgenol 164:581–588, 1995.

9. **How is a chest tube secured?**
Many clinicians secure the site with 2-0 silk sutures using a mattress stitch and then cover the wound with Vaseline gauze and a pressure dressing. Connections from the chest tube to the suction device should be taped carefully to avoid disconnection and air leak. A chest radiograph should be obtained to confirm tube position and to ensure that all side holes are within the pleural space.

KEY POINTS: PLACEMENT AND COMPLICATIONS OF CHEST TUBES

1. Chest tubes are generally placed in the fourth or fifth intercostal space along the anterior axillary line.

2. Tubes are directed inferiorly and posteriorly for drainage of fluid and apically for treatment of pneumothorax.

3. With wall suction off, the water level in the collecting chamber should fluctuate with respiration, indicating the chest tube is patent and communicating with the pleural space.

4. Air bubbles in the water seal chamber indicate an air leak, either inside or outside the pleural space.

5. Complications from chest tube placement include infection, malposition, bleeding, nerve damage, perforation of adjacent structures, and reexpansion pulmonary edema.

10. Should a trocar be used for chest tube placement?
Although a trocar may allow for rapid tube placement by an experienced operator, most clinicians avoid them because of increased risk of organ perforation.

11. What types of drainage devices are available? How do they work?
The most commonly used drainage systems are commercially available compartmentalized versions of the three-bottle system. The three compartments are a collection chamber, a water seal chamber, and a suction control chamber. The collection chamber traps pleural fluid or blood. The water seal chamber acts as a one-way valve, insuring that air does not return to the pleural space. The suction control chamber uses the height of the fluid in the chamber to control the amount of applied negative pressure. If the suction control chamber has water that is 20 cm high, then −20 cm of water pressure is generated.

12. How are function and patency confirmed?
Collection of pleural fluid or condensation on the tube during respiration helps confirm proper placement. Tube function can be assessed by turning off wall suction and observing the level of water in the water seal chamber. The water level should fluctuate with respiration, indicating that the tube is patent and communicating with the pleural space. If it does not fluctuate, the tube is obstructed or is not in the pleural space. In these situations, the tube should be examined to make sure it is not twisted or kinked and a chest radiograph should be ordered to check tube position. Saline irrigation, tube milking, or stripping can dislodge obstructing debris. If the tube is nonfunctional and cannot be cleared, it should be removed to decrease the risk of infection.

13. What is an air leak?
Air bubbles in the water seal chamber indicate air leak. Air can come from within the pleural space (e.g., pneumothorax or bronchopleural fistula) or from outside the pleural space (i.e., a loose connection in the tubing). The site of air leak can be determined by clamping the chest tube where it enters the thorax and observing the water seal chamber. If the leak continues, then the leak is outside the body and the tubing and connections should be checked. If the leak stops, the air is coming from the pleural space, assuming the side holes are in the pleural space and not in the chest wall, where they can suck air from outside the body.

14. **How and when should a chest tube be removed?**

If placed for pleural fluid, a chest tube can be removed once drainage is minimal (i.e., less than 150 mL/day). If placed for pneumothorax, it can be removed when the lung is fully reexpanded and there is no air leak for 24 hours. In mechanically ventilated patients, many clinicians leave the tube in until extubation. Before removing the tube, suction is discontinued and the tube is placed to water seal for up to 24 hours. The tube may then be clamped for several hours to further ensure stability. In the lateral decubitus position with the chest tube-side up, sutures are removed and the patient is instructed to take a deep breath. During a Valsalva maneuver, the tube is pulled out rapidly in one smooth motion. The wound is sutured and an occlusive dressing is reapplied. A chest radiograph should follow.

15. **List complications associated with chest tubes.**

Complications include infection; malposition; bleeding; nerve damage; perforation of the diaphragm, lung parenchyma, mediastinum, heart, or abdominal organs; pain; and reexpansion pulmonary edema.

Mahfood S, Hix WR, Aaron BL, et al: Reexpansion pulmonary edema. Ann Thorac Surg 45:340, 1988.

16. **When should a chest tube be placed for management of a malignant pleural effusion?**

Initial management of a malignant or paramalignant pleural effusion consists of thoracentesis and treatment of the underlying malignancy, often with chemotherapy. If fluid reaccumulates and the patient is symptomatic, other options include periodic palliative thoracentesis in patients with a short predicted survival. When the prognosis is not so grim, chest tube drainage and intrapleural instillation of a sclerosing agent may be considered. Various agents can be used to fuse the visceral and parietal pleurae, thereby obliterating the pleural space (called pleurodesis). Before pleurodesis is performed, the lung must be fully inflated and, because this is a palliative procedure, the patient should report symptomatic improvement after pleural fluid drainage.

Lynch TJ: Management of malignant pleural effusions. Chest 103:385S–389S, 1993.

17. **What is the recommended sclerosing agent for pleurodesis?**

A number of agents have been used for pleurodesis of malignant, paramalignant, and, less often, nonmalignant pleural effusions. The currently preferred agent is talc. Talc is available as a sterilized product free of asbestos. The recommended dose is 5 grams suspended in 50–100 mL of saline, instilled into the pleural space as a slurry through a chest tube. Alternatively, talc poudrage is performed through a thoracoscope or at the time of thoracotomy. Response rates as high as 90% have been reported in the treatment of malignant effusions. Side effects include pain, fever, dyspnea, empyema, arrhythmias, myocardial ischemia, and acute respiratory distress syndrome (ARDS).

Kennedy L, Sahn SA: Talc pleurodesis for the treatment of pneumothorax and pleural effusion. Chest 106:1215, 1994.

West SD, Davies RJ, Lee YC: Pleurodesis for malignant pleural effusions: current controversies and variations in practices. Curr Opin Pulm Med 10:305, 2004.

18. **Which parapneumonic effusions require chest tube drainage?**

Uncomplicated parapneumonic effusions generally resolve without chest tube drainage unless they occupy more than half of the hemithorax. Complicated parapneumonic effusions occur when bacteria invade the pleural space and there is fibrin deposition and anaerobic metabolism. A chest tube is indicated when these effusions result in a pleural pH < 7.20 and pleural glucose < 60 mg/dL. When pleural pH is between 7.20 and 7.30, repeat thoracentesis; chest tube placement may be required, depending on clinical course. Empyema is established by aspirating pus or by identifying bacteria on gram stain. Thickening of the parietal pleura on a contrast-enhanced chest computed tomograph (CT) also suggests empyema. Empyema is an indication for one or more chest tubes, depending on the presence of loculations.

Colice GL, Curtis A, Deslauriers J, et al: Medical and surgical treatment of parapneumonic effusions: An evidence-based guideline. Chest 118:1158, 2000.

Sahn SA: The sun should never set on a parapneumonic effusion. Chest 95:945, 1989.

Waite RJ, Carbonneau RJ, Balikian JP, et al: Parietal pleural changes in empyema: Appearances at CT. Radiology 175:145, 1990.

19. **When should a fibrinolytic agent be instilled through a chest tube?**

Inadequately drained loculated pleural fluid increases mortality and the need for late surgical decortication. Formation of a thick, fibrinous pleural peel may further limit lung expansion, causing a permanent restrictive defect. To curtail these complications, many experts recommend early instillation of a fibrinolytic agent through a chest tube, although the efficacy of this approach has not been established by large randomized trials. The most commonly used agents are streptokinase and urokinase. These agents break down the fibrin bands responsible for loculations and have reported success rates between 67% and 92%. Side effects include fever, pain, and the development of immunoglobulin G antistreptokinase antibodies when streptokinase is used.

Cameron R, Davies HR: Intra-pleural fibrinolytic therapy versus conservative management in the treatment of parapneumonic effusions and empyema. Cochrane Database Syst Rev CD002312, 2004

Sahn SA: Use of fibrinolytic agents in the management of complicated parapneumonic effusions and empyemas. Thorax 53(Suppl 2):S65, 1998.

CHAPTER 19

FLOW-DIRECTED PULMONARY ARTERY CATHETERS

John E. Heffner, MD

1. **What measurements does a pulmonary artery catheter provide in the intensive care unit (ICU)?**

   Flow-directed pulmonary artery (PA) catheters (or Swan–Ganz catheters) are placed in the central venous circulation to provide measurements of right ventricular (RV) and PA pressures. Inflation of a distal balloon allows blood flow to direct the catheter into an occlusion or wedge position for measurement of a pulmonary artery occlusion pressure (P_{PAO}) (or wedge pressure). The P_{PAO} is an indirect assessment of left atrial (LA) pressure. The PA catheter also allows sampling of mixed venous blood. Connected to a computer processor, the PA catheter facilitates the measurement and calculation of a variety of hemodynamic variables that include PA and systemic vascular resistance, cardiac output (CO), and cardiac stroke volume (SV). The last is the only volume assessed by the catheter, which is calculated by dividing the heart rate into the measured cardiac output.

   > Bridges EJ, Woods SL: Pulmonary artery pressure measurement: State of the art. Heart Lung 22:99, 1993.
   > Pinsky MR: Pulmonary artery occlusion pressure. Intens Care Med 29:19, 2003.

2. **What are the important design characteristics of a PA catheter?**

   Pulmonary artery catheters are 100 cm long with an inflatable balloon 1–2 mm from the distal end. Hash marks placed at 10-cm intervals from the tip assist the measurement of the depth of insertion. The most commonly used catheters are 7–8 Fr in diameter, with four ports. One port is at the catheter tip, a second port allows balloon inflation, a third proximal port exits 30 cm from the catheter tip, and a fourth port provides electronic access to a thermistor, which is located 4 cm proximal to the catheter tip and allows measurement of pulmonary artery flow for calculation of cardiac output. Some catheters have sensors that allow continuous monitoring of mixed venous oxygen saturation (Fig. 19-1).

3. **How is a PA catheter inserted?**

   The PA catheter is placed percutaneously using a modified Seldinger technique. The left internal jugular and left subclavian veins represent the least difficult insertion sites for passage of the catheter because they best accommodate the curvature of the catheter for its placement through the heart in a counterclockwise orientation. The right subclavian and right internal jugular veins and the femoral or antecubital veins provide acceptable insertion sites, however. Because catheter infections are one of the most common and important complications of PA catheter insertion, full barrier precautions with mask, gowns, gloves, and meticulous handwashing are mandatory.

   The operator cannulates the vessel with a needle and guidewire, allowing introduction of an introducer through which the PA catheter is passed to 15 cm under hemodynamic waveform monitoring. After inflation of the distal balloon with 1.5 cm of air, manual advancement of the catheter allows blood flow to "float" the balloon through the right cardiac chambers into the PA. The balloon should never be advanced without balloon inflation. The course of the catheter tip is monitored by noting the characteristic pressure waveforms during passage from the right atrium (RA) through the RV and into the PA. With a subclavian or internal jugular vein insertion site, the RA waveform usually appears after insertion of the catheter after 20 cm,

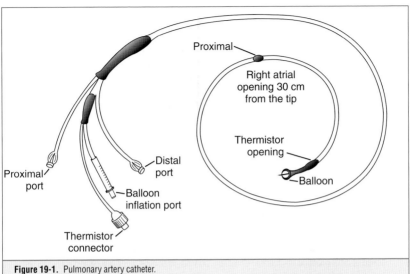

Figure 19-1. Pulmonary artery catheter.

the RV waveform after 30 cm, the PA waveform after 40 cm, and the P_{PAO} waveform after 50 cm, as measured with the catheter hash marks. After the detection of a P_{PAO} waveform, the balloon is deflated, which should result in return of a PA waveform to signify appropriate catheter positioning. Persistence of a P_{PAO} waveform with balloon deflation denotes a need to withdraw the catheter slightly to remove the tip from a wedged position (Fig. 19-2).

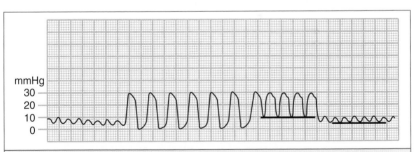

Figure 19-2. Typical waveforms obtained during passage of a PA catheter. Pulmonary artery wedge pressure (PAWP) should always be lower than mean pulmonary artery pressure (PAP). If it is higher than mean PAP, suspect an analytical error or that the catheter tip is not in zone 3 of the lung.

4. **What cardiac conditions complicate the placement of a PA catheter?**
   Severe tricuspid insufficiency causes a regurgitant flow from the RV to the RA, which can inter-fere with floating of the catheter into the RV. The presence of mitral regurgitation may compli-cate PA catheter placement because a large v wave detected with the catheter in the wedge position may simulate a PA nonwedged waveform. Simultaneous measurement of an electrocardiogram with the PA catheter waveform assists the discrimination between a v wave

(which occurs after the electrocardiogram [ECG] T wave) and a peak systolic PA pressure wave form (which occurs before the ECG T wave).

5. **How can correct catheter tip placement be confirmed?**
Before suturing a catheter to the skin adjacent to the insertion site, correct catheter placement must be confirmed after initial placement. If a P_{PAO} waveform is noted with inflation of the balloon with less than 1.5 cm of air, the catheter tip is too distal and should be withdrawn slightly. Inflation of the balloon in an overly distal position can cause vascular rupture. Inflation of the balloon with 1.5 cm should result in a P_{PAO} immediately. A 2- or 3-second delay indicates that the catheter tip is too proximal and that the catheter should be advanced.

6. **What are the indications for a PA catheter?**
Clinicians place PA catheters for diagnostic and therapeutic indications. Use of PA catheters has evolved since their initial introduction to the ICU in the 1970s, when they were first placed in unstable patients with acute myocardial infarctions and later were applied to patients with various forms of shock and respiratory failure. Despite extensive experience with these catheters, no data exist to definitively prove that they improve clinical outcome. Recommendations for their use rely largely on expert consensus, which has been marked by considerable controversy. A more judicious use of PA catheters has emerged, guided by published clinical practice guidelines. Clinicians should place a catheter only when a specific question exists that can be answered by placement of a catheter and when a specific course of action will be prompted by information the PA catheter can provide. Also, most unstable patients considered for PA catheter placement should first be observed for a response to initial therapy. Monitoring of central venous pressure can guide many therapeutic interventions previously managed with PA catheter placement.

American Society of Anesthesiologists Task Force on Pulmonary Artery Catheterization: Practice guidelines for pulmonary artery catheterization: A report by the American Society of Anesthesiologists Task Force on Pulmonary Artery Catheterization. Anesthesiology 78:380–394, 1993.

Bernard GR, Sopko G, Cerru F, et al: National Heart, Lung, and Blood Institute and Food and Drug Administration Workshop Report: Pulmonary Artery Catheterization and Clinical Outcomes (PACCO). JAMA 283:2568–2572, 2000.

Connors AF Jr, Speroff T, Dawson NV, et al: The effectiveness of right heart catheterization in the initial care of critically ill patients (SUPPORT Investigators). JAMA 276:889–897, 1996.

Dalen JE, Bone RC: Is it time to pull the pulmonary artery catheter? JAMA 276:916–968, 1996.

Eagle KA, Brundage BH, Chaitman BR, et al: Guidelines for perioperative cardiovascular evaluation for noncardiac surgery: Report of the American College of Cardiology/American Heart Association Task Force on Practice Guidelines (Committee on Perioperative Cardiovascular Evaluation for Noncardiac Surgery). J Am Coll Cardiol 27:910–948, 1996.

Mueller HS, Chatterjee K, Davis KB, et al: Present use of bedside right heart catheterization in patients with cardiac disease. J Am Coll Cardiol 32:840–864, 1998. Available at http://www.acc.org/clinical/consensus/catheter.htm/.

Pulmonary Artery Catheter Consensus Conference Participants: Pulmonary Artery Catheter Consensus Conference: Consensus statement. Crit Care Med 25:910–925, 1997.

Richard C, Warszawski J, Anguel N, et al: Early use of the pulmonary artery catheter and outcomes in patients with shock and acute respiratory distress syndrome: A randomized controlled trial. JAMA 290:2713, 2003.

Sandham JD, Hull RD, Brant RF, et al. A randomized, controlled trial of the use of pulmonary-artery catheters in high-risk surgical patients. N Engl J Med 348:5–14, 2003.

Yu DT, Platt R, Lanken PN, et al: Relationship of pulmonary artery catheter use to mortality and resource utilization in patients with severe sepsis. Crit Care Med 31:2734–2741, 2003.

KEY POINTS: INDICATIONS FOR PLACEMENT OF A PULMONARY ARTERY CATHETER

1. Diagnosis
   - Discriminating among different causes of hypotension
   - Discriminating between cardiogenic and noncardiogenic causes of pulmonary edema
   - Diagnosis of pericardial constriction and tamponade
   - Evaluation of severity and etiology of pulmonary hypertension
   - Detection of left-to-right intracardiac shunts

2. Management
   - Management of unstable cardiac patients or patients after cardiac surgery
   - Management of hypotensive patients receiving vasopressor, vasodilator, or inotropic therapy
   - Evaluation of severity and etiology of pulmonary hypertension
   - Monitoring of patients who require careful volume management (e.g., those with hemorrhage, burns, renal failure, sepsis, severe heart failure or cardiomyopathy, or cirrhosis with severe ascites)
   - Assistance with ventilator management to manage positive end-expiratory pressure

7. **Why is it important to note RA pressure waveforms with a PA catheter?**
RA pressures measured by a PA catheter in the setting of a normal tricuspid valve reflect RA venous return and RV end-diastolic pressure. An elevated RA pressure (normal = 0–7 mmHg) suggests the presence of volume overload, tricuspid regurgitation, pulmonary hypertension, right ventricular infarction, a left-to-right shunt, pericardial constriction or tamponade, or right ventricular infarction or cardiomyopathy.

8. **What do measurements of RV pressures tell the clinician?**
A PA catheter measures RV systolic pressure (normal = 15–25 mmHg) and RV end-diastolic pressure (normal = 3–12 mmHg). An elevated RV pressure indicates the presence of pulmonary hypertension (due to pulmonary vascular disease, such as as primary pulmonary hypertension or pulmonary embolism, or else due to left heart disease) or pulmonary valvular stenosis. An elevated RV end-diastolic pressure suggests the presence of right ventricular infarction, RV ischemia, cardiomyopathy, or cardiac constriction or tamponade.

9. **What is the significance of measured changes in PA pressures?**
A PA catheter can measure the PA systolic (normal = 15–25 mmHg) and diastolic (normal = 8–15 mmHg) pressures and assist in the calculation of mean PA pressure. Elevations of PA pressure occur in a wide variety of conditions.

10. **What is the clinical significance of measuring a P_{PAO}?**
Inflation of the distal catheter balloon causes the catheter to occlude a branch of the PA and stop blood flow through that branch (a "no flow" state). This results in a static column of blood with equalization of pressure from the catheter tip to the anatomic junction of the pulmonary vein downstream from the catheter and the other pulmonary veins with preserved blood flow. The pressure measured through the distal catheter port represents the pressure at the J point, which approximates in most settings the left ventricular (LV) end-diastolic pressure. Estimation of the LV end-diastolic pressure assesses myocardial performance and allows a further estimation of LV end-diastolic volumes and needs for diuresis (if volumes are high) or volume replacement (if volumes are low). If impedance to blood flow exists between the J point and the

KEY POINTS: CAUSES OF AN ELEVATED PULMONARY ARTERY PRESSURE

1. Volume overload

2. Left heart failure and left valvular disease

3. Pulmonary embolism

4. Hypoxia with pulmonary vasoconstriction

5. Pulmonary parenchymal disease (e.g., emphysema or interstitial lung disease)

6. Primary pulmonary vascular diseases (e.g., primary pulmonary hypertension or veno-occlusive disease)

7. Left-to-right intracardiac shunts

left ventricle, as occurs in mitral stenosis, the P_{PAO} will overestimate the LV end-diastolic pressure. Other causes of P_{PAO} overestimating LV end-diastolic pressure include mitral regurgitation, pulmonary embolism, and left atrial myxoma. P_{PAO} will underestimate LV end-diastolic pressure in the setting of aortic valvular insufficiency; decreased LV compliance, as occurs with an acute myocardial infarction and pericardial tamponade; and extreme increases in LV end-diastolic pressure (i.e., >25 mmHg).

Pinsky MR: Clinical significance of pulmonary artery occlusion pressure. Intens Care Med 29:175, 2003.

11. **What is the relationship between measured P_{PAO} and the actual pressure within the pulmonary capillaries?**
As evidenced by the fact that blood flows from the pulmonary capillaries through the J point toward the LA, a pressure gradient exists from the pulmonary capillaries and all downstream vascular points. Measurement of P_{PAO} with PA catheter inflation, however, occurs during a "no flow" state, at which time the pulmonary capillary pressure (P_{PC}) equals the J point pressure. It is important to recall, therefore, that the P_{PAO} does not reflect the actual pulmonary capillary pressure. Estimation of the pulmonary capillary pressures is often important in clinical practice because the capillary bed is a major site of fluid exchange in the lung and elevated pulmonary capillary pressures can induce or perpetuate pulmonary edema. Pulmonary capillary pressure can be estimated with the following equation, wherein P_{PA} is the mean PA pressure:

$$P_{PC} = P_{PAO} + 0.4 \times (\text{mean } P_{PA} - P_{PAO})$$

Weed HG: Pulmonary "capillary" wedge pressure not the pressure in the pulmonary capillaries. Chest 100:1138, 1991.

12. **How does a PA catheter measure CO?**
The thermistor attached to some PA catheters measures pericatheter fluid temperature and provides continuous monitoring of PA blood temperature, also termed core temperature. To calculate CO, a bolus of fluid cooler than blood temperature is injected through the proximal port. This cool injectate causes a transient reduction in blood temperature measured at the thermistor. The duration of the temperature drop makes possible determination of a temperature–time curve. If blood flow past the catheter is brisk (indicating high CO), the temperature rapidly returns to baseline. If blood flow is sluggish (indicating low CO), blood temperature returns more gradually. CO can be calculated by integration of the area under the temperature–time curve, factoring

in the injectate temperature and catheter calibration constants. Thermodilution CO is based on a theoretical model that assumes constant unidirectional blood flow. In patients with pulmonary or tricuspid valve regurgitation, the thermal tracer may recross the thermistor, resulting in an underestimation of true CO.

13. **What else is measured by a PA catheter?**
A PA catheter can collect blood from the central circulation, which allows measurement of mixed venous blood oxygen (MVO_2). This value allows calculation of arterial oxygen content (CAO_2). Other variables assessed by a PA catheter include cardiac index (CI), stroke volume, stroke volume index (SVI), systemic vascular resistance (SVR), systemic vascular resistance index (SVRI), pulmonary vascular resistance (PVR), pulmonary vascular resistance index (PVRI), left ventricular stroke work index (LVSWI), right ventricular stroke work index (RVSWI), oxygen delivery (D_{O2}), oxygen extraction ratio (O_2ER), and pulmonary shunt (Q_S/Q_T).

14. **Do pressures within the airways and alveoli affect measured values for P_{PAO}?**
Respiration causes biphasic fluctuations in alveolar and airway pressures that transmit to intrathoracic vasculature and cause an artifactual swing in the pressures measured by a PA catheter. During spontaneous breathing, a phasic inspiratory decrease in intrathoracic pressure causes associated dips in central venous pressure, P_{PA}, and P_{PAO}. During positive pressure breathing in patients undergoing mechanical ventilation, inspiration is associated with phasic increases in intrathoracic pressure and PA catheter pressure. PA catheter pressures should be measured at end-expiration to avoid this artifact.

15. **Does positive end-expiratory pressure (PEEP) affect the accuracy of PA catheter pressure measurements?**
PA catheters correctly placed in the most dependent regions of the lung (West zone 3) should not be affected by changes in airway pressures. If the respiratory fluctuation of a P_{PAO} is noted to be greater than that of a measured PA pressure, the catheter tip may not be in zone 3. In that circumstance, a portion of applied or instrinsic PEEP may transmit to the catheter and artifactually raise the measured P_{PAO}. The actual P_{PAO} can be estimated by subtracting one-half of the value of PEEP (in mmHg) from the measured P_{PAO} for patients with normal lung compliance and one-quarter of the PEEP value in patients with low lung compliance. (Dividing the measured PEEP in cmH_2O units by 1.36 converts PEEP values to units of mmHg.) In most circumstances, the actual artifactual increase in P_{PAO} is small.

Teboul JL, Besbes, M, Andrivet P, et al: A bedside index assessing the reliability of pulmonary artery occlusion pressure measurements during mechanical ventilation with positive end-expiratory pressure. J Crit Care 7:22, 1992.

16. **What are the catheter-related complications of PA catheter use?**
PA catheters require meticulous care to limit complications. They should always be removed when information from the catheter is no longer critical for patient care.

Ivanov R, Allen J, Calvin JE: The incidence of major morbidity in critically ill patients managed with pulmonary artery catheters: A meta-analysis. Crit Care Med 28:615, 2000.

17. **How can balloon malfunction be detected?**
Resistance to balloon inflation should prompt an evaluation to exclude catheter kinking, a closed valve to the balloon port, and catheter malposition in an overly distal position. When resistance to inflation is noted, attempts to inflate the balloon should be stopped so as to avoid rupturing a branch of the pulmonary artery. Signs of balloon rupture include loss of resistance to balloon inflation, lack of gas return into the syringe, and loss of ability to obtain a P_{PAO} tracing.

KEY POINTS: CATHETER-RELATED COMPLICATIONS OF PULMONARY ARTERY CATHETER USE

1. External bleeding from the insertion-site hemorrhage

2. Hemothorax

3. Pneumothorax

4. Infection

5. Venous thrombosis

6. Air embolism during insertion or from balloon rupture

7. Cardiac perforation

8. Catheter knotting

9. Atrial and ventricular arrhythmias or right bundle-branch block

10. Pulmonary infarction

11. Pulmonary artery rupture and pseudoaneurysm formation

12. Endocarditis

13. Injury to cardiac valves, papillary muscles, or chordae tendineae

CHAPTER 20

MEDIASTINOSCOPY

Francis C. Nichols, MD, and James R. Jett, MD

1. What are mediastinoscopy, anterior mediastinotomy, and video-assisted thoracic surgery (VATS)?

Cervical mediastinoscopy, first introduced by Carlens in 1959, is the endoscopic exploration of the superior and middle mediastinum utilizing a lighted rigid instrument, the mediastinoscope. It enables the surgeon to directly visualize and biopsy lymph nodes or other abnormal tissues in the mediastinal compartments within the instrument's reach.

Anterior mediastinotomy, described by McNeill and Chamberlain in 1966, allows the surgeon, through a small chest incision, to directly explore the anterior mediastinum and the aortopulmonary regions, which are not accessible by standard mediastinoscopy.

VATS is a surgical procedure performed in one hemithorax at a time utilizing the latest in both video and minimally invasive technology. VATS allows for visualization and biopsy of every nodal station, but only within the particular hemithorax being explored.

Carlens E: Mediastinoscopy: A method for inspection and tissue biopsy in the superior mediastinum. Dis Chest 36:343–352, 1959.

McNeill TM, Chamberlain JM: Diagnostic anterior mediastinotomy. Ann Thor Surg 2:532–539, 1966.

2. How is mediastinoscopy performed?

Mediastinoscopy is most commonly performed under general anesthesia. This permits maximal patient comfort, ease of surgery, and optimal management of potential complications. Knowledge of mediastinal anatomy is mandatory.

The patient is positioned supine on the operating table with the neck extended. A 2-cm transverse incision, 1 cm above the suprasternal notch, is performed. The neck strap muscles are divided in the midline, and the pretracheal fascia is incised. A plane anterior and lateral to the trachea is created with blunt finger dissection. Enlarged lymph nodes may be palpable. Using the anterior trachea's cartilaginous rings as a guide, the mediastinoscope is advanced into the superior and middle mediastinum. These mediastinal compartments are examined, and biopsies are obtained (Fig. 20-1).

3. How is anterior mediastinotomy (the Chamberlain procedure) performed?

Anterior mediastinotomy also requires general anesthesia. A 4-cm transverse incision in the second intercostal space is performed. Resection of the costal cartilage and ligation of the internal mammary artery are rarely required. The mediastinum is most easily approached by entering the pleural space and then entering the adjacent mediastinum in order to obtain appropriate biopsies. At the end of the procedure, a small catheter is used to evacuate air from the pleural space. This catheter is removed prior to the patient awakening from anesthesia. This procedure is most commonly done on the left, allowing access to the anterior mediastinal and aortopulmonary lymph nodes.

4. How is VATS performed?

VATS requires general anesthesia and a special double-lumen endotracheal tube that separately isolates the ventilation of each lung. Bronchoscopy is required to properly position this tube.

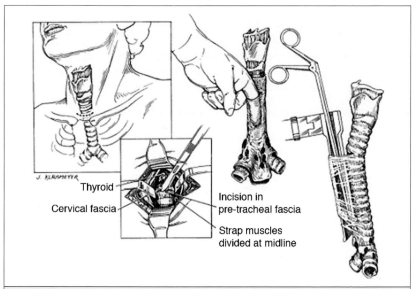

Figure 20-1. Technique of mediastinoscopy. (From Bocage JP, Mackenzie JW, Nosher JL: Invasive diagnostic procedures. In Shields TW [ed]: General Thoracic Surgery, 5th ed. Philadelphia, Lippincott Williams & Wilkins, 2000, pp 273–284, with permission.)

The video equipment consists of one or two monitors, a 5- or 10-mm diagnostic scope, and a special video camera head.

VATS is performed in a standard lateral thoracotomy position; it requires two to four 1- to 2-cm transverse incisions and special instrumentation for exposure and biopsies of the lymph node stations. Only biopsies of the ipsilateral nodal groups are possible (Fig. 20-2).

KEY POINTS: COMMON TESTS USED IN THE PATHOLOGIC STAGING OF LUNG CANCER

1. Noninvasive
   - Computed tomography (CT) scanning
   - Positron emission tomography (PET) scanning

2. Invasive
   - Bronchoscopy
   - Transbronchial needle aspiration and biopsy
   - CT-guided needle biopsy
   - Esophageal endoscopic ultrasound (EUS)
   - Mediastinoscopy
   - Anterior mediastinotomy (the Chamberlain procedure)
   - VATS

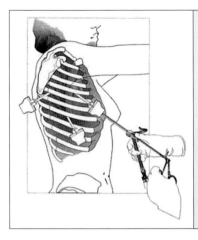

Figure 20-2. Right VATS lymph node staging. (From Gamliel Z, Krasna MJ: The role of video-assisted thoracic surgery in esophageal disease. In McKenna RJ [ed]: Video-Assisted Thoracic Surgery Update. Chest Surg Clin North Am 8:853–870, 1998, with permission.)

5. **Which lymph node groups are accessible to mediastinoscopy, anterior mediastinotomy, and VATS?**

   The anatomic locations of regional lymph nodes for lung cancer staging are shown in Figure 20-3 and are defined in Table 20-1.

   The following lymph node groups can be sampled during mediastinoscopy: the right and left upper and lower paratracheal lymph nodes (stations 2R, 2L, 4R, and 4L) and the subcarinal lymph nodes (station 7).

   Left anterior mediastinotomy provides access to the aortopulmonary window and the para-aortic lymph nodes (stations 5 and 6, respectively).

   VATS provides access to all lymph node stations within the particular hemithorax being explored, including the paraesophageal lymph nodes (station 8) and the inferior pulmonary ligament lymph nodes (station 9).

   Only mediastinoscopy allows for simultaneous biopsies of the right and left mediastinal lymph nodes through one small incision.

6. **What are the indications for mediastinoscopy?**

   Mediastinoscopy is most commonly used for the diagnosis and presurgical staging of lung cancer. It also may be valuable for diagnosing other mediastinal diseases such as sarcoidosis, lymphoma, various granulomatous disorders, and some mediastinal tumors. The need for mediastinoscopy in patients with lung cancer arises from the absence of reliable noninvasive methods for differentiating benign from malignant lymph nodes and also from the uniformly poor results of primary surgical resection in patients with lung cancer metastatic to the mediastinal lymph nodes.

7. **What is extended cervical mediastinoscopy?**

   Also called modified mediastinoscopy, this technique was described by Ginsberg in 1987. It involves the creation of a space between the left carotid artery and the innominate artery through a standard cervical mediastinoscopy incision. It can be used to access the aortopulmonary window and para-aortic lymph nodes. Experience with this approach is limited, and it has not been extensively studied or as routinely accepted as standard cervical mediastinoscopy (Fig. 20-4).

   Ginsberg RJ, Rice TW, Goldberg M, et al: Extended cervical mediastinoscopy. A single staging procedure for bronchogenic carcinoma of the left upper lobe. J Thorac Cardiovasc Surg 94:673–678, 1987.

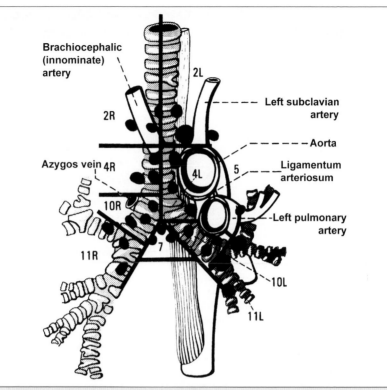

Figure 20-3. Regional lymph node stations for lung cancer staging. (From Mountain CF, Dresler CM: Regional lymph node classification for lung cancer staging. Chest 111: 1718–1723, 1997, with permission.)

TABLE 20-1. DEFINITIONS OF REGIONAL LYMPH NODE STATIONS FOR STAGING

Nodal Station	Anatomic Landmarks
N2 nodes: All N2 nodes lie within mediastinal pleural envelope.	
1. Highest mediastinal nodes	Above horizontal line at upper rim of brachiocephalic vein, where it ascends to left, crossing in front of trachea in its midline
2. Upper paratracheal nodes	Above horizontal line drawn tangential to upper margin of aortic arch and below inferior boundary of highest mediastinal nodes
3. Prevascular and retrotracheal nodes	May be designated 3A and 3P; midline nodes are considered to be ipsilateral
4. Lower paratracheal nodes* On the right	To right of midline of trachea between horizontal line drawn tangential to upper margin of aortic arch and line extending across right main bronchus

Continued

TABLE 20-1.   DEFINITIONS OF REGIONAL LYMPH NODE STATIONS FOR STAGING—CONT'D

Nodal Station	Anatomic Landmarks
On the left	To left of midline of trachea between horizontal line drawn tangential to upper margin of aortic arch and line extending across left main bronchus at level of upper margin of upper lobe bronchus, medial to ligamentum arteriosum
5. Subaortic (aortopulmonary window)	Lateral to ligamentum arteriosum or aorta or left pulmonary artery and proximal to first branch of left pulmonary artery
6. Para-aortic nodes	Anterior and lateral to ascending aorta and aortic arch or innominate artery, beneath line tangential to upper margin of aortic arch
7. Subcarinal nodes	Caudal to carina of trachea but not associated with lower lobe bronchi or arteries within lung
8. Paraesophageal nodes (below carina)	Adjacent to wall of esophagus and to right or left of midline, excluding subcarinal nodes
9. Pulmonary ligament nodes	Within pulmonary ligament, including those in posterior wall and lower part of inferior pulmonary vein
N1 nodes: All N1 nodes lie distal to mediastinal pleural reflection and within visceral pleura.	
10. Hilar nodes	Proximal lobar nodes, distal to mediastinal reflection and nodes adjacent to bronchus intermedius on right; on radiographs, hilar shadow may be created by enlargement of both hilar and interlobar nodes
11. Interlobar nodes	Between lobar bronchi
12. Lobar nodes	Adjacent to distal lobar bronchi
13. Segmental nodes	Adjacent to segmental bronchi
14. Subsegmental nodes	Around subsegmental bronchi

*For research purposes, lower paratracheal nodes may be designated as no. 4s (superior) and no. 4i (inferior) subsets. No. 4s nodes are defined by horizontal line extending across trachea and drawn tangential to cephalic border of azygos vein. No. 4i nodes are defined by lower boundary of no. 4s nodes, as described above.

Adapted from Mountain CF, Dresler CM: Regional node classification for lung cancer staging. Chest 111:1718–1723, 1997.

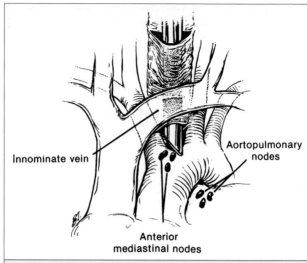

Figure 20-4. Extended mediastinoscopy. (From Bocage JP, Mackenzie JW, Nosher JL: Invasive diagnostic procedures. In Shields TW [ed]: General Thoracic Surgery, 5th ed. Philadelphia, Lippincott Williams & Wilkins, 2000, pp 273–284, with permission.)

8. **How does endoscopic ultrasound (EUS) help in the evaluation of the mediastinum?**
   The role of EUS in the diagnosis of both bronchial and mediastinal pathology is still under study. However, EUS can be used to evaluate lesions in proximity to the gastrointestinal tract. This includes adjacent lymph nodes. Lymph nodes that can be evaluated and biopsied with EUS include the left paratracheal lymph nodes, subcarinal lymph nodes, paraesophageal lymph nodes, and inferior pulmonary ligament lymph nodes (stations 7, 8, and 9, respectively).

   Wallace and colleagues reported on 121 patients who underwent esophageal EUS and fine-needle aspiration (FNA) for lung cancer staging. Advanced mediastinal disease was found in 77% of patients with enlarged mediastinal lymph nodes on computed tomography (CT). Further invasive staging was unnecessary.

   Wallace MB, Sivestri GA, Sahai AV, et al: Endoscopic ultrasound-guided fine needle aspiration for staging patients with carcinoma of the lung. Ann Thorac Surg 72:1861–1867, 2001.

9. **Which lymph nodes cannot be assessed with esophageal EUS?**
   EUS and FNA are unable to evaluate the right upper and lower paratracheal lymph nodes (stations 2R and 4R), aortopulmonary window and para-aortic lymph nodes (stations 5 and 6), and those in the pretracheal space. This limitation means that EUS should be considered complementary to other invasive staging techniques.

10. **Are there any contraindications to mediastinoscopy?**
    Conditions that preclude safe mediastinoscopy include permanent tracheostomy, huge thyroid goiter, and extensive calcification or aneurysm of the innominate artery or aortic arch.

11. **Besides these contraindications, what other factors may increase the difficulty of mediastinoscopy?**
    Other factors increasing the difficulty of mediastinoscopy include mediastinal irradiation, right-sided carotid bruit, prior mediastinoscopy, and superior vena caval obstruction.

Mediastinoscopy can be safely performed in the presence of superior vena caval obstruction. Repeat mediastinoscopy has also been safely performed and is usually done to determine the results of induction therapy for lung cancer.

Jahangiri M, Goldstraw P: The role of mediastinoscopy in superior vena caval obstruction. Ann Thorac Surg 59:453–455, 1995.

Mateu-Navarro M, Rami-Porta R, Bastus-Piulats R, et al: Remediastinoscopy after induction chemotherapy in non-small cell lung cancer. Ann Thorac Surg 70:391–395, 2000.

12. **What are the complications of mediastinoscopy and anterior mediastinotomy?**
The morbidity and mortality of both of these procedures has been well documented over the years. In several large series, the morbidity was between 1% and 2%. The most common complications include bleeding, pneumothorax (usually right-sided), and recurrent laryngeal nerve injury (usually left-sided). Less-frequent complications include cardiac dysrhythmias and injuries to the phrenic nerve, esophagus, and trachea. Tumor seeding is extremely rare. The mortality rate of both of these procedures is less than 0.1%, with several large series reporting no deaths.

Luke WP, Pearson FG, Todd TRJ, et al: Prospective evaluation of mediastinoscopy for assessment of carcinoma of the lung. J Thorac Cardiovasc Surg 91:53–56, 1986.

Trastek VF, Piehler JM, Pairolero PC: Mediastinoscopy. Br Med J 42:240–243, 1986.

13. **What are the findings at mediastinoscopy that would preclude initial curative surgical resection of bronchogenic carcinoma?**
   - Small cell carcinoma with any lymph node metastases
   - Contralateral mediastinal spread
   - Extranodal extension with invasion of vital structures such as the great vessels or the trachea
   - Extensive mediastinal lymph node metastases or involvement of high paratracheal (station 2) lymph nodes. These patients may be candidates for neoadjuvant therapy.

KEY POINTS: MEDIASTINOSCOPY

1. The most common indication is the staging of lung cancer.

2. It is the gold standard for mediastinal lymph node staging.

3. One small incision allows simultaneous biopsy of lymph nodes from both the right and left middle mediastinum.

14. **When should anterior mediastinotomy or VATS be used instead of cervical mediastinoscopy?**
Although some surgeons favor anterior mediastinotomy for staging of left-upper-lobe and hilar tumors, most begin with cervical mediastinoscopy first. If the patient is negative for metastasis, mediastinoscopy is followed by anterior mediastinotomy, especially if CT scanning shows pathologic lymphadenopathy in the aortopulmonary and hilar regions.

VATS allows for examination of all lymph node stations within a given hemithorax. VATS does not permit examination and sampling of contralateral mediastinal lymph nodes. Given the complexity and expense of VATS, it should not be considered an initial procedure.

Both anterior mediastinotomy and VATS are supplementary procedures to standard cervical mediastinoscopy.

15. **Describe the overall sensitivity and specificity of mediastinoscopy.**

$$\text{Sensitivity} = \frac{\text{True positive}}{\text{True positive} + \text{False negative}}$$

$$\text{Sensitivity} = \frac{\text{True negative}}{\text{True negative} + \text{False positive}}$$

In several reported series, the reported sensitivity and specificity of mediastinoscopy in the diagnosis of metastatic spread from bronchogenic carcinoma are 80–90% and 100%, respectively. The reported sensitivity of mediastinoscopy in the diagnosis of sarcoidosis is greater than 95%.

16. **What is positron emission tomography (PET)?**
PET takes advantage of the biologic activity of tumor cells. Cancer cells have an increased cellular uptake of glucose compared with normal cells. PET scanners can detect the radiolabeled glucose analogue fluorodeoxyglucose (FDG) trapped in cells. PET scans thus provide the clinician with information on the functional activity of a lesion rather than the anatomic information that a CT scan provides.

False positives can exist and are commonly due to infectious disorders or inflammatory lymphadenopathy.

17. **What is the role of PET scanning in the staging of lung cancer?**
Simply stated, PET is expensive and is not universally available, but it is assuming an increasing role in the diagnosis and staging of lung cancer. The overall accuracy of PET in lung cancer staging is high and surpasses CT. Patz and colleagues reported the sensitivity and specificity for mediastinal lymph nodes staged by PET scanning to be 92% and 100%, respectively, compared to 58% and 80% for CT scanning. Sasaki and colleagues reported somewhat worse results, with the sensitivity and specificity for PET scan staging of the mediastinum being 76% and 98%, respectively, compared with 65% and 87% for CT staging.

Patz EF, Lowe VJ, Goodman PC, et al: Thoracic nodal staging with PET imaging with 18-FDG in patients with bronchogenic carcinoma. Chest 108:1617–1621, 1995.

Sasaki M, Ichiya Y, Kuwabara Y, et al: The usefulness of FDG positron emission tomography for the detection of mediastinal lymph node metastases in patients with non-small cell lung cancer: A comparative study with x-ray computerized tomography. Eur J Nucl Med 23:741–747, 1996.

18. **What are the advantages of PET scanning in the staging of lung cancer?**
There is compelling evidence that PET scanning is superior to CT in terms of sensitivity, specificity, and overall accuracy in staging the mediastinum of lung cancer patients. However, the false-negative rate is 10–15%, which compares favorably with the 8–10% false-negative rate of mediastinoscopy. When compared to mediastinoscopy, PET scanning additionally evaluates for metastatic disease in organs outside the mediastinum such as the lung, liver, adrenal glands, and bone. However, since PET scanning does not provide histopathologic confirmation of metastatic disease, mediastinoscopy cannot be excluded from the evaluation of patients with lung cancer.

19. **Does mediastinoscopy play a role in making nonsurgical treatment decisions in lung cancer?**
The finding of mediastinal lymph node involvement is important in the decision about operability. It enables the physician to determine which patients are potential candidates for neoadjuvant therapy before thoracotomy. The role of neoadjuvant therapy for carefully selected Stage IIIA non-small-cell lung cancer patients continues to undergo careful evaluation. In most circumstances, patients with stage IIIB non-small-cell lung cancer are not offered neoadjuvant therapy.

20. **Should all patients with lung cancer undergo mediastinoscopy for staging?**
    Although there are some proponents who recommend mediastinoscopy routinely in all patients
    with lung cancer prior to thoracotomy, others consider it indicated only for selected patients.
    Regardless of their size, mediastinal lymph nodes that are positive on PET scan should be biop-
    sied prior to proceeding with thoracotomy. All patients with enlarged lymph nodes by CT scan
    should undergo mediastinoscopy to confirm or refute malignancy. The management of patients
    with normal-sized lymph nodes on CT scan is more controversial, especially if a PET scan shows
    no mediastinal involvement. In this latter subset of patients, we usually do not perform medi-
    astinoscopy prior to thoracotomy.

CHAPTER 21

THORACOSCOPY

Robert J. Karman, MD, and Praveen N. Mathur, MBBS

1. **Describe the differences between medical and surgical thoracoscopy.**
   - Medical thoracoscopy is used primarily for the diagnosis of pleural diseases and pleurodesis, whereas video-assisted thoracic surgery (VATS) is used for minimally invasive thoracic surgery and offers the opportunity to proceed with open thoracotomy if necessary.
   - VATS is performed in the operating room with the use of complex instruments, multiple ports of entry, double-lumen intubation, and general anesthesia; medical thoracoscopy is performed in the endoscopy suite with the use of local anesthesia, conscious sedation, and simple nondisposable instruments, and only one or two ports of entry are required.
   - In the appropriate clinical situations, medical thoracoscopy may be utilized instead of VATS at a substantial cost savings.

   http://www.aabronchology.org
   Seijo LM, Sterman DH: Interventional pulmonology. N Engl J Med 344:740, 2001.

2. **What is medical thoracoscopy?**
   Medical thoracoscopy, or pleuroscopy, is the endoscopic examination of the thoracic cavity. After thorough evaluation with pleural fluid analysis and closed pleural biopsy, the cause of up to 25% of pleural abnormalities or effusions remains indeterminate. Medical thoracoscopy enhances our diagnostic capability and has become a valuable tool in diagnosing and treating pleural and parenchymal lung diseases without the morbidity, mortality, or cost of open thoracotomy.

   Loddenkemper R: Medical thoracoscopy. In Light RW, Lee YCG (eds): Textbook of Pleural Diseases. London, Arnold, 2003, pp 498–512.
   Seijo LM, Sterman DH: Interventional pulmonology. N Engl J Med 344:740, 2001.

3. **What is the history of thoracoscopy?**
   In 1910, Jacobeus used a modified cystoscope to evaluate the pleural cavity and lyse adhesions to create pneumothoraces for the treatment of tuberculosis (TB). The use of thoracoscopy declined with the arrival of antituberculous therapy. However, recent technologic advances such as improved optical and video technology have revitalized the use of this procedure as a diagnostic and therapeutic tool.

   Loddenkemper R: Medical thoracoscopy—Historical perspective. In Beamis JF, Mathur P, Mehta A (eds): Interventional Pulmonary Medicine. New York, Marcel Dekker, 2004, p 411.

4. **What are the indications for thoracoscopy?**
   Thoracoscopy has both diagnostic and therapeutic indications. **Diagnostic thoracoscopy** should be considered only after careful routine evaluation of pleural abnormalities. Indications include exudative pleural effusions of unknown origin, suspected mesothelioma, cancer, TB, and benign or other pleural disorders including empyema and spontaneous pneumothorax. Exudative pleural effusions, caused by malignancy or TB, are diagnosed only 60–70% of the time after repeated thoracentesis and closed-needle pleural biopsy. Thoracoscopic evaluation, however, increases the sensitivity to 95–97%. In patients in whom adequate thoracoscopic visualization is possible, an unequivocal pathologic diagnosis of benign diseases can be made, with a specificity approaching 100%.

Therapeutic indications for thoracoscopy include lysis of adhesions and thoracoscopic talc pleurodesis for malignant pleural effusions, spontaneous pneumothorax, and recurrent nonmalignant pleural effusions.

Mares DC, Mathur PN: Medical thoracoscopy. The pulmonologist's perspective. Semin Respir Crit Care Med 18:603–615, 1997.

Menzies R, Charbonneau M: Thoracoscopy for the diagnosis of pleural disease. Ann Intern Med 114:271–276, 1991.

5. **What are contraindications to thoracoscopy?**
   Contraindications to thoracoscopy include the lack of a pleural space, respiratory insufficiency requiring ventilatory support, pulmonary arterial hypertension, and uncorrectable bleeding disorders. Relative contraindications include uncontrolled cough, unstable cardiovascular status, and hypoxemia that is not caused by a large pleural effusion.

   Mares DC, Mathur PN: Medical thoracoscopy. The pulmonologist's perspective. Semin Respir Crit Care Med 18:603–615, 1997.

6. **How is the patient evaluated before thoracoscopy?**
   Patient medical assessment before thoracoscopy should include a comprehensive review of the following:
   1. Chest x-ray, frequently supplemented with the bilateral decubitus view
   2. Chest computed tomography (CT) scan, to further assess pleural and parenchymal abnormalities
   3. Pleural fluid analysis
   4. Closed biopsies of the pleura
   5. Arterial blood gas analysis, to evaluate respiratory status
   6. Routine blood tests, including coagulation parameters
   7. Electrocardiogram (ECG)
   8. Pulmonary function tests (may be helpful)

   Loddenkemper R: Thoracoscopy under local anesthesia. Is it safe? J Bronchol 7:207–209, 2000.

7. **What equipment is used for thoracoscopy?**
   The rigid thoracoscope, rather than the flexible thoracoscope, is currently the most common and useful instrument in thoracoscopy. It provides both excellent optical quality and maneuverability within the pleural space. Additional instruments include the following:

Introduction trocars	Suction catheters
Xenon light sources	Video cameras
Probes for palpation	Forceps for coagulation or biopsy
Thoracostomy trays	Monitors

   A new flexirigid pleuroscope has been developed to improve viewing of the pleural cavity. The distal third is flexible, allowing it to reach all areas of the pleural cavity. It is also very similar in function to a bronchoscope; thus, pulmonary physicians use it with ease.

   Brandt HJ, Loddenkemper R, Mai J, Nehouse C: Atlas of Diagnostic Thoracoscopy: Indications—Technique. New York, Thieme, 1985, pp 1–46.

   Ernst A, Hersh CP, Herth F, et al: A novel instrument for the evaluation of the pleural space. An experience in 34 patients. Chest 122:1530–1534, 2002.

8. **How is thoracoscopy performed?**
   After continuous cardiac, hemodynamic, and pulse oximetry monitoring is instituted, the patient is placed in the lateral decubitus position, with the hemithorax to be inspected in the superior position. The entry point, which is the fourth or fifth intercostal space in the midaxillary line, is

prepared and draped in a sterile fashion. Local anesthetic is then injected into the site. The patient is consciously sedated by intravenous administration of a narcotic and midazolam. Blunt dissection at the point of entry is performed, and an artificial pneumothorax is created, allowing the lung to collapse. At this point, the trocar and thoracoscope can now be introduced safely. Pleural fluid is removed, and the thoracoscope is directed to systematically evaluate the entire chest cavity.

Thoracoscopy may be performed by the single puncture method, in which the instruments are introduced through the operating channel of the thoracoscope, or by the double puncture method, in which a second point of entry is made, through which instruments are introduced and manipulated. Biopsy forceps may be inserted through the working channel or through the second puncture site to perform biopsy or coagulation of the pleural space. Similarly, talc can be insufflated through the working channel or through the second point of entry under direct thoracoscopic visualization to ensure that the entire pleural space is covered with talc and pleurodesis is effective.

Brandt HJ, Loddenkemper R, Mai J, Nehouse C: Atlas of Diagnostic Thoracoscopy: Indications— Technique. New York, Thieme, 1985, pp 1–46.

Mathur PN: "How I do it." Medical Thoracoscopy. J Bronchol 1:144–151, 1994.

9. What structures are visualized by thoracoscopy?

During thoracoscopy, if no adhesions are present, the entire parietal surface of the thoracic cavity can be seen with the 0-degree telescope except for the immediate area of the hilum and the point of entry of the thoracoscope. However, with the additional use of the 50-degree telescope, these areas also can be visualized. Anatomic relationships and intrathoracic structures are well recognized by the location of the major parenchymal fissures. The diaphragm is identified by its anterior position and respiration-related movement. Major vascular structures are readily observed through the transparent pleura. Sometimes, however, distinguishing between pleural inflammation and malignancy may be difficult, and several biopsy samples may be needed. The surface of the normal lung is pink and soft. Atelectatic areas are purplish-red with a clear edge, whereas anthracotic areas are black and can be easily identified. Malignant nodules and emphysematous bullae may also be apparent, protruding from the surface. The inability of a lobe to collapse may indicate an obstructing endobronchial lesion or tumor mass.

Brandt HJ, Loddenkemper R, Mai J, Nehouse C: Atlas of Diagnostic Thoracoscopy: Indications— Technique. New York, Thieme, 1985.

Mathur PN: "How I do it." Medical Thoracoscopy. J Bronchol 1:144–151, 1994.

Menzies R, Charbonneau M: Thoracoscopy for the diagnosis of pleural disease. Ann Intern Med 114:271–276, 1991.

10. Is thoracoscopic talc pleurodesis superior to other methods of pleurodesis?

Talc pleurodesis by insufflation (i.e., poudrage) performed during thoracoscopy ensures complete drainage of fluid and distribution of talc over the entire pleural surface. Thoracoscopic talc pleurodesis is the most effective method of pleurodesis when compared with other modalities, including the administration of talc "slurry" by tube thoracostomy. Thoracoscopic talc pleurodesis has also proven to be superior to the intrapleural administration of either bleomycin or tetracycline (90% versus less than 60%, respectively).

Antony VB, Loddenkemper R, Astoul P, et al: Management of malignant pleural effusions. (ATS/ERS Statement). Am J Respir Crit Care Med 162:1987–2001, 2000.

Boutin C, Rey F: Thoracoscopy in pleural malignant mesothelioma: A prospective study of 188 consecutive patients. Cancer 72:389–404, 1993.

Mathur PN: Review: Thoracoscopic pleurodesis with talc may be the optimal technique in patients with malignant pleural effusions. ACP J Club 141(2):43, 2004.

Rodriguez-Panadero F, Antony VB: Pleurodesis. State of the art. Eur Respir J 10:1648–1654, 1997.

KEY POINTS: INDICATIONS FOR THORACOSCOPIC PLEURODESIS OF MALIGNANT EFFUSIONS

1. Malignancy has been established by positive cytologic studies, biopsy, or even examination of a frozen section at the time of thoracoscopy.

2. Pleural effusion rapidly reaccumulates and is the source of symptoms.

3. The lung is expandable after drainage of the effusion so that the visceral and parietal pleura will be in opposition for pleurodesis to occur.

4. The patient has a satisfactory functional clinical condition, is able to tolerate thoracoscopy, and has a relatively good performance status and life expectancy.

---

11. **What is the main reason for failure of thoracoscopic talc pleurodesis?**
    A trapped lung resulting from inability to expand because of an obstructing endobronchial lesion, adhesion, or a complicated pleural process is the main reason for failure of thoracoscopic talc pleurodesis.

12. **What care is required after thoracoscopy?**
    A chest tube is required after every procedure. The placement and duration of the chest tube varies with the indication for thoracoscopy. During a diagnostic procedure, when biopsy samples are taken from only the parietal pleura, a chest tube may be required for only a few hours. At the conclusion of the procedure, a chest tube is placed through the same incision as the thoracoscope and is directed cranially to evacuate the pneumothorax created for the procedure. If the lung has fully expanded and there is no air leak, the chest tube may be removed within 3–4 hours. Typically, patients undergoing diagnostic thoracoscopy are discharged from the hospital within 24 hours of the procedure. After talc pleurodesis, however, a second incision is required to place a chest tube at the lowest possible interspace for maximum drainage. It may take 3–6 days for the drainage to decrease to less than 150 cc/day, at which point the chest tube may be withdrawn, assuming no air leak exists. A daily chest radiograph is required to assess chest tube position, fluid reaccumulation, and lung reexpansion.

    Hartman DL, Gaither JM, Kesler KA, et al: Comparison of insufflated talc under thoracoscopic guidance with standard tetracycline and bleomycin pleurodesis for control of malignant pleural effusions. J Thorac Cardiovasc Surg 105:743–748, 1993.

13. **List the complications of thoracoscopy.**
    Although thoracoscopy is a safe procedure with relatively low morbidity and mortality rates, potential complications include:
    - Postoperative fever (16%)
    - Prolonged air leak (2%)
    - Oxygen desaturation (2%)
    - Subcutaneous emphysema (2%)
    - Infection (2%)
    - Hemorrhage (2%)

    No deaths were reported in one large study, whereas another review found one death in 8000 procedures.

    Colt HG: Thoracoscopy: A prospective study of safety and outcome. Chest 108:324–329, 1995.

14. **What is the role of thoracoscopy in the diagnosis and treatment of malignant mesothelioma?**

    Thoracoscopy has a valuable role in the diagnosis and management of malignant mesothelioma, a disease found in approximately 2000 patients per year in the United States. Thoracoscopy has also been useful in the staging of mesothelioma. In asymptomatic early-stage mesothelioma, nonspecific inflammation, fine granulations, lymphangitis, and local thickening of the parietal pleura by the costovertebral gutter and on the diaphragm are among the earliest thoracoscopic findings. Large samples of pleura obtained at thoracoscopy help to differentiate mesothelioma from metastatic adenocarcinoma and to stage mesothelioma if aggressive surgical intervention is being considered. Recent studies have shown that intrapleural chemotherapy may be useful in the treatment of mesothelioma. If intrapleural chemotherapy is being considered, thoracoscopy provides access to the pleural space and a way to directly evaluate therapeutic response.

    Boutin C, Rey F: Thoracoscopy in pleural malignant mesothelioma: A prospective study of 188 consecutive patients. Part 1: Diagnosis. Cancer 72:389–393, 1993.

    Boutin C, Rey F, Gouvernet J: Thoracoscopy in pleural malignant mesothelioma. Part 2: Prognosis and staging. Cancer 72:394–404, 1993.

    Boutin C, Schlesser M, Frenay C: Malignant pleural mesothelioma. Eur Respir J 12:972–981, 1998.

15. **What is the role of thoracoscopy in the treatment of chylothorax?**

    Patients with lymphoma and other malignancies metastatic to the mediastinum are occasionally troubled by dyspnea caused by recurrent accumulations of chylous pleural fluid, which is due to extrinsic compression or invasion of the thoracic duct. They require frequent thoracentesis for symptomatic control of dyspnea. Although treatment of the underlying disease process with either radiation therapy or chemotherapy may be of benefit, there are treatment failures, recurrences of the malignancy, and eventual resistance to these therapies. In these situations, more aggressive efforts are made to provide palliative symptomatic relief.

    Several therapies are currently available for the treatment of recurrent chylothorax refractory to chemotherapy and radiation therapies. These include multiple thoracentesis, tube thoracostomy, gastrointestinal rest, thoracic duct ligation, pleuroperitoneal shunt, and pleurodesis by thoracostomy tube or thoracoscopy. Recurrent thoracentesis and tube thoracostomy with gastrointestinal rest lead to severe protein malnutrition and lymphopenia. Thoracic duct ligation is frequently difficult due to massive mediastinal lymphadenopathy and may be too aggressive in this extremely debilitated population. Although pleuroperitoneal shunt placement may effectively treat dyspnea, it is contraindicated in the presence of chylous ascites. Pleurodesis by tube thoracostomy has been attempted using multiple agents and has been of limited effectiveness.

    Thoracoscopic talc pleurodesis is well tolerated and of high efficacy in treatment of other etiologies of recurrent pleural effusion. The procedure can be done in a bronchoscopy suite with conscious sedation and local anesthesia.

    Mares DC, Mathur PN: Medical thoracoscopic talc pleurodesis for chylothorax due to lymphoma: A case series. Chest 114:731–735, 1998.

16. **What are the complications of talc?**

    Talc can produce respiratory failure. Patients can develop adult respiratory distress syndrome, thus becoming critically ill. The usual culprit for this is the dose and size of the talc particle: the talc particle size should be large, and the dose should be less than 8 grams.

    Light RW: Talc should not be used for pleurodesis. Am J Respir Crit Care Med 162:2024–2026, 2000.

    Sahn SA: Talc should be used for pleurodesis. Am J Respir Crit Care Med 162:2023–2024, 2000.

CONTROVERSY

17. **Is there a role for thoracoscopy in the diagnosis and treatment of spontaneous pneumothorax?**

Some authorities advocate the use of thoracoscopy in all patients with a spontaneous pneumothorax to identify the type of pneumothorax and to initiate the appropriate therapy. The classification of pneumothoraces includes:

- **Type I:** Normal lung surface
- **Type II:** Adhesions
- **Type III:** Bullae less than 1.5 cm
- **Type IV:** Bullae larger than 2 cm

Thoracoscopic intervention has been suggested to cauterize or seal lesions or bullae of less than 1.5 cm. In addition, thoracoscopic pleurodesis with talc has been shown to decrease the recurrence rate of spontaneous pneumothorax.

In young individuals, however, talc pleurodesis is controversial because it may complicate any future thoracic procedures or surgery. Although talc is believed to be a safe agent, long-term complications are as yet unknown. In the context of uncertain recurrence rates of spontaneous pneumothoraces, unknown long-term sequelae of talc in benign disease, and the relative success of conservative management of pneumothoraces without thoracoscopy, further studies are needed to define the role of thoracoscopy, with or without talc pleurodesis, in spontaneous pneumothoraces.

When thoracoscopically viewed bullae are larger than 2 cm, coagulation is less successful, and the patient should be referred for surgical resection.

Boutin C, Astoul P, Rey F, et al: Thoracoscopy in the diagnosis and treatment of spontaneous pneumothorax. Clin Chest Med 16:497–503, 1995.

V. AIRWAY DISEASE

ASTHMA

Anne E. Dixon, MD

1. **What is the annual incidence of asthma?**
   The incidence of asthma, defined as an episode of asthma in the past 12 months, is approximately 4% in adults and 6% in children in the United States. The rate is higher in boys until adolescence, and in adults the rate is higher in women (Fig. 22-1). Asthma prevalence is particularly high in English-speaking countries, for reasons that are poorly understood.

   http://www.cdc.gov/nchs

2. **Are there any risk factors for developing asthma?**
   A family history of asthma is clearly a risk factor: a number of genes appear to be involved in conferring this increased susceptibility to asthma. Environmental risk factors are probably as important as genetics. These include exposure to tobacco smoke and indoor allergens (such as cockroaches, mold, and dust mites) and also exposure to infectious agents. In very young children, exposure to respiratory virus infections may trigger wheezing, but these infections may protect against the development of asthma in later life through effects on the developing immune system. Recent epidemiologic studies also suggest that obesity is a risk factor for asthma.

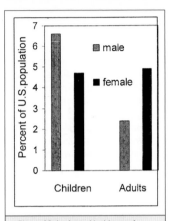

Figure 22-1. Annual incidence of asthma in the United States population by gender and age.

   Camargo CA, Weiss ST, Zhang S, et al: Prospective study of body mass index, weight change, and risk of adult-onset asthma in women. Arch Intern Med 159:2582–2588, 1999.

3. **Do patients "grow out" of asthma?**
   It is estimated that 30–70% of children diagnosed with asthma will not require treatment as adults, whereas adults with asthma typically have persistent disease. Persistence of asthma into adulthood is associated with female sex, smoking, airway hyperresponsiveness, atopy, and an onset of symptoms of wheezing at an early age.

   Sears MR, Greene JM, Willan AR, et al: A longitudinal, population-based, cohort study of childhood asthma followed to adulthood. N Engl J Med 349:1414–1422, 2003.

4. **Is a positive methacholine challenge test diagnostic of asthma?**
   Methacholine challenge testing can be useful to diagnose asthma in subjects with normal spirometry and atypical symptoms. The sensitivity of the test is reported as approximately 85%. However, false positives can occur in subjects with allergic rhinitis, cystic fibrosis, and chronic obstructive pulmonary disease (COPD), and so the clinical presentation must be considered when interpreting the test.

KEY POINTS: DIAGNOSIS OF ASTHMA

1. History of expiratory wheezing, cough, chest tightness, or dyspnea

2. Bronchodilator reversibility (12% and 200 cc improvement in the forced expiratory volume in 1 second [FEV_1] or the forced vital capacity [FVC])

3. Consider bronchoprovocation if atypical presentation

4. Consider vocal cord dysfunction if inspiratory abnormality noted

5. **What is vocal cord dysfunction?**
   Vocal cord dysfunction occurs when the vocal cords adduct on inspiration, obstructing inspiratory airflow. This causes inspiratory stridor, best heard over the neck. Often, patients with vocal cord dysfunction have been labeled with refractory asthma because they have not responded to asthma medication for their symptoms.

6. **How is vocal cord dysfunction diagnosed?**
   Vocal cord dysfunction is suspected from the clinical presentation and by the finding of inspiratory limb flattening on the flow-volume loop during spirometry (Fig. 22-2). The diagnosis is confirmed by flexible fiberoptic laryngoscopy.

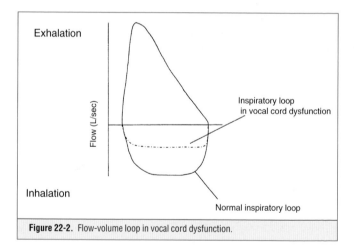

Figure 22-2. Flow-volume loop in vocal cord dysfunction.

7. **When should patients be started on controller therapy for asthma?**
   Patients who have symptoms more than once a week or nocturnal symptoms more than twice a month should be started on controller therapy, preferably an inhaled corticosteroid.

   http://www.nhlbi.nih.gov/guidelines/index.htm

8. **Do inhaled steroids have systemic side effects?**
   Yes. Twenty to forty percent of the inhaled dose of steroid may be absorbed. Decreased skin thickness and purpura may occur, particularly in the elderly. Inhaled corticosteroids may increase intraocular pressures in patients at risk of glaucoma and may also increase the risk of

cataracts, particularly in the elderly. In children, they appear to decrease growth velocity, but they do not appear to affect overall height. Inhaled steroids may decrease bone density and thereby increase risk of osteoporosis. Adrenal suppression with high doses of inhaled steroids can be detected by measurements of 24-hour urinary excretion of cortisol, and fluticasone appears to produce more adrenal suppression at equivalent doses than budesonide. Some individuals are particularly sensitive, and withdrawal of inhaled steroids has been reported to produce adrenal crisis.

9. **Do inhaled steroids prevent loss of lung function in asthma?**
   Asthmatics lose lung function at a faster rate then normal individuals. One of the goals of therapy is to prevent loss of lung function. Large trials show that inhaled steroids appear to have only a small effect on loss of lung function, although studies in very young children are ongoing to see if steroids initiated very early in the course of the disease can affect long-term outcomes. Inhaled steroids clearly benefit asthma control and prevent asthma exacerbations, so although the effect on lung function is only marginal, they have other clear benefits in asthma.

   Pauwels RA, Pedersen S, Busse WW, et al: Early intervention with budesonide in mild persistent asthma: A randomized, double-blind trial. Lancet 361:1071–1076, 2003.

   The Childhood Asthma Management Program Research Group: Long-term effects of budesonide or nedocromil in children with asthma. N Engl J Med 343:1054–1063, 2000.

10. **What symptoms indicate a patient's asthma is not well controlled?**
    Frequent symptoms (occurring three or more times a week), the increased use of rapidly acting bronchodilators, and the presence of symptoms at night or early in the morning all indicate poor control of asthma.

KEY POINTS: SIGNS OF POORLY CONTROLLED ASTHMA

1. Frequent nocturnal awakening

2. Frequent use of rescue inhaler

3. Frequent symptoms

4. High peak flow variability (i.e., >20%)

11. **How often should asthmatics get lung function tests?**
    Patients should get spirometry with bronchodilator testing initially to make the diagnosis of asthma. After that, the main goal of testing is to monitor response to therapy, but there is no ideal method or frequency for doing this. Daily home peak flow monitoring may be helpful in some individuals and is certainly advocated in asthma guidelines, but large studies suggest it lacks sensitivity and specificity for monitoring asthma severity. In a research setting, bronchial hyperreactivity (e.g., to methacholine), induced sputum cell counts, and exhaled nitric oxide have been used, but these tools are not readily available to most practitioners.

12. **Does the influenza vaccination cause asthma exacerbations?**
    Respiratory viruses trigger asthma exacerbations; therefore, all patients with asthma should receive the influenza vaccine unless they have a contraindication. The influenza vaccine is safe to use in asthmatics and does not trigger asthma exacerbations.

    The safety of inactivated influenza vaccine in adults and children with asthma. N Engl J Med 345: 1529–1536, 2001.

13. **When should asthmatics be started on anti-immunoglobulin E (anti-IgE)?**
Anti-IgE (omalizumab) is approved as an add-on therapy in patients with moderate to severe perennial allergic asthma with elevated IgE. Anti-IgE therapy does not yet have a clear place in any asthma guidelines, but it may be used as add-on therapy in an attempt to discontinue systemic steroids or in patients inadequately controlled despite appropriate inhaled corticosteroid therapy. It is normally given by subcutaneous injection every 2–4 weeks, with dosing based on weight and total IgE levels.

14. **Are antibiotics effective in asthma exacerbations?**
Antibiotics are not indicated for the routine treatment of asthma exacerbations except as needed to treat comorbid conditions when bacterial infection is also suspected (i.e., fever with purulent sputum, pneumonia, or bacterial sinusitis). Some authors have suggested that macrolide antibiotics may be useful in asthma exacerbations. Atypical infections (i.e., *Chlamydia pneumoniae* and *Mycoplasma pneumoniae*) may precipitate asthma exacerbations, and macrolide antibiotics are effective against these organisms and also have direct anti-inflammatory actions; however, there are no clinical trials to support using macrolide antibiotics in this setting (Table 22-1).

TABLE 22-1. TREATMENT FOR SEVERE ASTHMA EXACERBATIONS		
	First Line	**Second Line**
Beta agonists	+	
Systemic steroids	+	
Antibiotics	*	*
Anticholinergics		+
Magnesium		+
Methylxanthines		+
Heliox		+

*Antibiotics should be reserved for exacerbations with a coexisting bacterial infection (e.g., bacterial sinusitis or pneumonia).

15. **When should long-acting beta agonists be considered?**
Long-acting beta agonists should be used as add-on therapy in asthmatics not controlled on inhaled corticosteroids. Long-acting beta agonists should not be used as monotherapy in asthma. A large multinational trial of salmeterol found an increased risk of death in subjects in the salmeterol group compared with the placebo group: those at increased risk of death and adverse events were not taking inhaled steroids with the salmeterol.

16. **Can leukotriene-modifying drugs be used as monotherapy in asthma?**
Leukotriene modifying drugs are less effective than inhaled corticosteroids as monotherapy and so are recommended as add-on therapy.

Ducharme FM: Inhaled glucocorticoids versus leukotriene receptor antagonists as single agent asthma treatment: Systematic review of current evidence. BMJ 326:621, 2003.

17. **Is immunotherapy effective in asthma?**
The role of immunotherapy in asthma is controversial. It is not first-line therapy, but it may be considered as an add-on therapy in atopic subjects who have unavoidable exposure to an agent

to which they are sensitized and that clearly precipitates their asthma. However, patients with brittle, unstable, or steroid-dependent asthma are at increased risk of developing bronchospasm from immunotherapy and should not be considered for such treatment.

18. **When should you consider heliox in an asthma exacerbation?**
Substituting helium for nitrogen decreases gas density, thereby facilitating laminar flow, and so it should improve ventilation. Overall, there is no consensus on the role of heliox in asthma exacerbations. There are only small trials of heliox in acute asthma, and results have been conflicting. It may be useful early in the treatment of a severe exacerbation or in difficult-to-ventilate intubated patients.

19. **What strategies are effective for mechanically ventilating patients with status asthmatics?**
These patients have dynamic hyperinflation with air-trapping caused by bronchospasm and obstruction of airways with mucus and inflammatory cells; consequently, they have high airway pressures and are at risk of barotrauma. Adequate sedation to promote synchrony with the ventilator is crucial. On occasion, paralysis will be necessary, but these patients are at high risk of postparalytic myopathy because of concurrent use of high-dose steroids. A controlled mode of ventilation should be used, and airway pressures should be minimized by allowing permissive hypercapnia if necessary through reduction of minute ventilation. Expiratory time should be increased if possible, and inspiratory flow rates of 80–100 L/min are probably optimal.

20. **Is noninvasive ventilation effective in acute asthma?**
Noninvasive positive pressure ventilation is beneficial in respiratory failure from congestive heart failure with pulmonary edema and exacerbations of COPD. Noninvasive ventilatory support in the form of bilevel pressure ventilation increases tidal volume and adds positive end-expiratory pressure (PEEP): this will offset the intrinsic PEEP that occurs in a severe asthma exacerbation and so will decrease the work of the inspiratory muscles. In one study of 30 patients, there was a significant improvement in lung function and a decreased need for hospitalization in patients with acute asthma exacerbations treated in the emergency department. There are no large studies of noninvasive ventilation in acute asthma.

Soroksky A, Stav D, Shpirer I: A pilot prospective, randomized, placebo-controlled trial of bi-level positive airway pressure in acute asthmatic attack. Chest 123:1018, 2003.

CHAPTER 23

CHRONIC OBSTRUCTIVE LUNG DISEASE

Victor Pinto-Plata, MD, and Bartolome R. Celli, MD

1. **How is chronic obstructive pulmonary disease (COPD) defined?**

   COPD is a preventable and treatable disease state that is not fully reversible and is characterized by airflow limitation. The airflow limitation is usually progressive and is associated with an abnormal inflammatory response of the lungs to noxious particles or gases and is primarily caused by cigarette smoking. Although COPD affects the lungs, it also produces significant systemic consequences.

   Celli BR, MacNee W: Standards for the diagnosis and treatment of COPD. Eur Respir J 23:932–946, 2004.

2. **List the risk factors for COPD.**
   - **Tobacco smoking** accounts for an estimated 80–90% of the risk of developing COPD. In fact, many of the other risk factors simply represent modifiers of the host response to cigarette smoke. Age when smoking was started, total pack-years, and current smoking status are predictive of COPD mortality.
   - Both occupational and urban **pollution** are thought to play a role, but the significance of pollution remains unknown.
   - **Infection of lower respiratory tract** during childhood may increase the subsequent risk of COPD by affecting lung function, lung growth, or pulmonary defense mechanisms. Respiratory infection in patients with established COPD may accelerate subsequent functional deterioration, and established COPD may increase the incidence and severity of respiratory infection.
   - Asthma, atopy, and nonspecific **airway hyper-responsiveness** may play a role. Studies are underway to evaluate the importance of hyper-responsiveness.
   - In terms of **sex, race, heredity, and socioeconomic status**, men have a higher prevalence of respiratory symptoms, mortality rates are higher in whites than in nonwhites, and morbidity and mortality are inversely related to socioeconomic status. COPD may aggregate in families. Death from COPD is increasing in women much faster than in men: more than men died from COPD in the year 2000.
   - **Alpha$_1$ antitrypsin (α_1AT) deficiency** is the only known genetic abnormality that leads to COPD; it accounts for less than 1% of COPD in the United States. Normal M alleles occur in about 90% of persons of European descent with normal serum α_1AT level; the phenotype is designated PiMM. More than 95% of persons in the severely deficient category are homozygous for the Z allele, designated PiZZ. PiMZ heterozygotes have serum α_1AT levels that are intermediate between PiMM normals and PiZZ homozygotes. In population studies, PiMZ heterozygotes do not appear to be an increased risk for COPD.

     Celli BR, MacNee W: Standards for the diagnosis and treatment of COPD. Eur Respir J 23:932–946, 2004.
     Mannino DM, Homa DM, Akinbami LJ, et al: Chronic obstructive pulmonary disease surveillance—United States, 1971–2000. MMWR 51:1–16, 2002.

3. **What does the history often reveal in patients with COPD?**
   - **Cough** (usually chronic and productive): Hemoptysis is uncommon, and its presence should stimulate a careful search for other causes such as cancer or tuberculosis.
   - **Dyspnea** (progressive) is not closely related to abnormalities of arterial blood gases (ABGs).
   - **Smoking:** Most patients are heavy smokers.

- **Wheezing** is common.
- **Acute chest illness** is also frequent.

4. **Describe the findings on physical examination of patients with COPD.**
   Chest:
   - Airway obstruction is evidenced by wheezes during auscultation on slow or forced breathing and prolongation of forced expiratory time.
   - Severe emphysema is indicated by overdistention of lungs in stable state, low diaphragmatic position, and decreased intensity of breath and heart sounds.
   - Severe disease is suggested by pursed-lip breathing, by use of accessory respiratory muscles, and in drawing of lower interspaces. (These findings are characteristic, not diagnostic.)

   Other signs and symptoms:
   - Unusual positions to relieve dyspnea at rest
   - Digital clubbing (suggests lung cancer or bronchiectasis)
   - Mild dependent edema (may be seen in absence of right heart failure)

   Pauwels RA, Buist AS, Calverley PM, for the GOLD Scientific Committee: Global strategy for the diagnosis, management, and prevention of chronic obstructive pulmonary disease. NHLBI/WHO Global Initiative for Chronic Obstructive Lung Disease (GOLD) Workshop summary. Am J Respir Crit Care Med 163:1256–1276, 2001.

KEY POINTS: CHARACTERISTICS OF CHRONIC OBSTRUCTIVE PULMONARY DISEASE

1. A preventable and treatable disease

2. Primarily caused by cigarette smoking

3. An important cause of disability and death

4. Diagnosed by spirometry

---

5. **What are the radiographic changes in COPD?**
   - In **chronic bronchitis,** the chest radiograph may be normal, or tubular shadows (parallel or slightly tapering line shadows outside the boundary of hila) or prominent lung markings ("dirty lung") may be observed.
   - In **emphysema,** changes may include signs of *overinflation* (i.e., a low, flat diaphragm; increased retrosternal airspace; and a narrow heart shadow); *oligemia* (i.e., diminution in the caliber of pulmonary vessels with increased rapidity of tapering distally); and *bullae* (i.e., radiolucent areas larger than 1 cm in diameter and surrounded by hairline shadows). Bullae reflect only locally severe disease and are not necessarily indicative of widespread emphysema. With complicating pulmonary hypertension and right ventricular hypertrophy, the hilar vascular shadows are prominent, and the heart shadow encroaches on the retrosternal space as the right ventricle enlarges anteriorly. Emphysema is diagnosed on chest radiographs consistently when the disease is severe, never when the disease is mild, and in about 50% of cases when the disease is moderate.
   A chest radiograph is always indicated in the evaluation of patients with COPD, mainly to rule out other entities that may present with similar symptoms.

6. **What are the abnormalities in pulmonary function tests in COPD?**
   The measurement of forced vital capacity in one second (FEV_1) is necessary for the diagnosis and assessment of the severity of COPD. It is also helpful in following its progression. Airflow

obstruction is an important indicator of impairment of the whole person and the likelihood of blood gas abnormalities. FEV_1 is easily measurable, has less variability than other measurements of airway dynamics, and is more accurately predictable from age, sex, and height. Lung volume measurements show an increase in total lung capacity, functional residual capacity, and residual volume. The vital capacity may be decreased. The single breath-breath carbon monoxide diffusing capacity is decreased in proportion to the severity of emphysema because of the loss of alveolar capillary bed. The test is not specific, and it cannot detect mild emphysema. None of these tests can distinguish between chronic bronchitis and emphysema. Up to 30% of patients have an increase of 15% or more in FEV_1 after a beta agonist aerosol. The absence of a bronchodilator response during a single test never justifies withholding bronchodilator therapy. The determination of lung volumes or diffusion capacity is not routinely indicated in patients with COPD; these variables should be measured only in cases in which there is confusion about the physiologic nature of the disease causing the symptoms.

7. **How is the severity of COPD staged?**
   The severity of COPD may be staged on the basis of the degree of airflow obstruction using the criteria of the American Thoracic Society (ATS) statement on interpretation of lung function:

   - **At risk** (ratio of FEV_1 to forced vital capacity [FVC] higher than 0.7): Patients who smoke, patients exposed to high pollutant loads such as wood smoke or biomass fuel, and patients with respiratory symptoms such as cough, dyspnea, sputum, or repeated respiratory tract infections.
   - **Mild COPD** (FEV_1/FVC lower than 0.7 and FEV_1% predicted >80): includes the great majority of patients. The presence of severe dyspnea warrants additional studies and evaluation by a respiratory specialist.
   - **Moderate COPD** (FEV_1/FVC lower than 0.7 and FEV_1% predicted 50–80%): Includes the majority of patients under the care of primary care physicians. They do not usually require ABG analyses . They also account for a minority of patients who merit evaluation by a respiratory specialist and may receive continuing care by such a specialist.
   - **Severe COPD** (FEV_1/FVC lower than 0.7 and FEV_1 30–50% predicted): Also includes a minority of patients usually under the care of a respiratory specialist. These patients usually have abnormalities in ABGs and may be candidates for oxygen therapy if hypoxemia (i.e., PaO_2 <55 mmHg) is documented.
   - **Severe COPD** (FEV_1/FVC lower than 0.7 and FEV_1 30% predicted): These patients constitute a small minority, but they are the sickest of all. They usually present with frequent exacerbation of the disease, often require hospitalization, and consume a large portion of the resources needed to care for patients with COPD. They benefit the most from care by specialists with knowledge about the different forms of therapy available.

8. **How is the severity of disease assessed?**
   It is accepted that a single measurement of FEV_1 incompletely represents the complex clinical consequences of COPD. A staging system that could offer a composite picture of disease severity is highly desirable, although it is currently unavailable. However, spirometric classification is useful in predicting outcomes such as health status and mortality and should be evaluated. In addition to the FEV_1, body mass index (BMI) and dyspnea have proven useful in predicting outcomes such as survival. We recommend that they be evaluated in all patients. A recently published multidimensional disease severity grading system proved capable of predicting mortality better than the FEV_1.

   Celli BR, Cote CG, Marin JM, et al: The body mass index, airflow obstruction, dyspnea and exercise capacity index in chronic obstructive pulmonary disease. N Engl J Med 350:1005–1012, 2004.

   Celli BR, MacNee W: Standards for the diagnosis and treatment of COPD. Eur Respir J 23:932–946, 2004.

9. **List the elements needed to diagnose COPD.**
   - A complete **history and physical examination** should be performed. If history and physical findings are consistent with or suggest the diagnosis of COPD, the following supportive laboratory tests also should be performed.
   - **Chest radiography:** Diagnostic only of severe emphysema but essential to exclude other lung diseases.
   - **Spirometry** (prebronchodilator and postbronchodilator): Essential to confirm presence and reversibility of airway obstruction and to quantify maximum level of ventilatory function.
   - **ABGs:** Not needed in Stage 1 COPD but essential in Stages 2 and 3.

10. **What tests may help to stage the disease once the diagnosis is made?**
    - **Lung volumes:** Measurement of more than FVC is not necessary except in special circumstances (e.g., presence of giant bullae or evaluation for lung volume reduction surgery).
    - **Carbon monoxide diffusing capacity:** Not necessary except in special instances (e.g., dyspnea out of proportion to severity of airflow limitation).

    Pauwels RA, Buist AS, Calverley PM, for the GOLD Scientific Committee: Global strategy for the diagnosis, management, and prevention of chronic obstructive pulmonary disease. NHLBI/WHO Global Initiative for Chronic Obstructive Lung Disease (GOLD) Workshop summary. Am J Respir Crit Care Med 163:1256–1276, 2001.

11. **What is the natural history of COPD?**
    The FEV_1 in nonsmokers without respiratory disease declines by 25–30 mL per year, beginning at about age 35. The rate of decline of FEV_1 is steeper in COPD patients and smokers than in nonsmokers, and the heavier the smoking, the steeper the rate.
    The decline in function occurs along a slowly accelerating curvilinear path. There is a direct relationship between the initial FEV_1 level and the slope of FEV_1 decline. There is also a stronger association between a low FEV_1/FVC and subsequent decline in FEV_1 in men, but not in women. Age, the number of years of cigarette smoking, and the number of cigarettes currently smoked are the risk factors for more rapid decline of lung function. Acute chest illnesses generally decrease lung function for about 90 days in COPD patients. After cessation of smoking, a small amount of lung function is regained. Thereafter, the rate of decline in lung function approximates that seen in never-smokers of the same age. Smoking cessation improves prognosis, regardless of age.

    Anthonisen NR, Wright EC, Hodgkin JE, the IPPB Trial Group: Prognosis in chronic obstructive pulmonary disease. Am Rev Respir Dis 133:14–20, 1986.

12. **What are the prognostic factors in COPD?**
    Predictors of mortality in patients with COPD are advancing age, severity of airway obstruction as indicated by FEV_1, severity of hypoxemia, and the presence of hypercapnia and cor pulmonale. The presence of systemic manifestations of COPD, such as dyspnea, malnutrition, and decreased exercise capacity, adds to the prognostic value of a good medical evaluation. Marked reversibility of airway obstruction is a favorable prognostic factor. Persons with moderate obstruction but with FEV_1 greater than 1.0 L have a slightly higher mortality at 10 years than an age- and gender-matched population. In persons with FEV_1 less than 0.75 L, the approximate mortality rate at 1 year is 30%, and at 10 years it is 95%. However, some patients with severe airway obstruction may survive for as long as 15 years beyond the average. The reason appears to be that death in COPD generally occurs as a result of a medical complication such as acute respiratory failure, severe pneumonia, pneumothorax, cardiac arrhythmia, or pulmonary embolism.

    Celli BR, MacNee W: Standards for the diagnosis and treatment of COPD. Eur Respir J 23:932–946, 2004.

13. **How should stable COPD be managed?**

Once the diagnosis of COPD is established, the patient should be educated about the disease and encouraged to participate actively in therapy, especially in preventive care (e.g., immunization, including pneumococcal and annual influenza vaccines), and to maintain an active lifestyle. Above all, a patient who still smokes must be encouraged and supported in an effort to quit.

Airway obstruction should be managed with pharmacotherapy that includes bronchodilators, anti-inflammatory drugs, and mucokinetic agents. Hypoxia should be assessed, and supplemental oxygen must be administered if indicated. The response to therapy should be assessed periodically. A patient may benefit from a multidisciplinary rehabilitation program if severe symptoms or decreased functional capacity is observed over time or if there are more than two hospital or emergency department visits per year.

14. **What drug regimens are given for COPD?**

1. For mild, variable symptoms: selective beta$_2$ agonist metered dose inhaler (MDI) aerosol, 1–2 puffs every 6–12 hours as needed, not to exceed 8–12 puffs per 24 hours.

2. For mild-to-moderate continuing symptoms: long-acting inhaled bronchodilators such as tiotropium once daily or long-acting beta$_2$ agonists such as salmeterol or formoterol twice daily are the preferred forms of therapy. An alternative therapy may include ipratropium MDI aerosol, 2–6 puffs every 6–8 hours, not to be used more frequently, plus selective beta agonist MDI aerosol, 1–4 puffs as required 4 times daily for rapid relief, when needed or as regular supplement. The single canister providing a combination of a beta agonist (e.g., albuterol sulfate) and ipratropium bromide (Combivent) may help increase compliance.

3. If response to Step 2 is unsatisfactory or if there is a mild-to-moderate increase in symptoms, add sustained-release theophylline, 200–400 mg twice daily or 400–800 mg at bedtime for nocturnal bronchospasm (serum theophylline level must be monitored intermittently).

4. If control of symptoms is suboptimal, consider a course of oral steroids (i.e., prednisone), up to 40 mg/day for 10–14 days.
   - If improvement occurs, wean to low daily or alternate-day dose.
   - If no improvement occurs, stop abruptly.
   - If oral steroid appears to help, consider use of aerosol steroid MDI, particularly if the patient has evidence of bronchial hyperreactivity.

5. For severe exacerbation:
   - Increase beta$_2$ agonist dosage (e.g., MDI with spacer, 6–8 puffs every 30 minutes to 2 hours, or inhalant solution, unit dose every 30 minutes to 2 hours) or subcutaneous administration of epinephrine or terbutaline, 0.1–0.5 mL.
   - Increase ipratropium dosage (e.g., MDI with spacer, 6–8 puffs every 3–4 hours, or inhalant solution of ipratropium, 0.5 mg every 4–8 hours).
   - Provide theophylline dosage intravenously with a calculated amount to bring serum level to 10–15 mg/mL.
   - Provide methylprednisolone dosage intravenously, giving 50–100 mg immediately and then every 6–8 hours; taper as soon as possible (within 2 weeks).
   - Add an antibiotic, if indicated.

Celli BR, MacNee W: Standards for the diagnosis and treatment of COPD. Eur Respir J23:932–946, 2004.
Pauwels RA, Buist AS, Calverley PM, for the GOLD Scientific Committee: Global strategy for the diagnosis, management, and prevention of chronic obstructive pulmonary disease. NHLBI/WHO Global Initiative for Chronic Obstructive Lung Disease (GOLD) Workshop summary. Am J Respir Crit Care Med 163:1256–1276, 2001.

15. **What is the role of corticosteroids in severe stable COPD?**

In contrast to their value in asthma management, the role of steroids in COPD is less clear. Steroids may merit more careful evaluation in individual patients on adequate bronchodilator therapy who fail to improve sufficiently or whose disease worsens. At present, there is no evidence that patients with COPD who are being treated with regular bronchodilator therapy require the protective effects of added steroid therapy as used in asthma. Most studies suggest that only 20–30% of patients with COPD improve if given long-term oral steroid therapy. The dangers of steroids require careful documentation of the effectiveness of such therapy before a patient is put on prolonged dosing. It is possible that an aerosol steroid can be used in place of low-dose oral steroids, but again there is insufficient documentation to support such therapy. Two large trials have reported controversial results. More studies are needed to determine the real value of routine inhaled steroids. If the patient has frequent exacerbations and the lung function as represented by the FEV$_1$ is lower than 50%, inhaled steroids may decrease the rate of exacerbation and prevent deterioration of health status.

Burge PS, Calverley PM, Jones PW, et al: Randomised, double blind, placebo controlled study of fluticasone propionate in patients with moderate to severe chronic obstructive pulmonary disease: The ISOLDE trial. BMJ 320:1297–1303, 2000.

The Lung Health Study Research Group: Effect of inhaled triamcinolone on the decline in pulmonary function in chronic obstructive pulmonary disease. N Engl J Med 343:1902–1909, 2000.

16. **Is the nebulized inhaler superior to the MDI?**
    No. Inhaled bronchodilators delivered by MDI are as effective as those delivered by nebulizer. Inhaled bronchodilators can be administered as a wet aerosol from a jet or ultrasonic nebulizer, or they can be administered from an MDI as a propellant-generated aerosol or as a breath-propelled dry powder. The relative efficiencies of the nebulizer and metered-dose inhaler vary with the techniques used for each. With optimal technique, approximately 12% of the drug is delivered from the MDI to the lung; the remainder is deposited in the mouth, pharynx, and larynx. In general, the dose required in a nebulizer is 6–10 times that used in an MDI to produce the same degree of bronchodilation. Even in the emergency setting, supervised adrenergic therapy delivered by MDI with a spacer device is as effective as nebulizer treatment.

17. **What are the indications for long-term oxygen therapy in COPD?**
    Long-term oxygen therapy (LTOT) is indicated for patients whose disease is stable on a full medical regimen and who meet the following criteria:

    Continuous oxygen therapy (24 hours/day)
    - Resting PaO$_2$ less than 55 mmHg or SaO$_2$ less than 88%
    - Resting PaO$_2$ of 56–59 mmHg or SaO$_2$ less than 89% in the presence of any of the following: dependent edema suggesting congestive heart failure, P pulmonale on ECG (i.e., P wave more than 3 mm in inferior leads) or cor pulmonale, or erythrocytosis (i.e., hematocrit greater than 56)
    - Resting PaO$_2$ more than 59 mmHg or SaO$_2$ more than 89% (reimbursable only with additional documentation justifying the oxygen prescription and a summary of more conservative therapy that has failed)

    Noncontinuous oxygen therapy
    Oxygen flow rate and number of hours per day must be specified.
    - **During exercise:** PaO$_2$ less than 55 mmHg or SaO$_2$ less than 88% with a low level of exercise
    - **During sleep:** PaO$_2$ less than 55 mmHg or SaO$_2$ less than 88% with associated complications such as pulmonary hypertension, daytime somnolence, and cardiac arrhythmias

    O'Donohue WJ: Indications for long-term oxygen therapy and appropriate use. In O'Donohue WJ (ed): Long-Term Oxygen Therapy: Scientific Basis and Application. New York, Marcel Dekker, 1995, pp 53–68.

    Tarpy SP, Celli BR: Long-term oxygen therapy. N Engl J Med 333:710–714, 1995.

18. **What is the role of chest therapy with drainage and antibiotics in COPD?**
    The value of chest therapy with drainage in patients with COPD has not been documented. Trials of postural drainage in patients acutely ill with COPD have failed to show a positive effect on sputum volume, gas exchange, or spirometric measurements. Chest wall percussion and vibration used with postural drainage also lack scientific support. Furthermore, in patients acutely ill

with COPD, chest percussion and vibration can cause a transient decrease in FEV_1 and an increase in functional residual capacity as a result of acute bronchospasm. In patients with cystic fibrosis, the benefits of postural drainage are limited to patients who expectorate at least 25 mL of sputum per day. Extrapolating from those observations, it is recommended that postural drainage, with or without chest percussion or vibration, be limited to hospitalized patients with COPD whose sputum production also exceeds 25 mL/day. Patients with or without COPD whose course is complicated by mucus plugging with lobar atelectasis benefit from chest therapy. The value of antibiotics has not been proven in the prevention or treatment of COPD exacerbation unless there is evidence of infection (e.g., fever or leukocytosis) or a change in the radiograph. In cases of recurrent infection, particularly in winter, prolonged courses of continuous or intermittent antibiotics may be useful.

19. **When is intubation with mechanical ventilation indicated in acute exacerbation of COPD?**

Although no objective guidelines exist for determining the ideal time for intubation with assisted ventilation, this support will benefit two classes of patients: (1) those who have experienced progressive worsening of respiratory acidosis or altered mental status despite aggressive pharmacologic and nonventilatory support, and (2) those with clinically significant hypoxemia that has developed despite the provision of supplemental oxygen by usual techniques.

Intubation with mechanical support is indicated in the presence of one of the following major criteria or two minor criteria after the first hour of aggressive therapy:

Major criteria	Minor criteria
■ Respiratory arrest	■ A respiratory rate more than 35 breaths per minute and above the value on admission
■ Respiratory pauses with loss of consciousness or gasping for air	■ Arterial pH value less than 7.30 and below the value on admission
■ Psychomotor agitation making nursing care impossible and requiring sedation	■ PaO_2 less than 45 mmHg despite oxygen therapy
■ A heart rate less than 50 beats per minute with loss of alertness	■ Worsening mental status (e.g., asterixis, confusion, lethargy, agitation)
■ Hemodynamic instability with systolic arterial blood pressure less than 70 mmHg	

20. **What is the role of noninvasive ventilatory support in COPD exacerbation?**

Noninvasive ventilation—using both facial and nasal masks in conjunction with volume-cycled ventilation, bilevel positive airway pressure, and pressure support mode—can reduce the need for intubation, the length of the hospital stay, and the in-hospital mortality rate in selected patients with COPD exacerbation. Patient features that should discourage noninvasive ventilation include hemodynamic instability, copious secretions, an inability to defend the airway, poor cooperation with the technique, or impaired mental status. Noninvasive ventilation should be provided in settings where personnel are familiar with the techniques to be used and are able to manage the complications associated with this mode of ventilation, which include hypoventilation, hyperventilation, aspiration, and local discomfort.

Lightowler JV, Wedzicha JA, Elliot M, Ram SF: Noninvasive positive pressure ventilation to treat respiratory failure resulting from exacerbations of chronic obstructive pulmonary disease: chocrane systematic review and meta-analysis. BMJ 326:185–189, 2003.

Rossi A, Appendini L, Roca J: Physiological aspects of noninvasive positive pressure ventilation. Eur Respir Mon 16:1–10, 2001.

21. **How does the physician determine if intubation/ventilation is likely to be successful in a patient with severe COPD?**

Although subjective bedside judgment cannot accurately determine the likelihood of successful ventilation and survival, clinical data do indicate that outcome correlates with baseline function (i.e., the severity of underlying COPD when stable and the daily activity level) and the presence of nonpulmonary comorbid conditions such as gastrointestinal bleeding, pulmonary embolism, or coronary artery disease. Analysis of the typical clinical outcome of patients with COPD who present with acute respiratory failure can assist decision-making for intubation and mechanical ventilation. Between 75% and 90% of such patients who are mechanically ventilated survive to hospital discharge. Overall, short-term prognosis after intubation/ventilation for severe COPD is favorable, and the long-term prognosis is similar to that of patients with the same degree of underlying respiratory impairment who have not required mechanical ventilation.

22. **Is surgical therapy available for severe COPD?**
The following procedures may be contemplated for the patient with COPD:
- **Bullectomy** (resection of large bullae compressing normal lung) can be helpful in relieving severe dysfunction and dyspnea. Resection of bullae occupying more than one-third of the hemithorax produces the best result.
- **Lung volume reduction surgery** (pneumectomy of nonuniform emphysematous lung) has been encouraging. In selected patients, the improvements in symptoms, FEV_1, FVC, and ABGs have been significant. Studies are underway to evaluate the role of this procedure in patients with COPD.
- **Double lung transplantation** is the definitive procedure to improve COPD. Single lung transplantation can be life-saving. The procedure is costly, is hampered by lack of donor availability, and requires lifelong immunosuppression.

American Thoracic Society: International guidelines for the selection of lung transplant candidates. Am J Respir Crit Care Med 158:335–339, 1998.
National Emphysema Treatment Trial Research Group: A randomized trial comparing lung-volume-reduction surgery with medical therapy for severe emphysema. N Engl J Med 348:2059–2073, 2003.
Snider GL: Reduction pneumoplasty for giant bullous emphysema. Implications for surgical treatment of nonbullous emphysema. Chest 109:540–548, 1996.

KEY POINTS: THERAPIES FOR COPD THAT IMPROVE OUTCOMES

1. Long-acting inhaled bronchodilators and corticosteroids

2. Noninvasive ventilation during acute or chronic failure

3. Pulmonary rehabilitation

4. Surgery (for selected cases)

5. Oxygen therapy (if patient is hypoxemic)

23. **What elements are needed preoperatively to evaluate the risk for postoperative pulmonary complications?**
This process depends on the indications for surgery, the surgical site, the experience of the surgical team, the type of anesthesia, and the degree of respiratory impairment. When the nature and severity of a patient's lung disease are unclear, physiologic tests should be considered in addition to history and physical examination. Candidates for lung resection should have pulmonary function tests such as spirometry and diffusing capacity routinely performed. Routine preoperative spirometry in candidates for upper abdominal surgery can be useful in the preoperative evaluation of patients with symptoms of COPD, especially if the test has not been done previously. Preoperative ABG analysis in all patients with severe COPD is recommended

if a recent test is not available. A preoperative chest radiograph in patients about to undergo noncardiothoracic surgery is sensible because patients with COPD are at increased risk for pulmonary neoplasms. (The chest x-ray is always indicated in patients undergoing thoracic surgical procedures. The statement above supports the use of chest x-ray but does not mandate it since no data support its routine use.) Quantitative lung scintigraphy and exercise testing may be helpful in determining risk of postoperative complications, particularly in patients undergoing lung resection. In addition, exercise testing may reveal previously unexpected cardiovascular dysfunction and should be recommended often.

Martinez FJ, Iannettoni M, Paine III R: Medical evaluation and management of the lung cancer patient prior to surgery, radiation or chemotherapy. In Pass H, Mitchell J, Johnson D, Turrisi A (eds): Lung Cancer: Principles and Practice. Philadelphia, Lippincott Williams & Williams, 2000, pp. 649–681.

Trayner E Jr, Celli BR: Postoperative pulmonary complications. Med Clin North Am 85:1129–1139, 2001.

24. **How is a patient with COPD managed perioperatively?**
    - **Preoperative period:** General guidelines include preoperative risk evaluation, smoking cessation at least 8 weeks preoperatively, and aggressive treatment of lung dysfunction, using inhaled bronchodilators, theophylline, corticosteroids, and antibiotics as indicated. Patients with Stage 2 or Stage 3 COPD may be admitted to the hospital before surgery for multidisciplinary evaluation, patient education, and aggressive therapy.
    - **Intraoperative considerations**: The intraoperative period does not appear to pose major problems.
    - **Postoperative period**: In the immediate postoperative recovery period, a number of potential threats are present, including respiratory muscle dysfunction, acidemia, hypoxemia, and hypoventilation. In this delicate period, close monitoring and, if necessary, mechanical ventilatory support are crucial to the patient with COPD. The inability to overcome diaphragmatic dysfunction probably explains the failure of deep breathing, resulting in pulmonary complications. Intermittent positive-pressure breathing or incentive spirometry reduces postoperative complications after upper abdominal surgery. Continuation of the preoperatively prescribed antibiotics, bronchodilators, corticosteroids, and theophylline is standard therapy.

25. **Is pulmonary rehabilitation useful in COPD?**
    The available evidence indicates that pulmonary rehabilitation benefits patients with symptomatic COPD. The effect of pulmonary rehabilitation programs on health care utilization is promising but requires further investigation. In contrast, aerobic lower-extremity training is of benefit in several areas of importance to patients with COPD. These areas include exercise endurance, perception of dyspnea, quality of life, and self-efficacy. The exact role of upper-extremity exercise training programs requires further study. Education and psychological support improve the awareness of patients and increase their understanding of the disease, but when used alone, education and support are of limited value. Pulmonary rehabilitation, coupled with smoking cessation, optimization of blood gas levels, and medications, offers the best treatment option with symptomatic airway obstruction.

    Pulmonary rehabilitation: Official statement of the American Thoracic Society. Am J Respir Crit Care Med 159:1666–1682, 1999.

CHAPTER 24

CYSTIC FIBROSIS

Lori Shah, MD, and Michael C. Iannuzzi, MD

1. **What are the criteria for diagnosis of cystic fibrosis (CF)?**
   - Elevated sweat chloride ion concentration (>60 mEq/dL), *or*
   - Identification of mutations known to cause CF in both cystic fibrosis transmembrane conductance regulator (CFTR) genes, *or*
   - *In vivo* demonstration of characteristic abnormalities in ion transport across the nasal epithelium, *plus*
     - At least one of the following: (1) sinopulmonary disease, (2) characteristic gastrointestinal (GI) or nutritional disorders, (3) obstructive azoospermia, or (4) salt loss syndrome, *or*
     - Diagnosis of CF in a sibling, *or*
     - Positive newborn screening

   These criteria reliably diagnose more than 95% of children and adults with CF. False-positive sweat tests do occur, so the clinical history should also support the diagnosis of CF. About 1% of CF patients have normal sweat tests.

   Stern R: The diagnosis of cystic fibrosis. N Engl J Med 336(7):487–491, 1997.

2. **When should genetic testing (i.e., genotyping) be performed?**
   Genetic testing is not recommended routinely but may be useful in individuals in whom the diagnosis is considered but who do not meet classic diagnostic criteria. The sensitivity of genetic testing is limited because currently available commercial panels can only identify a minority of the >1000 identified CF mutations.

3. **Is a particular genotype associated with a worsened clinical course?**
   Genotype is highly predictive of pancreatic status, but it does not correlate with pulmonary or overall clinical severity. In the United States, the most common mutation, ΔF508, is present on about 70% of CF alleles. Patients homozygous for ΔF508 generally have an earlier onset of pulmonary disease and an increased likelihood of developing pancreatic insufficiency compared with heterozygotes. Additional genetic or environmental factors are also believed to influence these manifestations.

4. **What are the criteria for diagnosing pulmonary exacerbation in CF?**
   There are currently no universal criteria. However, a panel of experts has suggested that a pulmonary exacerbation be defined as the presence of at least *three* of the following:
   - Increased respiratory rate
   - Fever
   - Weight loss ≥1 kg
   - Increased cough
   - Increased sputum production or change in sputum appearance
   - New findings on chest examination (i.e., crackles or wheezing)
   - New finding on chest radiograph
   - Decreased exercise tolerance
   - Decrease in forced expiratory volume in 1 second (FEV_1) of ≥10% from a previous study that was obtained within 3 months
   - Decrease in oxygen saturation of ≥10% from a baseline that was obtained within 3 months

   Yankaskas JR, Marshall BC, Sufian B, et al: Cystic fibrosis adult care: Consensus conference report. Chest 125(1 Suppl):15–395, 2004.

5. **What is the significance of finding aspergillus on a sputum culture?**

Aspergillus species are important causes of morbidity in patients with CF. Allergic bronchopulmonary aspergillosis (ABPA), first described in patients with asthma, occurs in 10–15% of CF patients. Every CF patient admitted for pulmonary exacerbation should be screened for ABPA through immunoglobulin E (IgE) and sputum culture. ABPA may be difficult to diagnose in the CF patient because it shares many characteristics with atopy or other lung infections. Cultures can be falsely positive in the absence of significant clinical disease, but repeated isolation of the same species of *Aspergillus* is likely to be significant. Conversely, a consistent clinical picture—recurrent episodes of pulmonary infiltrates, segmental or lobar collapse, and eosinophilia—in the absence of a positive sputum culture should not exclude ABPA. In this situation, antibody tests (specifically, IgE and IgG) for aspergillus should be obtained. (*See* Chapter 28, Fungal Pneumonia.)

Stevens DA, Moss RB, Kurup VP, et al: ABPA in CF—State of the Art: Cystic Fibrosis Foundation Consensus Conference. Clin Infect Dis 37(Suppl 3):S225–264, 2003.

KEY POINTS: CHARACTERISTIC SINOPULMONARY FEATURES OF CYSTIC FIBROSIS

1. Chronic cough and sputum production

2. Persistent infection with characteristic pathogens

3. Airflow obstruction

4. Chronic chest radiographic abnormalities

5. Sinus disease or nasal polyps

6. **What is the significance of pneumothorax in patients with CF?**

Up to 5–8% of all CF patients and 20% of adult CF patients will eventually have pneumothorax. Pneumothorax should be suspected in patients who develop sudden-onset chest pain and respiratory distress. Every CF patient with pneumothorax, even those without symptoms, should be hospitalized and observed for at least 24 hours. Survival after the onset of pneumothorax is about 30 months, and the chance of recurrence is 50–70%. Whatever specific treatment for pneumothorax is undertaken, pulmonary infection should be assumed and antibiotic treatment instituted.

Flume PA: Pneumothorax in cystic fibrosis. Chest 123:217–221, 2003.

7. **How should CF patients with hemoptysis be managed?**

Blood streaking of sputum is common. If it persists, the diagnosis of a pulmonary exacerbation requiring antibiotic therapy should be considered. Major hemoptysis, defined as 240 cc in 24 hours or recurrent bleeding of more than 100 cc/day over 3–7 days, occurs in about 1% of all CF patients each year. The incidence is higher in patients over 16 years of age. Patients should be admitted for close observation. Hemoptysis can often be controlled with antibiotics, bed rest, correction of coagulopathy, vitamin K administration, cough suppressants, and discontinuation of vigorous airway clearance techniques. Bronchoscopy may be necessary to localize the site of bleeding. Angiography with bronchial arterial embolization to the hypertrophied bronchial circulation may be necessary if bleeding persists.

8. **Name some of the extrapulmonary manifestations of CF.**

   Exocrine pancreatic dysfunction leads to fat malabsorption, including the fat-soluble vitamins A, D, E, and K, which may lead to malnutrition. A body mass index (BMI) of less than 18 has been associated with worsened pulmonary function and survival in CF patients. Glucose intolerance and diabetes mellitus are present in a majority of older CF patients. The liver can be affected with biliary cirrhosis, which may lead to portal hypertension. Meconium ileus is seen in about 40% of infants with CF and is pathognomonic. A similar syndrome called distal intestinal obstruction syndrome (DIOS) occurs in older CF patients due to inspissated mucus in the GI tract. Osteopenia and osteoporosis are commonly seen in CF patients and are the result of factors including accelerated bone resorption, diminished bone formation, low vitamin D levels, and hypogonadism. About 95% of male CF patients are infertile, which may be due to congenital absence of the vas deferens or other undeveloped structures. Females with CF are not commonly infertile, although they may have difficulty conceiving due to thick cervical mucus or anovulation.

9. **Name the usual pathogens found in the lower airways of cystic fibrosis patients.**

   Bacterial infection of the airways is the major cause of morbidity and mortality in CF patients. Patients are initially colonized by *Haemophilus influenzae*, then with *Staphylococcus aureus*, later with *Pseudomonas aeruginosa*, and, in some cases, with *Burkholderia* (formerly *Pseudomonas*) *cepacia*. The presence of *P. aeruginosa* and *B. cepacia*, particularly genomovar III or *Burkholderia cenocepacia*, in sputum has been associated with poorer pulmonary status. By the age of 26 years, 80% of CF patients are infected with *P. aeruginosa*, compared with less than one-third in those younger than 5 years. Other pathogens, including *Aspergillus* and mycobacteria, should be considered when a patient's condition deteriorates without known cause.

   Gibson RL, Burns JL, Ramsey BW: Pathophysiology and management of pulmonary infections in cystic fibrosis. Am J Respir Crit Care Med 168:918–951, 2003.

10. **Describe the typical abnormalities noted on pulmonary function testing in patients with CF.**

    Early in the course of the disease, a decrease in midexpiratory flows may be noted. However, as the disease progresses, vital capacity diminishes and residual volume increases, reflecting hyperinflation. Later, FEV_1 values fall and DLCO may decrease. Hypoxemia may be present, as well as hypercapnia, in a minority of patients, largely due to shunting and V/Q mismatch.

KEY POINTS: PULMONARY COMPLICATIONS IN CYSTIC FIBROSIS

1. Bacterial Infections

2. ABPA

3. Pneumothorax

4. Hemoptysis

11. **Describe the typical radiographic features of CF.**

    Early in the course of the disease, the lungs may appear normal on radiographs. As the disease progresses, overinflation is seen, which represents bronchiolitis with small airway obstruction. Further progression includes bronchitis with thickened bronchial walls, which is seen as circular lesions when the bronchi are projected in cross section and as "tram lines" or parallel linear opacities when the bronchi project longitudinally. With further worsening, bronchiectasis develops, and small cysts and rounded opacities become evident (Fig. 24-1). For unknown reasons, the right upper lobe commonly is affected earlier and more severely than other lobes. Late findings are large blebs, most often found in the apices.

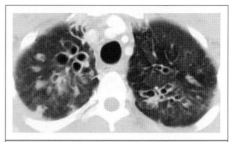

Figure 24-1. A high-resolution computed tomography scan demonstrates bronchiectasis and mucoid impaction.

Shah RM, Sexauer W, Ostrum BJ, et al: High-resolution CT in the acute exacerbation of cystic fibrosis: Evaluation of acute findings, reversibility of those findings, and clinical correlation. Am J Roentgenol 169:375–380, 1997.

12. **What intravenous antibiotics should be used to treat CF pulmonary exacerbations?**
   Antibiotic therapy should be guided by the patient's recent sputum culture and sensitivity testing. If a patient is colonized with *Pseudomonas*, aminoglycosides such as tobramycin and amikacin or antipseudomonal beta-lactams such as cefepime or piperacillin/tazobactam may be used in combination. Other choices include aztreonam, ceftazidime, imipenem/cilastatin, or ticarcillin/clavulanate. For patients colonized with methicillin-resistant *Staphylococcus aureus* (MRSA), vancomycin should be used. Some antibiotic dosages are weight dependent, and peak and trough levels may need to be followed. In addition, dosages may need to be adjusted based on renal function. In CF patients infected with multidrug-resistant organisms, specialized synergy studies can be useful.

13. **What is the role of an inhaled tobramycin solution in CF therapy?**
   Aerosolized tobramycin was studied in two large, multicenter, double-blind, placebo-control trials in patients with moderate to severe pulmonary disease, defined as an FEV_1 between 25% and 75% of predicted. It led to significant improvement in pulmonary function, decreased *Pseudomonas* concentration in sputum, and decreased hospitalizations. There was no increase in the prevalence of resistant organisms after inhaled tobramycin therapy.

   Ramsey BW, Pepe MS, Quan JM, et al: Intermittent administration of inhaled tobramycin in patients with cystic fibrosis. N Engl J Med 34:23–30, 1999.

14. **Which patients are most likely to benefit from dornase alfa? How should it be administered?**
   The high DNA content of sputum in CF patients contributes markedly to its stickiness and causes patients to have difficulty clearing secretions. Patients with abnormal lung function (i.e., a forced vital capacity <80% of predicted) and chronic purulent sputum are most likely to benefit from dornase alfa, a human recombinant deoxyribonuclease (rh DNase). Patients with normal lung function and uninfected or rarely infected sputum usually will not benefit. A once-daily dose of 2.5 mg of dornase alfa is standard; higher or twice-daily dosing has little additional benefit. A nebulizer that delivers particles in the respirable fraction (1–6 μm) should be used.

   Fuchs HJ, Borowitz DS, Christiansen DH, et al: Effect of aerosolized recombinant human DNAase on exacerbations of respiratory symptoms and on pulmonary function in patients with cystic fibrosis. NEJM 331(10):637–642, 1994.

15. **Does bronchodilator therapy have a role in CF?**
Bronchodilator treatment is helpful in 30% of patients, but many CF patients exhibit a paradoxi-cal response with worsening of expiratory flow rates. Investigators have hypothesized that the paradoxical response reflects excessive loss of large airway smooth muscle tone with upstream collapse, which limits effective emptying of the small airways. Because some may have reduced airflow in response to bronchodilator therapy, patients should be objectively evaluated and periodically monitored for improvement while receiving it.

16. **Should azithromycin be given to patients with CF?**
There is evidence suggesting that azithromycin may be beneficial for patients with CF. In a ran-domized, double-blind, placebo-control trial, treatment of CF patients chronically infected with *Pseudomonas aeruginosa* with azithromycin for 24 weeks resulted in improved pulmonary function and nutritional status, decreased pulmonary exacerbation rates, and slightly improved quality of life. Prior to the institution of azithromycin therapy and every 6 months thereafter, patients should be screened for mycobacteria to avoid the emergence of macrolide-resistant nontuberculous mycobacteria.

Saiman L, Marshall BC, Mayer-Hamblett N, et al: Azithromycin in patients with cystic fibrosis chronically infected with *Pseudomonas aeruginosa.* JAMA 290:1749–1756, 2003.

KEY POINTS: STANDARD THERAPIES IN CYSTIC FIBROSIS

1. Antibiotics

2. Mucolytic agents

3. Bronchodilators

4. Anti-inflammatory agents

5. Airway clearance

17. **Should anti-inflammatory drugs be used to treat CF patients?**
A large multicenter randomized trial of pediatric patients showed a higher percentage of pre-dicted FEV_1 in patients on alternate-day prednisone (1 mg/kg) compared with placebo. However, the steroid-treated group showed persistent growth retardation. As a result, long-term oral cor-ticosteroid use should be avoided if possible. In a double-blind, placebo-control trial of mildly affected patients with $FEV_1 > 60\%$, ibuprofen at a dose of 20–30 mg/kg slowed the progression of lung deterioration, particularly in children 5–12 years of age. Clinical trials are lacking to sup-port this therapy in patients with moderate to severe airway disease (i.e., $FEV_1 < 60\%$).

Eigen H, Rosenstein BJ, FitzSimmons S, et al: A multicenter study of alternate-day prednisone therapy in patients with cystic fibrosis. Cystic Fibrosis Foundation Prednisone Trial Group. J Pediatr 126:515–523, 1995.
Konstan MW, Byard PJ, Hoppel CL, et al: Effect of high dose ibuprofen in patients with cystic fibrosis. New Engl J Med 332:848–854, 1995.

18. **How important are airway clearance techniques in the management of CF patients?**
Airway clearance techniques are critical in the management of all CF patients. Secretions block airflow, may precipitate or worsen reactive bronchospasm, and likely contain proinflammatory substances. Some data suggest that exercise may be as effective as traditional chest physical therapy in keeping the airways clear, but until further studies are done, most experts encourage patients to incorporate both aerobic exercise and chest physical therapy into their daily routine.

Airway clearance techniques that may be performed without assistance include airway flutter, a handheld oral oscillator device, positive expiratory pressure devices, vests, or high-frequency chest wall oscillation systems. The optimal airway clearance device remains unclear, and each system has its advantages and disadvantages.

Langenderfer B: Alternatives to percussion and postural drainage. A review of mucus clearance therapies: Percussion and postural drainage, autogenic drainage, positive expiratory pressure, flutter valve, intrapulmonary percussive ventilation, and high-frequency chest compression with the ThAIRapy Vest: J Cardiopulm Rehabil 18:283–289, 1998.

19. **When should a patient with CF be referred for lung transplantation? What is the role of living lobar transplantation?**

CF is the most common indication for bilateral lung transplantation. Patients should be considered for transplantation if there is a decrease in FEV_1 to 30% of predicted, an increase in $PaCO_2$ or oxygen requirement, increased frequency or duration of hospitalizations, or a progressive decline in weight and lung function despite adequate nutritional support and therapy. Potential contraindications include liver disease with significant hepatocellular dysfunction or portal hypertension, airway colonization with *B. cepacia*, the presence of aspergilloma, malnutrition (i.e., BMI <18), or the lack of an appropriate social support network. In living lobar transplantation, two lower lobes are removed from two donors and are implanted into the recipient in place of the whole right and left lung. CF is currently the most common indication for this surgery.

Yankaskas JR, Mallory GB: Lung transplantation in cystic fibrosis: Consensus conference statement. Chest 113:217–226, 1998.

20. **Should pregnancy be discouraged in women with CF because of potential deterioration in lung function?**

A pregnancy in a woman with CF should be considered high-risk. However, pregnancy may be safe; patients with good nutritional status, pancreatic sufficiency, mild obstructive airway disease, and diagnosis at an older age are at lowest risk. Pregnancy in women with moderately severe or severe lung disease carries a substantial risk of morbidity and mortality.

21. **What genetic counseling should be offered to couples when either partner is affected with CF?**

If either partner has CF, a couple contemplating pregnancy should receive genetic counseling. In the American Caucasian population, assuming a negative family history, the odds of being a CF heterozygote are about 1 in 25. Thus, even if the genetic status in the non-CF partner is unknown, the odds of a CF patient having a child with CF are 1 in 50. If the non-CF partner is a heterozygous carrier, the risk is 1 in 2. The risk to a Caucasian child if both parents are of unknown CF status is 1 in 2500. Unfortunately, because there are >1000 CF mutations, negative results in the non-CF partner are not definitive. It is possible that the partner with negative results could be a carrier for a rare or unidentified CF mutation. However, the risk to the fetus can be lowered to 1 in 492 by testing for several of the common CF mutations.

CONTROVERSIES

22. **How should intravenous antibiotics be dosed in patients with CF? Is daily dosing appropriate?**

Aminoglycosides may be given in multiple doses, which is conventional, or once daily. Clinical data suggest efficacy comparable with traditional dosing; however, large, randomized, controlled trials are lacking. The advantages of once-daily dosing are that it may be less toxic in patients with normal renal function and that it is easier to give and monitor.

COMMUNITY–ACQUIRED PNEUMONIA

Michael S. Niederman, MD

CHAPTER 25

1. **Who is at high risk for developing community-acquired pneumonia (CAP)?**
   Patients at risk include those with coexisting medical conditions such as diabetes mellitus, chronic obstructive lung disease, and congestive heart failure; smokers; chronic alcohol abusers; and the elderly (i.e., those over age 65). These factors place individuals at high risk for pneumonia by impairing the normal host defense system, but even patients with normal host defenses can develop infection if they encounter a highly virulent pathogen (e.g., certain viruses and *Legionella*) or if the normal host defense system is overwhelmed by a large inoculum of organisms (as in massive aspiration). Coexisting medical illnesses and some of the therapies used to manage them (such as corticosteroids) can also cause defects in host defenses ranging from impaired mucociliary clearance to decreased immunoglobulin production or phagocytic function. Smoking can alter respiratory tract defenses by increasing mucus production and by interfering with mucociliary clearance, and smokers can be predisposed to more severe illness than nonsmokers. Altered immune function can occur in the elderly, but comorbid illness is a more important influence than aging itself.

KEY POINTS: RISK FACTORS FOR COMMUNITY-ACQUIRED PNEUMONIA

1. Coexisting illness: chronic obstructive pulmonary disease (COPD), heart failure, or diabetes

2. Advanced age

3. Cigarette smoking

4. Chronic alcohol abuse

5. Aspiration risks

2. **What is the 1-year mortality rate for hospitalized patients with CAP who are over age 65?**
   For hospitalized elderly patients with CAP, the immediate mortality in the hospital is approximately 10–12%, but the rate may be less than 5% in younger patients who are not admitted to the intensive care unit (ICU). Although most studies have focused on predictors of outcome for CAP, they have only examined the short-term impact of the disease. When those over age 65 are followed for up to 1 year after admission to the hospital, their mortality rate exceeds 40%, a rate that is higher than that for age-matched controls. These observations emphasize the importance of risk reduction and pneumonia prevention, especially in the elderly. These patients should receive yearly influenza vaccine and a pneumococcal vaccination at least once after the age of 65.

Kaplan V, Clermont G, Griffin MF, et al: Pneumonia: Still the old man's friend? Arch Intern Med 163: 317–323, 2003.

3. **What percentage of patients with CAP have a specific causative pathogen identified?**

Only 30–60% of patients have a specific causative pathogen identified, even with the use of extensive diagnostic testing such as serologic studies, sputum cultures and Gram stains, blood cultures, and microbial antigen assays. This testing is generally applied to inpatients, and the identification of an etiologic pathogen is less common in outpatients. This low diagnostic yield reflects the limited sensitivity—and perhaps clinical value—of available tests, but it also highlights the realization that we may not yet know all the pathogens that cause pneumonia. In recent years, we have seen the recognition of organisms that may have been present for years but not identified, such as Hantavirus, *Legionella pneumophila*, and *Chlamydia pneumoniae*. In addition, new pathogens have emerged, including the virus that causes severe acute respiratory syndrome (SARS). No differences exist, however, in clinical outcome for patients with or without an identified causative pathogen. These observations underscore the point that empirical therapy is necessary for most patients with CAP.

4. **What are the common pathogens that cause CAP?**

Streptococcus pneumoniae, Mycoplasma pneumoniae, respiratory viruses, *Legionella pneumophila, Chlamydia pneumoniae, Haemophilus influenzae*, occasionally *Moraxella catarrhalis*, and aerobic gram-negative bacilli represent the major pathogens that cause CAP. In some series, as many as 40% of all patients have mixed infections involving bacterial organisms and atypical pathogens (such as *Mycoplasma pneumoniae, Legionella pneumophila*, and *Chlamydia pneumoniae*). Aerobic gram-negative bacilli are becoming more prevalent as primary pathogens, possibly reflecting the changes in the population of patients who develop pneumonia. Although there is some debate about the prevalence of enteric gram-negatives in CAP, among hospitalized patients they account for at least 10% of episodes. Risk factors include pulmonary comorbidity, prior hospitalization, previous antibiotics, and aspiration. Although aspiration has long been considered a risk factor for anaerobic infection, recent data from nursing home patients with aspiration risks have shown that enteric gram-negatives are most common in this population. *Pseudomonas aeruginosa* may account for two-thirds of these episodes, especially in patients with pulmonary comorbidity and recent hospitalization. Staphylococcal pneumonia is relatively uncommon except in the setting of a postviral respiratory tract infection (as with influenza). The frequency of viral CAP has been poorly defined, but these pathogens can account for at least 20% of cases, with influenza virus, adenovirus, respiratory syncytial virus, and parainfluenza viruses being most common. The identity of the probable pathogens usually varies depending on patient age, comorbidity, and the severity of illness.

Arancibia F, Bauer TT, Ewig S, Mensa J, et al: Community-acquired pneumonia due to gram-negative bacteria and *Pseudomonas aeruginosa*: Incidence, risk and prognosis. Arch Intern Med 162:1849–1858, 2002.

De Roux A, Marcos MA, Garcia E, Mensa J, et al: Viral community-acquired pneumonia in nonimmunocompromised adults. Chest 125:1343–1351, 2004.

KEY POINTS: MOST COMMON PATHOGENS FOR CAP (IN DESCENDING ORDER)

1. *Pneumococcus* species

2. *Haemophilus influenzae*

3. Atypical pathogens (coinfection possible)

4. Enteric gram-negative organisms

5. *Staphylococcus aureus* (especially after influenza)

El-Solh AA, Pietrantoni C, Bhat A, et al: Microbiology of severe aspiration pneumonia in institutionalized elderly. Am J Respir Crit Care Med 167:1650–1654, 2003.

Marston BJ, Plouffe JF, File TM Jr, et al: Incidence of community-acquired pneumonia requiring hospitalization: Results of a population-based active surveillance study in Ohio. The Community-Based Pneumonia Incidence Study Group. Arch Intern Med 157:1709–1718, 1997.

5. **Can clinical, laboratory, or radiographic parameters predict the pathogen causing CAP?**

No. Most studies to date do not support the concept that the cause of pneumonia can be predicted by examination of clinical, laboratory, or radiographic data. For example, the "bulging fissure" sign of *Klebsiella pneumoniae*, the nonproductive cough of mycoplasmal pneumonia, the hyponatremia of *Legionella pneumophila*, and the atypical presentation of mycoplasmal pneumonia are not specific enough findings to rule out other pathogens. In fact, recent studies of CAP have shown that categorizing pneumonia as "atypical" versus "typical" based on patterns of clinical presentation in order to predict etiology is not accurate. Such classification may even lead to inaccurate management, as best evidenced by an elderly patient who may have pneumococcal pneumonia (a typical pathogen) with atypical clinical features because of age and disease-associated impairments in immune responses. In most patients, it is the immune status of the patient, not the identity of the etiologic pathogen, that defines the clinical features of illness.

6. **Can any data from the history be used to predict the likely pathogen in a CAP patient?**

Certain underlying illnesses lead to disease-specific immune impairments, and these can make infection with specific pathogens more likely. This type of information should be used to ensure that all likely pathogens are being treated, but it cannot be relied on to focus initial therapy to only a few organisms. Some specific associations to consider are listed in Table 25-1.

TABLE 25-1.   ASSOCIATIONS WITH SPECIFIC PATHOGENS

Condition	Commonly Encountered Pathogens
Alcoholism	*Streptococcus pneumoniae* (including penicillin-resistant *S. pneumoniae*), anaerobes, gram-negative bacilli
COPD/smoker	*S. pneumoniae, Haemophilus influenzae, Moraxella catarrhalis, Legionella* species
Nursing home residency	*S. pneumoniae*, gram-negative bacilli, *H. influenzae, Staphylococcus aureus*, anaerobes, *Chlamydia pneumoniae*
Poor dental hygiene	Anaerobes
Epidemic legionnaire's disease	*Legionella* species
Exposure to bats	*Histoplasma capsulatum*
Exposure to birds	*Chlamydia psittaci, Cryptococcus neoformans, H. capsulatum*
Exposure to rabbits	*Francisella tularensis*
Travel to southwestern United States	*Coccidioides immitis* and *C. posadasii*
Exposure to farm animals or parturient cats	*Coxiella burnetii* (i.e., Q fever)

Continued

TABLE 25-1. ASSOCIATIONS WITH SPECIFIC PATHOGENS—CONT'D	
Condition	**Commonly Encountered Pathogens**
Influenza active in community	Influenza, *S pneumoniae, S. aureus, H. influenzae*
Aspiration risks in the elderly	Enteric gram-negatives, anaerobes
Suspected large-volume aspiration	Anaerobes, chemical pneumonitis, obstruction
Structural disease of lung (e.g., bronchiectasis or cystic fibrosis)	*Pseudomonas aeruginosa, Pseudomonas cepacia, S. aureus*
Injection drug use	*S. aureus*, anaerobes, tuberculosis
Endobronchial obstruction	Anaerobes
Recent antibiotic therapy	Drug-resistant pneumococci, *P. aeruginosa*
Sickle cell disease, asplenia	*Pneumococcus, H. influenzae*
Suspected bioterrorism	Anthrax, tularemia, plague
Travel to Asia	SARS, tuberculosis, meloidosis

7. **How should the hospitalization decision be made for the patient with CAP?**

There is no set admission formula to establish when a patient with CAP should be hospitalized, and, ultimately, this still remains an "art of medicine" decision based on assessing multiple factors including the severity of acute illness, comorbidity, and social factors. In recent years, a number of scoring systems have been proposed to help guide the admission decision, but none is absolute.

The most commonly used scoring approach is the pneumonia severity index (PSI), a complex tool that considers multiple comorbidities and laboratory and clinical findings to predict a patient's risk of death. Some experts have advocated that patients with a low calculated risk of dying be treated out of the hospital and that the hospital only be used for patients with a high predicted mortality. Although this tool is accurate for predicting CAP mortality, there is often a disconnect between risk of dying and need for admission to the hospital, and many low-risk patients still need hospitalization. One recent study showed the limitations of the PSI when applied to an indigent population: many patients with low risk of death still needed hospitalization for CAP because of social factors such as homelessness, alcohol or drug intoxication, the need to rule out tuberculosis, or the inability to take medications by mouth.

Another prognostic tool has been used to avoid overlooking a seriously ill patient. This rule, named CURB-65, defines a patient as being ill (i.e., having at least a 10% risk of death) and probably needing hospitalization if at least two of five criteria are present:

- **C**onfusion
- Blood **U**rea > 7 mmol/L (i.e., blood urea nitrogen [BUN] of 19.6 mg/dL)
- **R**espiratory rate > 30 breaths/min
- **B**lood pressure of <90 mmHg systolic or <60 mmHg diastolic
- Age > **65** years

If three criteria are present, the patient is at an even greater risk of dying and may need admission to the ICU. This rule is simple to use and is based on clinical criteria that are generally available when the patient is first evaluated.

Goss CH, Rubenfeld GD, Park DR, et al: Cost and incidence of social comorbidities in low-risk patients with community-acquired pneumonia admitted to a public hospital. Chest 124:2148–2155, 2003.

Lim WS, van der Erden MM, Laing R, et al: Defining community acquired pneumonia severity on presentation to hospital: An international derivation and validation study. Thorax 58:377–382, 2003.

8. **What factors determine whether a patient with CAP needs admission to the ICU?**

As with the admission decision, there is no absolute rule to define who should be admitted to the ICU, but generally 10–20% of all hospitalized CAP patients require intensive care, with the highest rates being present in the elderly or in those with serious comorbid illness. ICU admission should be considered if patients have at least one of two major criteria or one of two minor criteria.

- The **major criteria**, which can be present on admission or later in the hospital course, include need for mechanical ventilation or septic shock.
- The **minor criteria** present on admission are systolic blood pressure < 90 mmHg, a PaO_2/FiO_2 ratio <250, or multilobar infiltrates.

As discussed above, another way to identify patients with more severe illness is to apply the CURB-65 criteria, considering ICU admission for patients with at least three of the five features present. There is some debate about the benefit of ICU care for patients with CAP, but the benefit seems most certain if patients are admitted early in the course of severe illness, thus emphasizing the need for sensitive criteria to define severe illness. The measurement of admission respiratory rate is a simple and reliable assessment, and in one study, investigators observed a linear relationship between admission respiratory rate (once it rose >30 breaths/min) and mortality.

Ewig S, De roux A, Bauer T, et al: Validation of predictive rules and indices of severity for community acquired pneumonia. Thorax 59:421–427, 2004.

9. **Is there a different pathogen profile in severe community-acquired pheumonia?**

Yes. As in all patients with community-acquired pneumonia, *Streptococcus pneumoniae* is still the most common pathogen, but in the clinical setting of severe infection, *Legionella* species or other atypical pathogens, *H. influenzae*, and enteric gram-negative bacilli play a greater role. This concept guides the selection of the initial antibiotic treatment regimen. *Legionella pneumophila* is more common in smokers, alcoholics, and patients presenting with multiorgan failure; it is particularly common in patients who present with acute respiratory failure requiring mechanical ventilation. Mortality from *Legionella pneumophila* is doubled if the disease is not treated rapidly and appropriately (i.e., with macrolide or quinolone).

The increased incidence of gram-negative bacilli may be, in part, caused by the patient population who are predisposed to severe community-acquired pneumonia, namely the elderly and the chronically ill. Patients who develop severe pneumonia while in a nursing home have a high frequency of infection with gram-negatives, especially if they have severe functional impairment. *Pseudomonas aeruginosa* has been identified as causing severe community-acquired pneumonia, accounting for 10–20% of all cases, but risk factors (i.e., bronchiectasis, prior antibiotics, or corticosteroids) are usually present.

Ruiz M, Ewig S, Marcos MA, et al: Etiology of community-acquired pneumonia: Impact of age, comorbidity, and severity. Am J Respir Crit Care Med 160:397–405, 1999.

Ruiz M, Ewig S, Torres A, et al: Severe community-acquired pneumonia: Risk factors and follow-up epidemiology. Am J Respir Crit Care Med 160:923–929, 1999.

10. **Once CAP is suspected, what diagnostic studies are appropriate and beneficial?**

- A thorough **history and physical examination** should be performed.
- **Standard posteroanterior and lateral chest radiographs** should be obtained. The chest radiograph is useful not only to diagnose the pneumonia but also to assess the severity of the disease by looking for complications such as multilobar disease, cavitation, or pleural effusion. A chest radiograph is necessary to establish the diagnosis of pneumonia, even in outpatients, but outpatients rarely need more testing unless they are evaluated for admission to the hospital.

- If there is any question about disease severity, an **assessment of oxygenation** (usually by oximetry, but an arterial blood gas is needed if carbon dioxide retention is suspected) is necessary for all patients, in or out of the hospital.
- Hospitalized patients should have two samples collected for **blood cultures** in addition to blood samples for the routine chemistries and blood counts. Although blood cultures are positive only 15–30% of the time, the presence of bacteremia can define bacteriology and the presence of resistant organisms. Blood cultures are more likely to be positive if the patient has not recently received antibiotic therapy and if severe illness is present. In the absence of signs of severe illness and if antibiotics are present, it may be unnecessary to collect blood cultures since the frequency of false positives may exceed the frequency of true positive results.
- Patients who have risk factors for drug-resistant organisms or unusual pathogens should have a **sputum culture** collected, and a **Gram stain** of the sample should be correlated with the culture data.
- **Routine chemistries and blood counts** can stratify hospitalized patients with regard to risk. For example, extremes of white blood cell count, renal failure, electrolyte abnormalities, and abnormal coagulation profiles (e.g., thrombocytopenia and elevated prothrombin time or partial thromboplastin time) may influence decisions about admission to the ICU.
- **Diagnostic thoracentesis** should be performed to evaluate for empyema in patients who have pleural effusion associated with pneumonia because this test defines a patient population who will have a complicated course and may require drainage procedures in addition to antibiotics.

Metersky ML, Ma A, Bratzler DW, Houck PM: Predicting bacteremia in patients with community-acquired pneumonia. Am J Respir Crit Care Med 169:342–347, 2004.

Niederman MS, Mandell LA, Anzueto A, et al: Guidelines for the management of adults with community-acquired lower respiratory tract infections: Diagnosis, assessment of severity, antimicrobial therapy and prevention. Am J Respir Crit Care Med 163, 1730–1754, 2001.

KEY POINTS: DIAGNOSTIC TESTS FOR INPATIENTS WITH CAP

1. **Chest radiograph**

2. **Assess oxygenation:** Oximetry or blood gas

3. **Routine blood work:** Complete blood cell count, chemistry

4. **Blood cultures:** If there is severe illness or no outpatient antibiotics

5. **Sputum culture:** If drug resistance or unusual pathogens are suspected

11. **Considering that no clear pathogen is identified in most patients with CAP, how is therapy initiated?**

Therapy should be empirical and based on the likelihood of certain pathogens being found in a given patient population (Table 25-2). There are four patient categories for empirical therapy (Table 25-3) based on the age of the patient, the need for hospitalization, the severity of pneumonia, and the presence of cardiopulmonary disease or modifying factors (i.e., the risk factors for specific pathogens, listed in Table 25-2).

Niederman MS, Mandell LA, Anzueto A, et al: Guidelines for the management of adults with community-acquired lower respiratory tract infections: Diagnosis, assessment of severity, antimicrobial therapy and prevention. Am J Respir Crit Care Med 163:1730–1754, 2001.

TABLE 25-2. MODIFYING FACTORS THAT INCREASE THE RISK OF INFECTION WITH SPECIFIC PATHOGENS

Penicillin-Resistant and Drug-Resistant Pneumococci	Enteric Gram-Negative Bacteria
Age > 65 years	Residence in a nursing home
Beta-lactam therapy within the past 3 months	Underlying cardiopulmonary disease
Alcoholism	Multiple medical comorbidities
Multiple medical comorbidities	Recent antibiotic therapy
Immune suppressive illness (including therapy with corticosteroids)	***Pseudomonas aeruginosa***
	Structural lung disease (i.e., bronchiectasis)
	Exposure to a child in a day-care center
	Corticosteroid therapy (>10 mg prednisone/day)
	Broad-spectrum antibiotic therapy for >7 days in the past month
	Malnutrition

TABLE 25-3. EMPIRICAL THERAPY FOR COMMUNITY-ACQUIRED PNEUMONIA

Outpatients with No Cardiopulmonary Disease and No Modifying Factors

Organisms	*S. pneumoniae* *M. pneumoniae* *C. pneumoniae* (alone or as mixed infection) *H. influenzae* Respiratory viruses Miscellaneous *Legionella* species, *Mycobacterium tuberculosis*, endemic fungi
Therapy	Advanced generation macrolide (azithromycin or clarithromycin) Doxycycline

Outpatients with Cardiopulmonary Disease or Modifying Factors

Organisms	*S. pneumoniae* (including drug-resistant *S. pneumoniae* [DRSP]) *M. pneumoniae* *C. pneumoniae* Mixed infection (bacteria plus atypical pathogen or virus) *H. influenzae* Enteric gram-negative organisms Respiratory viruses Miscellaneous

Continued

TABLE 25–3. EMPIRICAL THERAPY FOR COMMUNITY-ACQUIRED PNEUMONIA—CONT'D

	Moraxella catarrhalis, Legionella species, aspiration (anaerobes), *M. tuberculosis,* endemic fungi
Therapy (in no particular order)	Beta-lactam (i.e., oral cefpodoxime, cefuroxime, high-dose amoxicillin, amoxicillin/clavulanate, or parenteral ceftriaxone followed by oral cefpodoxime) plus macrolide or doxycycline
	Antipneumococcal fluoroquinolone (e.g., gatifloxacin, gemifloxacin, levofloxacin, moxifloxacin) used alone
	A ketolide (e.g., telithromycin) may be used as monotherapy if there is no concern for enteric gram-negative organisms

Inpatients Not in the ICU

(a) With cardiopulmonary disease or modifying factors (including residence in nursing home)

Organisms	*S. pneumoniae* (including DRSP)
	H. influenzae
	M. pneumoniae
	C. pneumoniae
	Mixed infection (bacteria plus an atypical pathogen)
	Enteric gram-negative organisms
	Aspiration (anaerobes)
	Viruses
	Legionella species
	Miscellaneous (*M. tuberculosis*, endemic fungi, or *Pneumocystis carinii*)
Therapy (in no particular order)	Intravenous beta-lactam (e.g., cefotaxime, ceftriaxone, ampicillin/sulbactam, or high-dose ampicillin) plus intravenous or oral macrolide or doxycycline
	Intravenous antipneumococcal fluoroquinolone alone (e.g., gatifloxacin, levofloxacin, or moxifloxacin)

(b) No cardiopulmonary disease and no modifying factors

Organisms	Same as above, but with DRSP, gram-negatives are less likely
Therapy	Intravenous azithromycin alone
	If macrolide allergic or intolerant, doxycycline and a beta-lactam or monotherapy with an antipneumococcal fluoroquinolone

Patients in the ICU

(a) No risks for Pseudomonas aeruginosa

Organisms	*S. pneumoniae* (including DRSP)
	Legionella species
	H. influenzae
	Enteric gram-negative bacilli

TABLE 25-3.   EMPIRICAL THERAPY FOR COMMUNITY-ACQUIRED PNEUMONIA—CONT'D

	S. aureus *M. pneumoniae* Respiratory viruses Miscellaneous (*C. pneumoniae, M. tuberculosis*, endemic fungi)
Therapy (in no particular order)	Intravenous beta-lactam (cefotaxime, ceftriaxone) plus either an intravenous macrolide (e.g., azithromycin) or intravenous fluoroquinolone (e.g., gatifloxacin, levofloxacin, or moxifloxacin)
(b) Risks for Pseudomonas aeruginosa	
Organisms	All of the above organisms plus *Pseudomonas aeruginosa*
Therapy (in no particular order)	*Combination therapy required* Selected intravenous antipseudomonal beta-lactam (i.e., cefepime, imipenem, meropenem, or piperacillin/tazobactam) plus intravenous antipseudomonal quinolone (i.e., ciprofloxacin) Selected intravenous antipseudomonal beta-lactam (i.e., cefepime, imipenem, meropenem, or piperacillin/tazobactam) plus aminoglycoside plus either intravenous macrolide (i.e., azithromycin) or intravenous nonpseudomonal fluoroquinolone

12. **Are there any benefits of one empirical antibiotic regimen over another?**
    In hospitalized elderly patients, a regimen that provides coverage for bacterial pathogens as well as atypical pathogens seems to lead to better outcomes, including reduced mortality, when compared to beta-lactam monotherapy. In a recent study of 12,945 inpatients aged 65 years or older, using a nonantipseudomonal third-generation cephalosporin as a comparator, three antimicrobial regimens were associated with a lower 30-day mortality rate: (1) a second-generation cephalosporin plus a macrolide, (2) a nonantipseudomonal third-generation cephalosporin plus a macrolide, or (3) monotherapy with a fluoroquinolone. Two other antibiotic regimens were associated with an increased 30-day mortality rate: (1) a beta-lactam/beta-lactamase inhibitor plus a macrolide, and (2) an aminoglycoside plus any other agent. These data applied only to elderly patients, but more recent studies have corroborated that the addition of a macrolide to therapy with a beta-lactam is associated with reduced mortality, even in younger hospitalized patients. The mechanism for benefit of such therapy is uncertain, but it may be related to therapy of atypical pathogen coinfection, a finding that is present, in some studies, in up to 40% of all hospitalized CAP patients.

    Brown RB, Iannini P, Gross P, Kunkel M: Impact of initial antibiotic choice on clinical outcomes in community-acquired pneumonia: Analysis of a hospital claims-made database. Chest 123:1503–1511, 2003.
    Gleason PP, Meehan TP, Fine JM, et al: Associations between initial antimicrobial therapy and medical outcomes for hospitalized elderly patients with pneumonia. Arch Intern Med 159:2562–2572, 1999.

13. **Which patient population can be treated with beta-lactam monotherapy?**
    According to recent North American guidelines, monotherapy with a beta-lactam is not recommended as empirical therapy for any outpatient or inpatient population with CAP. This is related to the finding that atypical pathogens, either as primary infectors or as coinfecting pathogens, are common in all patients with CAP. If monotherapy is done, it is generally in selected populations using either a macrolide, a ketolide, or quinolone, but not a beta-lactam (i.e., penicillin or cephalosporin).

There is still controversy about whether beta-lactam monotherapy can be used after a bacterial pathogen is identified with diagnostic testing. Several studies of pneumococcal pneumonia with bacteremia have shown that initial therapy with a combination regimen (generally including a macrolide or quinolone, along with a beta-lactam) leads to reduced mortality compared to monotherapy with a beta-lactam. The reason for this benefit has not been explained, and it is still unclear if changing from an initial combination regimen to monotherapy after the results of cultures are known is acceptable, or if this approach is also associated with increased mortality.

Martinez JA, Horcajada JP, Almela M, et al: Addition of a macrolide to a β-lactam-based empirical antibiotic regimen is associated with lower in-patient mortality for patients with bacteremic pneumococcal pneumonia. Clin Infect Dis 36: 389–395, 2003.

KEY POINTS: PRINCIPLES OF INPATIENT THERAPY

1. Give the first dose of antibiotics within 4 hours of arrival to the hospital.

2. No beta-lactam monotherapy as empirical therapy.

3. Limit macrolide monotherapy to patients without risks for drug-resistant pneumococcus or enteric gram-negative organisms.

4. No quinolone monotherapy for ICU-admitted patients.

5. For non-ICU patients, quinolone monotherapy is equivalent to a beta-lactam/macrolide combination.

14. **When is *S. pneumoniae* considered to be penicillin resistant?**
S. pneumoniae penicillin resistance is defined on the basis of a minimal inhibitory concentration (MIC), which is the lowest antibiotic concentration that inhibits visible growth after 18–24 hours of incubation. For infections caused by *S. pneumoniae* that do not involve the meninges, a penicillin MIC of 2.0 mg/L or more is considered to be highly resistant. If the MIC is 0.1–1.0 mg/L, *S. pneumoniae* is intermediately resistant to penicillin. Although as many as 40% of pneumococci are resistant, by these definitions, clinically relevant resistance has been defined as MIC values to penicillin of 4 mg/L or greater, and this degree of resistance is rare in the United States.

Patients at risk for penicillin-resistant pneumococci are those older than 65 years, those with a history of beta-lactam therapy in the past 3 months, those with a history of alcoholism or multiple medical comorbidities, and those with exposure to a child in day care. Penicillin resistance is often multidrug resistance, and recent usage of macrolides or quinolones can lead to macrolide-resistant or quinolone-resistant pneumococci, respectively.

Clavo-Sanchez AJ, Giron-Gonzalez JA, Lopez-Prieto D, et al: Multivariate analysis of risk factors for infection due to penicillin-resistant and multidrug resistant *Streptococcus pneumoniae*: A multicenter study. Clin Infect Dis 24:1052–1059, 1997.

15. **If penicillin-resistant *S. pneumoniae* is the cause of CAP, how should it be treated?**
Antibiotic treatment should be highly active, even if intermediate-level resistance is present, in order to rapidly and completely kill the organism. At current levels of resistance, many therapies (including penicillins and macrolides) may be effective, provided that high enough doses are used and provided that the drug penetrates well to the site of infection (as is the case with macrolides). In pneumococcal bacteremia, good outcomes can occur even if therapy is discordant with culture results, with a notable exception being therapy with cefuroxime. When empiric therapy includes a third generation cephalosporin (i.e., cefotaxime or ceftriaxone), outcome is generally good, even with *in vitro* resistance. With severe infection, ceftriaxone can be dosed up

to 2 grams every 12 hours. Another reliable therapy if resistance is suspected is monotherapy with a quinolone, with the agents ranking from least to most active (on an MIC basis) as follows: ciprofloxacin, levofloxacin, gatifloxacin, moxifloxacin, and gemifloxacin. If *S. pneumoniae* is highly resistant to both penicillins and cephalosporins, alternative therapy should be with a quinolone, vancomycin, or a carbapenem. The oxazolidinone linezolid may also be effective against resistant pneumococci, but this agent is best reserved for nosocomial infections due to resistant gram-positive organisms.

Lujan ML, Gallego M, Fontanals D, et al: Prospective observational study of bacteremic pneumococcal pneumonia: Effect of discordant therapy on mortality. Crit Care Med 32:625–631, 2004.

Yu VL, Chiou CC, Feldman C, Ortqvist A, et al: An international prospective study of pneumococcal bacteremia: Correlation with in vitro resistance, antibiotics administered, and clinical outcome. Clin Infect Dis 37:230–237, 2003.

16. **Is pneumococcal resistance to macrolides common in CAP? Is it clinically relevant?**

    More than 30% of pneumococci can be resistant to macrolides *in vitro,* but there are two types of resistance, each involving different mechanisms. In the United States, the most common type of resistance is due to an efflux mechanism, meaning that the drug enters the bacteria and then is pumped out. Usage patterns have increased this form of resistance, but it is generally a low level of resistance that does not lead to poor outcomes and can be overcome by good penetration of macrolides into respiratory sites of infection.

    The other form of resistance is due to altered binding to the ribosomal site of action, which results in a high level of resistance that may be clinically important and cannot be overcome by penetration or by proper dosing. In spite of these findings, reports of macrolide failures in CAP are uncommon, but currently these drugs are being used most often as part of a combination regimen rather than as monotherapy. Monotherapy should be limited only to patients with no risk factors for infection with resistant pneumococci or enteric gram-negatives.

    Lonks JR, Garau J, Gomez L, et al: Failure of macrolide antibiotic treatment in patients with bacteremia due to erythromycin-resistant Streptococcus pneumoniae. Clin Infect Dis 35:556–564, 2002.

17. **When a patient with CAP is admitted to the hospital, how rapidly should therapy be started?**

    Several studies have examined the impact of rapid therapy on the outcomes of patients with CAP. These studies have included only Medicare patients, but the findings have been extended to all hospitalized patients with CAP, and the data show a reduction in mortality if therapy is begun within 4 hours of the patient's arrival in the emergency department. If diagnostic testing is to be done, it should precede the initiation of therapy, but therapy should never be delayed to allow for testing. In general, therapy is given more rapidly when patients are more severely ill, but efforts at prompt therapy can reduce mortality. The best way to achieve rapid initiation of therapy is unclear, but ideally the diagnosis of pneumonia should be established rapidly by chest radiography in order to facilitate timely therapy.

    Houck PM, Bratzler DW, Nsa W, et al: Timing of antibiotic administration and outcomes for Medicare patients hospitalized with community-acquired pneumonia. Arch Intern Med 164:637–644, 2004.

18. **Can an admitted patient with CAP be treated with only oral antibiotics?**

    Most admitted patients are given initial therapy intravenously, and this should be the general practice since intravenous therapy is reliable when oral absorption is erratic (as can occur with hypotension or dehydration) and is potentially valuable if patients have bacteremia. However, oral therapy with a quinolone may be as effective as intravenous therapy, even with bacteremia, provided that the therapy is adequately absorbed, since these agents are highly bioavailable and can achieve the same serum levels orally and intravenously. When oral therapy has been used in place of intravenous therapy, it has led to good outcomes and a reduced length of stay. Candidates for exclusively oral therapy have generally been those with less severe illness who are younger and have fewer abnormalities in mental status than those treated with intravenous therapy.

Marras TK, Nopmaneejumruslers C, Chan CKN: Efficacy of exclusively oral antibiotic therapy in patients hospitalized with nonsevere community-acquired pneumonia: A retrospective study and meta-analysis. Am J Med 116:385–393, 2004.

19. How long should therapy for CAP be continued?

Traditionally, the duration of therapy has been 7–14 days, but many recent studies have suggested that shorter duration is possible and is equally effective. Most patients with CAP become clinically stable very rapidly, and in the hospital, vital sign abnormalities (i.e., in heart rate, respiratory rate, blood pressure, or temperature) usually normalize in 2–3 days, allowing a switch from intravenous to oral therapy. Prolonged therapy after reaching clinical stability is probably not necessary, and durations as short as 3 days with azithromycin in outpatients and 5 days with high-dose levofloxacin have been effective. Even with *Legionella* infection, quinolone therapy for 5–7 days has been effective.

Although the optimal duration of therapy has not been defined, a reasonable approach is to aim for a 5- to 7-day duration of therapy, assuring that medication is continued for at least 48–72 hours after the patient is afebrile and for a minimum of 5 days total. Even with bacteremia, short-duration therapy is possible if the patient has a good clinical response. Some pathogens may not be effectively treated with short-duration therapy, including *Staphylococcus aureus* and *Pseudomonas aeruginosa*. In addition, those with extrapulmonary infection (i.e., meningitis or empyema) may require longer durations of therapy.

Dunbar LM, Wunderink RG, Habib MP, et al: High-dose, short-course levofloxacin for community-acquired pneumonia: A new treatment paradigm. Clin Infect Dis 37:752–760, 2003.

Halm EA, Fine MJ, Marrie TJ, et al: Time to clinical stability in patients hospitalized with community-acquired pneumonia: Implications for practice guidelines. JAMA 279:1452–1457, 1998.

20. How are patients on empirical antibiotic therapy monitored?

Effective antibiotic therapy should improve clinical features of pneumonia in 48–72 hours. This is key to empiric therapy because antibiotics should not be changed within this time frame unless the patient has a marked clinical deterioration. Fever can continue for 2–4 days, and leukocytosis may persist until day 4, even with appropriate antibiotic therapy. With these concepts in mind, the clinician must try to determine the cause of the treatment failure. Several factors cause clinical deterioration in a patient on empirical antibiotics, including the presence of an unusual (e.g., tuberculosis or an endemic fungus) or drug-resistant pathogen, a disease process that mimics pneumonia (e.g., pulmonary embolus, congestive heart failure, bronchoalveolar cell carcinoma, or bronchiolitis obliterans with organizing pneumonia), the development of a complication (e.g., nosocomial infection, empyema, pulmonary embolus, or antibiotic-induced colitis), or the presence of a comorbid illness or therapy that leads to an inadequate host response (such as corticosteroid therapy).

In these patients, an aggressive diagnostic work-up is necessary, including further radiologic testing and, often, bronchoscopic sampling of the lower respiratory tract. A computed tomography (CT) scan of the chest may reveal cavities, effusions, or other findings that were not detectable by the standard chest radiograph. Microbiologic studies including sputum culture and possibly bronchoscopic quantitative cultures may define the presence of resistant and unusual pathogens.

Roson B, Carratala J, Fernandez-Sabe N, et al: Causes and factors associated with early failure in hospitalized patients with community-acquired pneumonia. Arch Intern Med 164:502–508, 2004.

21. Are invasive diagnostic tests indicated in the routine management of CAP?

Not usually. Invasive diagnostic tests include transtracheal aspiration, transthoracic needle aspiration, bronchoscopy, and open-lung biopsy. Only those patients who fail initial therapy should be considered for aggressive diagnostic testing, and more than 85% of patients respond to initial empirical therapy. Of the invasive tests mentioned, bronchoscopy with quantitative cultures is the most sensitive and most commonly performed test. Open-lung biopsy may be helpful but should be reserved only for nonresponding patients, especially when a pneumonia mimic is suspected.

Rello J, Bodi M, Mariscal D, et al: Microbiological testing and outcome of patients with severe community-acquired pneumonia. Chest 123:174-180, 2003.

22. **What are the causes of slowly resolving lung infiltrates in patients suspected of having CAP?**
See Table 25-4.

TABLE 25-4.	CAUSES OF SLOWLY RESOLVING LUNG INFILATRATES
Infectious	**Noninfectious (Pneumonia Mimics)**
Usual infectious causes	***Neoplasm***
Pneumococcus	Bronchogenic carcinoma
Legionella species	Lymphoma
H. influenzae	***Immunologic and idiopathic***
Virus	Lupus pneumonitis
Unusual infectious causes	Wegener's granulomatosis
Tuberculosis	Bronchiolitis obliterans-organizing
Atypical mycobacteria	pneumonia (BOOP)
Nocardia species	***Drug-induced lung injury***
Actinomyces species	Amiodarone toxicity
Aspergillus species	
Endemic fungi	

23. **When should a follow-up chest radiograph be done in a patient with CAP?**
If the patient is having a good clinical response to therapy, it is not necessary to repeat the chest x-ray for at least 4 weeks, but in a nonresponding patient, the radiograph should be repeated as soon as a failure to respond is identified. In the immunocompetent host, there should be at least a 50% clearing of the radiograph at 4 weeks if the the patient has had a symptomatic improvement on therapy. With pneumococcal pneumonia, 50% of patients have radiographic clearing at 5 weeks, and the majority clear in 2–3 months, but if bacteremia is present, it takes up to 9 weeks for 50% to have a clear chest radiograph, and most are clear by 18 weeks.

Factors that affect the rate of radiographic clearing include (1) underlying chronic diseases, with slower clearance in patients with chronic obstructive pulmonary disease (COPD), congestive heart failure, renal failure, or alcoholism; (2) the identity of the causative pathogens, with slower resolution being common with *Legionella, S. aureus,* and enteric gram-negative organisms; (3) the severity of pneumonia, with delayed clearing in patients with bacteremia or multilobar illness; (4) smoking history; and (5) age >55 years. Radiographic clearance decreases by 20% per decade after age 20.

El Solh AA, Aquilina AT, Gunen H, Ramadan F: Radiographic resolution of community-acquired bacterial pneumonia in the elderly. J Am Geriatr Soc 52:224–229, 2004.

CONTROVERSY

24. **Should sputum Gram stain be used routinely in the management of CAP?**

     Pros: The sputum Gram stain is a simple diagnostic test that can be performed easily and inter-
     preted more rapidly than any other diagnostic test used in pneumonia patients. It is relatively
     inexpensive and can be used to guide initial antibiotic therapy. If pneumococcus is identified on
     the stain, initial antibiotic therapy could possibly be focused, instead of broad-spectrum, giving
     the theoretical advantage of not promoting bacterial resistance. The Gram stain also can help
     indicate patients who may be infected by unsuspected, high-risk pathogens (e.g., *S. aureus* and
     gram-negative bacilli), thereby alerting the clinician early to their presence and guiding initial
     therapy.

     Cons: Although the sputum Gram stain can theoretically yield useful information in selected
     patients, its routine use has several limitations. One such limitation is the fact that 40% of
     patients with CAP cannot produce sputum. When sputum can be produced, specimens are
     almost always obtained by untrained individuals who collect nonpurulent samples that have little
     to no diagnostic usefulness. This sampling issue is further hindered by the fact that 30–45% of
     CAP patients are already on antibiotics before hospitalization. The diagnostic yield in this patient
     population is reduced. To illustrate these issues, in one recent study, the practical limitations of
     the test were clear: out of 116 patients with CAP, only 42 could produce a sputum sample. Of
     these, 23 were valid, and only 10 samples were diagnostic, with antibiotics directed to the diag-
     nostic result in only 1 patient.

     In the patient who has not been on antibiotics, another limitation to the Gram stain's useful-
     ness is in its interpretation. Unless collected and interpreted by skilled personnel, the sputum
     Gram stain lacks adequate sensitivity and diagnostic usefulness. In the majority of cases, the
     individual interpreting the sample is either inexperienced or has no clinical information to go
     with the sample. More recently, data have shown that even if bacterial infection is present, atypi-
     cal pathogen coinfection may exist, negating the ability of a Gram stain to help focus therapy.

     Ewig S, Schlochtermeier M, Goke N, Niederman MS: Applying sputum as a diagnostic tool in pneumonia:
     Limited yield, minimal impact on treatment decisions. Chest 121:1486–1492, 2002.

CHAPTER 26

NOSOCOMIAL PNEUMONIA

Richard G. Wunderink, MD

1. **Define nosocomial pneumonia.**
   Nosocomial pneumonia (NP), often called hospital-acquired pneumonia (HAP), is a pneumonia that develops 48 hours or more after admission to the hospital. It is the second-most-common hospital-acquired infection but is responsible for the highest mortality rate of all the nosocomial infections. Crude mortality rates range from 50–70%, and attributed mortality rates, or deaths resulting directly from infection, range from 30–50%.

   American Thoracic Society, Infectious Diseases Society of America: Guidelines for the management of adults with hospital-acquired, ventilator-associated, and healthcare-associated pneumonia. Am J Respir Crit Care Med 171:388–416, 2005.

2. **Are there different types of NP?**
   Most cases of NP occur in the intensive care unit (ICU). Those that occur outside the ICU may be different from those that occur in the ICU. Ventilator-associated pneumonia (VAP) refers specifically to pneumonia that develops in patients receiving mechanical ventilation. Most research has focused on NP in the ICU, especially VAP. The understanding of nosocomial pneumonia is derived mainly from VAP studies.

3. **What are the causative organisms of the various types of NP?**
   Two patterns of pathogens are seen in NP. The first group resembles the spectrum seen in community-acquired pneumonia (CAP), including *Streptococcus pneumoniae* and other streptococcal species, *Haemophilus influenzae*, methicillin-sensitive *Staphylococcus aureus* (MSSA), and, occasionally, anaerobes. The other group includes multidrug-resistant Enterobacteriaceae, *Acinetobacter* spp., *Pseudomonas aeruginosa*, and methicillin-resistant *S. aureus* (MRSA).

4. **How can you distinguish between the two groups of microorganisms?**
   Two factors are the primary determinants of the microbiologic spectrum of HAP. By far, the most important is prior exposure to antibiotics. Microorganisms in the first group are usually sensitive to most antibiotics, especially parenteral. However, even outpatient treatment with oral antibiotics can increase the risk of *Pseudomonas* and MRSA. The second-most-important risk factor is the duration of time in the hospital, especially the duration of time on mechanical ventilation. In addition to increasing the likelihood of antibiotic exposure, increasing the length of hospitalization increases the risk of cross-infection from other patients who are infected or colonized with these antibiotic-resistant pathogens.

5. **How can you prevent NP?**
   Understanding the pathogenesis is vital in attempts to prevent NP. Three factors are critical in the pathogenesis of VAP: colonization of the oropharynx with pathogenic microorganisms, aspiration of these secretions from the oropharynx into the lower respiratory tract, and the compromise of the normal host defense mechanisms. Most of the risk factors associated with nosocomial pneumonia affect one of these three factors.

   The most obvious is the use of an endotracheal tube (ETT), which bypasses the normal mechanical factors preventing aspiration, including closure of the vocal cords during swallowing and an effective cough. This factor alone explains much of the higher incidence of pneumonia in ventilated patients.

6. **Will placement of an ETT prevent aspiration?**
No. An ETT can prevent large-volume aspiration but allows microaspiration. The actual process of endotracheal intubation increases the risk of aspiration at the time of the procedure. This is felt to be a major mechanism in the pneumonias occurring in the first 48 hours of mechanical ventilation. The need for reintubation has also been found to be a risk factor for VAP, with the suggestion that aspiration at the time of reintubation is partially responsible.

7. **What is meant by microaspiration?**
An ETT predisposes the patient to microaspiration by holding open the vocal cords yet not totally occluding the airway, allowing small amounts of oral secretions to pass below the vocal cords. These infected secretions pool in the trachea above the inflated cuff of the ETT. Movement of the ETT allows small amounts of these secretions to pass around it. These movements of the ETT occur routinely in the usual care of patients, caused by movements such as turning the head from side to side or coughing. Since these secretions contain large numbers (i.e., 10^8–10^{10} colony-forming units [CFU] per milliliter) of bacteria, a large inoculum of bacteria actually enters the lower respiratory tract. If the normal host defense mechanisms are also compromised, this inoculum can rapidly develop into VAP.

8. **What can be done to prevent the microaspiration?**
Evidence that microaspiration is an important mechanism causing VAP comes from studies using a specially modified ETT with a suctioning port above the ETT cuff. Use of this special ETT for continuous aspiration of subglottic secretions has been proven to significantly decrease the incidence of early-onset VAP, although its use is not widespread. Additional evidence for the importance of aspiration around an ETT comes from a randomized controlled trial demonstrating that ventilating patients in the semirecumbent position is associated with fewer episodes of pneumonia than ventilating them in the supine position. Infrequent changing of ventilator tubing, use of heat and moisture exchangers rather than humidification systems, and avoiding transporting ventilated patients outside the ICU may also help.

  Kollef MH: The prevention of ventilator-associated pneumonia. N Engl J Med 340:627–634, 1999.

9. **How can colonization of the oropharynx be prevented?**
The most important factor preventing colonization of an individual patient is avoidance of antibiotic therapy. Many nosocomial pathogens require disruption of the normal flora to establish colonization. Management strategies that minimize antibiotic use consistently show lower associated mortality.
  In addition, colonization can occur by cross-contamination from another infected patient. Routine hand washing, barrier precautions, isolation precautions, and other infection control techniques are important in addressing this risk.
  Avoiding gastrointestinal hemorrhage prophylaxis agents that raise gastric pH, such as histamine$_2$ receptor blockers, appears to be less important than previously thought.

10. **What can be done about the problems with normal host defenses?**
This aspect of prevention has received the least investigation. Prudent strategies at this point include tight glycemic control and minimizing blood transfusions. The risk-to-benefit ratio of drugs with immunosuppressive properties, such as high-dose corticosteroids, should always be considered.

11. **Anything else?**
The risk of VAP increases almost linearly with the duration of ventilation. Therefore, anything that decreases the duration of ventilation, or even avoids the need for ventilation, decreases the

risk of VAP. Use of noninvasive ventilation has been shown to decrease the incidence of NP in patients admitted for chronic obstructive pulmonary disease (COPD) exacerbations or CAP. Sedation and ventilator weaning strategies that shorten the overall duration of ventilation have also been demonstrated to decrease VAP rates.

12. **How do you diagnose nosocomial pneumonia?**
Pneumonia is suspected by the presence of either new or changing radiographic infiltrates and evidence of systemic inflammation such as fever or leukocytosis. The presence of increased or purulent secretions directs attention to the lung as the source of fever. However, especially in the ventilated patient, these signs and symptoms are very nonspecific and consistently lead to over-diagnosis of pneumonia. This finding has led to tremendous uncertainty and controversy regarding the optimal way to confirm the presence of NP, especially VAP.

13. **Why is it difficult to accurately diagnose VAP?**
Because of the frequent use of other invasive devices, ventilated patients have multiple other potential sites of infection that can also lead to leukocytosis and fever. The aspiration mentioned above can lead to increased tracheal secretions. Oropharyngeal colonization by pathogenic organisms results in positive cultures of endotracheal aspirates. Even chest radiographic changes can be caused by multiple other clinical entities common in ventilated patients.

14. **List some noninfectious causes of pulmonary infiltrates that may mimic NP.**
   - Pulmonary edema
   - Lung contusion
   - Pulmonary hemorrhage
   - Acute respiratory distress syndrome (ARDS)
   - Atelectasis
   - Pulmonary embolus, with or without infarction
   - Pleural effusion
   - Acute eosinophilic pneumonia
   - Chemical pneumonitis from aspiration
   - Infiltrative tumor
   - Radiation pneumonitis

   In intubated patients, noninfectious causes of pulmonary densities can coexist with an extra pulmonary source of fever, thereby simulating pneumonia.

   Meduri GU, Maudlin GL, Wunderink RG, et al: Cases of fever and pulmonary densities in patients with clinical manifestations of ventilator-associated pneumonia. Chest 106:221–235, 1994.

15. **How can pneumonia be differentiated from all these other diseases?**
Several types of tests can confirm the presence of VAP. A positive blood or pleural fluid culture is strong confirmation. However, in up to 50% of ICU patients with a positive blood culture and an abnormal x-ray, another focus of infection is the source of the bacteremia. More importantly, the incidence of bacteremic VAP is $\leq$ 15%, and the incidence of empyema in nosocomial pneumonia is extremely low. Therefore, confirmation of NP usually relies on a lower respiratory tract culture. The unreliability of usual cultures of expectorated sputum and endotracheal aspirates has generated interest in the use of quantitative cultures (QCs), especially for the confirmation of the diagnosis of VAP. For nonintubated patients, bronchoscopic QCs or percutaneous lung aspirates are rarely used, and the majority of patients are treated empirically.

16. **What is the rationale for QCs?**
Simplistically, infection is more likely the higher the density of microorganisms in a particular space. Several studies have demonstrated that QCs of lower respiratory tract secretions increase for several days prior to the development of clinical manifestations of pneumonia, suggesting that a critical density must be reached in order to cause clinical infection. A certain

threshold, usually $>10^3$–10^4 CFU/mL, is therefore used in order to separate true infection from colonization.

17. **Do low QCs always mean that pneumonia is not present?**
The density of microorganisms in pneumonia is dynamic. The same inflammatory mediator release and alveolar capillary leak that lead to the clinical manifestations of fever and radiographic infiltrates are part of the normal host defense against infection. This host response can cause a dramatic decline in the density of microorganisms before even simple cultures can be obtained. Therefore, QC results are probably better thought of as a scorecard in the battle between the invading microorganisms and the normal host defenses—high QCs mean the pathogens are winning, and low colony counts suggest the defenders are mounting an adequate response.

18. **Are there any other advantages of QCs techniques?**
Many of the QC methods bypass the central airways in order to access the uncontaminated lower respiratory tract rather than tracheal secretions for culture. Bronchoscopic bronchoalveolar lavage (BAL) and protected specimen brush (PSB) accomplish this most reliably, but even studies of tracheal aspirate QCs emphasize obtaining specimens from as deep as possible in the respiratory tract.
Many of the techniques also employ a method to protect the sampling site from contamination by central secretions during passage to the peripheral airway. These can either be mechanical, such as the catheter within a catheter or the use of a distal plug with the PSB, or technical, such as the avoidance of suctioning through the channel for bronchoscopic BAL.

19. **List some of the most commonly used QC techniques.**
    1. Bronchoscopic
        Bronchoalveolar lavage
        Protected specimen brush
    2. Deep tracheal aspirates
    3. Nonbronchoscopic catheters
        Proximal sampling (e.g., BAL-Cath)
        Distal sampling, mini-BAL (e.g., Combicath)
    4. Nonbronchoscopic protected specimen brush

20. **What are the disadvantages of QC techniques?**
The greatest difficulty with QC methods is the effect of recent initiation of new antibiotics. If the new antibiotic regimen even partially covers the causative microorganism, the QC may be below threshold or even sterile. Optimal use of QCs therefore requires testing prior to any change of antibiotics. The nondirected, nonbronchoscopic techniques sample only the right lung in >85% of cases, potentially leading to sampling errors. VAP has a patchy distribution in many patients, and the limited sampling of the PSB may cause false-negative tests. Localizing pneumonia in a patient with the diffuse infiltrates of ARDS is also difficult and may require bilateral sampling. However, the greatest problem with QCs is when antibiotic therapy is not based on the results of the testing, exposing the patient to the minor risks (i.e., bleeding and hypoxemia) and costs of the QC without any of the potential benefits.

21. **Is there really any advantage of QCs compared with the usual clinical diagnosis of VAP?**
A large, multicenter, randomized trial of bronchoscopic QCs, compared to the strategy usually used in the United States (based on nonquantitative tracheal aspirate cultures), demonstrated a survival benefit with the use of QCs. QCs were also associated with significantly less antibiotic use, fewer inappropriate antibiotic choices, and a greater diagnostic rate for nonpulmonary sources of infection. This study confirms both the theoretical benefits of QCs and the findings of earlier nonrandomized trials.

Fagon JY, Chastre J, Wolff M, et al: Invasive and noninvasive strategies for management of suspected ventilator-associated pneumonia: A randomized trial. Ann Intern Med 132:621–630, 2000.

22. **Which is the best QC technique?**

Two randomized trials comparing diagnosis based on QCs of bronchoscopic specimens to QCs of tracheal aspirates did not show a clear advantage of bronchoscopic diagnosis. Therefore, although theoretically the more precise samplings of bronchoscopic techniques are more accurate, the practical differences are so slight that only a very large study could demonstrate a clinical difference between the sampling methods. One of the advantages of nonbronchoscopic sampling is that a trained bronchoscopist is not required, and studies have confirmed that respiratory care practitioners can effectively use nonbronchoscopic techniques.

23. **Is one bronchoscopic technique better than the other?**

Among bronchoscopic techniques, BAL is more sensitive, whereas PSB is more specific. When combined, these two procedures complement each other. Additional tests only available on BAL fluid, such as the percentage of neutrophils and the presence of intracellular bacteria, may increase its value. PSB is particularly valuable in lower-lobe infiltrates or in patients with emphysema, in whom return on BAL fluid is compromised.

24. **Does management of VAP then always require QC diagnosis?**

Principles developed based on the results of research on the diagnosis of VAP can also be used to improve management based on the usual clinical criteria. The first benefit is a greater realization of the possibility of alternative diagnoses in patients suspected of VAP. An aggressive search for alternative diagnoses is indicated in all patients suspected of VAP. The second improvement in clinical diagnosis is increased awareness of the high negative predictive value when no microorganisms are seen on Gram stain of a tracheal aspirate. The third modification is that patients who had a low probability of VAP could be safely treated with short courses (lasting 3 days) of antibiotics. Since it is the resultant antibiotic management, not the diagnostic test itself, that influences the outcome of VAP, use of these principles can improve the management of VAP, even using tracheal aspirate cultures, and potentially can decrease mortality.

Singh N, Rogers P, Atwood CW, et al: Short-course empiric antibiotic therapy for patients with pulmonary infiltrates in the intensive care unit: A proposed solution for indiscriminate antibiotic prescription. Am J Respir Crit Care Med 162:505–511, 2000.

25. **What is the optimal antibiotic treatment for NP?**

The key points in antibiotic therapy of NP start with broad-spectrum therapy to minimize the incidence of inappropriate initial therapy. Once cultures return, the antibiotic regimen should be streamlined to cover only the pathogens detected and should be stopped if no pathogen is cultured. The total course of treatment should also be shortened, especially if clinical signs have resolved. This strategy will address the two physician-controlled factors that have the greatest influence on mortality from VAP: (1) inappropriate initial antibiotic therapy and (2) excessive antibiotic therapy selecting for antibiotic-resistant pathogens.

KEY POINTS: ANTIBIOTIC THERAPY FOR VAP

1. Obtain lower respiratory tract culture.

2. Start broad-spectrum empiric antibiotic therapy.

3. Streamline the regimen to cover only pathogens present on culture.

4. Stop antibiotics if cultures are negative.

5. Stop all treatment after 7–8 days.

26. **What is meant by inappropriate antibiotic therapy?**

    With inappropriate therapy, the pathogen is not sensitive to the chosen antibiotic by in vitro testing. Antibiotic choices may still be inadequate despite being appropriate, based on tissue penetration, pharmacokinetics, and other factors. Using an aminoglycoside alone for *Pseudomonas* VAP is an example of appropriate yet inadequate therapy. These terms are often used synonymously in the literature.

27. **How significant is the problem of inappropriate initial antibiotic therapy for VAP?**

    Inappropriate initial therapy is consistently associated with higher mortality in patients with VAP. Correcting inappropriate initial therapy after culture results are available does not improve outcome. Therefore, broad-spectrum antibiotic therapy initially is recommended. The surprising issue is the frequency of inappropriate initial therapy, with most studies suggesting rates that are 20–50%. Use of a broad-spectrum three-drug regimen can decrease the inappropriate antibiotic rate to as low as 5%.

28. **What patients are at risk for inappropriate initial therapy?**

    Inappropriate antibiotic therapy occurs most often because of either unsuspected causative microorganisms or the presence of antibiotic-resistant strains of the usual suspected microorganisms. The factor most responsible for both is prior antibiotic therapy, especially broad-spectrum antibiotics. The most common causes of VAP in this setting are *Pseudomonas*, *Acinetobacter*, MRSA, and antibiotic-resistant clones of the Enterobacteriaceae family. The spectrum of causative microorganisms and resistance patterns will vary from hospital to hospital and even from ICU to ICU within the same hospital. Empiric antibiotic regimens should therefore be based on data from each individual ICU.

29. **What is the optimal duration of treatment for VAP?**

    A large multicenter trial demonstrated that clinical cure rates for 8 days of treatment were equivalent to those for 14 days of treatment. Caution should be used for *Pseudomonas* VAP since the recurrence rates were higher with shorter courses. However, it is likely that a change in antibiotics is needed anyway if more than 8 days of therapy are needed for *Pseudomonas* VAP. Other studies confirm that shorter courses are equivalent for efficacy and lead to lower superinfection rates, especially with drug-resistant pathogens.

    Chastre J, Wolff M, Fagon JY, et al: Comparison of 8 versus 15 days of antibiotic therapy for ventilator-associated pneumonia in adults: A randomized trial. JAMA 290:2588–2598, 2003.

30. **Should all patients with gram-negative VAP be treated with combination antibiotics?**

    Monotherapy in gram-negative pneumonia may be adequate if *P. aeruginosa* is not involved and if patients have only mild to moderate disease. Even for *Pseudomonas*, combination therapy has not been conclusively demonstrated to be superior. The main indication for combination therapy is avoidance of initial inappropriate empiric therapy. However, *P. aeruginosa* has a remarkable ability to develop resistance during therapy, and clinical failure rates for treatment remain approximately 50%. Many physicians therefore still use combination therapy.

31. **How common is treatment failure in VAP?**

    Because the accurate diagnosis of failure is even more complex than the original diagnosis of VAP, the exact incidence is difficult to determine. In addition to the 50% rate in *Pseudomonas* VAP, failure of therapy consistently occurs in ≥40% of MRSA pneumonias treated with vancomycin. Lower rates of clinical failure, with corresponding lower mortality, have been seen with linezolid treatment of MRSA VAP.

32. **What causes treatment failure in patients with NP?**

Unrecognized or inducible resistance to initial antibiotics, development of secondary resistance during therapy, and ineffective antibiotic therapy lead to persistence of the original organism. Ineffective therapy, despite being appropriate by sensitivity testing, may be due to lack of combination therapy when warranted, inadequate dosing, and use of antibiotics with poor penetration into the lungs. In addition, anatomic problems (e.g., lung abscess or empyema) or thrombosis in the area of infection limit antibiotic penetration. However, poor host defense in the chronically and critically ill patient is probably the greatest problem.

KEY POINTS: CAUSES OF APPARENT TREATMENT FAILURE IN VAP

1. Ineffective initial therapy

2. Superinfection pneumonia

3. Extrapulmonary infection, either concomitant or superinfection

4. Drug fever

5. Other noninfectious causes, such as ARDS or bronchiolitis obliterans-organizing pneumonia (BOOP)

33. **How easy is treatment failure to recognize?**

The most reliable clue that a patient is failing treatment of VAP is a lack of improvement in oxygenation. Sorting out the causes can be very difficult since treatment failure of NP can be confused with superinfection pneumonia with a different organism, concomitant infection with a different pathogen or in a closed space, extrapulmonary superinfection, such as pseudomembranous enterocolitis, or a noninfectious cause that clinically mimics failure to respond. Superinfection pneumonia occurs in approximately 12–15% of VAPs and increases the mortality rate. The pathogens causing superinfection are usually more drug resistant and are often more virulent than the initial causative organism. The overlap between VAP and sinusitis is particularly common.

Ioanas M, Ferrer M, Cavalcanti M, et al: Causes and predictors of nonresponse to treatment of intensive care unit-acquired pneumonia. Crit Care Med 32:938–945, 2004.

CHAPTER 27

ASPIRATION SYNDROMES

Rajesh Bhagat, MD, C. Hewitt McCuller, Jr., MD, and G. Douglas Campbell, Jr., MD

1. **What are aspiration syndromes?**

   Aspiration syndromes refer to the different clinical and pathophysiologic effects caused by physical introduction of foreign objects or substances into the lower respiratory tract. The inflammatory response that occurs in the lungs following aspiration injury is most correctly referred to as **aspiration pneumonitis**. Mendelson's syndrome is the chemical injury of the lungs secondary to aspiration of gastric contents. The early response (i.e., within 1–2 hours) is due to the caustic effect of aspirated gastric contents, and the late response (i.e., after 4–6 hours) is primarily neutrophilic in nature, with histologic characteristics of acute inflammation. **Aspiration pneumonia** refers to an infectious process of the lung parenchyma due to the introduction of pathogenic organisms into the lower respiratory tract. The two terms are often used interchangeably, but they are not necessarily synonymous.

   > DePaso WJ: Aspiration pneumonia. Clin Chest Med 12:269–284, 1991.
   > Marik PE: Aspiration pneumonitis and aspiration pneumonia. N Engl J Med 344:665–671, 2001.

KEY POINTS: ASPIRATION SYNDROMES

1. Aspiration pneumonitis: acute inflammation
   - Early response within 1–2 hours
   - Late response within 4–6 hours

2. Aspiration pneumonia: an infectious process

2. **How common is aspiration?**

   Microaspiration is seen in 45% of normal subjects in deep sleep. The incidence of aspiration post-stroke reportedly occurs in as many as 80% of patients, with almost 40% of these going on to develop aspiration pneumonia. One study observed silent aspiration occurs in almost 71% of elderly patients with community-acquired pneumonia (CAP), whereas in control subjects, it is seen in 10%. The two important risk factors for elderly subjects developing CAP are difficulty in swallowing food and use of sedative medicines. Several studies indicate that 5–15% of CAP are the result of aspiration. Aspiration pneumonia is the most common cause of death in patients with dysphagia and neurologic disorders. Aspiration pneumonitis is seen in almost 10% of hospital admissions due to drug overdose. It is a recognized complication of 1 in 3000 patients undergoing surgery with general anesthesia.

   > Doggett DL, Tapper KA, Mitchell MD, et al: Prevention of pneumonia in elderly stroke patients by systematic diagnosis and treatment of dysphagia: An evidence-based comprehensive analysis of the literature. Dysphagia 16:279–295, 2001.
   > Marik PE: Aspiration pneumonitis and aspiration pneumonia. N Engl J Med 344:665–671, 2001.
   > Marik PE, Kaplan D: Aspiration pneumonia dysphagia in the elderly. Chest 124:328–336, 2003.

3. **What are some of the major risk factors for aspiration?**
   See Table 27-1.

TABLE 27-1.   RISKS FACTORS FOR ASPIRATION

Altered level of consciousness
Drugs: general anesthesia, narcotic and sedative drugs, drug overdose
Postanesthetic recovery
Hypoxemia and hypercapnia
Central nervous system (CNS) infections
Seizures
Structural lesions of the CNS (i.e., tumors, cerebrovascular accident, or head trauma)
Metabolic encephalopathies (i.e., electrolyte imbalances, liver failure, uremia, or sepsis)

Gastrointestinal diseases
Alkaline gastric pH
Gastrointestinal tract dysmotility
Esophagitis (infectious or postradiation)
Hiatal hernia
Tracheoesophageal fistula
Scleroderma
Esophageal motility disorders (achalasia or megaesophageal)
Ascites
Gastrointestinal bleeding
Malignancy of the gastrointestinal tract
Intestinal obstruction or ileus

Neuromuscular diseases
Abnormal glottic closure
Guillain–Barré syndrome
Botulism
Muscular dystrophy
Parkinson's disease
Polymyositis
Amyotrophic lateral sclerosis
Multiple sclerosis
Myasthenia gravis
Poliomyelitis

Mechanical factors
Nasogastric or enteral feeding tubes
Emergent and planned airway mainpulation
Surgery to the neck and pharynx
Tracheostomy
Endotracheal intubation
Trauma to the neck and pharynx
Upper endoscopy
Tumors of the upper airway

Other factors
Extremes of age (infancy and old age)
Diabetes (functional gastric outlet obstruction)
Obesity
Pregnancy

- Elderly nursing home residents with poor orodental hygiene and difficulty swallowing
- Iatrogenic factors: use of sedative and anticholinergic medicines, prolonged mechanical ventilation, and tracheotomy
- Altered consciousness and neurologic and neuromuscular diseases
- Gastrointestinal dysfunction and disruption of the gastroesophageal junction
- Anatomic disruption of the upper aerodigestive tract, especially postsurgical (e.g., oropharyngeal resection and anterior cervical spine fusion)
- Miscellaneous: obesity, neck malignancies, and meconium aspiration

Green SM, Krauss B: Pulmonary aspiration risk during emergency department procedural sedation—An examination of the role of fasting and sedation depth. Acad Emerg Med 9:35–42, 2002.

Doggett DL, Tapper KA, Mitchell MD, et al: Prevention of pneumonia in elderly stroke patients by systematic diagnosis and treatment of dysphagia: An evidence-based comprehensive analysis of the literature. Dysphagia 16:279–295, 2001.

Marik PE: Aspiration pneumonitis and aspiration pneumonia. N Engl J Med 344:665–671, 2001.

4. **What factors affect pathogenesis and prognosis following the aspiration of gastric contents?**
   - **Agent:** The severity of injury that occurs after gastric aspiration is directly related to the pH, volume, and particulate nature of the aspirate. An aspirate with a low pH ($\leq$2.5), with large volume ($\geq$0.4 mL/kg), or with high particulate content has the worst prognosis. Aspiration of gastric contents at a more alkaline pH (>5) can also cause significant pulmonary inflammation and dysfunction, especially if particulate matter is suspended in the fluid.
   - **Environment:** Nursing home patients, patients hospitalized for over 72 hours, and patients recently discharged from the hospital are at higher risk for methicillin-resistant *Staphylococcus aureus* (MRSA) and gram-negative bacterial infection. This is due to changes in the bacteria colonizing the oropharynx.
   - **Host:** Elderly patients with poor swallowing and cough reflexes or poor orodental hygiene are at higher risk for developing aspiration pneumonia. Patients with dementia or neurologic brain obtundation and chronically bedridden patients are also obviously at risk.

   Marik PE: Aspiration pneumonitis and aspiration pneumonia. N Engl J Med 344:665–671, 2001.

5. **What are the clinical findings associated with foreign body aspiration syndrome?**
   The initial symptoms of foreign body aspiration vary according to the size of the aspirated object. Larger objects, such as poorly chewed food, can lodge in the larynx or trachea, leading to respiratory distress, aphonia, cyanosis, loss of consciousness, and sudden death (the so-called cafe coronary). With partial tracheal obstruction, biphasic stridor may be present, but as the object moves distally, inspiratory stridor becomes less prominent compared to expiratory wheezing. Impaction of a foreign body in a main-stem bronchus may lead to unilateral wheezing caused by both airway turbulence and reflex bronchospasm. Lobar or segment impaction can result in asymmetric breath sounds, localized wheezing, or diminished air entry. Smaller objects can descend farther into the tracheobronchial tree and can cause bronchial irritation, resulting in cough followed by varying degrees of dyspnea, chest pain, wheezing, fever, nausea, or vomiting. Recurrent pneumonias in the same segment should raise the suspicion of foreign body aspiration.

   DePaso WJ: Aspiration pneumonia. Clin Chest Med 12:269–284, 1991.
   Marik PE: Aspiration pneumonitis and aspiration pneumonia. N Engl J Med 344:665–671, 2001.

6. **What are the clinical findings that occur with acute gastric content aspiration?**
   Presence of gastric contents in the oropharynx and the respiratory tract clinically manifests as wheezing, coughing, cyanosis, fever, and hypoxemia, and sometimes is accompanied by shock

associated with profound hypoxemia due to ventilation-perfusion mismatching and intrapulmonary shunt. Initially, this may be caused by closure of small airways and atelectasis resulting
from loss of surfactant, which can be destroyed by acid or inactivated by plasma proteins.
Pulmonary capillary leak and edema also occur, worsening the shunt. This may then progress in
one of three ways: (1) rapid improvement within 1 week, (2) rapid death from progressive respiratory failure, or (3) initial improvement followed by deterioration and the development of acute
respiratory distress syndrome (ARDS) or bacterial superinfection (which may require further
evaluation).

DePaso WJ: Aspiration pneumonia. Clin Chest Med 12:269–284, 1991.
Marik PE: Aspiration pneumonitis and aspiration pneumonia. N Engl J Med 344:665–671, 2001.

KEY POINTS: MAJOR RISK FACTORS FOR ASPIRATION PNEUMONIA

1. Binge drinking or drug overdose

2. Use of sedation and anxiolytics

3. Intubation, mechanical ventilation, and extubation

4. Patients on tube feeds

5. Patients with stroke

6. Poor orodental hygiene

7. **What are the chronic diseases associated with aspiration?**
   Patients with esophageal disorders (e.g., achalasia, esophageal diverticula, tracheoesophageal
   fistula, or severe reflux) may develop acute recurrent or chronic pneumonitis. Chronic aspiration
   of particulate matter may cause granulomatous interstitial pneumonitis. Interstitial lung disease
   similar to idiopathic pulmonary fibrosis can be seen with chronic aspiration of small volumes of
   oropharyngeal or gastric contents. Aspiration may lead to chronic respiratory symptoms including cough, dyspnea, or hemoptysis. Acid regurgitation can stimulate bronchial hyperreactivity
   with or without true aspiration. Chronic bronchitis, with or without chronic airflow obstruction,
   has been associated with the presence of chronic aspiration.

   DePaso WJ: Aspiration pneumonia. Clin Chest Med 12:269–284, 1991.
   Marik PE: Aspiration pneumonitis and aspiration pneumonia. N Engl J Med 344:665–671, 2001.

8. **What are the typical roentgenographic findings seen with aspiration?**
   Foreign body aspiration: Typical roentgenographic findings depend on the type of object that
   is aspirated. Typically, the more dependent areas of the lungs are involved, such as the lower
   lobes when the patient is in the upright position or the posterior segment of the upper lobes
   and the superior segment of the lower lobes when the subject is supine. In adults, aspiration
   more frequently involves the right side because of the acute angle of the left mainstem
   bronchus, whereas in children aged less than approximately 15 years, the frequency of left-
   sided aspiration almost equals that of aspirate to the right side because of bronchial symme-
   try. Radiopaque objects can sometimes be visualized. Obstruction of segmental or larger
   airways may lead to lobar or, more rarely, complete lung collapse. Occasionally, inspiratory
   films may show no abnormalities, whereas expiratory films reveal air trapping on the involved
   side.

Gastric contents: The aspiration of large amounts of acidic material (i.e., gastric aspiration) usually leads to general involvement of both lungs by patchy airspace consolidation. The distribution is commonly bilateral and multicentric but usually favors perihilar or basal regions. Three basic patterns of disease can be seen: (1) extensive bilateral airspace consolidation (i.e., confluent acinar opacities), (2) widespread but fairly discrete acinar shadows, and (3) irregular opacities not fitting into either of these categories. The last is probably the most common pattern, accounting for slightly over 40% of cases. Worsening of the roentgenographic abnormalities after initial improvement is associated with the development of bacterial pneumonia, ARDS, or pulmonary embolism, and it requires further investigation.

DePaso WJ: Aspiration pneumonia. Clin Chest Med 12:269–284, 1991.

Landay MJ, Christensen EE, Bynum LJ: Pulmonary manifestations of acute aspiration of gastric contents. Am J Roentgenol 131:587–592, 1978.

Marik PE: Aspiration pneumonitis and aspiration pneumonia. N Engl J Med 344:665–671, 2001.

9. **How do you evaluate patients at risk for aspiration?**
   - Bedside history and physical exam for dysphagia screening
   - Clinical bedside swallow exam (e.g., trials of swallowing water)
   - Videofluoroscopic swallowing study
   - Modified barium swallow

   Other techniques include manometry, ultrasound, magnetic resonance imaging, an upper gastrointestinal series, esophagoscopy, and gastroscopy.

Doggett DL, Tapper KA, Mitchell MD, et al: Prevention of pneumonia in elderly stroke patients by systematic diagnosis and treatment of dysphagia: An evidence-based comprehensive analysis of the literature. Dysphagia 16:279–295, 2001.

Lind CD: Dysphagia: Evaluation and treatment. Gastroenterol Clin North Am 32:553–575, 2003.

10. **What is the treatment for foreign body aspiration?**
    Complete airway obstruction due to foreign body aspiration must be relieved immediately. In the United States, the Heimlich maneuver (i.e., subdiaphragmatic abdominal thrusts) usually accomplishes this, whereas the Canadian Heart Foundation recommends a combination of abdominal thrusts and back blows.

    If the foreign body remains in the lower respiratory tract, then the airway should be stabilized, including intubation if necessary, and depending on the size of the foreign body, rigid or fiberoptic bronchoscopy should be performed to remove the object. If these are unsuccessful, then thoracotomy may be necessary.

Dikensoy O, Usalan C, Filiz A: Foreign body aspiration: Clinical utility of flexible bronchoscopy. Postgrad Med J 78:399–403, 2002.

11. **What is the treatment for gastric aspiration?**
    In patients with massive gastric aspiration, the initial therapy involves establishing and maintaining adequate oxygenation. Occasionally, this may be accomplished with simple supplemental oxygen, but more often it requires intubation and mechanical ventilation with the application of positive end-expiratory pressure (PEEP) because of worsening of pulmonary edema and shunt. In severe cases, bronchoscopy may be helpful if there is particulate matter blocking the airways, but large-volume lavage is of little benefit in minimizing the effects of gastric acid since the acid is dispersed and rapidly neutralized. Hemodynamic and fluid management, adjusted to achieve the lowest pulmonary artery occlusion pressure (PAOP) consistent with an adequate cardiac output, should be instituted to reduce permeability edema and to improve shunt, hypoxemia, and lung compliance.

    Newer experimental modalities for the treatment of ARDS resulting from aspiration pneumonia, including extracorporeal membrane oxygenation (ECMO), alternate modes of mechanical ventilation, surfactant replacement therapy, and biochemical or immunologic intervention to treat cellular injury, remain under investigation.

DePaso WJ: Aspiration pneumonia. Clin Chest Med 12:269–284, 1991.

12. **What is the role of systemic corticosteroids in the treatment of aspiration?**
    Numerous studies in both animals and humans have shown inconsistent results when corticosteroids are administered prophylactically and therapeutically after aspiration. Additionally, steroids may be harmful, predisposing the patient to infection and causing fluid and electrolyte imbalance. Presently, there are no indications for the use of corticosteroids, either parenterally or by inhalation, in the treatment of aspiration pneumonia in adults. The only condition in which corticosteroids may have a role is in the early stages of meconium aspiration in newborn infants.

    Kaapa P: Corticosteroid treatment in meconium aspiration syndrome: A solution for better outcome? Acta Paediatr 93:5–7, 2004.

    Marik PE: Aspiration pneumonitis and aspiration pneumonia. N Engl J Med 344:665–671, 2001.

13. **Are prophylactic antibiotics indicated in aspiration?**
    The routine use of prophylactic antibiotics following a witnessed aspiration event is not recommended because of the hazard of selecting for antibiotic-resistant organisms. Unfortunately, the clinical manifestations of secondary bacteria infection can be confused with chemical injury to the lung tissue. Following all aspiration events, the patient should be closely observed. If clinical evidence compatible with pneumonia (i.e., new infiltrate, fever, or leukocytosis) is noted, empirical antibiotics, based upon the most probable spectrum of pathogens (*see* below), should be initiated for 24–48 hours, with the patient closely observed. Antibiotics should be discontinued if rapid improvement is noted (in <24–48 hours), but clinical worsening should prompt expansion of antibiotic coverage, with strong consideration given to obtaining respiratory secretions by bronchoscopy or tracheal suctioning.

    Marik PE: Aspiration pneumonitis and aspiration pneumonia. N Engl J Med 344:665–671, 2001.

14. **What are the infectious complications of aspiration syndrome?**
    Infectious complications of aspiration syndrome may present either as an acute or a chronic process, including acute pneumonitis, necrotizing pneumonia, lung abscess, bronchiectasis, and empyema. The probability of infectious complications is increased if there is a large volume of aspirated material, if the aspirate is contaminated by virulent pathogens, or if the host airway and lung defenses are ineffective.

    DePaso WJ: Aspiration pneumonia. Clin Chest Med 12:269–284, 1991.

    Marik PE: Aspiration pneumonitis and aspiration pneumonia. N Engl J Med 344:665–671, 2001.

15. **What are the clinical manifestations of aspiration pneumonia?**
    Acutely, aspiration pneumonia may be a primary event with clinical manifestations noted within the first 24–48 hours. Although primary pneumonia is noted in only 23–30% of all cases of aspiration, when it occurs, it is associated with increased morbidity and mortality. Fever, cough with phlegm, leukocytosis, and development of pulmonary infiltrates on chest radiograph frequently herald the onset of aspiration pneumonia. Many patients show initial improvement following aspiration, only to develop pneumonia 2–7 days later. These secondary pneumonias are the result of obstruction or inflammation in the lower respiratory tract that impairs the patient's host defenses. The risk of secondary infection may be increased by mechanical ventilation or the need for hospitalization for more than 5 days. In patients with aspiration pneumonia, predictors of mortality include ineffective initial antimicrobial therapy, a positive initial blood culture, hospital-acquired lower respiratory tract superinfections, and the use of inotropic support.

    Aspiration pneumonia may also present as a chronic indolent infection. In this setting, lung abscess may have developed. This presentation is more likely to occur in patients with particular risk factors, including swallowing dysfunction, gastroesophageal reflux, poor dentition, alcoholism, and seizure activity, and frequently it is manifested by low-grade fever and nonspecific findings, typically of 3 weeks' duration. The chest radiograph often reveals a rounded area of consolidation with or without an air-fluid level, but it may occasionally reveal patchy infiltrates or even interstitial changes. There may also be involvement of the pleural space with the development of a parapneumonic effusion or empyema.

DePaso WJ: Aspiration pneumonia. Clin Chest Med 12:269–284, 1991.

Marik PE: Aspiration pneumonitis and aspiration pneumonia. N Engl J Med 344:665–671, 2001.

16. **Which organisms are common causes of aspiration pneumonia?**

The etiology of aspiration pneumonia is frequently polymicrobial, reflecting the spectrum of pathogens seen in the oropharynx, and is affected by the same factors that affect oropharyngeal colonization (i.e., whether aspiration occurred in the community or hospital setting, recent antimicrobial therapy, and the presence of numerous dental caries). In aspiration pneumonia occurring in the community setting, the most frequent pathogens include *Staphylococcus aureus* and *Streptococcus pneumoniae* and anaerobic organisms such as *Bacterioides* spp., *Peptostreptococcus* spp., *Fusobacterium nucleatum*, and *Prevotella* spp.

Although the same spectrum of anaerobic organisms is frequently seen in aspiration pneumonia occurring in the hospital, the spectrum of aerobic pathogens differs, especially if the patient has been hospitalized for >4 days, has received prior antibiotics, or is being mechanically ventilated. *S. aureus* (which may be methicillin resistant), enteric gram-negative bacilli (i.e., *Escherichia coli, Klebsiella* spp., and *Proteus* spp.), and *Pseudomonas aeruginosa* are frequently isolated in this setting.

DePaso WJ: Aspiration pneumonia. Clin Chest Med 12:269–284, 1991.

Marik PE: Aspiration pneumonitis and aspiration pneumonia. N Engl J Med 344:665–671, 2001.

17. **How are the infectious complications of community-acquired aspiration syndrome treated?**

For aspiration pneumonia occurring in the community setting, high-dose penicillin is often the drug of choice. These relatively mild cases may also be treated with levofloxacin or ceftriaxone. But the presence of penicillin-resistant organisms, including *Bacteroides* spp. and *S. pneumoniae*, has resulted in the increased use of alternative therapy. Clindamycin may be more effective in shortening the duration of fever and sputum production and is associated with a lower failure rate. Metronidazole has activity against certain anaerobic organisms, but, because of its relative lack of efficacy against microaerophilic streptococci, it should be used in combination with penicillin. Imipenem-cilastatin or a beta-lactam antibiotic combined with a beta-lactamase inhibitor can also be used in this setting.

DePaso WJ: Aspiration pneumonia. Clin Chest Med 12:269–284, 1991.

Marik PE: Aspiration pneumonitis and aspiration pneumonia. N Engl J Med 344:665–671, 2001.

18. **Is there any difference in the spectrum of infecting organisms if aspiration pneumonia is seen in hospitalized or institutionalized patients?**

Selection of antimicrobial agents is affected by the probable spectrum of pathogens and the possibility of antibiotic-resistant organisms. Aspiration in the hospital setting is more likely to involve aerobic gram-negative bacilli, *S. aureus* (including MRSA), or anaerobic organisms. Empirical antibiotic therapy in the past included the use of third-generation cephalosporins, but with the growing emergence of resistant organisms, alternative therapies such as imipenem, meropenem, piperacillin-tazobactam, and fluoroquinolones combined with clindamycin are increasingly being used.

DePaso WJ: Aspiration pneumonia. Clin Chest Med 12:269–284, 1991.

Marik PE: Aspiration pneumonitis and aspiration pneumonia. N Engl J Med 344:665–671, 2001.

19. **What is the management of post-aspiration lung abscess or empyema?**

Lung abscess usually requires a prolonged course of antibiotics, generally for 6–8 weeks, depending on the clinical response. In patients whose medical management is unsuccessful (approximately 10% of patients) or if the abscess is very large, percutaneous drainage or lobectomy may be needed. Empyemas typically require drainage through a closed thoracostomy tube or by open surgical drainage, with or without decortication. Earlier surgical intervention for empyema is more practical because of the accessibility of video-assisted thoracic surgery (VATS) with drainage and directed placement of chest tubes.

DePaso WJ: Aspiration pneumonia. Clin Chest Med 12:269–284, 1991.

Marik PE: Aspiration pneumonitis and aspiration pneumonia. N Engl J Med 344:665–671, 2001.

20. **How can aspiration and some of its consequences be prevented?**
    - In neonates, careful antenatal and perinatal care can reduce the risk of aspiration.
    - In children, aspiration of foreign bodies is the leading cause of accidental death in the home for children under 1 year of age. When possible, attention to the consistency of food reduces the risk.
    - In young adults, aspiration usually follows substance and drug abuse, most commonly alcohol binge drinking.
    - In elderly patients, avoiding sedatives and ensuring that they follow aspiration precautions while swallowing carefully will help prevent aspiration pneumonia.
    - In critically ill patients, avoiding oversedation and keeping the head of the bed at a 45-degree angle have been shown to prevent aspiration events. If feeding tubes are being used, make sure that the distal end is beyond the ligament of Treitz. If the patients are intubated, use of sucralfate and aspiration of the suprabulb region may help.
    - In patients undergoing surgery, rapid-sequence induction of anesthesia will shorten the period between the loss of consciousness and tracheal intubation, hence reducing chances of aspiration. Likewise, the application of cricoid pressure (i.e., the Sellick maneuver) during intubation will help.
    - Obtunded patients at risk for large-volume aspiration should be closely observed and placed in the head-down lateral position to reduce the volume of material aspirated in the event of aspiration.
    - In patients requiring long-term nutritional support, surgical interventions such as gastrostomy or enterostomy, sometimes combined with an antireflux procedure such as a Nissen fundoplication, are often used; however, tube feedings do not necessarily reduce the risk of aspiration or pneumonia, and patients whose dysphagia is evident during feeding can continue to aspirate when nutrition is delivered directly to the stomach or lower in the gastrointestinal tract. Additionally, there are no irrefutable data comparing the safety of continuous versus bolus feeding, fine-bore versus wide-bore nasoenteric tubes, and jejunostomy versus gastrostomy.

DePaso WJ: Aspiration pneumonia. Clin Chest Med 12:269–284, 1991.

Marik PE: Aspiration pneumonitis and aspiration pneumonia. N Engl J Med 344:665–671, 2001.

McClave SA, Marsano LS, Lukan JK: Enteral access for nutritional support. Rationale for utilization. J Clin Gastroenterol 35:209–213, 2002.

CHAPTER 28

FUNGAL PNEUMONIA

Carol A. Kauffman, MD, and Joseph P. Lynch III, MD

ASPERGILLOSIS

1. **What is the appropriate treatment for invasive pulmonary aspergillosis (IPA)?**
    Voriconazole (4 mg/kg/day IV or 200 mg twice per day orally) is the treatment of choice for IPA.
    Amphotericin B (AMB), usually administered as a lipid formulation (5 mg/kg/day), is now sec-
    ond-line therapy. Caspofungin can be used in addition to voriconazole or amphotericin or for
    patients who are failing or are experiencing adverse effects from other agents. Surgical resection
    of a single cavitary lesion may be critical as adjunctive therapy in immunosuppressed patients.
    Even with aggressive antifungal therapy, mortality from IPA is high among patients with hemato-
    logic malignancies, hematopoietic stem cell transplant recipients, and patients with acquired
    immunodeficiency syndrome (AIDS).

    Herbrecht R, Denning DW, Patterson TF, et al: Voriconazole versus amphotericin B for primary therapy of
    invasive aspergillosis. N Engl J Med 347:408–415, 2002.

2. **How does allergic bronchopulmonary aspergillosis (ABPA) present? How
    should it be treated?**
    Both skin tests and serology are helpful in diagnosing ABPA, a hypersensitivity response to
    Aspergillus spp. Clinical manifestations of ABPA include asthma, eosinophilia, pulmonary infil-
    trates, and elevated serum IgE (both total [i.e., nonspecific] IgE and IgE antibodies directed
    against *Aspergillus fumigatus*). Skin tests are helpful. In patients with ABPA, intradermal chal-
    lenge with an *Aspergillus* antigen results in an immediate acute wheal-and-flare response
    (within 15–30 minutes); edema at the inoculation site occurs 3–6 hours later. Corticosteroids
    are the mainstay of therapy for ABPA. Oral itraconazole (200 mg twice daily) may have a
    steroid-sparing effect.

    Stevens DA, Schwartz HJ, Lee JY, et al: A randomized trial of itraconazole in allergic bronchopulmonary
    aspergillosis. N Engl J Med 342:756–762, 2000.

3. **What are the clinical features of pulmonary mycetoma?**
    Mycetomas are chronic masses of fungal mycelia (typically *Aspergillus* spp.) that develop within
    preexisting cavities in patients with chronic pulmonary disorders such as tuberculosis, sar-
    coidosis, histoplasmosis, bronchial cysts, bronchiectasis, or silicosis. Rarely, mycetomas
    develop subacutely in patients with hematologic malignancies and pulmonary aspergillosis. A
    round intracavitary mass that moves when the patient changes position and is surrounded by a
    crescent of air is characteristic. Hemoptysis occurs in approximately 50% of patients at some
    time in the course of the disease. Fatal, exsanguinating hemorrhage is the most dreaded
    complication.

    Judson MA: Non-invasive Aspergillus pulmonary disease. Semin Respir Crit Care Med 25: 203–219, 2004.

4. **How is pulmonary mycetoma treated?**
    Surgical resection is the only reliable cure, but this may be a formidable undertaking since
    extensive pleural adhesions and parenchymal scarring are usually present. In addition, many
    patients with mycetomas have severe, debilitating pulmonary disease and may not tolerate tho-
    racotomy. Surgical resection is reasonable for patients with mycetomas, hemoptysis, and no

contraindications to surgery. Intravenous AMB or voriconazole should be given perioperatively to reduce surgical complications such as empyema or bronchopleural fistulae. Medical therapy is rarely effective for mycetomas, but anecdotal successes were noted after intracavitary instillation of AMB.

5. **What is the role of antibody and antigen assays in diagnosis of aspergillosis?**
Antibody assays are of value in the diagnosis of ABPA and pulmonary mycetomas but are not useful for invasive aspergillosis. An assay specific for *Aspergillus* galactomannan in serum was validated when serial samples from stem cell transplant patients at high risk for invasive aspergillosis showed increasing readings. The utility of this assay in other populations (e.g., solid-organ transplant recipients) has not been defined. False-positive reactions may occur with administration of piperacillin-tazobactam and ampicillin-sulbactam.

Adam O, Auperin A, Wilquin F, et al: Treatment with piperacillin-tazobactam and false-positive *Aspergillus* galactomannan antigen test results for patients with hematological malignancies. Clin Infect Dis 38:917–920, 2004.

KEY POINTS: TREATMENT OF ASPERGILLOSIS

1. The treatment of choice of invasive aspergillosis is voriconazole.

2. Second-line treatments for invasive aspergillosis are amphotericin B and caspofungin.

3. Mycetoma is best treated by surgical resection.

4. Allergic bronchopulmonary aspergillosis is treated primarily with corticosteroids; itraconazole can decrease the amount of corticosteroids required.

6. **What is the significance of *Aspergillus* spp. in the sputum or bronchoalveolar lavage (BAL) fluid?**
Isolation of *Aspergillus* spp. may reflect contamination, colonization, or invasive infection. The significance of positive cultures strongly depends on the presence of risk factors for IPA. Risk factors for IPA include severe and sustained granulocytopenia, organ or hematopoietic stem cell transplantation, graft-versus-host disease (GVHD), hematologic malignancy, and corticosteroid or immunosuppressive therapy. In patients with one or more of these risk factors and a pulmonary infiltrate, isolation of *Aspergillus* spp. in respiratory secretions often reflects tissue invasion and warrants more aggressive diagnostic studies, if possible, and specific antifungal therapy. Detecting hyphae on sputum smears or in BAL fluid increases the likelihood of invasive infection. In contrast, *Aspergillus* spp. frequently colonize the respiratory tract in patients with solid tumors or chronic pulmonary diseases but rarely cause invasive disease. Unless focal pneumonia or cavitary lesions are present, isolation of *Aspergillus* spp. in these less-immunocompromised hosts does not require further evaluation or treatment.

BLASTOMYCOSIS

7. **When should blastomycosis be treated, and what drug should be used?**
Except for rare cases of acute self-limited pulmonary blastomycosis, all patients with blastomycosis require treatment with an antifungal agent. Even one localized cutaneous lesion implies disseminated blastomycosis that requires therapy. Itraconazole (200 mg once or twice daily) is the treatment of choice for non–life-threatening, nonmeningeal blastomycosis. Treatment should be continued for a minimum of 6–12 months, until all lesions have resolved. Fluconazole

is less effective than itraconazole. Data regarding voriconazole are sparse. AMB (0.7–1.0 mg/kg/day) is the drug of choice for acute life-threatening or meningeal blastomycosis. After improvement, treatment can be changed to itraconazole.

Chapman SW, Bradsher RW, Campbell GD, et al: Practice guidelines for the management of patients with blastomycosis. Clin Infect Dis 30:679–683, 2000.

8. **Are serologic assays helpful in the diagnosis of blastomycosis?**
No. The commercially available serologic assays (e.g., complement fixation and immunodiffusion) are neither sensitive nor specific and should not be used. The diagnosis of blastomycosis is best made by histopathologic study (the organism has a distinctive appearance) and cultures from involved sites.

CANDIDIASIS

9. **What is the significance of isolating *Candida* spp. in the sputum?**
Isolation of *Candida* spp. in sputum or respiratory secretions almost always reflects colonization, rarely warrants additional diagnostic interventions, and does not require therapy. Primary pneumonia caused by *Candida* spp. is rare, even among immunocompromised hosts, but can occur in the context of disseminated candidiasis or in patients with profound, sustained impairment of host defenses (e.g., in patients with prolonged granulocytopenia). Repetitive isolation of *Candida* spp. in immunosuppressed patients with pulmonary infiltrates refractory to broad-spectrum antibiotics should prompt a more aggressive diagnostic evaluation for candidiasis.

El-Ebiary M, Torres A, Fabrega N, et al: Significance of the isolation of Candida species from respiratory samples in critically ill, non-neutropenic patients. Am J Respir Crit Care Med 156:583–590, 1997.

Kontoyiannis, DP, Reddy, BT, Torres, HA, et al: Pulmonary candidiasis in patients with cancer: an autopsy study. Clin Infect Dis 34:400, 2002.

COCCIDIOIDOMYCOSIS

10. **What is the most appropriate treatment for coccidioidomycosis?**
Acute pulmonary coccidioidomycosis usually does not require treatment. However, patients with persistent symptomatic pulmonary coccidioidomycosis, asymptomatic cavitary lesions on chest radiograph, or disseminated disease should be treated. Itraconazole and fluconazole, 400 mg daily, have shown similar efficacy; voriconazole has not been tested. Life-threatening coccidioidomycosis mandates treatment with AMB (0.7–1.0 mg/kg/day); this regimen is frequently required in immunosuppressed patients. Fluconazole or itraconazole can be substituted for AMB after the clinical condition improves. For meningeal coccidioidomycosis, oral fluconazole (800 mg/day) is the drug of choice but must be continued for life because the relapse rate is exceedingly high.

Galgiani JN, Ampel NM, Catanzaro A, et al: Practice guidelines for the treatment of coccidioidomycosis. Clin Infect Dis 30:658–661, 2000.

Galgiani JN, Catanzaro A, Cloud GA, et al: Randomized double-blind comparison of oral fluconazole and itraconazole for progressive non-meningeal coccidioidomycosis. Ann Intern Med 133:676–686, 2000.

11. **Do skin tests and serologic assays have a role in the diagnosis of coccidioidomycosis?**
Skin tests are most useful in patients who are not from but have recently traveled through endemic regions and present with a clinical syndrome compatible with coccidioidomycosis. A positive skin test for *Coccidioides immitis* should prompt further workup. A negative skin test does not rule out active coccidioidomycosis, especially in immunocompromised hosts.

Complement fixation and immunodiffusion assays are helpful in both diagnosis and assessment of prognosis. High antibody titers, especially combined with anergy-to-skin test antigens, usually portend a worse prognosis.

These tests should be performed by laboratories with special expertise in fungal serologic assays. *Coccidioides immitis* is easily grown in the laboratory and has a distinctive appearance in tissues.

CRYPTOCOCCOSIS

12. **What is the appropriate diagnostic evaluation for pulmonary cryptococcosis?**
    The diagnosis of pulmonary cryptococcosis is best made by bronchoscopy, yielding BAL fluid for cytological examination and culture. Cryptococcal antigen, measured by a latex agglutination assay, can be detected in BAL fluid but is rarely positive in serum unless the patient has diffuse pulmonary infection or disseminated disease. Meningeal spread occurs in more than two-thirds of patients with pulmonary cryptococcosis. Because of the avidity of *Cryptococcus neoformans* for the central nervous system (CNS), a lumbar puncture must be obtained in patients with pulmonary cryptococcosis, even when no CNS symptoms are apparent.

    Aberg JA, Mundy LM, Powderly WG: Pulmonary cryptococcosis in patients without HIV infection. Chest 115:737–740, 1999.

    Pappas PG, Perfect JR, Cloud GA, et al: Cryptococcosis in HIV-negative patients in the era of effective azole therapy. Clin Infect Dis 33:690–699, 2001.

13. **What is the best treatment for cryptococcosis?**
    AMB (0.7 mg/day) combined with flucytosine (100 mg/kg/day in 4 divided doses) is optimal therapy for cryptococcal meningitis and disseminated cryptococcosis. Therapy should continue for at least 2 weeks, until improvement has been achieved and colony-stimulating factor (CSF) cultures are negative, and then can be changed to oral fluconazole (400 mg/day), continued for a minimum of 10 weeks. Severely immunocompromised patients at risk for relapse should be maintained on fluconazole (200 mg/day) indefinitely. For localized pulmonary cryptococcosis in nonimmunocompromised patients, oral fluconazole (400 mg/day) is recommended.

    Saag MS, Graybill JR, Larsen RA, et al: Practice guidelines for the management of cryptococcal disease. Clin Infect Dis 30:710–718, 2000.

HISTOPLASMOSIS

14. **When should histoplasmosis be treated?**
    Acute pulmonary histoplasmosis usually does not require treatment. However, treatment is indicated for the following conditions: (1) severe or progressive pulmonary involvement after exposure to a point source of *Histoplasma capsulatum* (i.e., "epidemic histoplasmosis"), (2) chronic cavitary pulmonary histoplasmosis, (3) symptomatic acute disseminated histoplasmosis, (4) histoplasmosis in immunocompromised hosts, and (5) chronic progressive disseminated histoplasmosis.

15. **What antifungal agent should be used for histoplasmosis?**
    Itraconazole (200 mg once or twice daily) is the preferred drug for non–life-threatening, non-meningeal histoplasmosis. Most patients with acute pulmonary or disseminated infection can be treated for 3–6 months. Treatment should be ≥12 months for patients who respond slowly to therapy and those with chronic progressive disseminated and chronic cavitary pulmonary infections. Fluconazole (800 mg daily) is less effective for histoplasmosis. Data regarding voriconazole for histoplasmosis are lacking. AMB (0.7 mg/kg/day) is the initial

treatment for life-threatening infection. After stabilization, therapy can be switched to oral itraconazole.

Wheat J, Sarosi G, McKinsey D, et al: Practice guidelines for the management of patients with histoplasmosis. Clin Infect Dis 30:688–695, 2000.

16. **Do serologic assays have a role in the diagnosis of histoplasmosis?**
Complement fixation (CF) and immunodiffusion (ID) assays can be useful to diagnose pulmonary histoplasmosis. Tests should be performed by laboratories proficient in fungal serologic assays and are most useful in patients with acute and chronic pulmonary histoplasmosis. A fourfold rise in CF titer or development of an M band by ID in a patient with an acute pneumonia and a possible environmental exposure is strong evidence for acute histoplasmosis. In chronic cavitary infections, CF titers $\geq 1:32$, and an M band or H and M bands are strong evidence for histoplasmosis. Detection of a *Histoplasma* antigen in urine or serum by enzyme immunoassay is a sensitive test that has proven very useful in disseminated histoplasmosis.

Wheat LJ: Laboratory diagnosis of histoplasmosis: Update 2000. Semin Respir Infect 16:131–140, 2001.

ZYGOMYCOSIS (MUCORMYCOSIS)

17. **What are the clinical manifestations of zygomycosis? How is the diagnosis made?**
Clinical forms of zygomycosis include rhinocerebral, pulmonary, gastrointestinal, cutaneous, and disseminated infection. Risk factors for zygomycosis include granulocytopenia, hematologic malignancies, corticosteroid or immunosuppressive therapy, burn wounds, diabetes mellitus with ketoacidosis, and iron chelator (i.e., deferoxamine) therapy. The Zygomycetes, most commonly *Rhizopus* spp. and *Mucor* spp., are angioinvasive. Black eschars overlying ulcers or areas of necrosis are clues to the diagnosis. Antemortem cultures are positive in a minority of cases. The presence of broad, ribbon-like, nonseptated hyphae that branch at right angles is diagnostic.

Kontoyiannis DP, Wessel VC, Bodey GP, Rolston KV: Zygomycosis in the 1990s in a tertiary-care cancer center. Clin Infect Dis 30:851–856, 2000.

18. **What is the best treatment for zygomycosis?**
Invasive disease should be treated with lipid formulation AMB (5–10 mg/kg/day), combined with surgical resection or debridement of all involved tissue, when possible. Posaconazole, a new oral azole, is useful as salvage therapy in patients who have failed AMB. Control of the underlying disease or reduction in the level of immunosuppression is critical to optimize outcome.

KEY POINTS: CHARACTERISTICS OF ANGIOINVASIVE FUNGI

1. The most common organisms are *Aspergillus, Fusarium,* and *Scedosporium* spp and Zygomycetes.

2. These organisms invade through blood vessels and cause hemorrhage and necrosis.

3. Computed tomography (CT) scans typically reveal nodules surrounded by a halo sign, indicating hemorrhage; cavitation (indicated by a crescent sign) may evolve later.

4. Mortality with angioinvasive fungal infections is high (typically >40%).

5. Identification by cultures is essential because organisms may be resistant to standard antifungal agents.

DIAGNOSTIC AND TREATMENT PEARLS

19. **Which fungus causes pulmonary infiltrates that mimic those of invasive aspergillosis and looks like *Aspergillus* on histopathologic examination? Why is this important?**

    Scedosporium apiospermum, also called *Pseudallescheria boydii* when it assumes the sexual stage, mimics the clinical, radiographic, and histopathologic picture seen with invasive aspergillosis. This common environmental mold causes infection mostly in immunocompromised patients, as do *Aspergillus* spp. The most important difference between these fungi is that *P. boydii* is resistant to AMB and should be treated with voriconazole. Thus, cultures (not just histopathology or cytology) are critically important.

    Castiglioni B, Sutton DA, Rinaldi MG, et al: *Pseudallescheria boydii* (anamorph *Scedosporium apiospermum*) infection in solid organ transplant recipients in a tertiary medical center and review of the literature. Medicine (Baltimore) 81:333–348, 2002.

20. **What is the role of high-resolution CT scanning in the diagnosis of pulmonary angioinvasive fungal infections?**

    Angioinvasive fungi include *Aspergillus, Scedosporium (Pseudallescheria), Fusarium* spp., and the Zygomycetes. They cause infections in immunosuppressed hosts, exhibit a propensity to invade blood vessel walls, may cause tissue infarction and hemorrhage, and are associated with high mortality rates. Early and aggressive therapy is critical. High-resolution CT scanning facilitates early diagnosis of angioinvasive fungal infections. Typical features include multiple macroscopic nodules, often with cavitation. A halo sign (i.e., a ground-glass appearance surrounding a nodule) implies tissue hemorrhage. A crescent sign or cavity formation (indicating tissue necrosis) is a late sign. Bronchoscopy or percutaneous needle aspiration should be performed if focal infiltrates, nodules, or halo signs are noted on a CT scan. However, empirical antifungal therapy should be initiated while awaiting culture results.

    Caillot D, Casasnovas O, Bernard A, et al: Improved management of invasive pulmonary aspergillosis in neutropenic patients using early thoracic computed tomographic scan and surgery. J Clin Oncol 15:139–147, 1997.

    Caillot D, Couailler J-F, Bernard A, et al: Increasing volume and changing characteristics of invasive pulmonary aspergillosis on sequential thoracic computed tomography scans in patients with neutropenia. J Clin Oncol 19:253–259, 2001.

21. **What is the safest antifungal agent to use in pregnant women?**

    Although amphotericin B is the antifungal agent with the most side effects, it is the safest agent with regard to its effects on the fetus. Azoles are teratogenic in animals, and birth defects have occurred in pregnant women taking fluconazole. Flucytosine is associated with birth defects in

---

KEY POINTS: THE MAJOR ENDEMIC MYCOSES— HISTOPLASMOSIS, BLASTOMYCOSIS, AND COCCIDIOIDOMYCOSIS

1. Serology is helpful to diagnose histoplasmosis and coccidioidomycosis but not blastomycosis.

2. Self-limited pulmonary infection does not require antifungal therapy.

3. The treatment for mild to moderate disease is itraconazole. Fluconazole is as effective for coccidioidomycosis, but not for histoplasmosis and blastomycosis.

4. The treatment for severe disease is amphotericin B (or a liposomal form).

both animals and humans. The echinocandins are teratogenic in animals and are contraindicated in pregnancy.

22. **What side effects are common with azole antifungal agents?**

Fluconazole has few adverse effects. Skin rash, nausea, and elevated liver enzymes are the most common. Alopecia may occur in 12–20% of patients receiving high dosages for ≥2 months; it reverses with cessation of the drug or a reduction in dose.

The principal side effects of **itraconazole** are nausea, abnormalities in liver enzymes, hypokalemia, hypertension, and edema. Myocardial dysfunction may occur; itraconazole should not be used in patients with a history of congestive heart failure if other options exist.

Voriconazole has the highest incidence of rash; besides the typical maculopapular rash, severe blistering photosensitivity has been noted. Hepatotoxicity may be dose related. There is generally no reason to increase the dosage above that recommended, but if that should be done, liver enzymes must be watched closely. Up to 30% of patients will experience photopsia, described as wavy lines, flashing lights, or other visual distortions, for about an hour after taking voriconazole. This is not associated with any serious or lasting visual problems.

Johnson LB, Kauffman CA: Voriconazole: A new triazole antifungal agent. Clin Infect Dis 36:630–637, 2003.

23. **What important points should you tell patients for whom you prescribe oral azoles?**

Each oral formulation has specific requirements to ensure adequate absorption. Fluconazole is 100% bioavailable; absorption is not influenced by food or gastric acidity. The capsule formulation of itraconazole requires both gastric acid and food for adequate absorption; histamine (H_2) blockers, antacids, and proton pump inhibitors should not be used. The oral suspension of itraconazole is given on an empty stomach; food and gastric acid are not needed for absorption. Voriconazole is 95% bioavailable on an empty stomach. Food reduces bioavailability; gastric acid is not needed for absorption.

24. **What is the role of echinocandins in the treatment of fungal infections? What adverse effects occur with echinocandins?**

This new class of antifungal agents is active against all *Candida* spp. and *Aspergillus* spp. but not against other fungi. The echinocandins are most useful for treating candidiasis or as adjunctive therapy for invasive aspergillosis. Echinocandins are administered once daily. Side effects are uncommon and include rash and flushing when the infusion is given too quickly.

Deresinski SC, Stevens DA: Caspofungin. Clin Infect Dis 36:1445–1457, 2003.

CHAPTER 29

PARASITIC INFECTIONS

Samer Saleh, MD, and Om P. Sharma, MD, FRCP

1. **Why is it important for health care professionals to be familiar with parasitic diseases?**

   Social and political upheavals, economic catastrophes, and technologic advances have blurred natural boundaries, and increasing travel and intercontinental migration have made the world a smaller place. Consequently, physicians and other health care workers can expect to encounter previously unfamiliar diseases and exotic medical syndromes that once occurred only in tropical and subtropical areas. Several of these diseases manifest primarily in the lungs; others involve the respiratory apparatus only in conjunction with other tissue systems. The possibility of a parasitic or imported illness should be considered in every visitor, tourist, political refugee, student, businessperson, or diplomat who presents with an unexplained pulmonary illness.

2. **Name the common symptoms of pulmonary parasitic diseases.**

   See Table 29-1.

TABLE 29-1.	PRINCIPAL SYMPTOMS OF PULMONARY PARASITIC DISEASES					
Disease	Cough	Wheezing	Dyspnea	Pneumonitis	Hemoptysis	Chronic
Ascariasis	+++	+++	++	+++	+	−
Hookworm	+++	+++	++	++	−	−
Strongyloides	+++	+++	++	+++	−	−
Visceral larva migrans	+++	+++	++	++	−	−
Toxoplasmosis (neonatal)	+	−	+++	+++	−	−
Amebiasis	++	−	+++	+++	−	−
Filariasis	++	++	++	++	−	−
Schistosomiasis	++	−	++	++	−	−
Paragonimiasis	++	+	++	++	+++	+++
Echinococcosis	−	−	−	−	++	+++

−, +, ++, +++ = usually absent to key symptom
Adapted from Jones JE: Signs and symptoms of parasitic diseases. Prim Care 18:153–165, 1991.

3. **Which of the following parasitic diseases is caused by eating raw or undercooked freshwater crustaceans such as crabs and crayfish: amebiasis, melioidosis, paragonimiasis, or malaria?**

   Paragonimiasis. Paragonimiasis is a helminthic zoonosis caused by a lung fluke of the genus *Paragonimus*. Human disease is caused by ingestion of undercooked crabs and crayfish infected with metacercarial larvae. Although found in Africa and Latin America, paragonimiasis is endemic in Korea, Thailand, Laos, the Philippines, China, and Japan.

Amebiasis, usually considered a tropical disease, exists in every country in the world. It is transmitted from human to human and is caused mainly by *Entamoeba histolytica*.

Melioidosis is endemic in Vietnam, Laos, Cambodia, Thailand, the Philippines, and Malaysia. It is caused by *Burkholderia pseudomallei*, a gram-negative aerobe and facultative anaerobe that lives in muddy water and soil in endemic areas. Wound contamination, inhalation, and aspiration are the most likely modes of transmission.

Malaria is caused predominantly by the four species of *Plasmodium*: *P. vivax*, *P. falciparum*, *P. ovale*, and *P. malariae*. The disease is transmitted by the bite of an *Anopheles* sp. mosquito.

4. **What are the clinical features of paragonimiasis?**
Ninety percent of patients have blood-stained, coffee-colored, or rusty sputum. Sputum production is greatest in the morning and after brisk exercise. There are usually no constitutional symptoms, so fever or weight loss is uncommon. Physical examination is usually unremarkable; however, hemiparesis, paraplegia, or convulsions may be seen. The diagnosis is established by low-power microscopic identification of operculated eggs in morning sputum specimens or in the stool. Enzyme-linked immunosorbent assay (ELISA) testing may also be helpful. Praziquantel is the treatment of choice.

Nakamura-Uchiyama F, Mukae H, Nawa Y: Paragonimiasis: A Japanese perspective. Clin Chest Med 23:409–420, 2002.

KEY POINTS: CLINICAL FEATURES OF PARAGONIMIASIS

1. Sputum production with blood-stained sputum

2. Fever and weight loss are uncommon; disease mimics tuberculosis

3. Diagnosed by detecting the eggs in sputum or stool

4. Praziquantel is the treatment of choice

5. **What are the pulmonary manifestations of trichinosis?**
Trichinosis is caused by the nematode of the genus *Trichinella*; there are five species that infect humans. The infection is acquired by eating inadequately cooked meats, including pork, walrus, bear, wild boar, and horse. Pulmonary involvement includes pneumonitis caused by direct larval invasion, myositis of respiratory muscles, and pleural effusion. The diagnosis is made by demonstrating nematode larvae in biopsied muscle.

Gilles HM: Soil transmitted helminths (geohelminths). In Cook GC, Zumla A (eds): Manson's Tropical Diseases, 21st ed. London, Saunders, 2003, pp 1553–1557.

6. **Name the pleuropulmonary manifestations of amebiasis.**
The different forms of pleuropulmonary amebiasis include:
- Direct extension of the liver abscess into the lung, pleural space, or pericardium
- Hematogenous pulmonary involvement without liver disease
- Independent pulmonary and hepatic involvement
- Rarely, inhalation of dust containing cysts of *Entamoeba histolytica* may cause primary lung disease

The lung and pleura appear to be involved in 6–40% of patients with amebic abscess of the liver. Most cases of thoracic involvement originate by extension of liver lesions through the diaphragm. If the abscess ruptures into free pleural space, amebic empyema is formed. Because the most common site of an amebic abscess is the right lobe of the liver, extension is usually to the right lower lobe of the lung. The diagnosis of pleuropulmonary amebiasis should always be considered in an individual with an unexplained right lower lobe pneumonia, mass, or empyema.

Shamsuzzaman SM, Hashiguchi Y: Thoracic amebiasis. Clin Chest Med 23:479–492, 2002.

7. **Describe the typical clinical and laboratory features of a patient with tropical pulmonary eosinophilia.**

The endemic areas for tropical eosinophilia include India, Pakistan, Sri Lanka, Burma, Thailand, and Malaysia. The disease has a predilection for individuals, mostly men, from the Indian sub-continent. It results from immunologic hyper-responsiveness to *Wuchereria bancrofti* and *Brugia malayi*. Symptoms include dry cough, malaise, fever, and wheezing. Typically, cough, dyspnea, and wheezing are most prominent at night. The chest radiograph may reveal a diffuse nodular (i.e., miliary) or an interstitial pattern. The erythrocyte sedimentation rate (ESR) is almost always elevated. The following criteria are used to make the diagnosis:

- Peripheral blood eosinophilia in excess of 3000 μL
- Absence of microfilaria in day and night blood samples
- Raised total serum immunoglobulin E (IgE) level (>1000 U/mL)
- Elevated titers of filarial antigen
- Favorable response to the drug diethylcarbamazine

Ong RKC, Doyle RL: Tropical pulmonary eosinophilia. Chest 113:1673–1679, 1998.

KEY POINTS: COMMON FEATURES OF TROPICAL PULMONARY EOSINOPHILIA

1. Chest x-ray may show diffuse nodular or interstitial pattern.

2. ESR is almost always elevated.

3. Eosinophilia and elevated IgE levels are characteristic findings.

4. Responds to diethylcarbamazine.

8. **Which parasites cause pulmonary granulomas?**

Parasitic causes of lung granulomas include visceral leishmaniasis (i.e., kala-azar), metazoan tissue parasites such as *Trichinella* spp., nematodes such as *Ascaris lumbricoides* and *Toxocara canis*, and trematodes such as *Schistosoma mansoni*.

9. **List the parasitic causes of pulmonary eosinophilic syndromes.**

The association between pulmonary infiltrates and blood eosinophilia is recognized as pulmonary eosinophilia, or pulmonary infiltration with eosinophilia (PIE). The parasitic causes of pulmonary eosinophilias include *Filaria* (i.e., tropical eosinophilia), *Strongyloides, Schistosoma, Ascaris, Trichinella, Ancylostoma*, and *Paragonimus* spp. The pulmonary infiltrates appear during larval migration through the lung and are usually transitory.

10. **What is visceral larva migrans, or toxocariasis?**

Infection with the dog roundworm, *Toxocara canis*, and the cat roundworm, *Toxocara cati*, produce the clinical syndrome of visceral larva migrans. Pulmonary symptoms include wheezing, dyspnea, and cough caused by pneumonitis. The diagnosis is suspected in a patient with marked eosinophilia and hypergammaglobulinemia. The diagnosis is made by demonstration of larvae in biopsied tissue or by serology (i.e., ELISA).

Gilles HM: Soil transmitted helminths (Geohelminths). In Cook GC, Zumla A (eds): Manson's Tropical Diseases, 21st ed. London, Saunders, 2003, pp 1536–1538.

11. **List the common parasitic lung infections in the immunocompromised host.**
Toxoplasmosis, although commonly a disseminated infection, can cause pneumonitis. *Strongyloides stercoralis* may cause life-threatening pulmonary disease. Although *Cryptosporidium* spp. have been found in the sputum, bronchoalveolar lavage fluid, and lung biopsy samples of immunodeficient patients with gastrointestinal disease, these parasites are not believed to cause lung infection.

12. **Describe the manifestations of strongyloidiasis.**
Uncomplicated infections in the immunocompetent patient are minimally symptomatic. Altered cellular immunity, such as long-term steroid therapy, malignancies (e.g., lymphoma), and kidney allograft recipients, may cause disseminated disease. Strongyloidiasis is not an important opportunistic infection associated with AIDS. In disseminated disease, gastrointestinal and respiratory symptoms predominate. Pulmonary manifestations include cough, sputum production, hemoptysis, dyspnea, bronchospasm, and respiratory insufficiency. Disruption of gastrointestinal mucosal integrity by penetrating filariform larvae may facilitate the entry of gram-negative bacteria, resulting in septicemia.

Siddiqui AA, Berk SL: Diagnosis of strongyloides stercoralis infection. Clin Infect Dis 33:1040–1047, 2001.

13. **What are the common lung changes in Chagas' disease?**
American trypanosomiasis is an endemic disease of rural populations caused by a protozoan, *Trypanosoma cruzi*, that is transmitted to humans by a blood-sucking bug of the subfamily Triatominae. It is a widespread human infection that is reported from the southwestern United States to Argentina. Except for bronchiectasis, which results from direct infection by *T. cruzi*, lung manifestations are uncommon and only occur secondary to infection of other organs (e.g. the heart or esophagus). Aspiration pneumonia is a common problem in patients with megaesophagus. In patients with congestive cardiomyopathy, pulmonary congestion or pulmonary thromboembolism may occur.

Magill AJ, Reed SG: American trypanosomiasis. In Strickland GT (ed): Hunter's Tropical Medicine and Emerging Infectious Diseases, 8th ed. London, W.B. Saunders, 2000, pp 653–664.

14. **How are hydatid cysts of the lung managed?**
Surgery is still the mainstay of management. In the natural history of hydatid disease, there is a latent period of several years. Once the cyst becomes symptomatic, however, deterioration is rapid. The type of surgery depends upon the extent of lung disease and the presence or absence of symptoms. Surgical procedures include cystectomy and capitonnage or wedge or other resections. Rupture of the cyst and spillage of its contents during surgery are feared complications that may lead to anaphylactic shock or result in spread of disease. Various methods of cyst sterilization are available before surgery. Mebendazole and albendazole are anthelmintic drugs that have been found to be effective.

Gottstein B, Reichen J: Hydatid lung disease. Clin Chest Med 23:397–408, 2002.

15. **Name the most serious complication of schistosomiasis.**
From a clinical standpoint, chronic cor pulmonale secondary to diffuse arteriolar disease represents the most important pulmonary complication of schistosomiasis. The pulmonary disease has been reported with *Schistosoma mansoni, Schistosoma hematobium,* and *Schistosoma japonicum.* Pulmonary injury may start during the invasive stage of the disease, when the circulating cercariae cause patchy congestion in the lungs; however, the more important pulmonary lesions, granulomas and obliterative arteritis, are caused by embolization of ova from the normal habitat of the worms.

Morris W, Knauer M: Cardiopulmonary manifestations of schistosomiasis. Semin Respir Infect 12:159–170, 1997.

16. **How does leishmaniasis affect the lung?**

Coughing as a symptom of visceral leishmaniasis has been well documented. It appears early in the disease, persists throughout the course, and disappears with cure. Interstitial pneumonitis is seen in patients with visceral leishmaniasis. Cells of the reticuloendothelial system present in the lung can become infected with the flagellate *Leishmania donovani*. After the bite of an infected sandfly, *Phlebotomus ovani*, the infective amastigotes are taken up by the mononuclear phagocytes, including alveolar macrophages, where they multiply. Interstitial pneumonitis is thought to facilitate bacterial growth, leading to a bronchopneumonia in some patients.

Duarte MIS, Matta VLR, Corbett CEP, et al: Interstitial pneumonitis in human visceral leishmaniasis. Trans R Soc Trop Med Hyg 83:73–76, 1989.

17. **What are the drugs commonly used to treat parasitic infections?**

Mebendazole is used to treat ascariasis and hookworms. Praziquantel is used for paragonimiasis and schistosomiasis. Diethylcarbamazine is used to treat tropical pulmonary eosinophilia. Ivermectin and thiabendazole are used to treat strongyloidiasis.

18. **What is pentastomiasis?**

Pentastomiasis is a disease caused by the larvae of several species of bloodsucking parasites. The majority of human infections are caused by *Armillifer armillatus* and *Linguatula serrata*; both are found in carnivorous animals. Most infections are asymptomatic and occur by ingesting eggs in contaminated food or water. Larvae mostly affect the abdomen and rarely the lung.

Drabick JJ: Pentastomiasis. Rev Infect Dis 9:1087–1094, 1987.

19. **How does malaria affect the lung?**

Noncardiogenic pulmonary edema is the most serious pulmonary manifestation of malaria. Out of the four species of malaria mentioned, *Plasmodium falciparum* is the most common culprit; however, *Plasmodium vivax* and *Plasmodium ovale* have occasionally caused pulmonary edema. Other pulmonary manifestations of malaria include iatrogenic pulmonary edema from fluid overload and pneumonia. Pulmonary edema can occur anytime during the illness: it can occur at presentation, after several days of treatment, with clinical improvement, or when the parasitemia has fallen or cleared. Pregnant women are at higher risk. It is usually associated with cerebral malaria.

Taylor WRJ, White NJ: Malaria and the lung. Clin Chest Med 23:457–468, 2002.

WEBSITE

http://www.biosci.ohio-state.edu/~parasite/home.html

CHAPTER 30

VIRAL PNEUMONIA

Carlos E. Girod, MD

1. **How frequently are viral pathogens identified as the cause of community-acquired pneumonia (CAP)?**
   Viral pathogens are especially common causes of pneumonia in infants and children. In children under the age of 3 years, viral pneumonia (e.g., caused by the respiratory syncytial virus [RSV]) may account for as many as 50% of all cases of pneumonia. In contrast, viruses are less-common causes of CAP in adults. Studies performed during the past 3 decades have identified viruses as the cause of 5–34% of CAPs in adults. A recent study by de Roux and colleagues detected a respiratory virus in 18% of CAPs using acute and convalescent serology.

   de Roux A, Marcos MA, Garcia E, et al: Viral community-acquired pneumonia in nonimmunocompromised adults. Chest 125:1343–1351, 2004.

   Monto AS: Viral respiratory infections in the community: Epidemiology, agents, and interventions. Am J Med 99(Suppl 6B):24S–27S, 1995.

2. **Which patients are at risk for the development of viral pneumonia?**
   Immunocompetent persons with viral pneumonia are usually children. Infants under the age of 6 months appear to be at the highest risk for viral pneumonia, especially RSV and parainfluenza. In children, epidemiologic studies have identified day-care center or school attendance as a risk factor. In the immunocompetent adult, the main risk factor for the development of viral pneumonia is the presence of congestive heart failure or pulmonary disease.

   Immunocompromised patients are at increased risk for viral infection with cytomegalovirus (CMV) and herpes simplex virus (HSV). Other risk factors for development of viral pneumonia include human immunodeficiency virus (HIV) and acquired immunodeficiency syndrome (AIDS), cancer, radiation, chemotherapy, malnutrition, skin breakdown, and burns.

   Chien JW, Johnson JL: Viral pneumonias: Infection in the immunocompromised host. Postgrad Med 107:67–80, 2000.

   de Roux, A, Marcos MA, Garcia E, et al: Viral community-acquired pneumonia in nonimmunocompromised adults. Chest 125:1343–1351, 2004.

   Monto AS: Viral respiratory infections in the community: Epidemiology, agents, and interventions. Am J Med 99(Suppl 6B):24S–27S, 1995.

3. **What clinical features suggest a viral cause of pneumonia?**
   There is no specific or sensitive clinical or radiologic feature that distinguishes viral from bacterial pneumonia. The absence of sputum expectoration has been reported to be a useful criterion for distinguishing viral pneumonia from pneumococcal infection. Nonspecific clinical symptoms and signs include cough, fever, myalgias, headaches, fatigue, tachypnea, and low oxygen levels. The presence of a rash characteristic of varicella, measles, or herpes can aid in diagnosing viral pneumonia. Findings on chest radiograph are not specific and include unilateral or bilateral alveolar or interstitial infiltrates. Thus, the diagnosis of viral infection requires a high index of suspicion. A viral pathogen should be highly suspected during the winter months.

   Chien JW, Johnson JL: Viral pneumonias: Epidemic respiratory viruses. Postgrad Med 107:41–52, 2000.
   Chien JW, Johnson JL: Viral pneumonias: Multifaceted approach to an elusive diagnosis. Postgrad Med 107:67–72, 2000.

   de Roux, A, Marcos MA, Garcia E, et al: Viral community-acquired pneumonia in nonimmunocompromised adults. Chest 125:1343–1351, 2004.

KEY POINTS: IMPORTANT CLINICAL FEATURES THAT SUGGEST VIRAL PNEUMONIA

1. Children under the age of 3 years

2. History of chronic heart failure (CHF) or chronic obstructive pulmonary disease (COPD)

3. Bone marrow transplant or AIDS patients

4. Disease occurring during the winter months

5. Absence of sputum expectoration

6. Rash

7. Bilateral patchy infiltrates

4. **What are the most commonly available laboratory diagnostic tools for viral pneumonia?**

   The specimens that should be obtained in patients with suspected viral pneumonia include nasal washes, nasopharyngeal swabs, throat swabs, tracheal aspirates, and sputum cultures. Respiratory samples are also obtained with bronchoscopy or open lung biopsy. There are four main laboratory techniques used for detecting viral pathogens:

   - **Culture** of viruses is performed by inoculation of the sample into various tissue culture cell lines with direct observation of viral cytopathogenic activity. Viruses known to grow rapidly in culture include influenza and rhinovirus. Diagnosis by culture can be delayed in slow-growing viruses such as CMV and varicella-zoster virus (VZV). For these slow-growing viruses, the shell-vial culture system allows for rapid identification.

   - **Rapid antigen detection by immunofluorescence and enzyme-linked immunosorbent assay (ELISA)** of various viral antigens is especially useful in rapidly diagnosing influenza, CMV, respiratory syncytial virus (RSV), adenovirus, herpes simplex, and varicella pneumonia.

   - **Serologic studies** are commonly available for the diagnosis of influenza, parainfluenza, RSV, and CMV pneumonitis. A fourfold increase in titer from acute to convalescent serum of viral-specific antibodies is consistent with a recent viral infection.

   - **Polymerase chain reaction (PCR) and *in situ* hybridization** has successfully demonstrated the presence of viral pathogens in respiratory secretions, cells, and blood early in the course of viral infections.

       Chien JW, Johnson JL: Viral pneumonias: Multifaceted approach to an elusive diagnosis. Postgrad Med 107:67–72, 2000.
       Greenberg SB: Viral pneumonia. Infect Dis Clin North Am 5:615, 1991.

5. **How successful are antiviral agents in the treatment of viral pneumonia?**

   The treatment of viral pneumonias has been enhanced by the development of various agents with virucidal activity (Table 30-1). Nevertheless, the cornerstone of treatment is supportive care consisting of oxygen therapy, mechanical ventilation (in severe cases), and adjunctive antimicrobial therapy to treat bacterial superinfection. Antiviral agents either block viral replication or boost the host's immune response and are very successful *in vitro*, but response is less encouraging in the treatment of viral pneumonia.

       Chien JW, Johnson JL: Viral pneumonias: Epidemic respiratory viruses. Postgrad Med 107:41–52, 2000.
       Chien JW, Johnson JL: Viral pneumonias: Infections in the immunocompromised host. Postgrad Med 107:67–80, 2000.
       Greenberg SB: Viral pneumonia. Infect Dis Clin North Am 5:615, 1991.

TABLE 30-1. ANTIVIRAL AGENTS WITH POTENTIAL BENEFIT IN VIRAL PNEUMONIA

Agent	Virus
Ganciclovir, foscarnet, intravenous immunoglobulin	Cytomegalovirus
Acyclovir	Herpes simplex virus, varicella-zoster
Amantadine, rimantadine	Influenza A
Zanamivir	Influenza A and B
Oseltamivir	Influenza A and B
Ribavirin	Respiratory syncytial virus (RSV)*, parainfluenza*, adenovirus*, measles*, severe acute respiratory syndrome (SARS)-associated coronavirus*

*The use of ribavirin for these viruses remains controversial except for hospitalized infants with RSV.

6. **Is respiratory isolation required for patients with suspected or documented viral pneumonia?**
   Viral pneumonia may spread to other patients or hospital personnel even when patients are being treated with antiviral therapy. It is imperative that patients be placed in respiratory isolation rooms, and visitors and hospital personnel must wear disposable gloves, gowns, and masks. This is particularly important during the treatment of RSV in children.

   Hall CB: Respiratory syncytial virus and parainfluenza virus. N Engl J Medicine 344:1917–1928, 2001.

7. **What vaccines are available for the prevention of viral pneumonia?**
   The most common viral vaccination program is directed to the influenza virus. The **influenza vaccine** has been available for more than 50 years and is prepared yearly based on expected or predicted major and minor mutations in viral capsular antigens. Influenza vaccine should be administered in the early fall to provide enough time for a specific antibody response. The **varicella vaccine** is recommended for all children at 12–18 months of age, those older than 13 years of age without prior varicella infection, and women of childbearing age. It is contraindicated in pregnancy. Work is ongoing for developing vaccines directed to RSV, parainfluenza virus, severe acute respiratory syndrome (SARS)-associated coronavirus, and avian influenza viruses. Passive immunity through administration of immunoglobulin is another way of preventing viral infection. It has been limited to patients at risk for RSV, CMV, VZV, and measles viruses.

   Couch RB: Prevention and treatment of influenza. N Engl J Med 343:1778–1787, 2000.
   Feldman S: Varicella-zoster virus pneumonitis. Chest 106 (Suppl):22S–26S, 1994.
   Greenberg SB: Viral pneumonia. Infect Dis Clin North Am 5:603–621, 1991.

8. **How effective is vaccination in preventing influenza infection?**
   Yearly immunization for prevention of influenza is recommended for healthy adults aged 50 years and older and all age groups with high risk factors or chronic medical illness. During years of vaccine shortage, the recommendation for healthy adults is changed to ≥65 years of age. This vaccine is also recommended for nursing home residents and health care workers. Various studies involving healthy adults and children have demonstrated a vaccination efficacy of 77–80% in preventing laboratory-confirmed influenza infection. Studies that have included elderly patients have shown decreased efficacy of 52–60% during influenza outbreaks.

Couch RB: Prevention and treatment of influenza. N Engl J Med 343:1778–1787, 2000.

Mandell LA, Bartlett JG, Dowell SF, et al: Infectious Diseases Society of America guidelines. Update of practice guidelines for the management of community-acquired pneumonia in immunocompetent adults. Clin Infect Dis 37:1405–1433, 2003.

Nicholson KG, Wood JM, Zambon M: Influenza. Lancet 362:1733–1745, 2003.

Niederman MS, Mandell LA, Anzueto A, et al: Guidelines for the management of adults with community-acquired pneumonia. Diagnosis, assessment of severity, antimicrobial therapy, and prevention. Am J Respir Crit Care Med 163:1730–1754, 2001.

KEY POINTS: GROUPS FOR WHOM INFLUENZA VACCINATION IS RECOMMENDED

1. Adults aged ≥50 years (during vaccine shortage, ≥ 65 years)

2. Residents of nursing homes or chronic care facilities

3. Patients with chronic cardiovascular or pulmonary disease

4. Chronic medical illness (e.g., diabetes, renal insufficiency, or hemoglobinopathies)

5. Patients with HIV or AIDS

6. Immunosuppressed individuals

7. Pregnant women with their second or third trimester coinciding with flu season

8. Physicians, nurses, health care providers, and employees of nursing homes or chronic care facilities

9. Household contacts of high-risk persons

10. Breast-feeding mothers

11. Travelers during influenza season

9. **Are there new therapies for prophylaxis or treatment of influenza pneumonia?**

The use of amantadine or rimantadine has proven to be effective in the **prophylaxis** of laboratory-confirmed influenza infection. Various studies have demonstrated a 61–90% efficacy for these agents in preventing clinical illness by influenza A. However, these medications are associated with side effects, predominantly neurologic complaints.

Amantadine and rimantadine are also effective in the **treatment** of influenza A infection. These agents reduce the duration of clinical illness by 1–2 days when started within the first 24–48 hours from the onset of symptoms. For adults, amantadine is given orally at 200 mg/day, and for children under the age of 10, 4 mg/kg/day is given. Zanamivir and oseltamivir are approved by the Food and Drug Administration (FDA) for the prophylaxis and treatment of both influenza A and B. Both agents provide 69–81% protection against symptomatic laboratory-confirmed influenza infection. When administered within 48 hours from the onset of influenza, both agents shorten duration of symptoms and the time needed for the patient to return to normal activities. Zanamivir is an inhaler delivered at 20 mg/day for 5 days. Oseltamivir is given orally at 75 mg twice a day for 5 days.

Couch RB: Prevention and treatment of influenza. N Engl J Med 343:1778–1787, 2000.

Nicholson KG, Wood JM, Zambon M: Influenza. Lancet 362:1733–1745, 2003.

Niederman MS, Mandell LA, Anzueto A, et al: Guidelines for the management of adults with community-acquired pneumonia. Diagnosis, assessment of severity, antimicrobial therapy, and prevention. Am J Respir Crit Care Med 163:1730–1754, 2001.

10. **What is the most common cause of upper respiratory tract infection and pneumonia in children? How is it diagnosed?**

RSV is the leading cause of bronchiolitis (50–90%) and pneumonia (5–40%) in young children. Epidemics usually occur during the spring and winter months. Infections can be severe in children under the age of 2, sometimes requiring mechanical ventilation. The chest radiograph patterns of air-trapping or patchy consolidation are suggestive of but not specific for RSV infection. Some reports suggest that right-upper-lobe consolidation and collapse are characteristic of RSV infection. Diagnosis can be made by identification of RSV antigens using immunofluorescence or ELISA of nasopharyngeal epithelial cells obtained by swab. The test is readily available in most hospitals and outpatient clinics. Reverse transcriptase-polymerase chain reaction (RT-PCR) has a much higher sensitivity.

Hall CB: Respiratory syncytial virus and parainfluenza virus. N Engl J Med 344:1917–1928, 2001.

11. **What therapy is available for the treatment of RSV infection?**

Although controversial, children hospitalized with RSV infection have been treated with ribavirin (6 grams in 300 cc of sterile water nebulized continuously for 18–22 hours per day for 3–7 days). Studies with infants infected with RSV have demonstrated improved oxygenation. Nebulization has to be supervised and requires a closed room to prevent aerosolation of RSV and contagious spread to hospital personnel or patients. Recent studies have not demonstrated a significant reduction in respiratory deterioration or mortality. Ribavirin has also been used in adults with severe RSV infection without prior controlled studies. Bone marrow transplant recipients infected with RSV have a high mortality (60–78%), and it appears that rapid detection and early antiviral therapy may improve outcome. RSV hyperimmune globulin and the monoclonal antibody have been utilized with marginal results.

Hall CB: Respiratory syncytial virus and parainfluenza virus. N Engl J Med 344:1917–1928, 2001.
Rodriguez WJ, Gruber WC, Groothius JR, et al: Respiratory syncytial virus immune globulin treatment of RSV lower respiratory tract infection in previously healthy children. Pediatrics 100:937–942, 2000.

12. **Which patients are at risk of CMV infection and pneumonia?**

CMV is a herpesvirus. Herpesviruses are prone to attack susceptible patients, especially recent recipients of organ transplantation and patients with AIDS. CMV infection is an important complication of bone marrow, renal, heart, and lung transplants. Infection occurs from transmission by a CMV-positive transplanted organ or from reactivation in recipients with evidence of prior CMV infection. CMV is also recognized as the most common viral pathogen affecting AIDS patients. The rate of infection, based on autopsy studies, is as high as 49–81% of AIDS patients. It is common for CMV to be isolated in respiratory secretions of AIDS patients **without** clear evidence of lung involvement.

Greenberg SB: Respiratory herpesvirus infections. An overview. Chest 106(Suppl):1S–2S, 1994.
McGuinness G, Scholes JV, Garay SM, et al: Cytomegalovirus pneumonitis: Spectrum of parenchymal CT findings with pathologic correlation in 21 AIDS patients. Radiology 192:451–459, 1994.
Tamm M, Traenkle P, Grilli B, et al: Pulmonary cytomegalovirus infection in immunocompromised patients. Chest 119:838–843, 2001.
Yen KT, Lee AS, Krowka MJ, Burger CD: Pulmonary complications in bone marrow transplantation: a practical approach to diagnosis and treatment. Clin Chest Med. 25:189–201, 2004.

13. **How soon after organ transplantation should CMV infection be suspected? What clinical clues suggest CMV pneumonitis?**

CMV infection usually occurs 6–12 weeks after transplantation, which suggests that the cause is reactivation of prior infection or infection borne by the transplanted organ. Thus, pulmonary infiltrates occurring within the first month after transplantation are almost never the result of

CMV. No specific sign or symptom is associated with CMV infection. Patients usually manifest fever, malaise, dry cough, dyspnea, diminished exercise tolerance, and hypoxia. Most patients have diffuse interstitial infiltrates by chest radiography.

Yen KT, Lee AS, Krowka MJ, Burger CD: Pulmonary complications in bone marrow transplantation: A practical approach to diagnosis and treatment. Clin Chest Med. 25:189–201, 2004.

14. **What agents are indicated for prophylaxis against CMV infection in transplant recipients?**
CMV pneumonitis occurs in 10–40% of transplant patients and is associated with a high morbidity and mortality (40–90%). Routine CMV prophylaxis utilizing acyclovir or ganciclovir has been used in many transplant centers. Most recently, transplant centers prefer not to use routine CMV prophylaxis and use a CMV surveillance approach with serial blood antigenemia assays and PCR. The detection of CMV antigen or DNA in blood leads to empirical antiviral therapy with ganciclovir. The use of CMV hyperimmune globulin or immune globulin for CMV prophylaxis remains controversial.

Yen KT, Lee AS, Krowka MJ, Burger CD: Pulmonary complications in bone marrow transplantation: A practical approach to diagnosis and treatment. Clin Chest Med. 25:189–201, 2004.

15. **Is isolation of CMV in bronchoalveolar lavage (BAL) or sputum sufficient to document active CMV pneumonitis?**
CMV culture and isolation from BAL has been documented in as many as 8–29% of HIV-positive patients and bone marrow transplant recipients. Of those, only 16–20% have an active CMV pneumonitis. For this reason, evaluation of lung tissue for the diagnosis of CMV pneumonitis remains the gold standard. With the advent of serum CMV antigenemia assays and PCR, patients are receiving early treatment for CMV viremia, thus reducing the need for BAL or lung biopsy. Furthermore, positive CMV immunostaining in respiratory cells retrieved by BAL has high sensitivity and specificity (89% and 99%, respectively) for CMV pneumonitis.

Tamm M, Traenkle P, Grilli B, et al: Pulmonary cytomegalovirus infection in immunocompromised patients. Chest 119:838–843, 2001.
Yen KT, Lee AS, Krowka MJ, Burger CD: Pulmonary complications in bone marrow transplantation: A practical approach to diagnosis and treatment. Clin Chest Med. 25:189–201, 2004.

16. **When and how should treatment of CMV pneumonitis be initiated in transplant patients?**
In transplant patients, treatment for CMV pneumonitis is usually begun when symptoms suggestive of lung involvement occur and pulmonary infiltrates or nodules develop on chest

KEY POINTS: IMPORTANT FEATURES OF CYTOMEGALOVIRUS PNEUMONITIS

1. Common in transplant patients and AIDS.

2. Affects 10–40% of transplant patients.

3. Usually occurs 6–12 weeks after transplantation.

4. BAL for CMV is positive in 28–29% of AIDS patients and bone marrow transplant recipients.

5. Approximately 80% of the patients with positive CMV BAL do not have CMV pneumonitis.

6. The gold standard for diagnosis is tissue biopsy with confirmed cytopathic changes.

7. CMV immunostaining in respiratory cells may be diagnostic for pneumonitis without a need for tissue biopsy.

radiograph or computed tomography (CT) scan or when surveillance blood, BAL, or lung biopsy samples become CMV-positive. Early, combined therapy with ganciclovir and immunoglobulin has been demonstrated to improve survival. Most patients need maintenance antiviral therapy for as long as 120 days after transplantation.

Enright H, Haake R, Weisdorf D, et al: Cytomegalovirus pneumonia after bone marrow transplantation. Risk factors and response to therapy. Transplantation 55:1339–1346, 1993.

Yen KT, Lee AS, Krowka MJ, Burger CD: Pulmonary complications in bone marrow transplantation: A practical approach to diagnosis and treatment. Clin Chest Med. 25:189–201, 2004.

17. **Which patients are at increased risk for developing varicella pneumonia?**
Varicella is usually limited to children. Recently, infection is being increasingly identified in adults with an associated high risk for pneumonia and a high mortality. The following individuals are at risk for varicella pneumonia:

Immunocompromised patients

AIDS patients

Inhaled corticosteroid users

Cancer patients

Organ transplant recipients

Patients with chronic obstructive pulmonary disease (COPD)

Newborns, especially premature newborns

Elderly patients

Pregnant women

Smokers

Patients with varicella with numerous lesions or severe skin eruption

Feldman S: Varicella-zoster virus pneumonitis. Chest 106 (Suppl):22S–26S, 1994.

Harger JH, Ernest JM, Thurnau GR, et al: Risk factors and outcome of varicella-zoster virus pneumonia in pregnant women. J Infect Dis 185:422–427, 2002.

18. **What are the clinical features of varicella pneumonia?**
Pneumonia usually develops 1–6 days after the onset of a characteristic rash. Symptoms include shortness of breath and cough. The chest radiograph usually shows diffuse bilateral infiltrates with some nodular pattern. Microcalcifications ranging from 2–3 mm detected in the chest radiograph can be a late sequelae.

Feldman S: Varicella-zoster virus pneumonitis. Chest 106 (Suppl):22S–26S, 1994.

Harger JH, Ernest JM, Thurnau GR, et: Risk factors and outcome of varicella-zoster virus pneumonia in pregnant women. J Infect Dis 185:422–427, 2002.

19. **Is there a role for acyclovir prophylaxis in varicella infection? What is the treatment for varicella pneumonia?**
Prophylaxis with oral acyclovir or varicella zoster immunoglobulin (VZIG) should be considered for patients at risk for progression to varicella pneumonia. When given within 3–4 days of exposure to varicella, VZIG has been documented to reduce by 50% the incidence of infection and disease. Treatment for varicella pneumonia includes the administration of intravenous acyclovir (10 mg/kg, three times a day for 7–10 days). The use of adjunctive therapy with corticosteroids has been reported. With the use of acyclovir, the mortality of varicella pneumonia in the general population is 9%. A mortality as high as 14% has been reported in pregnant patients.

Harger JH, Ernest JM, Thurnau GR, et al: Risk factors and outcome of varicella-zoster virus pneumonia in pregnant women. J Infect Dis 185:422–427, 2002.

Mer M, Richards GA: Corticosteroids in life-threatening varicella pneumonia. Chest 114:426–431, 1998.

Potgieter PD, Hammond JMJ: Intensive care management of varicella pneumonia. Respir Med 91:207–212, 1997.

20. **What viral outbreak led to the first pandemic of the 21st century and accounted for 774 deaths?**

This viral pandemic was called severe acute respiratory syndrome (SARS) and emerged in a province of China. It affected as many as 8000 patients in 26 countries and 5 continents and created widespread panic. The viral pathogen was identified as the SARS-associated coronavirus and is suspected to be an animal virus that, for unclear reasons, crossed over to humans. It is suspected that the initial human infection occurred in individuals involved in the trade of wild, exotic animals.

This virus is highly contagious and was contained thanks to aggressive public health measures consisting of rapid identification, isolation, and quarantine of suspected infected individuals. The incubation period is usually 2–14 days from exposure and patients are contagious for 5–10 days after the onset of symptoms. Common presenting symptoms of SARS include fever, myalgias, chills, cough, shortness of breath, tachypnea, and pleurisy. Lung examination may be negative in two-thirds of patients, but the chest radiograph is abnormal in most patients. Laboratory data commonly reveal lymphopenia and, in some patients, thrombocytopenia, as well as elevated D-dimers, liver function tests, creatinine kinase, and lactate dehydrogenase (LDH). Approximately 20–30% of patients deteriorate and require admission to the intensive care unit for mechanical ventilation. Diagnosis requires a high level of suspicion; RT-PCR for the SARS-associated coronavirus in fecal and respiratory secretions confirms the diagnosis. Treatment is largely supportive. Ribavirin has been utilized in anecdotal reports. High-dose intravenous methylprednisolone has been used early in the SARS course with the hope of modulating lung injury. Isolation of hospitalized patients is paramount and requires respiratory and contact isolation with the use of disposable gowns and gloves. Mortality rate for patients older than 65 years of age is about 50%.

Peiris JSM, Yuen KY, Osterhaus ADME, Stöhr K: The severe acute respiratory syndrome. N Engl J Med 349:2431–2441, 2003.

21. **What is avian influenza, and why has it been called a global threat?**

Three of the most deadly influenza pandemics of the last century (1918, 1957, and 1968) were caused by a newly identified influenza type A virus originally classified as an avian flu virus. The total mortality of the last two pandemics of 1957 and 1968 was more than 2 million people. Avian influenza viruses are found in poultry, migratory birds, and waterfowl and usually have low pathogenicity. Transmission from chickens to humans of a highly virulent H5N1 avian influenza has led to two outbreaks (1997 and 2004) with 44 total cases. After a 2–10 day incubation period, avian influenza leads to an acute respiratory illness with a mortality quoted at 72%. Most recently, human-to-human transmission of avian influenza was reported in Thailand. Many experts believe that these sentinel outbreaks serve as strong warnings of possible future pandemics likely to originate in an Asian country. The World Health Organization (WHO) has advocated and supported the rapid development and testing of an H5N1 avian flu vaccine. Oseltamivir, a neuramidase inhibitor, is active against H5N1 viruses, and many countries are stockpiling this agent for treatment and prophylaxis.

Hien TT, de Jong M, Farrar J: Avian influenza—A challenge to global health care structures. N Engl J Med 351:2363–2365, 2004.

Monto AS: The threat of an avian influenza epidemic. N Engl J Med 352:323–325, 2005.

Ungchusak K, Auewarakul P, Dowell S, et al: Probable person-to-person transmission of avian influenza A (H5N1). N Engl J Med 352:333–340, 2005.

CHAPTER 31

PNEUMONIA PREVENTION

Kala Davis, MD, Ann Weinacker, MD, and Steve Nelson, MD

COMMUNITY-ACQUIRED PNEUMONIAS

1. **What vaccines are recommended to prevent viral and bacterial community-acquired pneumonia (CAP)?**
   - **Influenza vaccine:** For prevention of viral pneumonias caused by influenza A and B. It is available in the United States as an inactivated split-product vaccine administered intramuscularly or as a live cold-attenuated intranasal vaccine. The vaccine is reformulated each year to correlate with strains that are expected to circulate in the upcoming flu season.
   - **Pneumococcal vaccine:** For prevention of invasive *Streptococcus pneumoniae* infections. It is most commonly administered as a 23-valent vaccine. A conjugate vaccine is also available and is recommended for use in children less than 2 years in age.

2. **Who should receive the influenza vaccine, and how often?**
   - The influenza vaccine is administered annually prior to and throughout the flu season.
   - Children < 9 years old who have never received the flu vaccine should receive two vaccine doses, 1 month apart (Table 31-1).

TABLE 31-1. INFLUENZA VACCINE	
Indications	**Side Effects and Adverse Reactions**
<ul><li>Age 50 years and above</li><li>Chronic illness (e.g., diabetes; chronic cardiovascular, pulmonary, renal, or hepatic disease; or hemoglobinopathies)</li><li>Immunocompromised persons</li><li>Children aged 6–23 months</li><li>Children aged 2–18 years on long-term aspirin therapy</li><li>Pregnant women</li><li>Residents of nursing homes or chronic care facilities</li><li>Health care workers or persons caring for patients who are in any of the above high-risk groups</li></ul>	<ul><li>Injection site tenderness and induration</li><li>Fever and malaise (may start within 6–12 hours and last 1–2 days)</li><li>Allergic or anaphylactoid reactions</li><li>Guillain–Barré syndrome (GBS): patients with a history of GBS have a greater likelihood of developing GBS than those without</li><li>Intranasal vaccine has been associated with the additional side effects of headaches, nasal congestion, and sore throat</li></ul>
http://www.cdc.gov/flu/protect/whoshouldget.htm	

3. **When is the influenza vaccine contraindicated?**
   Absolute contraindications: Hypersensitivity to the influenza vaccine or any of its components (i.e., allergies to egg or chicken proteins or to thimerosal)

Relative contraindications: in the presence of an acute respiratory illness or active neurologic disorder, immunization should be delayed. Caution should be used in patients with a history of febrile seizures because of the risk for a febrile reaction.

4. **Are there any special considerations or contraindications for the live cold-attenuated intranasal influenza vaccine?**
   Antiviral medications should be discontinued for at least 48 hours prior to administering this vaccine and for 2–3 weeks after. Contraindications include the following:
   - Persons <5 years or >49 years old
   - History of anaphylaxis to egg proteins or gentamicin
   - Known or suspected immune deficiency
   - History of Guillain–Barré syndrome, asthma, or reactive airway disease
   - Children on long-term salicylate therapy (because of increased risk for Reye's syndrome)
   - Household members or persons caring for immunocompromised patients

5. **What alternatives are available for patients who are unable to take the influenza vaccine?**
   The Food and Drug Administration (FDA) has approved the drugs listed in Table 31-2 for influenza chemoprophylaxis. Chemoprophylaxis should not replace vaccination in individuals for whom it is indicated.

TABLE 31–2.   INFLUENZA CHEMOPROPHYLAXIS

Indications	Drug and Treatment Profile	Serious Adverse Reactions
• High-risk persons who cannot be immunized • Protection of high-risk individuals during the 2 weeks following immunization (while immune response is developing)	*Amantadine/Rimantadine* • >1 year of age • 70–90% effective against influenza A • Not effective against influenza B	*Amantadine*: Arrhythmias, pulmonary edema, neuroleptic malignant syndrome, and psychosis *Rimantadine*: Seizures, ataxia, hallucinations, hypertension, heart block, and bronchospasm
• Immunocompromised persons who may not mount an adequate response to the vaccine • Control of influenza outbreaks in a closed setting	*Oseltamivir* • >13 years of age • 70–90% effective against influenza A and B • Must be taken within 48 hours of flu symptom onset	*Oseltamivir*: No known serious adverse reactions. Common side effects include nausea, vomiting, and diarrhea

http://www.cdc.gov/flu/ professionals/treatment/0405antiviralguide.htm

6. **How effective are herbal remedies in preventing influenza?**
   There is no scientific evidence that herbal or homeopathic remedies (e.g., Echinacea, vitamin C, or zinc supplements) have any benefit in preventing influenza.

7. **Who should receive the pneumococcal vaccine, and how often?**
   See Table 31-3.

TABLE 31-3. PNEUMOCOCCAL VACCINE

Indications for Pneumococcal Vaccine	Revaccination
<ul><li>Persons >65 years of age</li><li>Persons aged 2–64 years with chronic illnesses (e.g., diabetes, pulmonary or cardiovascular disease, alcoholism, hepatic dysfunction, chronic cerebrospinal fluid leak, or sickle cell disease)</li><li>Persons aged 2–64 years who reside in chronic care facilities</li><li>Alaskan natives and certain Native American populations</li><li>Immunocompromised persons (e.g., those with HIV, malignancy, chronic renal failure, or asplenia; patients on long-term immunosuppressive therapy; and transplant recipients)</li></ul>	<ul><li>Routine revaccination of immunocompetent persons is not recommended</li><li>Single revaccination is recommended for those persons aged 65 years and older who received their first dose at <65 years, with more than 5 years elapsing since then</li><li>Single revaccination if, in immunocompromised persons, >5 years have elapsed since receiving the first dose</li><li>For patients under 10 years of age, consider revaccination after 3 years</li></ul>

http://www.cdc.gov/mmwr/preview/mmwrhtml/00047135.htm

8. **Why is the pneumococcal vaccine needed when antibiotics that are effective against *Streptococcus pneumoniae* are available?**
The increasing prevalence of drug-resistant strains and the appreciable morbidity and mortality associated with invasive pneumococcal infections make primary prevention with vaccination an attractive option, especially in patients who are at high risk.

9. **What are the side effects of the pneumococcal vaccine? When is it contraindicated?**
Side effects include the following:
- Injection site tenderness and induration (~72%)
- Low-grade fever, myalgias, or rash
- Anaphylaxis (<1%)
- Guillain–Barré syndrome (<1%)

Contraindications: Hypersenitivity to the pneumococcal vaccine or the component.
Pneumococcal polysaccharide vaccine is not recommended for use in children <2 years of age.

10. **How effective are the available vaccines?**
Influenza vaccine:
- Inactivated intramuscular vaccine: 30–90% efficacy
- Live cold-attenuated vaccine: 34–100% efficacy

Pneumococcal vaccine:
- Efficacy of 59% over all risk categories, 75% efficacy in persons >65 years of age
- The pneumococcal conjugate vaccine (PCV) has an efficacy of 97%, but cost and limited supplies have restricted its use to children under 2 years of age.

Greenberg HB, Piedra PA: Immunization against viral respiratory disease: A review. Pediatr Infect Dis J 23(11 Suppl):S254–261, 2004.
Levy J, Swennen B: Pneumococcal conjugate vaccine in children. Rev Med Brux 25(4):A219–222, 2004.

11. **What is SARS? How can it be prevented?**
Severe acute respiratory syndrome (SARS) is a viral respiratory illness caused by a coronavirus. SARS was first reported in Asia in February 2003. It is spread by respiratory droplets and direct contact of infected secretions with the eyes or nasal or oral mucosa. SARS presents clinically with flu-like symptoms including high fevers, headaches, myalgias, diarrhea, and dry cough. Most patients develop pneumonia. SARS is prevented by avoiding travel to cities in which there are SARS outbreaks, by limiting contact with infected individuals, and by frequent hand washing.

    http://www.cdc.gov/ncidod/sars

KEY POINTS: PNEUMONIA PREVENTION STRATEGIES

1. Universal precautions such as frequent hand washing and the use of antiseptic hand lotions or rubs

2. Avoidance of sick contacts

3. Proper disposal of tissues contaminated with infected respiratory secretions

4. Covering the nose and mouth when sneezing or coughing to prevent aerosolization of infected respiratory droplets

5. Use of influenza and pneumococcal vaccines in at-risk populations

HOSPITAL-ACQUIRED PNEUMONIAS

12. **What measures should be used to prevent ventilator associated pneumonia (VAP)?**
    - Diligent airway cuff management to minimize aspiration
    - Aspiration of subglottic secretions and use of oscillatory beds in selected patients
    - Prevention of aerodigestive tract colonization
    - Routine drainage of ventilator circuit condensate
    - Use of a closed endotracheal suctioning system
    - Semirecumbent body positioning, to minimize aspiration risk
    - Distal placement of feeding tubes and use of prokinetic agents
    - Use of weaning protocols to shorten duration of mechanical ventilation

    Kollef MH: Prevention of hospital-associated pneumonia and ventilator-associated pneumonia. Crit Care Med 32(6):1396–1405, 2004.

13. **How does body positioning affect the risk of nosocomial pneumonia (NP)?**
Supine positioning is associated with an increased incidence of gastric content aspiration and pneumonia in mechanically ventilated patients.

14. **Is there a difference in NP risk with nasotracheal intubation versus orotracheal intubation?**
An increased incidence of nosocomial sinusitis and pneumonia has been observed with nasotracheal intubation.

15. **Do histamine (H_2) blockers, proton pump inhibitors, and antacids increase susceptibility to NPs?**
Medications used for stress ulcer prophylaxis increase gastric pH, which has been associated with gastric bacterial colonization and an increased risk of VAP. Restricted use of these medications in

patients who are at risk for stress ulcers or who have a history of peptic ulcer disease can limit the risk of VAP. Sucralfate for stress ulcer prophylaxis decreases the incidence of VAP but should not be used in patients at high risk for gastrointestinal bleeding.

16. **Is selective decontamination of the digestive tract (SDD) effective in preventing NP in critically ill patients?**
   - SDD has been shown to decrease the incidence of NP but has not been shown to reduce mortality.
   - SDD prevents NPs by decreasing the colonization of the oropharynx and aerodigestive tract with potential pathogens that could be aspirated in critically ill patients.
   - Commonly used regimens include an intravenous cephalosporin (cefotaxime) for the first 4 days and nonabsorbable antibiotic agents against gram-negative bacilli (aminoglycoside plus polymyxin) and *Candida* (nystatin or amphotericin B).
   - In intensive care units (ICUs) with high incidences of methicillin-resistant *Staphylococcus aureus* (MRSA), oral vancomycin should also be considered.
   - The routine use of SDD has not been shown to lead to the emergence of resistant organisms.

   de la Cal MA, Cerda E, van Saene HK, et al: Effectiveness and safety of enteral vancomycin to control endemicity of methicillin-resistant *Staphylococcus aureus* in a medical/surgical intensive care unit. J Hosp Infect 56(3):175–183, 2004.

   van Saene HK, Petros AJ, Ramsay G, et al: All great truths are iconoclastic: Selective decontamination of the digestive tract moves from heresy to level 1 truth. Intens Care Med 29(5):677–690, 2003.

KEY POINTS: PREVENTING AN INFLUENZA EPIDEMIC

1. The influenza vaccine can be up to 100% effective in healthy populations—use it!

2. Individuals at high risk for influenza complications should be vaccinated.

3. Outbreaks in close settings (e.g., nursing homes) should be limited with chemoprophylaxis.

4. Use universal precautions to prevent spread from infected individuals.

IMMUNOCOMPROMISED HOST

17. **What is the utility of pneumococcal and influenza vaccines in patients who are immunocompromised?**
   Although immunocompromised patients mount a diminished immune response to the vaccines compared to immunocompetent persons, vaccination does confer a variable amount of protection for persons who are at high risk for morbidity and mortality from a viral or bacterial pneumonia. Recent studies have shown pneumococcal vaccine efficacy approaching 65% in HIV-positive individuals when a 9-valent pneumococcal conjugated vaccine was used.

   Klugman KP, Madhi SA, Huebner RE, et al: A trial of a 9-valent pneumococcal conjugate vaccine in children with and those without HIV infection. N Engl J Med 349(14):1341–1348, 2003.

18. **What additional measures should be taken to prevent pneumonia in immunocompromised adults?**
   - HIV-infected patients with CD4 counts < 200, patients on long-term corticosteroid and immunosuppressive therapies, patients with hematological malignancies, patients with solid tumors, and transplant recipients are at risk for the development of *Pneumocystis* pneumonia (PCP). These patients should receive prophylaxis against *Pneumocystis jirovecii,* which has

recently been identified as the etiologic agent responsible for PCP.

- Transplant recipients who are cytomegalovirus (CMV)-seropositive or who receive organs from a seropositive donor should receive prophylaxis against CMV.

Lung transplant recipients with a history of *Aspergillus* colonization prior to transplant should be considered for prophylaxis against *Aspergillus*.

19. **What is the most effective agent for prophylaxis against PCP?**
   - Trimethoprim-sulfamethoxazole (TMP-SMZ) is the most effective agent for prophylaxis against *Pneumocystis jirovecii,* although its use has been limited by poor tolerance and toxicity.
   - A recent study showed a similar level of efficacy with an atovaquone-azithromycin combination.

   Aerosolized pentamidine, dapsone alone, dapsone–pyrimethamine, and atovaquone alone are also used but have proven less efficacious in preventing PCP in randomized controlled trials.

   Rodriguez M, Fishman JA: Prevention of infection due to Pneumocystis spp. in human immunodeficiency virus-negative immunocompromised patients. Clin Microbiol Rev 17(4):770–782, 2004.

MISCELLANEOUS

20. **What can be done to prevent pneumonias in patients who chronically aspirate (e.g., the elderly, patients with neuromuscular disease, or patients who have recently had a stroke)?**
   - Dietary modifications, using foods of modified consistency that are easier to swallow
   - Use of compensatory swallowing techniques such as chin tucks, multiple swallows, and head-turn techniques
   - Maintaining an upright position during eating
   - Feeding through a gastric or jejunal tube for patients who are unable to swallow or who have severe aspiration
   - Surgical laryngotracheal separation can be considered in select cases

21. **Do gastric or jejunal feeding tubes decrease the risk for aspiration?**
   Feeding tubes decrease the risk of oropharyngeal aspiration since patients receive their nutrition directly into the stomach or jejunum instead of by mouth. However, this does not completely eliminate the risk of aspiration of oral secretions and gastric or duodenal contents.

CHAPTER 32

EMPYEMA AND LUNG ABSCESS

John E. Heffner, MD

1. **What is a parapneumonic effusion? What is an empyema?**

   A **parapneumonic effusion** is an inflammatory pleural effusion that occurs in association with a pneumonia. Although most of these effusions are sterile and resolve with antibiotic therapy alone, 5–10% of patients with parapneumonic effusions develop an intrapleural infection, as defined by the presence of bacteria in the pleural space.

   An **empyema** is defined by the presence of intrapleural pus. Patients without pneumonia can also develop an empyema by introduction of bacteria into the pleural space, as occurs with trauma, chest surgery, bacteremia, or extension of infection from the mediastinum or chest wall.

2. **What are the common pathogens associated with parapneumonic effusions and empyemas?**

   A wide range of bacterial, viral, parasitic, and fungal pneumonias cause parapneumonic effusions. The most common bacterial pathogens are those that most often cause community-acquired pneumonia (CAP): *Streptococcus pneumoniae*, *Staphylococcus aureus*, *Haemophilus influenzae,* and *Klebsiella pneumoniae*. Patients with parapneumonic effusions acquired in the hospital have gram-negative bacilli, *Staphylococcus aureus*, and antibiotic-resistant bacteria as etiologic pathogens. The bacterial profile of patients with established empyemas, however, differs. These patients most often have anaerobic bacteria. They typically have a history of aspiration and clinical factors that promote aspiration of bacteria-laden oral secretions, as occurs with alcoholism, seizures, or stroke in the setting of poor dentition. These empyemas tend to be polymicrobial, with a mixture of aerobic and anaerobic pathogens.

   Chapman SJ, Davies RJ: Recent advances in parapneumonic effusion and empyema. Curr Opin Pulm Med 10:299–304, 2004.

3. **What are the stages of an empyema?**

   Parapneumonic effusions begin as neutrophil-rich inflammatory exudates. These early effusions represent the **exudative** phase of empyema formation, wherein pleural fluid is free-flowing and nonviscous. Patients with exudative effusions usually respond to antibiotics alone.

   If left untreated, exudative effusions can progress to the **fibrinopurulent** stage, characterized by the deposition of fibrin along pleural membranes. Fibrin induces the formation of pleural loculations and pleural peels, which can encase the lung. Fibrin also forms lattice-like stranding in the pleural space that promotes the influx of fibroblasts. These cells deposit collagen, which causes thickening of pleural membranes. Most patients in the fibrinopurulent stage require drainage of pleural fluid before extensive loculations occur.

   Eventually, membranes undergo further thickening, and pleural fluid becomes purulent and highly viscous in this **organized** stage of empyema formation. These patients need an open surgical drainage procedure to resolve sepsis and to recover full lung function.

4. **What are the clinical signs of a parapneumonic effusion?**

   The signs and symptoms of a parapneumonic effusion and empyema often merge with those of the underlying pneumonia. Patients present with fever, cough, purulent sputum, and shortness of breath. Some patients experience pleuritic chest pain, which may evolve to dull pain in patients who progress to a frank empyema. Failure to respond to antibiotic therapy of a pneumonia also suggests the possibility of an empyema. Patients with anaerobic empyemas may present with weight loss, foul breath, fatigue, and inanition simulating a cancer.

Signs of a parapneumonic effusion include decreased breath sounds, dullness, egophony, and decreased fremitus over the region of pleural fluid collection. A pleural friction rub denotes pleurisy.

5. **How is a parapneumonic effusion or empyema diagnosed?**
Every patient with pneumonia requires careful assessment to detect the presence of a pleural effusion. A standard chest radiograph can exclude a clinically important effusion if the diaphragm appears distinct on posterior–anterior and lateral views and if the nondependent regions of the pleural space appear free of fluid loculations. Lower-lobe consolidation from a pneumonia adjacent to the diaphragm can obscure the presence of dependent fluid collections. Such patients require chest ultrasonography or a lateral decubitus chest radiograph to exclude a parapneumonic effusion. The presence of more than 10 mm of layering on the decubitus view indicates the need for a thoracentesis. Delaying a thoracentesis and subsequent pleural fluid drainage when indicated are associated with increased morbidity and likelihood that a parapneumonic effusion will progress to an organized empyema. Results of the thoracentesis, combined with the clinical and radiologic presentation, determine the likelihood that the patient will require pleural fluid drainage.

6. **What is the proper method for performing a thoracentesis?**
Patients with free-flowing parapneumonic effusions in the exudative stage can undergo thoracentesis with a needle and small-bore catheter introduced into the pleural space by a Seldinger technique after first localizing the fluid by physical examination. Patients with radiographic evidence of pleural loculation benefit from ultrasonographic guidance of thoracentesis to ensure a successful sampling of pleural fluid and avoidance of puncture of the lung, diaphragm, and intra-abdominal organs. More extensive loculations may require computed tomography (CT)-guided thoracentesis by an interventional radiologist. Because of the availability of portable ultrasonographic equipment, we now use image guidance for performing thoracentesis for even free-flowing parapneumonic effusions.

Attempt to remove as much pleural fluid as possible during thoracentesis. If the patient's thoracentesis results return later with borderline evidence of a need of chest tube insertion, complete drainage during thoracentesis allows avoidance of chest tube placement by monitoring the patient for pleural fluid reaccumulation.

Beckh S, Bolcskei PL, Lessnau KD; Real-time chest ultrasonography: A comprehensive review for the pulmonologist. Chest 122:1759–1773, 2002.

Villena V, Lopez-Encuentra A, Garcia-Lujan R, et al: Clinical implications of appearance of pleural fluid at thoracentesis. Chest 125:156–159, 2004.

7. **What determines the need for pleural fluid drainage?**
The goals of the initial clinical evaluation of a patient with a parapneumonic effusion center on determining which patients require pleural fluid drainage. Patients with pleural fluid pus have progressed to the late stage of empyema formation and require drainage. The detection of bacteria by pleural fluid Gram stain or culture establishes a need for drainage. The presence of extensive pleural loculations as detected by chest CT scanning also indicates that a patient requires drainage (Fig. 32-1). Other clinical, radiologic, and laboratory results estimate the extent of pleural inflammation and the likelihood that patients will not recover with antibiotic therapy alone. These markers are not absolute indicators of the need for drainage, but their presence increases the probability that drainage will be required. These markers include the estimated volume of pleural fluid, the free-flowing nature of the fluid, the degree of pleural thickening, and the pleural fluid pH. The American College of Chest Physicians has proposed a staging system that guides clinicians in selecting patients for pleural fluid drainage (Table 32-1).

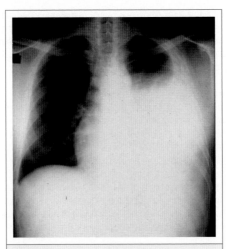

Figure 32-1. Large, free-flowing left-sided parapneumonic effusion in a patient with *Streptococcus pneumoniae* pneumonia. The patient responded to antibiotics and chest tube drainage.

TABLE 32-1. AMERICAN COLLEGE OF CHEST PHYSICIANS STAGING SYSTEM FOR SELECTING PATIENTS FOR PLEURAL FLUID DRAINAGE

Pleural Space Anatomy		Pleural Fluid Bacteriology		Pleural Fluid Chemistry	Risk of Poor Outcome	Drainage
Minimal, free-flowing effusion (<10 mm on lateral decubital)	AND	Culture and Gram stain results unknown	AND	pH unknown	Very low	No
Small to moderate free-flowing effusion (>10 mm and < ½ the hemithorax)	AND	Negative culture and Gram stain	AND	pH ≥ 7.20	Low	No
Large, free-flowing effusion (≥ ½ the hemithorax), loculated effusion, or effusion with thickened parietal pleura	OR	Positive culture or Gram stain	OR	pH < 7.20	Moderate	Yes
Any finding	OR	Pus	OR	Any finding	High	Yes

8. **Why is pleural fluid pH used to determine need for drainage?**
   Pleural fluid pH mirrors the degree of pleural inflammation and the likelihood that pleural fluid requires drainage. Intrapleural bacteria and polymorphonuclear leukocytes metabolize glucose to lactic acid and carbon dioxide. Organization of pleural membranes into a thick pleural peel

blocks the diffusion of carbon dioxide and hydrogen ions out of the pleural space. Together, these processes lower the pH of pleural fluid. A pleural fluid pH less than 7.20 indicates an increased likelihood that pleural fluid drainage will be required.

One should note, however, that studies supporting the clinical utility of pleural fluid pH are small and are limited by weak study designs. Consequently, pleural fluid pH is considered adjunctive in determining the need for drainage. Also, the single cutoff point of 7.20 should not be overinterpreted because many patients with pleural fluid pH values slightly below and above this value may be misclassified regarding their need for drainage. Patients with extremely low pH values are more likely to need pleural drainage.

Heffner JE, Brown LK, Barbieri C, et al: Pleural fluid chemical analysis in parapneumonic effusions. A meta-analysis. Am J Respir Crit Care Med 151:1700–1708, 1995.

9. **What are the risks of leaving infected pleural fluid undrained?**
Infected pleural fluid can rapidly undergo loculation, making simple drainage with a chest tube unlikely. Such patients may be initially easily managed with a few days of chest tube drainage but may later be more difficult to treat if loculations occur. The presence of loculations may require surgical drainage with attendant morbidity and prolonged hospitalizations.

10. **What antibiotics are used for treatment of a parapneumonic effusion and empyema?**
Initial selection of antibiotics is directed by published guidelines for treatment of the underlying pneumonia. These guidelines are based on epidemiologic observations that certain pathogens are more likely in different clinical settings and patient populations. Anaerobic coverage is added when patients have a history of aspiration or sufficient risk factors that increased the likelihood that aspiration would occur. Patients with nosocomial pneumonia (NP) and parapneumonic effusions are treated with broad-spectrum antibiotic regimens designed to cover the etiologic pathogen for the pneumonia. The microbiologic results of thoracentesis allow the refinement of the antibiotic regimen.

11. **How long should patients be treated?**
For most patients with exudative parapneumonic effusions that do not require pleural fluid drainage, the duration of antibiotic therapy is dictated by the needs of the underlying pneumonia. Patients with fibrinopurulent effusions who require drainage can also be treated for a duration determined by the pneumonia as long as the pleural fluid is adequately drained. Patients with frank empyemas or poorly draining fibrinopurulent parapneumonic effusions may require longer periods of antibiotic therapy until systemic signs of infection resolve.

Davies CW, Gleeson FV, Davies RJ: BTS guidelines for the management of pleural infection. Thorax 58(Suppl 2):18–28, 2003.

12. **How should a parapneumonic effusion or empyema be drained?**
Once the need for drainage is established, several methods should be considered for pleural fluid drainage. Free-flowing exudative effusions can be drained with insertion of a small-bore (i.e., 7–12 Fr) chest catheter. As pleural fluid viscosity increases, the caliber of the chest tube may also need to increase. Many centers place chest tubes under ultrasonographic or CT image guidance to ensure proper placement within the region of fluid and to detect areas of loculation. Repeated imaging studies are required to determine adequacy of drainage. Patients who do not quickly drain require a subsequent procedure to enhance drainage.

Patients with loculated effusions in the fibrinopurulent stage usually fail chest tube insertion. Such patients require drainage with video-assisted thoracic surgery (VATS) or a limited, muscle-sparing thoracotomy. Either procedure can break down adhesions and loculations, allowing drainage through a chest tube placed during surgery.

Organized empyemas require thoracotomy with decortication. The decortication removes the pleural peel that limits reexpansion of the lung and prevents obliteration of the empyemal space. Poor operative candidates for decortication who have a chronic, organized empyema may require an Eloesser flap. This procedure removes segments of several ribs overlying the empyema sac, promoting long-term open drainage.

Petrakis I, Katsamouris A, Drossitis I, et al: Usefulness of thoracoscopic surgery in the diagnosis and management of thoracic diseases. J Cardiovasc Surg (Torino) 41(5):767–771, 2000.

Ulmer JL, Choplin RH, Reed JC: Image-guided catheter drainage of the infected pleural space. J Thorac Imag 6(4):65–73, 1991.

Waller SM, Rajesh PB: Delayed referral reduces the success of video-assisted thoracoscopic surgery for spontaneous pneumothorax. Respir Med 92:246–249, 1998.

13. **Do fibrinolytics have a role in the treatment of empyema?**
For patients with parapneumonic effusions and empyemas, many clinical studies suggest that the intrapleural instillation of fibrinolytic drugs, such as streptokinase, urokinase, or tissue plasminogen activator, through a chest tube promotes pleural fluid drainage and decreases the need for subsequent surgical drainage. These studies, however, are small and suffer from flaws in their experimental designs. A large, multicenter clinical trial of streptokinase has shown no clinical benefit. This study, however, treated many patients who probably had organized empyemas with extensive fibrosis and who would not be expected to respond to fibrinolytic drugs.

To date, no strong evidence supports the role of fibrinolytic agents in this clinical setting. Proceed to VATS or thoracotomy for patients who cannot be drained effectively with chest tubes, and reserve the intrapleural instillation of fibrinolytic agents for patients with inadequate chest tube drainage who are poor surgical candidates and for those patients who refuse surgery.

Diacon AH, Theron J, Schuurmans MM, et al: Intrapleural streptokinase for empyema and complicated parapneumonic effusions. Am J Respir Crit Care Med:49–53, 2004.

Maskell NA, Davies CWH, Cunn AJ, et al: A controlled trial of intra-pleural streptokinase in pleural infection. N Engl J Med 352(9):865–874, 2005.

14. **What is the clinical course of patients who are successfully treated for an empyema?**
After removal of a chest tube, some patients may have residual pleural thickening that may restrict pulmonary function. After several weeks, however, this pleural thickening resolves and, several months later, no abnormalities on measured pulmonary function are apparent. Some residual blunting of the costophrenic area may be present on chest radiographs.

KEY POINTS: FACTORS THAT SUPPORT THE DECISION TO DRAIN AN EMPYEMA

1. The presence of intrapleural pus, or evidence thereof, by pleural fluid Gram stain or culture of bacteria in the pleural space

2. Loculated effusions

3. Large effusions (i.e., ≥50%) of a hemithorax

4. A pleural fluid pH < 7.20

15. **What is the definition of a lung abscess?**
A lung abscess is defined by the presence of necrosis within the pulmonary parenchyma that results from an infection. Lung abscesses are classified as **acute** or **chronic**. Chronic lung abscesses have been present for 4 or more weeks. Lung abscesses can also be categorized as **primary** or **secondary**. A primary lung abscess occurs in previously healthy patients who

aspirate oral contents and develop a localized pneumonitis that progresses to a lung abscess. These abscesses are usually caused by anaerobic bacteria, which do not grow well in culture. Primary lung abscesses with negative sputum cultures are termed **nonspecific lung abscesses**. A secondary lung abscess develops in patients with an underlying predisposition for pulmonary infection, such as in a patient with a cavitating lung cancer that becomes infected or in a patient with an immunocompromising condition such as acquired immunodeficiency syndrome (AIDS).

16. **How do primary lung abscesses form?**
   Primary lung abscesses develop as a result of aspiration of bacteria-laden oral contents. Etiologic pathogens are those bacteria that populate gingival crevices. Patients with poor oral hygiene, therefore, are at increased risk, as are patients with a predisposition to aspiration. Such patients include the elderly, alcoholics, patients with seizure disorders, and patients with dysphagia. Aspirated particles most commonly transit through the right bronchus because it comes off of the trachea at a more vertical angle than the left bronchus. Particles lodge in dependent bronchi because most aspiration events occur in the supine position. Consequently, lung abscesses most often develop in the posterior segments of the right upper lobe and the superior segment of the right lower lobe. An area of pneumonitis develops and progresses to tissue necrosis and lung abscess formation.

17. **How do secondary lung abscesses form?**
   Lung abscesses can occur when septic emboli reach the pulmonary circulation. A special example of septic emboli with multiple lung abscesses is Lemierre syndrome. This condition is characterized by suppurative thrombophlebitis from local spread of pharyngitis or tonsillitis. Right-sided endocarditis can also seed the lung with bacteria and cause multiple lung abscesses. Cavitating conditions, such as lung cancer or pulmonary infarction, can become secondarily infected and can form lung abscesses. Endobronchial lesions, such as bronchial carcinoma and aspirated foreign bodies, can produce postobstructive pneumonitis and lung cavitation.

18. **What are the most common pathogens that cause lung abscesses?**
   Anaerobic bacteria that inhabit the mouth are the most common cause of primary lung abscesses. These pathogens include *Peptostreptococcus*, *Prevotella*, *Bacteroides* (but usually not *B. fragilis*), and *Fusobacterium* spp. Aerobic bacteria may contribute to polymicrobial anaerobic lung infections. These bacteria include *Streptococcus milleri* and other microaerophilic streptococci. Other causes of lung abscess include *Klebsiella pneumoniae*, *S. aureus*, *Streptococcus pyogenes*, *Haemophilus influenza*, *Actinomyces* spp., and *Nocardia* spp. Lung abscesses can also be caused by a broad array of fungal, parasitic, and mycobacterial pathogens (Table 32-2).

   Hammond JM, Potgieter PD, Hanslo D, et al: The etiology and antimicrobial susceptibility patterns of microorganisms in acute community-acquired lung abscess. Chest 108:937–941, 1995.

19. **How do patients with lung abscesses present?**
   Most patients with a primary lung abscess due to anaerobic pathogens present in an indolent manner with nonspecific symptoms that progress over several weeks. These symptoms include cough with sputum and hemoptysis, low-grade fever, night sweats, weight loss, chest pain, hypoalbuminemia, and anemia. Patients with anaerobic lung abscesses may have putrid sputum. Patients with acute lung abscesses due to nonaerobic pathogens present in a more acute manner, often with signs of sepsis.

20. **How are lung abscesses diagnosed?**
   A classic clinical presentation of lung abscess, with indolent symptoms in a patient with risk factors for aspiration and a radiographic appearance of a cavitary lesion, is sufficient to make a

TABLE 32-2.   MICROBIAL CAUSES OF LUNG ABSCESSES

Bacterial

- Anaerobes: *Peptostreptococcus, Prevotella, Bacteroides* (usually not *B. fragilis)*, and *Fusobacterium* spp.
- Aerobes: Microaerophilic streptococci (i.e., *Streptococcus milleri*), *Klebsiella pneumoniae, Staphylococcus aureus, Streptococcus pyogenes, Haemophilus influenza, Actinomyces* spp., *Nocardia* spp., and *Rhodococcus equi*
- *Mycobacterium* spp.

Fungal

- *Cryptococcus neoformans, Aspergillus* spp., *Mucor* spp., *Blastomyces dermatitidis, Histoplasma capsulatum,* and *Coccidioides immitis*

Parasitic

- *Paragonimus westermani* and *Entamoeba histolytica*

diagnosis of a primary lung abscess (Fig. 32-2). Some patients require a CT scan to differentiate a lung abscess adjacent to the pleura from an empyema. CT scanning can also demonstrate cavitation that may not be apparent on a standard radiograph. Patients with more acute or atypical presentations have a broader differential diagnosis that includes noninfectious etiologies such as Wegener's granulomatosis. These patients require a more extensive evaluation to confirm the infectious nature of the cavitary lesion and the source of infection.

21. **When should bronchoscopy be considered in a patient with a lung abscess?**
   Patients with typical presentations for a primary lung abscess and risk factors for

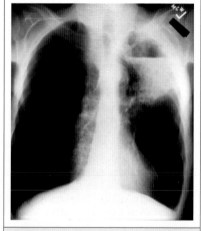

Figure 32-2. A left-upper lobe nonspecific lung abscess in an alcoholic.

KEY POINTS: INDICATIONS FOR BRONCHOSCOPY IN PATIENTS WITH PRESUMED LUNG ABSCESS

1. Atypical presentation of a patient who has no risk factors for aspiration

2. Clinical or radiographic signs of an endobronchial lesion

3. Massive hemoptysis

4. A differential diagnosis that includes noninfectious causes of a cavitary lesion

5. An immunocompromised host suspected of having unusual etiologic pathogens

aspiration do not require bronchoscopy unless other signs of an endobronchial lesion are present. Bronchoscopy is also not required to obtain microbiologic samples because antibiotic therapy is empirical. Patients with atypical presentations, however, may require bronchoscopy to obtain specimens for microbiologic evaluation and tissue samples to exclude alternative diagnoses such as cancer.

22. **What is the treatment for lung abscesses?**

Primary lung abscesses are usually due to polymicrobial anaerobic and aerobic pathogens. Clindamycin has been demonstrated to be effective when given intravenously, followed by a course of oral therapy until the chest radiograph is normal or stable with a small residual lesion. Other effective drugs and drug combinations are also effective as long as they cover the anaerobic and aerobic pathogens usually involved. Metronidazole, although an effective agent against anaerobes, has poor efficacy in treating lung abscesses, probably because it does not treat microaerophilic streptococci. Therapy for other lung abscesses is directed toward the etiologic pathogen.

23. **What are the indications for surgery in the treatment of lung abscess?**

Most patients respond to antibiotic therapy, and surgery is rarely required. Indications for lobectomy include massive hemoptysis unresponsive to bronchial artery embolization, failure to respond to antibiotics, underlying cavitary cancer, and abscesses distal to an obstructing lesion that cannot be resolved. Extremely large lung abscesses (i.e., >6 cm) may not respond to medical management and require resection. Patients who cannot tolerate surgery but who are not responding to antibiotic therapy may benefit from percutaneous catheter drainage.

CHAPTER 33

TUBERCULOSIS

Neil W. Schluger, MD

1. **What is a positive tuberculin test?**

   A properly administered tuberculin test, consisting of five tuberculin units (TUs) of new tuberculin, injected intradermally (usually on the volar forearm), should be read 48–72 hours after placement, and the amount of induration (not erythema) should be recorded. Reactions that consist solely of erythema usually reflect an immunoglobulin E (IgE) response and do not indicate a true delayed hypersensitivity response. The American Thoracic Society's (ATS) guidelines for the amount of induration that should be considered positive are as follows:

   - **5 mm:** Patients with human immunodeficiency virus (HIV) infection, close contacts of patients with infectious disease, and those with fibrotic lesions on a chest radiograph
   - **10 mm:** Other high-risk patients, including infants and children under age 4, health care workers, recent immigrants from countries with a high prevalence of tuberculosis, recent converters (i.e., patients whose skin tests were negative within the past 2 years), medically underserved low-income populations, residents of long-term care facilities (i.e., nursing homes, mental institutions, and correctional facilities), patients with medical conditions known to increase risk of reactivation of tuberculosis (i.e., end-stage renal disease, silicosis, diabetes mellitus, injection drug use, malnutrition, and prolonged immunosuppressive therapy), and patients with certain hematologic or reticuloendothelial cell malignancies
   - **15 mm:** All other patients (i.e., those generally considered to be at low risk for developing tuberculosis)

   The ATS recommends that "persons who are not likely to be infected with *Mycobacterium tuberculosis* should generally not be skin tested because the predicted value of a skin test in low-risk populations is poor." This cannot be stressed enough. In general, testing should only be performed on patients for whom a positive test will result in administration of treatment for latent infection.

   American Thoracic Society: Targeted tuberculin testing and treatment of latent tuberculosis infection. Am J Respir Crit Care Med 161:S221–S247, 2000.

2. **When is skin testing with second-strength tuberculin indicated?**

   The standard tuberculin test contains 5 TUs of purified protein derivative (PPD). This dose of tuberculin has been shown to have a dose-response relationship to prior exposure to tuberculosis, so the majority of patients with no prior history of tuberculosis exposure will have a negative test. Furthermore, radiographic evidence of previous tuberculosis correlates with a positive skin test using the 5-TU dose. For these reasons, the 5-TU dose has replaced the 1-TU dose (the so-called first-strength dose) in routine testing.

   If a second-strength tuberculin dose of 250 TUs is used for skin testing, the frequency of positive reactions seems unrelated to prior tuberculosis exposure, and there is no correlation between radiographic evidence of prior tuberculosis and skin test results. Additionally, there is significant cross-reactivity between *M. tuberculosis* and other mycobacterial species. For these reasons, the 250-TU second-strength tuberculin should no longer be used.

3. **How should a positive tuberculin test be interpreted in a person who has received vaccination with bacille Calmette–Guérin (BCG) ?**

   Vaccination with *Mycobacterium bovis*, strain BCG, is used to prevent tuberculosis in many countries despite long-standing controversy about its efficacy. A recent meta-analysis concluded that the vaccine has 50% efficacy in preventing mortality from tuberculosis and also may reduce the number of cases of miliary disease and meningitis. Because of the frequent immigration to the United States of persons from countries where immunization with BCG is practiced, it is likely that many health care providers will see patients with positive tuberculin tests who have also received BCG.

Both protective immunity and the cutaneous delayed hypersensitivity response associated with BCG vaccination disappear 5–10 years after immunization. For persons vaccinated in childhood, therefore, a positive tuberculin skin test as an adult is overwhelmingly likely to represent true tuberculosis infection rather than an effect of BCG. Thus, current recommendations are to ignore any prior history of BCG administration in the interpretation of a tuberculin skin test. This is certainly the case for persons known to be close contacts with those of active disease and persons with a large area of induration. Such patients should receive preventive isoniazid therapy. If a person has been vaccinated recently and has no recent tuberculosis contacts, a positive tuberculin skin test of 5–10 mm of induration may reflect BCG administration.

A new diagnostic test for latent tuberculosis infection (QuantiFERON-TB Gold, Cellestis Inc.) has been approved for use in the United States by the Food and Drug Administration (FDA). The test is a whole-blood interferon gamma-release assay that stimulates peripheral blood mononuclear cells with secreted proteins specific to only *M. tuberculosis* and not *M. bovis*, strain BCG. Theoretically, this test should distinguish more accurately between true latent infection and prior vaccination with BCG, although there has not yet been extensive clinical use of the new assay. Another similar assay based on the enzyme-linked immunosorbent spot-forming cell (ELISPOT) technique, T SPOT-TB (Oxford Immunotec), is available in Europe. The Centers for Disease Control and Prevention (CDC) has recently issued guidelines for use of these tests.

American Thoracic Society: Targeted tuberculin testing and treatment of latent tuberculosis infection. Am J Respir Crit Care Med 161:S221–S247, 2000.

4. **Who should receive preventive therapy for tuberculosis infection?**
Recommendations for treatment of latent tuberculosis infection have changed recently to reflect both epidemiologic trends in tuberculosis and clinical trials that have evaluated new drug regimens. Recently revised guidelines of the ATS and the CDC recommend that skin testing and treatment be offered to groups at highest risk for recent infection with *M. tuberculosis* (and therefore at highest risk of developing active tuberculosis), *regardless of age*. Thus, tuberculin-skin-test–positive persons who are HIV infected, close contacts of active cases, documented skin-test converters, recent (within 5 years) immigrants from high-prevalence countries, and those with medical conditions that increase the risk of developing active disease (e.g., prolonged immunosuppression, end-stage renal disease, malnutrition, diabetes mellitus, silicosis, rapid unexplained weight loss, and postgastrectomy patients) should all be tested and treated if positive. In most instances, 9 months of treatment with isoniazid is now the preferred regimen for latent tuberculosis infection, rather than 6 months.

5. **What is the initial diagnostic approach in a patient with suspected tuberculosis?**
Clinical symptoms, chest radiography, and sputum smear examination are the mainstays of rapid diagnosis. Ultimate diagnosis rests on identification of *M. tuberculosis* in culture or demonstration of a definite clinical response to therapy. In most reported series, sputum smear examination is positive in 50–75% of patients with tuberculosis. Smears are more often positive in patients with cavitary disease and less often positive in patients with HIV infection, who often present with manifestations of primary tuberculosis.

Thus, when managing patients with suspected tuberculosis whose sputum examination is negative, the clinician has two choices: institute therapy empirically and wait for either sputum culture results (which take 2–12 weeks) or clinical improvement (also 2–12 weeks), or else pursue further testing. Nucleic acid amplification assays can provide incremental diagnostic yield and should be ordered in patients with a high clinical likelihood of tuberculosis but whose sputum smear examination is negative. The test most commonly employed next is flexible bronchoscopy.

Schluger N: The diagnosis of tuberculosis: What's old, what's new. Semin Resp Infect 18:241–248, 2003.

6. **Should bronchoscopy be performed in patients with suspected tuberculosis who have negative sputum smears?**

Bronchoscopy seems to be able to diagnose tuberculosis immediately in 35–50% of cases of smear-negative tuberculosis. The highest yield during bronchoscopy appears to come not from bronchoalveolar lavage, which infrequently shows acid-fast bacilli, but from transbronchial biopsy specimens, which show acid-fast bacilli or necrotizing granulomata.

The benefits of bronchoscopy must be weighed against its risks, which include bleeding and pneumothorax for the patient and possible nosocomial transmission of tuberculosis for the bronchoscopist. In view of these risks, a prudent approach to the diagnosis of sputum-smear-negative patients with suspected tuberculosis is as follows: if expectorated sputum smears are negative, induced sputum samples should be obtained. If those are negative, empirical therapy should be instituted and clinical response assessed while cultures are awaited. Bronchoscopy should be reserved for patients in whom the risks of empirical therapy are significant or in whom the differential diagnosis is wide and includes entities requiring early and specific treatment. Many patients with HIV infection fall into the latter group. When bronchoscopy is performed, it should be done in a setting with proper environmental and personal respiratory controls.

Schluger N: The diagnosis of tuberculosis: What's old, what's new. Semin Respir Infect 18:241–248, 2003.

7. **Which patients with tuberculosis should be admitted to the hospital?**

The decision to admit a patient with tuberculosis to the hospital is more often based on social factors than medical ones. Most patients with tuberculosis are not physically sick enough to require hospitalization, although patients with hemoptysis, meningitis, pericarditis, severe malnutrition, or impending respiratory failure should be admitted to the hospital for evaluation and treatment. In the absence of these features, the decision to admit a patient with tuberculosis usually rests with a judgment regarding in which setting, in or out of the hospital, the patient is likely to pose a greater infectious hazard.

Admission may be beneficial for patients who would otherwise expose large numbers of vulnerable individuals such as children or persons with illness or immunosuppression. Admission may also be justified to initiate a course of therapy if there is concern about adherence or adverse effects from medication.

If a decision not to admit a patient with tuberculosis is made, the treating physician must take steps to ensure adherence to therapy and must have a strategy of monitoring that adherence.

8. **How long should patients with tuberculosis be isolated?**

Patients are kept in isolation until they are no longer infectious. Although infectiousness of a tuberculosis patient is difficult to quantify, several clinical characteristics are correlated with a high degree of infectiousness. These include a positive sputum smear showing acid-fast bacilli, cavitary lesions on chest radiograph, coughing, and no treatment. Patients with laryngeal tuberculosis are believed to be highly infectious. Prompt institution of therapy is certainly the mainstay of reducing infectiousness; after 2 weeks of effective chemotherapy, most patients will no longer be infectious to any great degree, particularly if cough has subsided and clinical improvement is evident. Conversion to sputum smear negativity, as documented by 3 consecutive days of no demonstrable organisms on smear, also provides evidence of a low infectious risk and should be a minimum criterion for discontinuing isolation. It may be prudent to isolate patients with multidrug-resistant tuberculosis for longer periods, such as the time needed for sputum cultures to become negative.

Siddiqui AH, Perl TM, Conlon M, et al: Preventing nosocomial transmission of pulmonary tuberculosis: When may isolation be discontinued for patients with suspected tuberculosis? Infect Control Hosp Epidemiol 23:141–144, 2002.

9. **Should patients with extrapulmonary tuberculosis be isolated?**

Patients with extrapulmonary tuberculosis are not infectious and do not require isolation. On rare occasions, some of these patients pose an infectious risk, and infection control procedures become important. For example, patients with tuberculous septic arthritis who require open irrigation of the joint space may present an infectious risk because of aerosolization of organisms. Additionally, a few patients with tuberculosis lymphadenitis will have spontaneous drainage, and infectious material also may become aerosolized. Covering the wound with a dressing is important in such cases.

10. **What is the infectious risk to health care providers caring for patients with tuberculosis?**

The risk to health care providers of infection with *M. tuberculosis* depends on the intensity and duration of exposure to infectious patients. Those performing procedures during which respiratory droplet nuclei are likely to be created (i.e., bronchoscopy, endotracheal intubation and suctioning, or sputum induction) have the highest risk. Several recent studies have indicated that in hospitals with up-to-date infection control procedures, the annual rate of skin test conversion among employees is about 1% overall. However, earlier studies indicated that up to 11% of pulmonary fellows in training become tuberculin skin test positive during their training, as compared with 1% of infectious disease trainees; the disparity is caused partly by exposure during bronchoscopy.

Occupational risk of tuberculosis infection can be reduced by using a hierarchy of control measures. Administrative controls aimed at prompt isolation of tuberculosis suspects and prompt institution of therapy for known cases are undoubtedly the most important measures. Environmental controls, such as the use of germicidal ultraviolet irradiation, high-efficiency air filters, and proper ventilation, constitute the next level of control. Finally, proper use of personal particulate respirators (standard surgical masks provide no real protection when worn by health care workers) may provide additional benefit, particularly for those at highest risk of exposure.

11. **How should patients with tuberculosis be transported through the hospital?**

Most exposures during transport through the hospital are likely to be brief and are not associated with an increased risk of tuberculosis transmission. However, several precautions that are prudent and easy to carry out should be used. First, the patient should not leave the room except for tests and procedures that are absolutely necessary, and the patient should wear a mask whenever outside the room. The area to which the patient is to be transported should be notified in advance so that exposure to other patients and personnel can be minimized. Whenever possible, tuberculosis patients should be scheduled at the end of the day. A private elevator should be used for transport. If the patient being transported wears a mask continually, it is probably not necessary for the personnel transporting the patient or performing a test to wear particulate respirators. Finally, if certain tests or procedures are being performed commonly on tuberculosis patients (e.g., sputum induction), those locations should be renovated to ensure adequate ventilation and filtration of air, and an ultraviolet germicidal irradiation device should be installed.

12. **What type of contact investigation should be done when a case of tuberculosis is detected?**

Contact investigations are important public health measures because they can identify those persons at greatest risk for developing active tuberculosis after infection, and they can lead to the institution of effective chemopreventive therapy. Contact investigation should follow the concentric circle model; in other words, the initial investigation should focus on those persons with the closest and most intense exposure to the index case, and the investigation should be expanded until a level of contact is reached that has no persons with evidence of recent infection. The concentric circle model applies to a contact investigation either inside or outside the hospital.

All persons being investigated should have a tuberculin test, and if the test is negative, it should be repeated 12 weeks after the contact was known to have occurred. Contacts should also be questioned closely for symptoms, and any person with a positive tuberculin test or symptoms suggestive of tuberculosis should be evaluated clinically and with a chest radiograph. Persons known to have had a positive tuberculin skin test before exposure to the index case do not need chest radiographs unless they have symptoms suggestive of active tuberculosis.

13. **What is the standard therapy for pulmonary tuberculosis?**
Current therapy for pulmonary tuberculosis is based on several short-course regimens developed in the 1970s and 1980s. The induction phase of chemotherapy consists of 2 months of isoniazid, rifampin, and pyrazinamide followed by 4 months of continuation therapy with isoniazid and rifampin. A recent study by the Tuberculosis Trials Consortium (TBTC), a CDC-funded international research group, indicates that for certain low-risk patients, once-weekly therapy with isoniazid and rifapentine in the continuation phase is an effective strategy. In areas where isoniazid resistance is found in more than 4% of isolates, ethambutol or streptomycin should be added to the initial regimen until drug susceptibility results are known. Strong consideration should be given to treating all patients with programs of directly observed therapy (DOT), and this approach is mandatory if intermittent therapy is to be used. Use of the regimens discussed above to treat drug-susceptible pulmonary disease should be associated with a 100% cure rate and a relapse rate of no more than 3.5%.

The Tuberculosis Trials Consortium: Rifapentine and isoniazid once a week versus rifampicin and isoniazid twice a week for treatment of drug-susceptible pulmonary tuberculosis in HIV-negative patients: A randomised clinical trial. Lancet 360:528–534, 2002.

14. **How should antituberculosis therapy be monitored?**
Properly administered, antituberculosis therapy should be extremely effective. A bacteriologic response (i.e., conversion of sputum cultures to negative) can be expected in essentially 100% of patients with tuberculosis caused by susceptible strains of *M. tuberculosis*. The most common reason for treatment failure is lack of adherence to the prescribed regimen. The following steps are critical for monitoring therapy:
1. At the initiation of therapy, efforts should be made to ensure that the mycobacteriology laboratory has received an adequate specimen for culture and sensitivity testing, particularly in regions where drug resistance has been noted.
2. Once therapy has begun, sputum smears should be followed until negative, and the clinical response (e.g., fever or weight change) should also be noted.
3. After discharge, patients should be seen at least monthly by the treating physician. The following should be done at each visit:
   - Careful symptom review
   - Record of the patient's weight
   - Sputum collected for smear and culture
   - Blood count, serum electrolyte levels, and liver function tests obtained to monitor for adverse effects of medications
4. Chest radiographs need not be obtained frequently; a chest radiograph at the 3-month mark can be considered optional if the patient's clinical and bacteriologic responses have been good, and a chest radiograph should be obtained at the completion of therapy.

Failure to respond to what should be an adequate drug regimen is overwhelmingly likely to be the result of poor patient adherence to this medical regimen.

15. **Should serum levels of antituberculous drug be obtained routinely?**
Dosing of antituberculous medications is usually based on body weight; none of the major chemotherapy trials relied on serum levels to adjust dosages. Therefore, in routine cases of tuberculosis, there is no reason to obtain serum levels. In addition, studies in which serum

levels have been obtained have failed to demonstrate a close correlation between serum drug levels and patient outcome. Under certain circumstances, serum drug levels may be helpful, for example, if a patient has been prescribed an adequate regimen but fails to have a clinical response, and malabsorption of drugs is suspected. Malabsorption rarely occurs, but might be more common in patients with HIV infection. However, the most common reason for treatment failure in patients with tuberculosis caused by susceptible organisms is lack of adherence to the prescribed regimen.

A second scenario in which drug levels may be helpful is in managing patients with multidrug-resistant tuberculosis. In this circumstance, experts advocate obtaining drug levels and using high doses so that patients are kept at the upper end of the therapeutic range. This requires extremely close monitoring for side effects, particularly when aminoglycosides are used and ototoxicity is a major concern.

16. **How should patients be monitored after completion of therapy?**
Standard short-course (i.e., 6-month) chemotherapy regimens are associated with low relapse rates. Most relapses occur in the first 2 years after completion of therapy. Patients who have a prompt and complete response to therapy (i.e., sputum cultures become negative within the first 2 months of therapy) do not need routine follow-up when treatment is completed. Patients whose response to therapy was slower or in whom radiographic abnormalities persist after completion of therapy should be evaluated at 6-month intervals and encouraged to report promptly any symptoms of recurrent cough, fever, or weight loss. Follow-up should be closer and more routine in patients who completed treatment for drug-resistant tuberculosis.

17. **What steps should be taken with patients who do not adhere to their treatment regimens?**
Adherence to medical regimens is a complex and poorly understood phenomenon; it is likely that only about 50% of patients take medications exactly according to physician instructions. In relation to tuberculosis, individual noncompliance or erratic self-administration of drugs can lead to spread of infection and the development of drug-resistant strains of mycobacteria.

The chief causes of nonadherence to antituberculous regimens are the fact that treatment continues for a long time after symptomatic improvement occurs, the side effects caused by the polypharmacy required for tuberculosis treatment, and several social factors and comorbid conditions common among tuberculosis patients. Patient counseling and education are crucial first steps in ensuring adherence. Attention to other factors such as substance abuse, mental illness, and housing is also critical. DOT programs are the best venues in which to address these issues, and DOT should be the standard approach to tuberculosis therapy in the United States. Such programs promote adherence in a wide variety of patient groups and reduce the incidence of drug-resistant tuberculosis.

If patients fail to adhere to a regimen of DOT, more restrictive steps are required to protect the public health. Long-term enforced detention in tuberculosis wards is an option available in many states in the United States, although good DOT programs will obviate the need for detention in all but a few persons with tuberculosis.

Schluger N, Ciotoli C, Cohen D, et al: Comprehensive tuberculosis control for patients at high risk for non-compliance. Am J Respir Crit Care Med 151:1486–1490, 1995.

18. **Do patients with HIV infection require a longer duration of therapy?**
Yes. It is recommended that patients with HIV infection receive 9 months of isoniazid preventive therapy when being treated for latent tuberculosis infection. A previously recommended regimen for latent tuberculosis infection, rifampin and pyrazinamide given together for 2 months, has been withdrawn because of a high incidence of severe and often fatal hepatitis. This regimen should not be used in any patient with latent infection, regardless of HIV status.

The current ATS and CDC guidelines state that patients with active tuberculosis may receive standard short-course therapy if their infection is caused by a susceptible organism and if clinical response is prompt, as manifested by rapid improvement in symptoms and sputum culture conversion within the first 2 months of therapy.

For HIV-infected patients who are slow to respond to therapy, a prudent approach would be to continue therapy for at least 6 months after the last positive sputum culture and then to monitor very closely for relapse after termination of therapy. Extensive bilateral or cavitary disease, significant weight loss, or failure to convert sputum cultures to negative after 2 months of therapy are clinical indicators of a high risk of relapse. All patients with these findings, whether HIV infected or not, should be considered candidates for at least 9 months of therapy.

19. **How should a pregnant woman with a positive tuberculin (PPD) skin test be managed?**

Pregnant women with positive tuberculin skin tests should be evaluated in exactly the same manner as any other patient, in other words, with a thorough symptom review, physical examination, and chest radiograph. Done with adequate abdominal shielding, a standard single chest radiograph in pregnancy poses no risk to the developing fetus. Delaying a chest radiograph to the postpartum period is a serious error that can result in exposure of the newborn to active tuberculosis, which may have disastrous consequences. When active tuberculosis is detected in a pregnant woman, therapy should be instituted promptly with isoniazid, rifampin, and ethambutol, none of which poses a danger to the developing fetus. Aminoglycosides and quinolones should be avoided. Few data are available regarding the safety of pyrazinamide in pregnancy, although it is used in Europe in this situation.

For pregnant women with only tuberculosis infection, isoniazid preventive therapy is recommended only if the woman is HIV seropositive, is known to be a recent skin test converter, or is a close contact of an individual with active tuberculosis. In all other situations, therapy can be postponed until after delivery. Because of concern about a possible higher incidence of isoniazid hepatotoxicity in the peripartum period, preventive therapy should begin 8–12 weeks after delivery.

20. **When are steroids indicated in the treatment of tuberculosis?**

Under certain circumstances, adjunct therapy with corticosteroids may be indicated to decrease morbidity in patients with tuberculosis. Steroids should be used only in conjunction with an adequate antituberculous drug regimen; otherwise, disastrous results may occur. The two most common indications for steroids in patients with tuberculosis are tuberculous meningitis and pericarditis. Although most patients with extrapulmonary tuberculosis recover without incident, patients with meningitis may develop cerebrospinal fluid block and focal findings, such as hearing loss, which can be permanent. For these reasons, patients with central nervous system

KEY POINTS: TUBERCULOSIS

1. Screening for latent tuberculosis infection should be performed only in persons at high risk for reactivation.

2. Ignore any history of BCG vaccination when interpreting a tuberculin skin test result.

3. The previously recommended regimen of 2 months of rifampin and pyrazinamide for latent tuberculosis infection should not be used because severe hepatitis may occur.

4. Negative sputum smears do not rule out tuberculosis in patients in whom there is a high clinical suspicion for the disease.

5. It is the responsibility of the treating physician, as well as the patient, to ensure adherence to therapy for active tuberculosis.

tuberculosis or with tuberculous meningitis with focal findings should receive corticosteroids as adjunctive therapy.

Patients with tuberculous pericarditis are at risk for development of constrictive pericarditis and sudden death early in their course. Although steroids have long been used in the treatment of tuberculous pericarditis, exact indications for their use remain unclear. Creation of a pericardial window through a subxiphoid approach and complete pericardial stripping are probably more important therapeutic maneuvers than steroid administration. If these maneuvers are not used, steroids should be given. Some physicians use steroids even if the pericardium has been stripped.

A rare indication for steroids in tuberculosis is the patient who presents with tuberculosis and hypoxic respiratory failure mimicking acute respiratory distress syndrome (ARDS). In this case, steroids may decrease the inflammatory response and improve gas exchange, allowing clinical improvement before antibiotics would be expected to have an effect.

21. **How should patients receiving isoniazid preventive therapy be monitored?**
The most feared complication of isoniazid preventive therapy is fulminant hepatitis and hepatic failure, which may result in death. Fortunately, this is a rare complication. Isoniazid-induced hepatitis seems related to age and coexisting liver injury. For persons under age 35 who have normal liver function tests at baseline and no history of prior liver disease, a monthly symptom review alone, without liver function testing, is adequate. Patients who are HIV positive, patients who are pregnant or in the early (i.e., first 3 months) postpartum period, patients with chronic liver disease, or patients who use alcohol regularly should receive baseline liver function tests. Older individuals need not have baseline tests routinely, but such a decision should be made on a case-by-case basis. If baseline tests are abnormal, monthly follow-up liver function tests are indicated.

Patients should be educated about the symptoms of hepatitis and instructed to discontinue isoniazid immediately and to seek medical attention if such symptoms occur. Patients must be counseled to avoid alcohol completely, and no more than 1 month's supply of isoniazid should be dispensed to any patient. If symptomatic hepatitis results from isoniazid preventive therapy, the drug should be stopped and not reinstituted.

Transient small increases in transaminase levels are common in patients receiving isoniazid; abnormalities are observed in 15–20% of patients. These elevations in transaminase level usually resolve without discontinuation of isoniazid, and the drug need not be stopped in asymptomatic patients whose transaminase levels are within 3–5 times the normal limit. Such patients should be followed closely, however.

22. **What type of preventive therapy should be given to persons exposed to cases of drug-resistant tuberculosis?**
Few data exist about the efficacy of preventive regimens other than the commonly used 6- to 12-month course of isoniazid for latent tuberculosis infection. Persons exposed to isoniazid-resistant tuberculosis should receive 6 months' therapy with rifampin, in the usual daily dose. This approach should have a high degree of efficacy. Some advocate adding a second drug, such as ethambutol, to the preventive regimen, although there are no data on which to base this decision.

No data are available about the efficacy of any preventive regimen for patients exposed to tuberculosis resistant to isoniazid and rifampin. Many advocate observation alone in this setting, but therapy seems prudent in persons at high risk for developing active tuberculosis (including children, those with HIV infection, and so forth). In such cases, a combination of ethambutol and pyrazinamide may be used, or a combination of pyrazinamide and a quinolone may seem logical. (Most authorities consider quinolones to be contraindicated in children because of potential arthropathy.) These regimens may be given for 6 months, and careful attention should be paid to excluding active disease before these preventive regimens are employed. If a person has been exposed to multidrug-resistant tuberculosis and no adequate regimen can be constructed for preventive therapy, vaccination with BCG should be considered if the patient is at high risk for development of active disease. BCG vaccine should not be given to persons with HIV infection, as it has been reported to cause disseminated disease in such cases.

Centers for Disease Control: Management of persons exposed to multidrug-resistant tuberculosis. MMWR 41:61–70, 1992.

Iseman MD: Treatment of multidrug-resistant tuberculosis. N Engl J Med 329:784–790, 1993.

CONTROVERSY

23. **Should anergy testing be performed in patients with a negative tuberculin skin test and HIV infection?**

Patients with coexisting HIV and tuberculosis infection are at high risk of developing active tuberculosis. For this reason, identification and treatment of persons with HIV and tuberculosis coinfection are public health priorities. However, the standard tuberculin skin test (TST) may be less helpful in HIV-infected persons because the ability to mount a delayed hypersensitivity response depends upon intact cellular immunity, which is precisely the part of the immune system most affected by advanced HIV infection.

Some have advocated that patients with HIV infection and negative TSTs receive anergy testing to further assess the integrity of their cell-mediated immunity. If patients do not respond to the anergy panel, the negative TST would be considered a false-negative test, and isoniazid preventive therapy would be given.

This approach presents several problems. First, anergy is a complex and poorly understood phenomenon, and methods for assessing it are not well standardized and often are not reproducible. It is well known that many healthy individuals do not develop a reaction to one or more of the commonly used skin-test antigens (i.e., tetanus, mumps, trichophytin, or *Candida* spp.); also, positive reactions may become negative when repeated and vice versa. Second, although it is generally true that persons with advanced HIV infection are more likely to display cutaneous anergy to common antigens, this is not always the case. Third, the risk of tuberculosis is not the same among all HIV subgroups, and not every tuberculin-negative, anergic patient with HIV can be assumed to have tuberculosis infection. For example, the recently concluded Pulmonary Complications of HIV Infection Study found that cases of tuberculosis in acquired immunodeficiency syndrome (AIDS) patients varied greatly with geographic distribution. For these reasons, the case to perform anergy testing on all tuberculin-negative HIV-infected patients is not a compelling one.

A recently performed decision analysis suggested that all HIV-infected patients receive 12 months of isoniazid preventive therapy, regardless of TST status. However, this approach has not been empirically verified. At present, decisions to institute isoniazid preventive therapy in TST-negative patients should be made on an individual basis after careful assessment of the patient's risk for tuberculosis infection.

WEBSITES

http://www.cdc.gov/nchstp/tb/

http://www.nationaltbcenter.edu/

http://www.stoptb.org/

http://www.umdnj.edu/ntbcweb/

BIBLIOGRAPHY

Iseman M: A Clinician's Guide to Tuberculosis. Philadelphia, Lippincott, Williams & Wilkins, 2000.

Rom WN, Garay S (eds): Tuberculosis, 2nd ed. Philadelphia, Lippincott, Williams & Wilkins, 2004.

CHAPTER 34

ATYPICAL MYCOBACTERIA

Milene T. Saavedra, MD, and Michael E. Hanley, MD

1. **What are atypical mycobacteria?**
   These are mycobacteria that are biologically distinct from *Mycobacterium tuberculosis*, *Mycobacterium bovis,* and *Mycobacterium leprae.* Traditionally, these acid-fast bacilli (AFBs) were thought to be primarily saprophytic organisms that were not pathologic in humans. However, many are now commonly recognized human pathogens, in both immunosuppressed patients and normal hosts. They are also referred to as the "environmental mycobacteria."

2. **How are atypical mycobacteria classified?**
   The **Runyon classification system** categorizes these organisms into four groups based on growth characteristics, colonial morphology, and pigmentation:

Group I: Photochromogens	**Group III:** Nonchromogens
Group II: Scotochromogens	**Group IV:** Rapid growers

   Although the Runyon system has significant laboratory utility, it is of limited clinical useful-ness. The **Bailey system** is an alternative schema that classifies the organisms by their response to therapy:

Easier to Treat	**More Difficult to Treat**
Mycobacterium kansasii	*Mycobacterium avium* complex (MAC)
Mycobacterium xenopi	*Mycobacterium scrofulaceum*
Mycobacterium szulgai	*Mycobacterium simiae*
Mycobacterium marinum	*Mycobacterium chelonae* and *Mycobacterium abscessus*
Mycobacterium ulcerans	*Mycobacterium fortuitum*

   Brown-Elliott B, Wallace R: Clinical and taxonomic status of pathogenic nonpigmented or late-pigmenting rapidly growing mycobacteria. Clin Micro Rev 15:716–746, 2002.

3. **Which atypical mycobacteria are clinically significant in humans?**

Group I (photochromogenic)	**Group III** (nonchromogenic)
M. kansasii	MAC
M. marinum	*M. ulcerans*
M. simiae	*M. xenopi*
Group II (scotochromogenic)	**Group IV** (rapid growers)
M. szulgai	*M. chelonae*
M. scrofulaceum	*M. fortuitum*
	M. abscessus

   Human pulmonary disease most commonly results from infection with either MAC, *M. kansasii,* or the rapidly growing mycobacteria. One review indicated the following frequency of mycobacteria isolated in state public health laboratories:
   - 65% *Mycobacterium tuberculosis*
   - 21% MAC
   - 6.5% *M. fortuitum-chelonei*
   - 3.5% *M. kansasii*

- 2.3% *M. scrofulaceum*

  However, many of the isolates may have reflected colonization as opposed to true disease, and the review was published before the human immunodeficiency virus (HIV) epidemic.

4. **What are the most common sites of infection by atypical mycobacteria?**
   See Table 34-1.

TABLE 34-1. MOST COMMON SITES OF INFECTION BY ATYPICAL MYCOBACTERIA			
Pulmonary	**Lymphadenitis**	**Cutaneous**	**Disseminated**
MAC	MAC	*M. marinum*	MAC
M. kansasii	*M. scrofulaceum*	*M. fortuitum*	*M. kansasii*
M. abscessus	*M. malmoense*	*M. chelonae*	*M. chelonae*
M. xenopi	*M. abscessus*	*M. haemophilum*	
M. malmoense	*M. ulcerans*		

5. **Discuss the epidemiology of atypical mycobacteria.**
   Atypical mycobacteria are common saprophytes that can be readily isolated from soil, water, and milk. The likely route of entry is inhalation (except for *M. marinum*), with acquisition directly from environmental reservoirs. Although atypical mycobacteria cause disease in many animals, animal-to-human and human-to-human transmission have not been proven and probably do not occur. Routine isolation of patients with pulmonary infections is therefore not warranted.

6. **What conditions predispose patients to pulmonary disease from atypical mycobacteria?**
   Pulmonary infections are more common in immunosuppressed patients and in patients with preexisting pulmonary disorders, including bronchiectasis, chronic obstructive pulmonary disease (COPD), lung cancer, and silicosis. They may also occur in patients with no previous history of lung disease.
   - **HIV:** Highly active antiretroviral therapy (HAART) decreases the incidence of disseminated MAC fivefold. Risk factors for disseminated MAC include a CD4 count < 40 at the time of diagnosis. Toxoplasmosis prophylaxis also decreases the incidence of MAC.
   - **Cystic fibrosis (CF):** The prevalence of atypical mycobacteria in patients with CF is 13%, far higher than the prevalence in the general population. MAC and *M. abscessus* are the most common pathogens. The increase in prevalence may be due to an increase in lifespan in CF patients and suggests that screening for these organisms may be valuable in older patients. The diagnosis can be difficult to make given overlap of symptoms and findings between the two diseases. Once an atypical mycobacteria species is identified in the sputum of a patient with CF, serial cultures should be obtained and treatment considered, particularly if American Thoracic Society (ATS) criteria for disease are met and if clinical decline is noted despite treatment of common bacterial pathogens.
   - **Normal hosts with postoperative infections from rapidly growing mycobacteria:** Corneal infections after laser *in situ* keratomileusis (LASIK) surgery with *M. chelonae* and *M. abscessus* are well described. Catheter infections, sternal wound infections after cardiac surgery, and infections following plastic surgery, liposuction, tympanostomy tube placement, and hemodialysis also occur, usually from rapidly growing atypical mycobacteria.

   Aksamit TR: *Mycobacterium avium* complex pulmonary disease in patients with pre-existing lung disease. Clin Chest Med 23:643–653, 2002.

John T, Velotta E: Nontuberculous (atypical) mycobacterial keratitis after LASIK: Current status and clinical implications. Cornea 24:245–255, 2005.

Olivier KN, NTM in CF study group: The natural history of nontuberculous mycobacteria in patients with cystic fibrosis. Paediatr Resp Rev 5(SupplA):S213–216, 2004.

7. **Which atypical mycobacteria cause pulmonary disease?**
The lungs are the most common site of infection by atypical mycobacteria. Although pulmonary disease may result from infection with *M. scrofulaceum, M. szulgai, M. xenopi, M. fortuitum,* or *M. chelonae*, it is most commonly due to either MAC, *M. kansasii*, or *M. abscessus*.

Daley CL, Griffith DE: Pulmonary disease caused by rapidly growing mycobacteria. Clin Chest Med 23:623–632, 2002.

Han D, Lee KS, Koh WJ: Radiographic and CT findings of nontuberculous mycobacterial pulmonary infection caused by *Mycobacterium abscessus*. Am J Roentgenol 181:513–517,2003.

Heifets L: Mycobacterial infections caused by nontuberculous mycobacteria. Sem in Resp Crit Care Med 25:283–296, 2004.

KEY POINTS: MOST COMMON ATYPICAL MYCOBACTERIA PULMONARY PATHOGENS

1. MAC

2. *Mycobacterium kansasii*

3. *Mycobacterium abscessus*

8. **Are pulmonary infections with atypical mycobacteria more common in specific demographic patient groups?**
MAC disease traditionally occurred as apical fibrocavitary lung disease in middle-aged to older males with a history of tobacco abuse and COPD. A newer phenotype has emerged in middle-aged to elderly nonsmoking females characterized by asthenic body type, scoliosis, and mitral valve prolapse. Disease in these patients appears as nodular interstitial lung disease, frequently found in the right middle lobe and lingula, with slower progression (5–10 years vs. 1–2 years) than the disease previously described in elderly male smokers.

9. **How is the diagnosis of pulmonary infection with atypical mycobacteria established?**
Diagnosis generally requires fulfillment of several criteria:
1. Radiographically apparent and clinically compatible lung disease without another evident cause. Radiographically compatible findings include infiltrative, nodular, or cavitary changes on chest roentgenogram or multifocal bronchiectasis or multiple small nodules on high-resolution computed tomography. This diagnostic criterion is strengthened if there is evidence of progressive radiographic changes or clinical deterioration.
2. Isolation of the suspected organism from pulmonary secretions (i.e., sputa, bronchial wash, or bronchoalveolar lavage):
   - **If three sputa or bronchial wash results are available from the previous 12 months:** Three positive cultures with negative AFB smear results *or* two positive cultures and one positive smear
   - **If only one bronchial wash is available:** Positive culture with a 2+, 3+, or 4+ smear *or* 2+, 3+, or 4+ growth on solid media

3. If sputum or bronchial wash results are nondiagnostic or if another disease cannot be excluded:
   - Transbronchial or lung biopsy yielding an atypical mycobacterium, *or*
   - Biopsy demonstrating mycobacterial histologic features (i.e., granulomatous inflammation or AFB) with one or more sputa or bronchial washings positive for atypical mycobacteria (even in low numbers).

Whether *Mycobacterium abscessus* is ever a true pulmonary colonizer is controversial. Some experts believe that all patients with *M. abscessus* in their sputa have some degree of disease.

Wallace R, Glassroth J, Griffith D, et al: Diagnosis and treatment of disease caused by nontuberculous mycobacteria. Am J Respir Crit Care Med 156:S1–S25, 1997.

10. **What is hot tub lung?**
    This term refers to a hypersensitivity pneumonitis-like syndrome that occurs in healthy adults exposed to aerosolized MAC. Many of these cases have been described in users of indoor hot tubs, where high levels of infectious aerosols may be found. Whether the syndrome represents hypersensitivity pneumonitis, infection, or both is controversial. Treatment consists of discontinuation of hot tub use, corticosteroids, antimycobacterial therapy, or a combination thereof.

    Aksamit TR: Hot tub lung: Infection, inflammation or both? Semin Respir Infect 18:33–39, 2003.
    Marras TK, Wallace RJ, Koth LL, et al: Hypersensitivity pneumonitis reaction to Mycobacterium avium in household water. Chest 127:664–671, 2005.

11. **How does pulmonary infection from *M. kansasii* differ clinically from that due to *M. tuberculosis*?**
    Although lung disease from *M. kansasii* closely resembles that from *M. tuberculosis*, *M. kansasii* tends to result in thin-walled cavities and a paucity of pleural disease or effusions. In addition, extrapulmonary disease rarely complicates infection with *M. kansasii*, usually occurring only in immunocompromised hosts.

12. **How are pulmonary infections from *M. kansasii* managed?**
    M. kansasii is susceptible to most standard antituberculous chemotherapeutic agents, although some resistance to isoniazid exists. A cornerstone to therapy is rifampin. Inclusion of this drug in a multidrug regimen is associated with more rapid conversion of sputum and with lower relapse rates. Standard treatment recommendations include the use of isoniazid, rifampin, and ethambutol. (Clarithromycin or rifabutin should be substituted for rifampin in HIV seropositive patients on protease inhibitors.) In some circumstances, streptomycin may be added or substituted for ethambutol for the first 2 months. Although the optimum duration of therapy is unknown, most regimens are continued for 18–24 months or for 1 year past sputum culture negativity. This approach has resulted in response rates nearing 100%, with virtually no relapses.

13. **Do all patients in whom MAC is isolated from sputum require treatment?**
    Patients with bronchiectasis and progressive lung disease, who have evidence of systemic dissemination, or who meet the diagnostic criteria outlined in Question 9 should be promptly treated. Patients with positive cultures whose symptoms or radiographic findings appear to be minimal or stable may be observed without specific therapy. However, they should be followed closely with regular chest imaging studies and frequent cultures of respiratory secretions. Therapy should be initiated at any suggestion of disease progression. In this regard, it should be emphasized that patients with MAC may experience prolonged periods of stable lung function punctuated with periods of sudden, significant decline.

    Watanabe K, Fujimura M, Kasahara K: Characteristics of pulmonary *Mycobacterium avium-intracellulare* complex (MAC) infection in comparison with those of tuberculosis. Respir Med 97:654–659, 2003.

14. **How is pulmonary disease from MAC managed?**
    Successful management of pulmonary infection from MAC involves both medical and surgical strategies. MAC is resistant *in vitro* to most of the traditional antituberculous

chemotherapeutic agents, limiting the efficacy of these agents. Although the initial sputum conversion rate with multidrug therapy involving these agents is good, subsequent relapses are common. However, the newer macrolides (clarithromycin and azithromycin) and rifabutin (an analog of rifampin that is significantly more active against MAC than rifampin) have good activity against MAC and have become the cornerstone of therapy. Initial therapy usually consists of a macrolide (preferably clarithromycin), rifabutin (rifampin may be substituted in patients who are intolerant of rifabutin), and ethambutol. The optimal duration of therapy is unclear; however, continuing therapy for 10–12 months beyond conversion of sputa culture results may be adequate for most patients. Chemotherapy followed by surgical resection should be considered in patients with limited disease who are good surgical candidates. Although it is preferable that sputum conversion occur prior to resection, some authors have advocated resection after 3–4 months of therapy, regardless of sputa status.

Iseman MD: Medical management of pulmonary disease caused by *Mycobacterium avium* complex. Clin Chest Med 23:633–641, 2002.

15. **Is susceptibility testing a necessary adjunct to therapy?**
Although controversial, routine susceptibility testing of MAC with rifabutin and other antituberculous drugs is not recommended, in part because such testing has not been demonstrated to consistently predict clinical response. Clarithromycin testing should not be performed routinely except on those patients who have failed previous therapy or who have received prior macrolide therapy.

16. **List the common side effects of drugs used to treat MAC.**
- **Clarithromycin:** Nausea, vomiting, bitter taste, hepatitis, diarrhea, and impaired hearing
- **Azithromycin:** Diarrhea, nausea, vomiting, hepatitis, and impaired hearing
- **Rifabutin:** Nausea, vomiting, hepatitis, leukopenia, thrombocytopenia, polymyalgia or polyarthralgia, uveitis, and hyperpigmentation
- **Rifampin:** Nausea, vomiting, hepatitis, flu-like syndrome, hypersensitivity, renal failure
- **Ethambutol:** Impaired visual acuity, loss of red/green color discrimination

17. **What are indications for surgery in patients with pulmonary MAC infection?**
Criteria for surgery of mycobacterial diseases in general include presence of a persistent cavity with a high organism burden, a destroyed or trapped lung, massive hemoptysis, bronchopleural fistula, and bronchostenosis. In the setting of MAC infection, surgery should be considered in patients whose disease is limited to one lung and who have either resistant organisms or poor response to drug therapy. The morbidity of surgery is considerable: 21–47% of patients who undergo lung resection develop postoperative bronchopleural fistulae. Patients being considered for surgical resection should receive at least 3 months of antimycobacterial chemotherapy prior to surgery.

18. **What are the clinical manifestations of disseminated MAC in HIV-seropositive patients?**
Disseminated MAC infection is usually a consequence of severe immune suppression and is rare in HIV-seropositive patients with CD4 lymphocyte counts > 100. However, clinicians should have a high index of suspicion regarding this diagnosis in appropriately symptomatic patients with CD4 lymphocyte counts < 50. Although the symptoms may be nonspecific, more than 90% of patients with disseminated MAC present with fever of unknown origin. Fever is frequently high and accompanied by night sweats. Weight loss with cachexia, abdominal pain, and diarrhea is also common; physical examination may reveal hepatosplenomegaly and lymphadenopathy. The most common laboratory abnormalities include anemia, which may be profound (i.e., hematocrit < 25%), and elevated alkaline phosphatase.

19. **How is the diagnosis of disseminated MAC infection in HIV-seropositive patients established?**

    This diagnosis can be difficult to establish. Pulmonary involvement in disseminated disease is uncommon, so demonstration of MAC in pulmonary secretions of HIV-seropositive patients alone rarely confirms the diagnosis. The diagnosis is most commonly confirmed from blood cultures, which have a sensitivity of 90%. HIV-seropositive patients with MAC-positive sputum cultures and low CD4 lymphocyte counts should be followed vigilantly. In a prospective study, 67% of HIV-seropositive patients with CD4 counts < 50 and MAC-positive sputum or stool cultures developed disseminated disease within 1 year. However, since only a third of those with disseminated disease had prior positive stool or sputum cultures, routine screening of stool and sputum in patients with low CD4 counts is not recommended.

KEY POINTS: CLINICAL PATTERNS IN PATIENTS WITH PULMONARY *M. AVIUM* COMPLEX

1. Solitary pulmonary nodule

2. Cavitary bronchitis or bronchiectasis with granuloma on biopsy or sputum repeatedly positive for MAC

3. Cavitary lung disease with scattered pulmonary nodules

4. Diffuse pulmonary infiltrates in immunocompromised patients

20. **How is pulmonary disease from *M. abscessus* managed?**

    Eighty percent of chronic lung disease caused by rapidly growing atypical mycobacteria is due to *M. abscessus*. *In vitro* susceptibility testing is recommended. Treatment usually is initiated with amikacin and cefoxitin or imipenem for 2–6 weeks in combination with clarithromycin. Most patients improve with this regimen, but tolerance of the drugs is poor over longer time periods. Permanent sputum conversion is rare, and, on occasion, surgical resection of localized pulmonary disease results in long-term sputum conversion.

INFECTIOUS PULMONARY COMPLICATIONS OF HIV INFECTION

CHAPTER 35

Mark J. Rosen, MD, and Mangala Narasimhan, DO

1. **Why are patients with human immunodeficiency virus (HIV) susceptible to infections?**

   Infection with HIV leads to viral replication in the pool of helper-T-lymphocytes (CD4+ lymphocytes), depleting their numbers and ability to function. This leads to reduced cell-mediated immunity, which in turn reduces humoral immune function. The best available surrogate marker for immune function is the blood CD4+ lymphocyte count; in general, patients with <200 cells/μL are considered to have moderate immunosuppression, and those with <100 cells/μL have severe immunosuppression.

2. **What are the most common pulmonary infections in patients with HIV infection?**

   Although a wide variety of pulmonary infections are associated with HIV-associated immune suppression, the most common infections diagnosed in the United States are bacterial pneumonia and *Pneumocystis* pneumonia (PCP). Endemic fungi commonly cause pneumonia in areas of the world in which they are prevalent, and tuberculosis is very common in HIV-infected persons in Africa and Asia. The strongest predictor of the likelihood of developing a specific pulmonary infection is the degree of immunosuppression, as assessed by measurement of the blood CD4+ lymphocyte count.

   Wallace JM, Rao AV, Glassroth J, et al: Respiratory illness in persons with human immunodeficiency virus infection. Am Rev Respir Dis 148:1523–1529, 1993.

3. **How have respiratory illnesses changed since the development of highly active antiretroviral therapy (HAART)?**

   Successful use of combination antiretroviral therapy leads to suppression of HIV replication and restoration of immune function. With the increasing use of HAART, the incidence of most pulmonary complications of HIV infection has declined, including lower rates of PCP, bacterial pneumonia, and tuberculosis. However, many persons with AIDS are not in care or are not compliant with these regimens, or, in some cases, these agents are not effective.

   Dore GJ, Li Y, McDonald A, et al: Impact of highly active antiretroviral therapy on individual AIDS-defining illness and survival in Australia. J Acquir Immune Defic Syndr 29:388–395, 2002.

   Wolff AJ, O'Donell AE: Pulmonary manifestations of HIV infection in the era of highly active antiretroviral therapy. Chest 120:1888–1893, 2001.

4. **What information should be obtained in the assessment of an HIV-infected person with suspected pulmonary infection?**

   - Degree of immune dysfunction, as assessed by CD4+ lymphocyte count or evidence of impaired immunity such as a history of weight loss, thrush, or previous opportunistic infections
   - How the patient developed HIV infection. Injection drug users are at higher risk for tuberculosis and bacterial pneumonia; gay or bisexual men are at increased risk for pulmonary Kaposi sarcoma (KS)

- Use of HAART and prophylactic drugs for PCP or tuberculosis and compliance with these regimens. Patients who are taking trimethoprim-sulfamethoxazole (TMP-SMZ) are unlikely to have PCP
- Exposure to a person with tuberculosis or a positive tuberculin skin test (TST)
- Residence in an area endemic for tuberculosis, fungi, or parasites
- Clinical presentation (i.e., acute or subacute)
- Assessment of oxygenation by pulse oximetry or arterial blood gas (ABG) analysis (determines urgency of evaluation and treatment for PCP)
- Serum lactate dehydrogenase (LDH) (may be helpful for the diagnosis of PCP)
- Radiographic pattern (Table 35-1)

TABLE 35-1. HIV INFECTION: CHEST RADIOGRAPHIC PATTERNS AND COMMON ETIOLOGIES

Focal opacity	**Mediastinal lymphadenopathy**
Bacteria	*Pneumocystis tuberculosis*
Mycobacterium tuberculosis	*Mycobacterium avium–intracellulare*
Pneumocystis jiroveci	Kaposi sarcoma
	Lymphoma
Diffuse opacities	Fungi
Pneumocystis carinii	
Mycobacterium tuberculosis	**Pleural effusion**
Kaposi sarcoma	Bacteria (parapneumonic effusion, empyema)
Bacteria	*Mycobacterium tuberculosis*
Fungi	Kaposi sarcoma
Cytomegalovirus	Lymphoma
Hypoproteinemia	Fungi
	Cardiomyopathy
Diffuse nodules	
Kaposi sarcoma (large)	**Cavitation**
Mycobacterium tuberculosis (miliary)	*M. tuberculosis* (high CD4)
Fungi (small)	*Pneumocystis carinii* (low CD4)
	Pseudomonas aeruginosa (low CD4)
Pneumothorax	*Rhodococcus equi*
Pneumocystis jiroveci	Fungi
	Lymphoma

5. **What are the most common bacterial respiratory infections associated with HIV infection?**

Regardless of the severity of immunosuppression, bacterial bronchitis and pneumonia are the most common causes of lower respiratory tract infection. Bronchitis and pneumonia may be recurrent, especially in patients with severe immunosuppression, and some patients develop bronchiectasis. The incidence of bacterial pneumonia is highest among patients with severe immunosuppression, injection drug users, and patients with CD4+ lymphocyte counts < 200/μL.

6. **How does bacterial pneumonia present?**
The clinical presentation of bacterial pneumonia is similar in patients with and without HIV infection, although bacteremia is more common with HIV disease. The onset is usually rapid (i.e., hours to days), with fever, productive cough, dyspnea, and, often, chest pain. Leukocytosis is common, and the serum LDH is usually normal or slightly elevated. Chest radiographs show segmental or lobar infiltrates, but diffuse patterns may be seen in severe pneumonia, particularly with *Haemophilus influenzae.* Cavitation may occur with *Staphylococcus aureus, Pseudomonas aeruginosa,* and *Rhodococcus equi.*

Afessa B, Green B: Bacterial pneumonia in hospitalized patients with HIV infection. Chest 117:1017–1022, 2000.

7. **Are CT scans useful in the diagnosis of bacterial pneumonia in HIV-infected patients?**
CT scans are especially useful when the chest radiographic findings are typical and when culture or serology has failed to identify an organism. Nodules, cavities, and fluid collections are better delineated on CT than on conventional radiographs. CT is also better for diagnosing and treating complications of infection such as abscess or empyema.

Aviram G, Boiselle PM: Imaging features of bacterial respiratory infections in AIDS. Curr Opin Pulm Med 10:183–188, 2004.

8. **Which organisms cause bacterial pneumonia in HIV-infected persons?**
The most common pathogens are *Streptococcus pneumoniae* and *H. influenzae,* and initial empirical therapy is usually directed against these pathogens. Interestingly, infections with *Mycoplasma pneumoniae* and *Chlamydia pneumoniae,* common in the general population, seem to be unusual in patients with HIV infection except, perhaps, those with good immune function. *S. aureus* and gram-negative organisms also should be considered in seriously ill patients. *P. aeruginosa* may cause community- or hospital-acquired pneumonia, usually when the CD4+ count is < 50/μL. Unusual causes of pneumonia are *R. equi, Nocardia asteroides,* group B streptococci, *Moraxella catarrhalis,* and *Legionella pneumoniae.*

Hirschtick RE, Glassroth J, Jordan MC, et al: Bacterial pneumonia in patients infected with human immunodeficiency virus. N Engl J Med 333:845–851, 1995.

9. **Which antibiotics should be used in the initial treatment of presumed bacterial pneumonia in HIV?**
With increasing concerns about drug-resistant pneumococci, a third-generation cephalosporin (e.g., ceftriaxone or cefotaxime) or a newer quinolone (e.g., levofloxacin or gatifloxacin) is usually given as initial empirical therapy. Antibiotics may be changed after the results of cultures are

KEY POINTS: BACTERIAL PNEUMONIA IN HIV-POSITIVE PATIENTS

1. Presentation is similar in patients with and without HIV infection.

2. CT scans are useful when no organism has been identified.

3. The most common pathogens are *S. pneumoniae* and *H. influenzae.*

4. Initial empirical treatment the same as in patients without HIV infection.

available or if the patient is not responding to treatment. Broader antimicrobial coverage may be appropriate in selected cases. Although TMP-SMZ is the treatment of choice for PCP, concerns about bacterial resistance make it undesirable as empirical monotherapy in patients with bacterial pneumonia.

10. **What is the organism that causes PCP in immunosuppressed patients?**
The organism that causes pneumonia is *Pneumocystis jiroveci*, formerly named *Pneumocystis carinii*. Studies of the *Pneumocystis* genome show that the *Pneumocystis carinii* organism only causes disease in rats and that the organism found in humans exists only in human hosts. Also, the organism was thought to be a parasite, but studies of the genome have indicated that it is in fact a fungus. Regardless, the term "PCP" is still used in common clinical parlance, standing for *Pneumocystis* **p**neumonia (instead of *Pneumocystis* **c**arinii **p**neumonia).

11. **Which patients with AIDS are at risk of developing PCP, and how often does it occur?**
PCP usually occurs in patients with CD4+ lymphocyte counts < 200/μL, and the risk increases as the CD4+ count declines. PCP is still the most common HIV-associated opportunistic infection, but its incidence has declined dramatically with the wide use of HAART and with use of prophylaxis against this pathogen in patients at risk for the disease.

12. **How does PCP present clinically?**
The onset is usually subacute or insidious, over days to weeks, but some patients present with the rapid onset of fulminant disease. Patients usually have fever, nonproductive cough, and dyspnea. The typical chest radiographic pattern shows bilateral diffuse ground glass opacities, but some have thin-walled cysts, upper-lobe infiltrates, focal infiltrates, nodules, or even no visible abnormalities. Spontaneous pneumothorax may be the presenting feature. In fact, a patient with known or suspected AIDS who presents with a spontaneous pneumothorax should be considered to have PCP until proven otherwise.

13. **How is PCP diagnosed?**
The diagnosis of PCP should be suspected in patients with advanced HIV disease and respiratory symptoms, especially if the patient is not using antipneumocystis prophylaxis (particularly TMP-SMZ). The serum LDH is elevated in more than 90% of cases, but this finding is nonspecific and is also seen in tuberculosis, fungal infections, and patients with liver disease. The PaO_2 or oxygen saturation measured by pulse oximetry is usually low and decreases further with exercise. The organism cannot be cultured, so confirming the diagnosis depends on identifying it with Gram–Weigert, methenamine silver, toluidine blue, or immunofluorescent stains from sputum induced after inhalation with 3% saline or from bronchoalveolar lavage (BAL) fluid or transbronchial lung biopsy specimens obtained by bronchoscopy.

14. **Should patients with suspected PCP who have negative sputum studies be treated empirically, or should bronchoscopy be done routinely to confirm the diagnosis?**
Most patients suspected of having PCP actually have that diagnosis, but the risks of empirical therapy, including treating patients with a potentially harmful regimen (including corticosteroids for severe disease) for an infection they do not have, leads many clinicians to confirm the diagnosis. There are no studies comparing one approach to the other, but a retrospective study of patients diagnosed with PCP shows no difference in outcomes between patients treated empirically and those in whom the diagnosis is confirmed with bronchoscopy.

Parada JP, Deloria-Knoll M, Chmiel JS, et al: Relationship between health insurance and medical care for patients hospitalized with human immunodeficiency virus-related *Pneumocystis carinii pneumonia*, 1995–1997: Medicaid, bronchoscopy and survival. Clin Infect Dis 37:1549–1555, 2003.

15. **What is the yield of bronchoscopy in diagnosing PCP?**
Appropriate stains of BAL fluid yield the diagnosis of PCP in around 90% of cases. Many clinicians also perform transbronchial biopsy, which enhances the diagnostic yield of the procedure but carries the added risks of pneumothorax and bleeding.

16. **How is PCP treated?**
The proper treatment of PCP depends upon disease severity and whether the patient is allergic or intolerant of certain agents. The options for treatment are outlined in Table 35-2. The drug of choice is TMP-SMZ, 15 mg/kg/day orally or intravenously in divided doses. Some patients do not respond because they have resistant organisms, and others, because their immune system is profoundly suppressed. The drugs used for PCP have a high incidence of toxicity, and a switch to an alternative agent is often necessary. Desensitization to TMP-SMZ has been successful in some patients allergic to the drug.

TABLE 35-2. TREATMENT OF PNEUMOCYSTIS PNEUMONIA

Drug	Dose	Comments
Moderate to severe disease (PaO$_2$ $\leq$ 70 mmHg or D(A-a)O$_2$ $\geq$ 35–45 mmHg, breathing room air)		
Trimethoprim-sulfamethoxazole (TMP/SMZ)	15–20 to 75–100 mg/kg IV or PO in 3 divided doses	Drug of choice, but toxicity (e.g., rash, fever, or nausea) is frequent
Pentamidine isethionate	3–4 mg/kg IV daily	Toxicity can include dysglycemia, renal failure, neutropenia, Q-T prolongation, arrhythmias, pancreatitis, and orthostatic hypotension
Trimetrexate-folinic acid	45 mg/m^2 IV daily 20 mg/m^2 IV or PO q6h	Not as effective as trimethoprim-sulfa-methoxazole, but better tolerated
Prednisone	40 mg PO b.i.d., days 1–5 20 mg PO b.i.d., days 6–10 20 mg PO daily, days 11–21	Recommended as adjunctive therapy, along with an antipneumocystis agent for all patients with PCP who meet criteria for moderate to severe disease
Mild to moderate disease (PaO$_2$ $\geq$ 70 mm Hg or D(A-a)O$_2$ $\leq$ 35 mmHg, breathing room air)		
TMP-SMZ	Same as above	Most likely to cause hepatotoxicity of all oral regimens
Dapsone-trimethoprim	100 mg PO daily *or* 5–6 mg/kg PO t.i.d.	Methemoglobinemia and hemolysis in patients with G6PD deficiency
Clindamycin/primaquine	600 mg IV or PO t.i.d. *or* 15 mg base PO daily	Rash, leukopenia, nausea, diarrhea-methemoglobinemia, and hemolysis in patients with G6PD deficiency
Atovaquone suspension	750 mg b.i.d.	Less effective than TMP-SMZ, but better tolerated

b.i.d. = twice a day, PO = orally, q6h = every 6 hours, t.i.d. = three times a day.

17. **Why are corticosteroids used in treatment of PCP?**

    Corticosteroids reduce progression to respiratory failure and death in moderate to severe cases of PCP, defined as $PaO_2 < 70$ mmHg or an alveolar-to-arterial (A-a) gradient ≥ 35 mmHg on room air. Treatment of PCP leads to lung inflammation and clinical deterioration in the first few days of treatment, and this inflammatory response is attenuated by corticosteroids.

    The National Institutes of Health-University of California Expert Panel for Corticosteroid as Adjunctive Therapy for Pneumocystis Pneumonia: Consensus statement on the use of corticosteroid as adjunctive therapy for *Pneumocystis* pneumonia in the acquired immunodeficiency syndrome. N Engl J Med 323:1500–1504, 1990.

18. **Can PCP be prevented?**

    The best preventive strategy is restoration of immune function with HAART. Prophylaxis should be given to any patient with a $CD4^+$ count ≤ 200 cells/μL or with 2 weeks of unexplained fever (>37.8°C), malaise, or thrush. However, it can be stopped successfully in patients who maintain $CD4^+$ lymphocyte counts > 200/μL in response to HAART. The agent of choice is TMP-SMZ (1 double strength orally per day or 1 single-strength per day). Alternative drugs are listed in Table 35-3.

TABLE 35-3. PROPOSED U.S. PUBLIC HEALTH SERVICE AND INFECTIOUS DISEASE SOCIETY OF AMERICA GUIDELINES FOR THE PRIMARY AND SECONDARY PROPHYLAXIS OF PCP IN ADULTS AND ADOLESCENTS

Indication	First Choice	Alternative Regimens
CD4 count < 200/μL, oropharyngeal candidiasis, unexplained fever ≥ 2 weeks, or prior PCP	TMP-SMZ (1 DS PO qd, 1 SS PO qd)	Dapsone (50 mg PO b.i.d. *or* 100 mg qd) Dapsone (50 mg qd) *plus* pyrimethamine (50 mg PO qw) *plus* leucovorin (25 mg PO qw)
		Dapsone (200 mg PO) *plus* pyrimethamine (75 mg PO qw) *plus* leucovorin (25 mg PO qw)
		Aerosolized pentamidine (300 mg qm by Respirgard II nebulizer)
		Atovaquone (1500 mg PO qd)
		TMP-SMZ (1 DS PO tiw)

DS = double-strength, PO = orally, qd = once daily, qm = once monthly, qw = once weekly, SS = single strength, tiw = three times per week, b.i.d. = twice a day.
From Masur H, Kaplan J, Holmes K, et al: Guidelines for preventing opportunistic infections among HIV-infected persons—2002: Recommendations of the U.S. Public Health Service and the Infectious Diseases Society of America. MMWR Recomm Rep 51(RR-8):1–52, 2002.

19. **What is the relationship of tuberculosis to HIV infection?**

    HIV-infected persons may develop active tuberculosis (TB) following new infection (i.e., primary tuberculosis) or by activation of latent disease in the presence of impaired cell-mediated immunity. In developed nations, injection drug users and persons in lower socioeconomic groups are at especially high risk of developing tuberculosis, probably because the disease is more prevalent in their communities and because they are less likely than others to access health care and to use antituberculosis prophylaxis. TB may be rapidly progressive in HIV-infected patients with very low $CD4^+$ cell counts who are exposed to *Mycobacterium tuberculosis*. Tuberculosis also accelerates the course of HIV infection because patients with TB experience more rapid declines in CD4+ cell counts than others.

KEY POINTS: *PNEUMOCYSTIS* PNEUMONIA IN HIV-POSITIVE PATIENTS

1. It usually occurs in patients with CD4+ lymphocyte counts < 200/μL.

2. It usually presents with insidious onset with fever, cough, and dyspnea.

3. Most cases have an elevated LDH and hypoxemia.

4. It is diagnosed by finding the organism in induced sputum or with bronchoscopy (i.e., bronchoalveolar lavage or lung biopsy).

5. The drug of choice is TMP-SMZ, and adjunctive steroids improve mortality in patients with moderate or severe disease.

20. **When should tuberculosis be suspected?**
    Tuberculosis should be suspected in any HIV-infected patient with a respiratory infection in geographic areas in which *M. tuberculosis* is prevalent. In underdeveloped countries, especially sub-Saharan Africa and Southeast Asia, tuberculosis is the leading cause of AIDS-associated mortality. In the United States, tuberculosis is more common in HIV-infected persons who have resided in jails, prisons, homeless shelters, or chronic care facilities.

21. **What is the clinical presentation of tuberculosis in HIV-infected persons?**
    The most common presenting symptoms are fever, cough, and weight loss. The lungs are involved in most patients, but the incidence of extrapulmonary tuberculosis increases as the CD4+ count falls. The most common extrapulmonary site is the lymph nodes, but brain abscesses, meningitis, pericardial disease, and gastric and bone tuberculosis are also seen. Disseminated disease occurs in around 10% of cases, and mycobacteremia is common.

22. **What are the radiographic manifestations of TB in HIV-infected persons?**
    When tuberculosis occurs relatively early in the course of HIV infection, the chest radiographic features are similar to those of non-HIV-infected patients, with predominantly upper lobe fibrocavitary opacities. As the CD4+ count drops to < 200 cells/μL, focal or diffuse consolidation, reticulonodular or miliary patterns, pleural effusions, and intrathoracic adenopathy are commonly seen. Norma radiographs are seen in up to 20% of cases of active tuberculosis in HIV-infected persons. The presence of intrathoracic lymphadenopathy on routine radiographs or CT strongly suggests this diagnosis.

23. **Is the TST helpful in the diagnosis of tuberculosis?**
    A TST with a purified protein derivative (PPD) in HIV-positive persons is less reliable than it is in the general population because of a higher likelihood of false-negative tests in patients with reduced cell-mediated immunity. A PPD skin test in an HIV-infected patient is considered positive if there are 5 mm or more of induration; persons with a positive TST should be treated to prevent the emergence of active disease.

    American Thoracic Society, Centers for Disease Control: Targeted tuberculin testing and treatment of latent tuberculosis infection. Am J Respir Crit Care Med 161:S221–247, 2000.

24. **What is the role of sputum examination in the diagnosis of tuberculosis?**
    Examination of sputum is usually the first and best test. Cultures are positive in 85–100% of patients, but results may take 3–6 weeks. Smears are positive in 30–90% of patients. A major

problem in diagnosing tuberculosis is failure to consider the diagnosis and to send adequate sputum specimens (i.e., three to five samples). Identification of *M. tuberculosis* using nucleic acid amplification (NAA) techniques is possible, but this is recommended only to confirm the diagnosis in persons with positive acid-fast bacillus (AFB) smears or to dismiss the diagnosis in smear-negative persons. When there is a discrepancy between the smear and the NAA test, other tests are necessary.

25. **What is the role of invasive tests in the diagnosis of tuberculosis?**
Bronchoscopy is used if sputum smears are negative, if an immediate result is needed, or if diagnoses other than tuberculosis are being considered. Biopsies show granulomas in some cases, which leads to a rapid diagnosis. Culture of BAL, washing, and biopsies also increase the yield for tuberculosis over sputum alone. When pleural fluid is present, cultures are positive in approximately 90% of cases, and smears in 15%. A closed pleural biopsy that shows granulomas suggests tuberculosis or fungal disease. Blood cultures are useful as they are positive in up to 40% of cases of disseminated tuberculosis in advanced HIV infection. Cultures of urine, stool, bone marrow, and sites such as the liver, the pericardium, and the central nervous system also may be helpful in some patients.

26. **What is multidrug-resistant tuberculosis? How is it treated?**
Multidrug resistance (MDR) refers to organisms that are resistant to two or more drugs, including isoniazid and rifampin. Treatment is difficult and requires the use of other drugs based on patterns of sensitivity in a given community.

CHAPTER 36

NONINFECTIOUS PULMONARY COMPLICATIONS OF HIV INFECTION

Mangala Narasimhan, DO, and Mark J. Rosen, MD

1. **Are people with human immunodeficiency virus (HIV) infection predisposed to lung diseases other than opportunistic infections?**

   Yes. HIV-infected persons are predisposed to the development of the following:

   - **Neoplastic diseases that affect the lung:** Kaposi sarcoma (KS), lymphoma, and primary lung cancer
   - **Noninfectious inflammatory disorders:** Nonspecific and lymphocytic interstitial pneumonitis
   - **Pulmonary hypertension**
   - **Immune reconstitution inflammatory syndrome:** A disease complex of increased inflammatory activity after starting highly active antiretroviral therapy (HAART)

2. **What causes KS?**

   KS has been etiologically linked to human herpesvirus-8 (HHV-8), also known as Kaposi sarcoma herpesvirus (KSHV), because viral DNA is detected in sarcomatous lesions. KS is the most common malignancy related to acquired immunodeficiency syndrome (AIDS), and usually it affects skin with typical violaceous or red plaques.

   Sarid R, Klepfish A, Schattner A: Virology, pathogenetic mechanisms, and associated diseases of Kaposi's sarcoma-associated herpesvirus (HHV-8). Mayo Clin Proc 77:941–949, 2002.

3. **How do patients with pulmonary KS present clinically?**

   Patients with pulmonary KS usually have skin disease but often have no pulmonary symptoms. The most common complaint is chronic cough, and some patients have hemoptysis, infection related to bronchial obstruction, and dyspnea with extensive parenchymal involvement or large pleural effusions. Weight loss and fever are also common.

4. **Do patients with pulmonary KS always have cutaneous involvement?**

   No. Patients with pulmonary KS usually have cutaneous disease, which is an important clinical clue. However, up to 15% of patients with pulmonary KS have no cutaneous involvement. Oropharyngeal lesions are also seen commonly on physical examination.

5. **What are the typical chest radiographic findings in pulmonary KS?**

   The most common radiographic findings in pulmonary KS are:

   - Linear opacities that follow septal lines (i.e., Kerley's B lines)
   - Nodular opacities that are ill defined and of various sizes; coalescence may occur with areas of patchy consolidation
   - Pleural effusions, which may be unilateral or bilateral
   - Hilar or mediastinal lymphadenopathy
   - Bronchial thickening

   Chest computed tomography (CT), particularly high-resolution CT (HRCT), may be useful in the diagnosis of patients who have indistinct findings on standard radiographs.

6. **How is the diagnosis of pulmonary KS established?**

In most patients with pulmonary KS, the diagnosis is usually inferred by visualizing typical lesions in the pharynx or the tracheobronchial tree. Cytology of sputum bronchoalveolar lavage fluid is rarely diagnostic, and histologic diagnosis of bronchoscopic lung biopsy specimens have a low (26–60%) diagnostic yield because endobronchial lesions are deep below the mucosa and parenchymal lesions are patchy in distribution. Pleural fluid cytology and pleural biopsy are also rarely helpful in the diagnosis. Open-lung biopsy has the highest diagnostic yield but is rarely performed because bronchoscopy is usually adequate to visualize airway lesions and to rule out the possibility of infection.

Aboulafia DM: The epidemiologic, pathologic, and clinical features of AIDS-associated pulmonary Kaposi's sarcoma. Chest 117:1128–1145, 2000.

Antman K, Chang Y: Kaposi's sarcoma. N Engl J Med 342:1027–1038, 2000.

7. **How is pulmonary KS treated?**

The treatment must be individualized, depending on the site and the extent of involvement. Patients with disseminated disease may benefit from cytotoxic chemotherapy with vinca alkaloids, etoposide, and bleomycin. Liposomal anthracyclines, paclitaxel, angiogenesis inhibitors, thalidomide, interferon alpha (IFNA), and retinoic acids have all been used.

Toschi E, Sgadari C, Monini P, et al: Treatment of Kaposi's sarcoma—An update. Anticancer Drugs 13:977–987, 2002.

8. **What is the effect of HAART on the prognosis of KS?**

The most promising approach, which should always be offered to patients with KS, is the use of HAART, which may lead to regression of KS lesions. Protease inhibitor-based and non-nucleoside reverse transcriptase inhibitor–based antiviral regimens may lead to an undetectable KSHV load, and an undetectable KSHV load is associated with KS regression. *In vivo* and *in vitro* clinical studies show that protease inhibitors are able to block angiogenesis, KS lesion formation, and tumor growth.

Gill J, Bourboulia D, Wilkinson J, et al: Prospective study of the effects of antiviral therapy on Kaposi sarcoma-associated herpesvirus infection in patients with and without Kapsoi sarcoma. J Acquir Immune Defic Syndr 31:384–390, 2002.

KEY POINTS: PULMONARY KAPOSI SARCOMA

1. KS is etiologically linked to human herpesvirus 8.

2. Patients with pulmonary KS usually have concomitant skin lesions.

3. Radiographic findings: linear opacities, nodules, bronchial thickening, pleural effusions, and lymphadenopathy.

4. Diagnosis is usually established by bronchoscopic visualization of lesions in the upper airway, trachea, or bronchi.

5. May improve with chemotherapy or treatment with HAART.

9. **How often does lymphoma affect the lung in persons with HIV infection?**

Although non-Hodgkin lymphoma (NHL) is an HIV-associated disorder, most patients with lymphoma do not have prominent pulmonary complaints. Thoracic involvement occurs in up to 31% of cases of patients with NHL and HIV infection. Typically, it is found along with systemic symptoms or is discovered as part of the staging process. HIV-associated primary pulmonary lymphoma is usually a high-grade B-cell tumor occurring in the setting of advanced HIV infection. "B" symptoms are often present, and latent Epstein–Barr virus infection of these tumor cells has been demonstrated.

10. **What are the typical radiographic findings in AIDS patients with pulmonary NHL?**
Chest radiographs most commonly show parenchymal infiltrates (including interstitial and air space disease) and single or multiple nodules. These nodules may grow rapidly (doubling in size in days or weeks), and cavitation within these nodules may occur. Rare cases of endobronchial lesions have also been reported. Pleural effusions (unilateral or bilateral) occur in up to 70% of cases and are often noted in the absence of parenchymal disease. In contrast to non-AIDS patients, mediastinal and hilar lymphadenopathy is generally not prominent in patients with NHL and HIV infection.

11. **How is pulmonary or pleural NHL diagnosed?**
Diagnosis depends on biopsy of involved lymph nodes, pleura, or lung tissue or cytologic analysis of pleural fluid. The diagnosis is sometimes inferred in patients with known NHL and clinical and radiographic findings consistent with NHL, but clinicians should try to establish the diagnosis and to rule out opportunistic infectious etiologies.

12. **What is the prognosis for HIV-infected patients with NHL?**
In general, the prognosis is poor, with median survival of only 4–6 months. Respiratory involvement causing significant morbidity or mortality is unusual. Factors associated with a poor prognosis include a history of an AIDS-defining illness before the diagnosis of lymphoma, bone marrow involvement, and a low Karnofsky performance status. In the absence of these factors, prognosis is more favorable. Complete remission is attained after therapy in up to 75% of patients, and median survival is 11.3 months.

13. **Is the incidence of lung cancer increased in HIV-infected patients?**
In the pre-HAART era, several studies reported an increase in lung neoplasms in HIV-infected men. They were usually adenocarcinomas and were associated with aggressive courses with short survival. In later years, the use of HAART led to a dramatic decrease in morbidity and mortality associated with opportunistic infections, with a concurrent increase in mortality due to non-AIDS-defining malignancies. The reason for this increase in malignancies is not known, but it has been suggested that patients with impaired immune systems may be more predisposed to developing malignancy.

There has also been an increase in the incidence of lung cancer in the post-HAART era. The incidence in the pre-HAART era was 0.8 per 10,000 patient-years, and, in the post-HAART era, it has risen to 6.7 per 10,000 patient-years. One of the possible reasons is that the prolonged immunosuppression that patients experience on HAART and the increased survival time may predispose them to lung cancer; lung cancers develop when patients at risk for lung cancer live to develop it because they do not succumb to infection.

Bower M, Powles T, Nelson M: HIV-related lung cancer in the era of highly active antiretroviral therapy. AIDS 17:371–375, 2003.

Herida M, Mary-Krause M, Cadranel J, et al: Incidence of non-AIDS-defining cancers before and during the highly active antiretroviral therapy era in a cohort of human immunodeficiency virus-infected patients. J Clin Oncol 21:3447–3453, 2003.

14. **What is the clinical course in HIV-infected patients with lung cancer?**
Some studies have suggested that HIV-infected patients with lung cancer have a more fulminant, rapidly declining course (resulting from the lung cancer) when compared with others.

15. **Is the incidence of pulmonary hypertension increased in patients with HIV infection?**
Yes. HIV infection is associated with an increased prevalence of pulmonary hypertension, ranging up to 0.5%, a rate significantly higher than the 1 in 200,000 found in the general population. Pulmonary hypertension in patients with HIV infection resembles idiopathic pulmonary arterial hypertension (IPAH) in the general population. Like IPAH, pulmonary hypertension associated with HIV infection is likely to be linked to HHV-8 infection, the same virus that causes KS. The diagnosis should not be made without evaluating for common secondary causes of pulmonary hypertension, including thromboembolism, left-sided heart disease, congenital heart disease, severe lung disease, and obstructive sleep apnea.

Cool CD, Rai PR, Yeager ME, et al: Expression of human herpesvirus-8 in primary pulmonary hypertension. N Engl J Med 349:1113–1122, 2003.

McGoon M, Gutterman D, Steen V, et al: Screening, early detection, and diagnosis of pulmonary arterial hypertension: ACCP evidence-based clinical practice guidelines. Chest 126:14S–34S, 2004.

16. **What are the clinical features of pulmonary hypertension in patients with HIV infection?**
Most patients present with dyspnea on exertion. They may also present with syncope, heart murmurs, or other symptoms of heart failure. Patients should be graded according to their New York Heart Association score, which is the only parameter that significantly correlates with survival. There has been no correlation with the stage of AIDS (as defined by the Centers for Disease Control and Prevention [CDC]), the CD4+ lymphocyte count, or the plasma HIV viral load.

Mehta NJ, Khan IA, Metha RN, et al: HIV-related pulmonary hypertension: Analytic review of 131 cases. Chest 118:1133–1141, 2000.

Opravil M, Pechere M, Speich R, et al: HIV-associated primary pulmonary hypertension. A case control study. Swiss HIV cohort study. Am J Respir Crit Care Med 155:990–995, 1997.

17. **How is pulmonary hypertension treated in patients with HIV infection?**
Treatment is the same as in patients with IPAH, with anticoagulation and vasodilator therapy, and these patients usually have similar responses to treatment. However, HIV infection is considered a contraindication to lung transplantation.

18. **What is the prognosis for HIV-associated pulmonary hypertension?**
Survival is significantly decreased in HIV-infected patients with pulmonary hypertension compared with those without pulmonary hypertension. Successful treatment of the HIV disease with HAART does not seem to alter the clinical course of pulmonary hypertension.

Recusani F, Di Matteo A, Gambarin F: Clinical and therapeutical follow-up of HIV-associated pulmonary hypertension: Prospective study of 10 patients. AIDS 17(S1):S88–S95, 2003.

KEY POINTS: PULMONARY HYPERTENSION IN HIV DISEASE

1. The incidence of pulmonary hypertension is increased in patients with HIV infection.

2. The clinical features, pathologic findings, diagnostic evaluation, and treatment are the same in patients with idiopathic pulmonary arterial hypertension as with non-HIV-infected persons.

3. The incidence of pulmonary hypertension is unrelated to the CD4+ lymphocyte count.

4. Secondary causes of pulmonary hypertension should be ruled out.

19. **What is immune reconstitution inflammatory syndrome (IRIS)?**

IRIS is defined as a paradoxical deterioration in clinical status attributable to the recovery of the immune system during HAART. Diagnostic criteria include:

- Diagnosis of AIDS
- Current treatment with anti-HIV medications
- Symptoms consistent with an infectious or inflammatory condition that appeared while on antiretroviral therapy
- Symptoms that cannot be explained by a newly acquired infection, by the expected clinical course of the disease, or by side effects of therapy

Autran B, Carcelaint G, Li TS: Restoration of the immune system with antiretroviral therapy. Immunol Lett 66:207–211, 1999.

Shelbourne SA, Hamill RJ, Rodrguez-Barradas MC, et al: Immune reconstitution inflammatory syndrome: Emergence of a unique syndrome during highly active antiretroviral therapy. Medicine 81(3):213–227, 2002.

20. **Which diseases have been associated with IRIS?**

Cases of paradoxical deterioration of a variety of disorders have occurred after initiation of HAART. These include *Mycobacterium avium* complex (MAC), *Mycobacterium tuberculosis*, cryptococcosis, cytomegalovirus, herpes zoster, sarcoidosis, KS, Graves' disease, *Pneumocystis* pneumonia (PCP), hepatitis B and C viruses, and progressive multifocal leukoencephalopathy.

Connick E, Lederman MM, Kotzin BL, et al: Immune reconstitution it the first year of potent antiretroviral therapy and its relationship to virologic response. J Infect Dis 181:353–363, 2000.

21. **Has IRIS been associated with thoracic disease?**

Yes. Paradoxical worsening of tuberculosis may occur; after an appropriate response to antituberculous therapy and starting HAART, patients may develop fever, pulmonary infiltrates, thoracic lymphadenopathy, and pleural effusions. In patients recovering from PCP, administration of HAART may lead to deterioration and respiratory failure.

Narita M, Ashkin D, Hollender ES, Pitchenik AE: Paradoxical worsening of tuberculosis following antiretroviral therapy in patients with AIDS. Am J Respir Crit Care Med 158:157–161,1998.

Wislez M, Bergot E, Antoine M, et al: Acute respiratory failure following HAART introduction in patients treated for *Pneumocystis carinii* pneumonia. Am J Respir Crit Care Med 164:847–851, 2001.

22. **How is IRIS diagnosed?**

IRIS is a diagnosis of exclusion, suggested by a compatible clinical syndrome in a patient recovering from an infection who was begun on HAART in the previous several months. Plasma HIV loads invariably improve. The CD4+ lymphocyte count usually improves compared to prior measurements, but this may not be the case in all patients because these cells may compartmentalize to sites of active inflammation. Opportunistic infection is usually a diagnostic consideration, but in patients without life-threatening symptoms who are likely to have IRIS, invasive diagnostic procedures can usually be avoided, with the patient remaining under observation.

23. **How is IRIS treated?**

Most patients should just receive palliative therapy for symptoms such as antipyretics for fever. Systemic corticosteroids can be used for severe inflammatory disease that is causing significant end-organ damage.

DeSimone JA, Pomeantz RJ, Babinchak TJ: Inflammatory reactions in HIV-1 infected patients after initiation of highly active antiretroviral therapy. Ann Intern Med 133:447–454, 2000.

VIII. PULMONARY VASCULAR DISEASES

THROMBOEMBOLIC DISEASE

Harold I. Palevsky, MD

CHAPTER 37

1. **What are the signs and symptoms of pulmonary embolism (PE)?**

   The clinical presentation of PE varies with the size of the embolus and the patient's underlying cardiopulmonary functional status (Table 37-1). Large pulmonary emboli that occlude the main pulmonary artery may present as an acute, fatal event. Somewhat smaller clots may present as a syncopal event. Very small pulmonary emboli that occlude the distal pulmonary vasculature may cause only transient dyspnea with pleuritic pain. The extent of hemodynamic and gas exchange abnormalities observed may be disproportionate to the size of the clot as a result of the release of humoral factors, possibly serotonin, occurring after clots interrupt flow in the pulmonary vascular bed.

   In the Urokinase–Streptokinase Pulmonary Embolism Trials (USPET) and Prospective Investigation of Pulmonary Embolism Diagnosis (PIOPED) studies, the most common complaint, regardless of clot size, was dyspnea (75–85%). Pleuritic chest pain was the second-most-common complaint (57–87%), followed by cough (40–53% of patients), hemoptysis, and syncope. Hemoptysis was more commonly observed in patients in the USPET study and was most often associated with smaller clots.

   Bell WR, Simon TL, DeMets DC: The clinical features of submassive and massive pulmonary emboli. Am J Med 62:355–360, 1977.

   PIOPED Investigators: Value of the ventilation/perfusion lung scan in acute pulmonary embolism: Results of the Prospective Investigation of Pulmonary Embolism Diagnosis. JAMA 263:2753–2759, 1990.

   Quinn DA, Thompson BT, Terrin ML, et al: A prospective investigation of pulmonary embolism in men and women. JAMA 268:1689–1696, 1992.

2. **What are the typical chest radiographic findings in patients with pulmonary emboli?**

   The standard chest radiograph may be helpful in the diagnostic evaluation of patients with suspected PE. However, a normal chest radiograph does not eliminate the possibility of PE, and the radiographic findings associated with the disease are nonspecific.

   Of the associated findings, decreased vascularity in one lung, causing a unilateral increase in radiographic lucency (Westermark's sign), suggests the presence of a large pulmonary embolus. This finding may be associated with prominence of the central pulmonary artery shadows. A wedge-shaped peripheral infiltrate (Hampton's hump) may be seen after a pulmonary embolus that occludes distal vessels in the pulmonary arterial tree. Most wedge-shaped pulmonary infiltrates resolve over time, and, although historically the infiltrate has been ascribed to a pulmonary infarction, it probably represents hemorrhagic edema. The most frequently seen radiographic pattern in patients with PE, however, is a combination of nonspecific parenchymal infiltrates, atelectasis, and pleural effusions. Only 12% of chest radiographs in patients with pulmonary emboli are interpreted as normal.

   The presence of radiographic abnormalities does not obviate the value of the ventilation-perfusion (V/Q) lung scan. Finding unmatched perfusion defects, especially in areas where the chest radiograph is relatively normal, warrants further consideration of PE. Also, the lung scan retains its diagnostic accuracy in patients with diffuse, relatively symmetrical radiographic abnormalities such as those seen in interstitial lung disease, congestive heart failure,

TABLE 37-1. FREQUENCY OF SIGNS AND SYMPTOMS OF PULMONARY EMBOLISM IN WOMEN VERSUS MEN AND MASSIVE VERSUS SUBMASSIVE PULMONARY EMBOLISM

Symptom or Sign	PIOPED Data		USPET Data	
	Women	Men	Massive	Submassive
Dyspnea	80%	78%	85%	82%
Pleuritic chest pain	60%	57%	64%	85%
Cough	41%	40%	53%	52%
Hemoptysis	10%	21%	23%	40%
Leg pain	23%	30%		
Leg swelling	24%	36%		
Pleural rub	2%	7%		
Crackles	60%	57%		
Mean heart rate ± SD (beats/min)	98 ± 19	93 ± 18		
Mean respiratory rate ± SD (breaths/min)	24 ± 8	23 ± 7		
Syncope	—	—	20%	4%

SD = standard deviation from the mean, PIOPED = Prospective Investigation of Plumonary Embolism Diagnosis, USPET = Urokinase–Steptokinase Plumonary Embolism Trials.

and obstructive pulmonary disease. It has been proposed that in patients with abnormal chest radiographs, computed tomography (CT) scanning is more appropriate as an initial diagnostic study to evaluate for pulmonary emboli; however, this has never been fully evaluated.

Stein PD, Terrin MC, Hales CA, et al: Clinical, laboratory, roentgenographic and electrocardiographic findings in patients with acute pulmonary embolism and no pre-existing cardiac or pulmonary disease. Chest 100:598–603, 1991.

3. **Do patients with PE always have hypoxemia or an increased alveolar-arterial gradient?**
No. Patients with pulmonary emboli frequently have tachypnea and may present with hyperventilation and a resulting respiratory alkalosis. The partial pressure of oxygen (pO_2) may be variably elevated, normal, or low, but the alveolar-arterial (A-a) gradient is most often increased. No absolute value of pO_2 or A-a gradient, however, can reliably exclude the diagnosis of PE in a patient with a clinical presentation suggestive of the disease. Furthermore, it was shown in a group of 64 patients with angiographically proven PE that A-a gradients ranged from 11.6–83.9 mmHg. Three patients who had strongly suggestive histories of PE and confirmed disease presented with a pO_2 of less than 85 and a normal A-a gradient. Although normal A-a gradient and pO_2 values may reassure the clinician that the thromboemboli are not severe or extensive, these findings do not obviate a further work-up in a patient with clinical presentation suggestive of the disease.

Overton DT, Bocks JJ: The alveolar-arterial oxygen gradient in patients with documented pulmonary embolism. Arch Intern Med 148:1610–1617, 1988.

Stein PD, Terrin MC, Hales CA, et al: Clinical, laboratory, roentgenographic and electrocardiographic findings in patients with acute pulmonary embolism and no pre-existing cardiac or pulmonary disease. Chest 100:598–603, 1991.

4. **What is the significance of severe hypoxemia in a patient with PE?**
    Large or multiple pulmonary emboli can lead to obstruction in a substantial portion of the pulmonary vascular bed, resulting in an increase in dead space ventilation, an increase in pulmonary artery pressures, and an increase in the A-a gradient. These are associated with decreased PO_2 and evidence of right heart failure (e.g., peripheral edema, distended neck veins, tricuspid regurgitation, a right-sided fourth heart sound [S_4], and a loud pulmonic second sound [P_2]). In patients who have a patent foramen ovale, atrial septal defect, or ventricular septal defect, however, increases in pulmonary artery pressure may result in unloading of the right ventricle by shunting blood flow to the left side of the heart, bypassing the pulmonary bed. When this extrapulmonary shunt occurs, signs of right heart failure are absent and arterial pO_2 is low, typically less than 60 mmHg, and fails to improve with the patient breathing supplemental 100% oxygen. Activation of a right-to-left shunt in patients with pulmonary emboli may promote paradoxical embolization and result in embolic strokes or occlusion of other systemic arterial vascular beds.

    Patients with suspected pulmonary emboli who present with very low pO_2 should undergo V/Q lung scans with additional images obtained over the brain and kidneys. Normally, the technetium-labeled microaggregated albumin used for the perfusion scan is trapped in the lungs and never enters the systemic circulation. In the setting of an extrapulmonary shunt, however, the radiolabeled particles cross directly to the left side of the heart and are trapped in systemic capillary beds. Images taken over the brain or kidneys, therefore, show radioactivity. Additionally, the shunt fraction can be calculated from the ratio of counts measured systematically to total counts.

    Morthy SS, Losasso AM, Gibbs PS: Acquired right-to-left intracardiac shunts and severe hypoxemia. Crit Care Med 6:28–31, 1978.

5. **What is the D-dimer assay? What is its utility for the diagnosis of deep venous thrombosis (DVT) and PE?**
    D-dimer is a degradation product that is released into the systemic circulation by endogenous fibrinolysis of cross-linked fibrin (i.e., a thrombus). The use of D-dimer assays is most useful as an exclusionary test; it has an excellent negative predictive value for PE and DVT in outpatients

---

KEY POINTS: D-DIMER DETERMINATION

1. D-dimer determination has become a key test in the assessment of outpatients suspected of DVT or PE.

2. Advances in technology have improved reliability and have shortened the time until results are available.

3. When combined with low pretest clinical probability of disease, a negative D-dimer can exclude DVT or PE with approximately 99% negative predictive value.

4. Negative D-dimer in patients with intermediate or high probability of disease does not exclude disease with sufficient negative predictive value.

5. A negative D-dimer in conjunction with a negative duplex ultrasound study (for DVT) or a negative helical CT scan (for PE) can be used to exclude disease.

6. D-dimer is less reliable in inpatients because values increase with age and in the presence of multiple medical conditions (e.g., malignancy, recent surgery, infection, vascular disease, or trauma).

with low pretest probability for thromboembolic disease. A study of 1177 consecutive patients suspected of PE found that a negative D-dimer (using the SimpliRED technique) had a negative predictive value of 85%. However, in the 703 patients with a low clinical probability of PE, the negative predictive value of the negative D-dimer test increased to 99%. Thus, a negative D-dimer can be used to exclude DVT or PE in patients with low pretest clinical probability of disease; in patients with higher pretest clinical probability of disease (i.e., malignancy), a negative D-dimer assay is insufficient as a single diagnostic test to exclude disease.

Ginsberg JS, Well PS, Kearon C, et al: Sensitivity and specificity of a rapid whole-blood assay for D-dimer in the diagnosis of pulmonary embolism. Ann Intern Med 129:1006–1011, 1998.

Kutinsky I, Blakley S, Roche V: Normal D-dimer levels in patients with pulmonary embolism. Arch Intern Med 159:1569–1572, 1999.

Lee AY, Julian JA, Levine MN, et al: Clinical utility of a rapid whole-blood D-dimer assay in patients with cancer who present with suspected acute deep venous thrombosis. Ann Intern Med 131:417–423, 1999.

Stein PD, Hull RD, Patel KC, et al: D-dimer for the exclusion of acute venous thrombosis and pulmonary embolism: A systematic review. Ann Intern Med 140:589–602, 2004.

6. **What tools can a clinician use to aid in assigning a pretest clinical probability of PE to an individual patient?**

The pretest clinical probability of PE was very useful in the PIOPED study, in combination with the V/Q scan results, for determining a patient's likelihood of PE. Subsequently, a clinical scoring system has been developed and validated for clinical use in assessing the likelihood of PE:

History:
- History of DVT or PE (1.5 pts)
- Active malignancy (1.5 pts)
- Hemoptysis (1 pt)
- Recent (i.e., <4 weeks) immobilization or surgery (1.5 pts)

Physical exam:
- Signs or symptoms of DVT (3 pts)
- Tachycardia (1.5 pts)

Clinical judgment:
- PE as the most likely diagnosis (3 pts)

Probability of PE is based on the total points assigned to the patient:
- Low: <2 pts
- Intermediate: 2–6 pts
- High: >6 pts

PIOPED Investigators: Value of the ventilation/perfusion scan in acute pulmonary embolism: Results of the Prospective Investigation of Pulmonary Diagnosis (PIOPED). J Am Med Assoc 263:2753–2759, 1990.

Wells PS, Ginserg JS, Anderson Dr, et al: Use of a clinical model for safe management of patients with suspected pulmonary embolism. Ann Intern Med 129:997–1005, 1998.

7. **Why is the D-dimer assay of less utility in inpatients compared with outpatients?**

Although D-dimer levels of greater than 500 mg/mL are present in most patients with acute DVT or PE, the assay is nonspecific. D-dimer values are elevated in a number of conditions frequently found in hospitalized patients (e.g., recent surgery, malignancy, active infection, vascular disease, and trauma) and may increase with age.

Crowther MA, Cook DJ, Griffith LE, et al: Neither baseline tests of molecular hypercoagulability nor D-dimer levels predict deep venous thrombosis in critically ill medical-surgical patients. Intensive Care Med 31:48–55, 2005.

Rathbun SW, Whitsett TL, Vesely SK, Raskob GE: Clinical utility of D-dimer in patients with suspected pulmonary embolism and nondiagnostic lung scans or negative CT findings. Chest 125:851–855, 2004.

Righini M, Goehring C, BoFunameaux H, Perrier A: Effects of age on the performance of common diagnostic tests for pulmonary embolism. Am J Med 109:357–361, 2000.

8. **What laboratory or imaging techniques are helpful in identifying patients with PE at risk for complicated courses or mortality?**

Serum brain natriuretic peptide levels of > 90 pg/mL (drawn within 4 hours of presentation) have a sensitivity of 85% and a specificity of 75% for predicting adverse clinical outcomes such as death or thrombolysis or the need for cardiopulmonary resuscitation, mechanical ventilation, vasopressor therapy, or embolectomy.

Echocardiographic evaluation of the right ventricle can identify dilation and hypokinesis, which, even in the absence of systemic hypotension, suggest the need for aggressive intervention. An echocardiogram (ECG) may also identify additional thrombus in the right heart or the presence of a patent foramen ovale, each of which may influence the treatment required.

Recently, helical CT scans have been used to identify high-risk patients with PE. Computer reconstructions are used to look for evidence of right ventricular enlargement on four-chamber views. Evidence of right ventricular enlargement, defined as a ratio of the diameter of the right ventricle to the diameter of the left ventricle of greater than 0.9, predicts a fivefold increase in mortality. Further assessment of the utility of the additional information obtained from a helical CT scan obtained to assess for pulmonary embolization is currently ongoing.

Goldhaber SZ: Echocardiography in the management of pulmonary embolism. Ann Intern Med 136:691–700, 2002.

Grifoni S, Olivotto I, Cecchini P, et al: Short-term clinical outcome of patients with acute pulmonary embolism, normal blood pressure, and echocardiographic right ventricular dysfunction. Circulation 101:2817–2822, 2000.

Kucher N, Goldhaber SZ: Cardiac biomarkers for risk stratification of patients with acute pulmonary embolism. Circulation 108:2191–2194, 2003.

Kucher N, Printzen G, Goldhaber SZ: Prognostic role of brain natriuretic peptide in acute pulmonary embolism. Circulation 107:2545–2547, 2003.

Quiroz R, Kucher N, Schoepf UJ, et al: Right ventricular enlargement on chest computed tomography: prognostic role in acute pulmonary embolism. Circulation 119:2401–2404, 2004.

KEY POINTS: INDICATORS OF RISK IN PATIENTS WITH PULMONARY EMBOLISM WHO APPEAR INITIALLY STABLE

1. Serum brain natriuretic peptide (BNP) (drawn within 4 hours of presentation) of greater than 90 pg/mL

2. An echocardiogram demonstrating right ventricular dilation or dysfunction, residual thrombus within the right atrium or right ventricle, or the presence of a patent foramen ovale

3. A helical CT scan demonstrating right ventricular enlargement (i.e., the ratio of the diameter of the right ventricle to the diameter of the left ventricle is greater than 0.9)

9. **How does PE present in patients undergoing mechanical ventilation?**
The ventilated critically ill patient is at greatly increased risk for pulmonary emboli because of immobilization, long-term intravenous lines, infections, and recent trauma or surgery. Unfortunately, the presentation and evaluation of thromboembolic disease may be hampered by a lack of suggestive complaints from a sedated and possibly paralyzed patient. Tachycardia often may be the only immediate manifestation of distress available to prompt a clinical evaluation of primary thromboembolic disease.

Other signs result from the physiologic changes that occur when a PE obstructs blood flow to pulmonary segments distal to a clot. In these lung regions, perfusion decreases, but ventilation remains unchanged. The resulting increase in dead space ventilation causes an increase in the partial pressure of carbon dioxide (pCO_2), which results in an increase in minute ventilation. An unexplained rise in minute ventilation, therefore, may suggest the presence of a PE. In weak or paralyzed patients who cannot trigger the ventilator, the respiratory rate and tidal volume are fixed at the level of the ventilator settings. An increase in dead space ventilation, therefore, may cause an increase in pCO_2 and possibly a decrease in the partial pressure of oxygen (pO_2) without a change in lung compliance.

The combination of tachycardia, an increase in pCO_2, a decrease in pO_2, and an unchanged lung compliance may warrant further investigation. The diagnostic accuracy for PE of a drop in pO_2 with an unchanged lung compliance has been examined in ventilated trauma patients. Of 583 ventilated patients cared for in a trauma service, 48 developed a decrease in pO_2 without a change in lung compliance. Forty-four percent of these patients had positive pulmonary angiograms for pulmonary emboli. No other instances of pulmonary emboli were identified in this population of patients who had the diagnosis pursued off of the study protocol. However, this study may overestimate the utility of this clinical presentation for the diagnosis of PE because patients who did not have a change in lung compliance did not undergo pulmonary angiography.

Braithwaite CEM, O'Malley KF, Ross CE, et al: Continuous pulse oximetry and the diagnosis of pulmonary embolism in critically ill trauma patients. J Trauma 33:528–531, 1992.
Geerts W, Cook D, Selby R, et al: Venous thromboembolism and its prevention in critical care. J Crit Care 17:95–104, 2002.

10. **How are lung scans used to diagnose pulmonary emboli?**
The V/Q lung scan can be the initial study for the specific diagnosis of PE in patients with suggestive clinical findings. A normal perfusion lung scan excludes the diagnosis with more than 98% confidence. A high-probability lung scan (revealing multiple segmental defects that ventilate but do not perfuse) in the setting of high clinical suspicion (i.e., an estimated likelihood of PE greater than 80%) has a 96% positive predictive value. Unfortunately, the PIOPED study showed that 59% of patients with angiographically documented PE have an abnormal lung scan that is not of high probability. These intermediate-, indeterminate-, and low-probability lung scans offer less diagnostic accuracy compared with normal or high-probability scans. Some investigators pool these results into the category of "nondiagnostic."

A low-probability lung scan associated with a low clinical suspicion (i.e., an estimated likelihood of PE less than 20%) has a 96% negative predictive value. However, a low-probability scan in association with a high clinical suspicion has an estimated likelihood of PE of approximately 40%. An intermediate-probability scan (which represent 42% of all lung scan results in the PIOPED study) requires further diagnostic evaluation.

Further evaluation is also indicated for patients who have a lung scan result that does not agree with the physician's clinical impression. In unstable patients who require urgent diagnosis or in those with underlying cardiopulmonary disease, a pulmonary angiogram may be indicated. Conversely, in stable patients, evaluation of the lower extremities may detect venous thrombosis and establish an indication for anticoagulation or placement of an inferior vena caval filter. However, it is important to recognize that 50% of patients with proven pulmonary emboli may have normal noninvasive studies of the lower extremity.

Kelly MA, Carson JL, Palevsky HL, et al: Diagnosing pulmonary embolism: New facts and strategies. Ann Intern Med 114:300–306, 1991.

Miniati M, Pediletto R, Formichi B, et al: Accuracy of clinical assessment in the diagnosis of pulmonary embolism. Am J Respir Crit Care Med 159:864–871, 1999.

PIOPED Investigators: Value of the ventilation/perfusion scan in acute pulmonary embolism: Results of the Prospective Investigation of Pulmonary Diagnosis (PIOPED). JAMA 263:2753–2759, 1990.

11. **Can high-probability lung scans be the result of diagnoses other than acute PE?**
The PIOPED study provides data and a method of reasoning that allow clinicians to improve the predictive value of a V/Q lung scan by taking into account the patient's clinical presentation. The combination of a high index of suspicion (i.e., more than 80% likelihood of PE on clinical grounds) and high-probability lung scan has a 96% positive predictive value for PE. Conversely, a low (i.e., less than 20% likelihood) clinical suspicion combined with a high-probability lung scan drops the positive predictive value to 56%. This means that almost 50% of patients with this clinical presentation will have a false-positive lung scan.

Furthermore, the PIOPED study indicates that the diagnostic accuracy of a high-probability lung scan is reduced to 74% in patients with a history of prior thromboembolic disease. Lung scan abnormalities in this setting probably represent unresolved defects from a previous embolic event. Lung scans represent the cornerstone study in the diagnostic algorithm for PE but should not be interpreted in isolation. If the index of suspicion is low but the scan is high probability, confirmation of the diagnosis with further diagnostic studies is needed.

Three major disease categories other than thromboembolism that can cause defects on perfusion scans are listed below:
1. Prior PE (residual organized thrombotic material, not an acute clot)
2. Compression or entrapment of pulmonary vasculature
   - Mass lesion (i.e., malignancy, especially lung cancer)
   - Adenopathy (malignant, sarcoid, tubercular, or broncholithiatic)
   - Mediastinal fibrosis (idiopathic or post-radiation therapy)
   - Compression by adjacent vascular structure (i.e., aortic aneurysm)
3. Intraluminal obstruction of pulmonary vasculature
   - Congenital vascular anomaly: agenesis, hypoplasia, coarctation, stenosis, or branch stenosis
   - Malignancy: metastatic (i.e., renal cell, myxoma, or cardiac sarcoma) or primary tumor of pulmonary artery (i.e., sarcoma)
   - Arteritis (i.e., Takayasu's disease or schistosomiasis)

Palevsky HL, Cone L, Alavi A: A case of "false-positive" high probability ventilation-perfusion lung scan due to tuberculosis mediastinal adenopathy with a discussion of other causes of "false-positive" high probability ventilation-perfusion lung scans. J Nucl Med 32:512–517, 1991.

12. **Describe the diagnosis of PE based on CT and MRI technology.**
Helical (i.e., spiral) CT and electron-beam CT (EBCT) have increased image acquisition speed and resolution compared with conventional CT and have been reported to detect central-to-segmental pulmonary emboli with 95% sensitivity and 80% specificity. In one study, EBCT was compared with lung scanning in patients with angiographically proven pulmonary emboli. The study results indicated that EBCT was more sensitive and specific than lung scans in 38 of 60 patients.

CT scanning has an added advantage in that it may reveal pathology other than or in addition to embolic disease to explain clinical symptoms. A recent review evaluated the sensitivity and specificity of helical CT compared to pulmonary angiography. The sensitivity of helical CT ranged from 53–100%. The specificity ranged from 81–100%. Helical CT appears comparable to

V/Q scan for large central or segmental clots. However, its sensitivity appears to lessen with small subsegmental clots. Pulmonary angiography remains the gold standard for the diagnosis of PE.

MRI scanning technology can demonstrate interruptions in flow across the pulmonary arterial bed in patients with PE and, at the same time, can obtain images of the deep veins of the pelvis and lower extremities. These studies were previously limited by cardiac and respiratory motion artifact. Scan times are decreasing, however, and computer assistance allows for respiratory gating of scans so that imaging is not limited to patients who can hold their breath. MRI has the advantage of not needing iodinated contrast, and the time saved by imaging lower extremity veins and the pulmonary bed simultaneously may make this modality a cost-effective means of diagnosing clinically significant thromboembolic disease.

Newer MRI technologies, such as the advent of arterial-spin-labeled perfusion MRI, offer the advantage of the use of no contrast material. These new technologies, however, remain investigational and require larger clinical studies to determine their role in patients with suspected pulmonary emboli.

Ohno Y, Higashino T, Takenaka D, et al: MR Angiography with sensitivity encoding (SENSE) for suspected pulmonary embolism: Comparison with MDCT with ventilation-perfusions scintigraphy. Am J Roentgenol 183:91–98, 2004.

Perrier A, Roy PM, Sanchez O, et al: Multidetector-row computed tomography in suspected pulmonary embolism. N Engl J Med 352:1760–1768, 2005.

Stein PD, Woodard RK, Hull RD, et al: Gadolinium-enhanced magnetic resonance angiography for detection of acute pulmonary embolism: An in-depth review. Chest 124:2324–2328, 2003.

13. **Does it matter who reads your helical CT scan?**
Yes. There is a learning curve to reading helical CT scans done to evaluate for acute PE. The experience of the reading radiologist clearly influences the reliability of the interpretation. In one study comparing the CT readers at two institutions, at the first institution, helical CT had 60% sensitivity, 81% specificity, a 60% positive predictive value, an 81% negative predictive value, and 75% overall accuracy. At the second institution, helical CT had a 53% sensitivity, 97% specificity, an 89% positive predictive value, an 82% negative predictive value, and 83% accuracy.

Drucker EA, Rivitz SM, Shepard JAO, et al: Acute pulmonary embolism: Assessment of helical CT for diagnosis. Radiology 209:235–241, 1988.

14. **Can literature regarding the use of helical CT scanning be directly applied to your patient?**
No. Helical CT scan technology has been changing rapidly. It is essential to know the generation of the CT scanner you are using (i.e., single-slice vs. multidetector-row spiral CT scanner) in order to assess the applicability of the published study to your patients and your institution.

Perrier A, Roy P-M, Sanchez O, et al: Multidetector-row computed tomography in suspected pulmonary embolism. N Engl J Med 352:1760–1768, 2005.

Schoepf NJ, Goldhaber SZ, Costello P: Spiral computer tomography for acute pulmonary embolism. Circulation 109:2160–2167, 2004.

15. **Can anticoagulation be withheld on the basis of a negative helical CT scan in patients with suspected PE?**
Studies have suggested that, with newer-generation helical CT scanners, the clinical validity of using a CT scan to rule out PE is similar to that reported for conventional contrast pulmonary angiography. However, there are false-negative helical CT scans, particularly in patients with a high clinical probability of PE. Combining a negative helical scan with a negative D-dimer test gives a 99% negative predictive value for PE lung scan and clearly supports withholding anticoagulation.

Musset D, Patent F, Meyer G, Maitre S: Diagnostic strategy for patients with suspected pulmonary embolism: A prospective multicenter outcome study. Lancet 360:1914, 2002.

Perrier A, Roy P-M, Sanchez O, et al: Multidetector-row computed tomography in suspected pulmonary embolism. N Engl J Med 352:1760–1768, 2005.

Quiroz R, Kucher N, Zou KH, et al: Clinical validity of a negative computed tomography scan in patients with suspected pulmonary embolism. A systematic review. JAMA 293:2012–2017, 2005.

16. Does upper-extremity DVT result in PE?

More than 90% of pulmonary emboli arise from the deep venous system of the lower extremities. Occasionally, however, patients with upper-extremity DVT experience thromboembolic events. Deep venous thrombosis of the axillary or subclavian veins occurs in three clinical settings:

- Spontaneous thromboses, which may be idiopathic or associated with strenuous upper-arm work or athletic efforts
- Thromboses associated with central venous cannulation
- Miscellaneous occurrences related to trauma, intravenous drug use, and intrathoracic tumors

A review of 71 case reports and 17 patient series indicates that up to 10% of these patients may experience an associated PE. Embolic phenomena associated with upper-extremity DVT have a clinical importance similar to that of pulmonary emboli from lower-extremity sources: 10% of patients with pulmonary emboli related to upper-extremity DVT die from their thromboembolic event. However, this is likely an overestimate, as many pulmonary emboli from upper-extremity sites are smaller and are less likely to be diagnosed than those from proximal lower-extremity sites.

Becker DM, Philbrick JT, Walker FBIV: Axillary and subclavian venous thrombosis. Arch Intern Med 151:1934–1943, 1991.

Hingorani A, Ascher E, Markevich N, et al: Risk factors for mortality in patients with upper extremity and internal jugular deep venous thrombosis. J Vasc Surg 41:476–478, 2005.

Joffe HV, Kucher N, Tapson VF, et al: Upper-extremity deep vein thrombosis: A prospective registry of 592 patients. Circulation 110:1605–1611, 2004.

Thomas IH, Zierler BK: An integrative review of outcomes in patients with acute primary upper extremity deep venous thrombosis following no treatment or treatment with anticoagulation, thrombolysis or surgical algorithms. Vasc Endovascular Surg 39:163–174, 2005.

17. Should impedance plethysmography or duplex ultrasonographic studies of the lower extremities be used for the initial diagnostic evaluation of patients with PE?

No. In the initial evaluation of a patient with a suspected PE, it is critically important to establish the presence of pulmonary emboli with a lung scan to determine prognosis, the need for thrombolytic therapy, and the explanation for respiratory systems. Lung scans or helical CT scans, therefore, remain the initial and pivotal diagnostic test for patients with cardiopulmonary symptoms compatible with PE.

Lower-extremity studies cannot be the initial test of the diagnosis of PE. In one study, only 29% of 149 patients with diagnosed PE had a positive compression ultrasound for DVT. Explanations include false-negative leg studies, emboli from sources other than the proximal legs, and embolization of all of the detectable DVTs in one clinical event.

Noninvasive studies of the lower extremity may serve to establish the diagnosis of DVT in patients with nondiagnostic V/Q or CT scans. They can also evaluate the likelihood of recurrent pulmonary emboli by demonstrating the presence of remaining lower extremity clots in patients who have already experienced a thromboembolic event.

Turkstra R, Kuijer PM, van Beck EJ, et al: Diagnostic utility of ultrasonography of leg veins in patients suspected of having pulmonary embolism. Ann Intern Med 126:775–781, 1997.

18. **Can anticoagulation be withheld in suspected DVT after initial negative compression ultrasonography?**
    In outpatients with suspected DVT and initial negative (i.e., normal) compression ultrasonography, a negative D-dimer test or a normal repeat ultrasound study supports withholding anticoagulation, with only a 2% risk of DVT during 6 months of follow-up.

    Stein PD, Hull RD, Patel KC, et al: D-dimer for the exclusion of acute venous thrombosis and pulmonary embolism: A systematic review. Ann Intern Med 140:589–602, 2004.

19. **How can the available tests be used to make a diagnosis of PE?**
    The following algorithm outlines an evidence-based approach to the diagnosis of PE based on recent data:
    - A normal lung scan effectively excludes the possibility of PE.
    - A high-probability scan strongly supports the diagnosis of PE and justifies the initiation of therapy unless the patient has had a previous PE or clinical suspicion of PE.
    - A low-probability lung scan combined with low clinical suspicion has less than a 5% likelihood of PE; observation without therapy is warranted with this combination of results.
    - Positive noninvasive studies of the lower extremities can identify the presence of DVT and can establish the need for anticoagulation.
    - Patients with negative results of leg studies and nondiagnostic lung scans can be followed with serial leg studies in the absence of cardiopulmonary disease or can proceed to pulmonary angiography if they have sufficiently severe cardiopulmonary disease, such that a recurrent PE would be life threatening.

    Kelley MA, Carson JL, Palevsky HI, et al: Diagnosing pulmonary embolism: New facts and strategies. Ann Intern Med 114:300–306, 1991.

20. **Are low-molecular-weight heparins (LMWHs) equivalent and interchangeable?**
    No. The available LMWHs are prepared by different methods of depolymerizing unfractionated heparin. They have different weight ranges, and the ratios of antifactor Xa to antifactor IIa activity differ. They are not equivalent, nor are they interchangeable.

    Hirsh J, Warkentin TE, Shaughnessy SG, et al: Heparin and low-molecular-weight heparin: Mechanisms of action, pharmacokinetics, dosing, monitoring, efficacy, and safety. CHEST, 119(1 suppl):63S–94S, 2001.

    White RH, Ginsberg JS: Low-molecular-weight heparins: Are they all the same? Br J Haematol 121:12–20, 2003.

    Zakarija A, Bennett CL: Low-molecular-weight heparins. Arch Intern Med 165:722–723, 2005.

21. **What are the data regarding the use of LMWH for venous thromboembolism or PE?**
    Unfractionated heparin (UFH) and LMWH are glycosaminoglycans consisting of chains of alternating residues of D-glucosamine and either glucuronic acid or iduronic acid. UFH is a heterogeneous mixture of polysaccharide chains that range from 3000–30,000 daltons in molecular weight. Controlled enzymatic or chemical depolymerization of UFH produces LMWH, smaller chains with average molecular weights of about 5000 daltons. LMWH preferentially inhibits Factor Xa, compared to UFH.

    The size characteristics, protein binding, and ratio of activity of Factor Xa to Factor IIa vary between the different LMWHs. It is not appropriate to generalize findings from one particular agent to other LMWHs.

    In 1996, two large studies compared the use of LMWH with UFH in the treatment of venous thromboembolism (VTE). There was no difference between the groups with respect to death, recurrent thromboembolism, or major bleeding; however, the length of hospital stay was sharply reduced in the LMWH groups. These results have been confirmed by several large, well-designed studies. It appears that no one LMWH is superior in terms of efficacy or safety in the treatment of VTE.

More recently, a large study randomized over 1000 patients with symptomatic thromboembolism, of which 27% had PE, to treatment with UFH or LMWH. There was no difference between the two groups with respect to death, recurrence, or major hemorrhage. Other studies have come to similar conclusions. Studies have supported the outpatient treatment of DVT with LMWH. Some authors have suggested moving the care of patients with PE to the outpatient setting using LMWH. At the present time, in the absence of large controlled trials, we do not routinely recommend this approach.

Boccalon H, Elias A, Cahle JJ, et al: Clinical outcome and cost of hospital vs. home treatment of proximal deep vein thrombosis with low-molecular-weight-heparin: The Vascular Midi-Pyrenees Study. Arch Intern Med 160:1769–1773, 2000.

Columbus Investigators: Low-molecular-weight heparin in the treatment of patients with venous thromboembolism. N Engl J Med 337:657–662, 1997.

Dolovich LR, Ginsberg JS, Douketis JD, et al: A meta-analysis comparing low-molecular-weight heparins with unfractionated heparin in the treatment of venous thromboembolism: Examining some unanswered questions regarding location of treatments, product type, and dosing frequency. Arch Intern Med 160:181–188, 2000.

Hirsh JS, Raschke R: Heparin and low-molecular-weight heparin. Chest 124:188S–203S, 2004.

Hirsh J, Warkentin TE, Shaughnessy SG, et al: Heparin and low-molecular-weight heparin: Mechanism of action, pharmacokinetics, dosing, monitoring, efficacy and safety. Chest 119:64S–94S, 2001.

Hyers TM: Management of venous thromboembolism: Past, present and future. Arch Intern Med 163:759–768, 2003.

Simonneau G, Sors H, Charbonnier B, et al: A comparison of low-molecular-weight heparin with unfractionated heparin for acute pulmonary embolism. N Engl J Med 337:663–669, 1997.

22. **Can patients with hemoptysis caused by PE be treated with full-dose heparin?**

Although no studies have specifically addressed this question, our practice has been to anticoagulate patients with a confirmed diagnosis of PE despite the presence of hemoptysis. Hemoptysis, however, may warrant additional diagnostic studies (e.g., bronchoscopy) to rule out accompanying lesions (e.g., endobronchial malignancies) because significant hemoptysis as a presenting manifestation of PE is unusual.

23. **What thrombolytic agents are available? What are their therapeutic and pharmacologic differences?**

The Food and Drug Administration has approved three thrombolytic agents for the treatment of PE: streptokinase, urokinase, and recombinant tissue plasminogen activator (rt-PA) (Table 37-2). Only streptokinase has been approved for the treatment of DVT. When administered systemically, all of these agents lower fibrinogen, plasminogen, and alpha$_2$ antiplasmin levels and generate a systemic lytic state. In clinical practice, the theoretic fibrin selectivity of rt-PA has not proven to be of clinical importance in distinguishing among the available agents, and it has not been associated with a lower rate of bleeding complications.

According to the standard protocols for treatment of venous thromboembolism, streptokinase is administered by continuous peripheral IV infusion for 24–72 hours, and urokinase for 12–24 hours, whereas tissue plasminogen activator is given in a 100-mg dose over 2 hours. These standard dosing protocols for PE or DVT (or both) do not include the concurrent use of antithrombotic medications such as aspirin or heparin. Only after the completion of a course of thrombolytic therapy is standard anticoagulation instituted.

We question whether the standard time-based dosing protocols for thrombolytic therapy are optimal. In our practice, once thrombolytic therapy is initiated, we continue treating until all of

	Plasma	Loading	Hourly	Recommended
Agent	Clearance	Dose	Dose	Duration
Streptokinase	12–18 min	250,000 IU over 30 min	100,000 IU	PE: 24 hr DVT: 48–72 hr
Urokinase	12 min	2000 U/lb	2000 U/lb	PE: 12-24 hr DVT: not approved
rt-PA	2–6 min	None	50 mg	PE: 2 hr DVT: not approved

TABLE 37-2. AVAILABLE THROMBOLYTIC THERAPY FOR VENOUS THROMBOEMBOLISM

DVT = deep venous thrombosis, IU = international units, PE = pulmonary embolism, rt-PA = recombinant tissue plasminogen activator.

the thrombus is lysed or until serial imaging shows that the remaining thrombus is resistant to further lysis. Often, this requires treatment for longer than the recommended period.

24. **Which patients with PE should be treated with thrombolytic agents?**
Thrombolytic therapy should be used in the treatment of patients with pulmonary emboli that obstruct a substantial portion of the pulmonary vascular bed. It is generally accepted that occlusion of more than 50% of the pulmonary vascular bed warrants thrombolysis, although some clinicians consider thrombolytic therapy in younger patients who have obstruction of 25–33% of the pulmonary circulation. Regardless of the degree of pulmonary obstruction, thrombolytic therapy should be considered whenever pulmonary emboli result in hemodynamic instability or respiratory compromise.

In addition, some investigators have proposed evaluating stable patients with large pulmonary emboli by echocardiography; any evidence of right ventricular dysfunction or dilation is used as a rationale for treating with thrombolytic agents. Thrombolytic therapy is likely most effective when given within 24 hours of symptom onset, yet its benefit may extend up to 2 weeks after symptom onset. A recent meta-analysis revealed pulmonary perfusion increased by 16% in 86% of patients presenting within 24 hours of symptom occurrence. Only 65% of patients improved an average of 8% when treated > 6 days after onset of symptoms.

Arcasoy SM, Kreit JW: Thrombolytic therapy of pulmonary embolism: A comprehensive review of current evidence. Chest 115:1695–1707, 1999.

Daniels LB, Parker JA, Patel SR, et al: Relation of duration of symptoms with response to thrombolytic therapy in pulmonary embolism. Am J Cardiol 80:184–188, 1997.

Thabut G, Thabut D, Myers RP, et al: Thrombolytic therapy of pulmonary embolism: A meta-analysis. J Am Coll Cardiol 40:1660–1667, 2002.

Wan S, Quinlan DJ, Agnelli G, Eikelboom JW: Thrombolysis compared with heparin for the initial treatment of pulmonary embolism: A meta-analysis of the randomized controlled trials. Circulation 110:744–749, 2004.

Wood KE: Major pulmonary embolism: Review of a pathophysiologic approach to the gold hour of hemodynamically significant pulmonary embolism. Chest 121:2888, 2005.

25. **What are the major complications of thrombolytic therapy?**
The most concerning complication of thrombolytic therapy for PE is intracranial hemorrhage (ICH). A recent review evaluated the data from 312 patients undergoing PE thrombolysis in five

different studies. The frequency of intracranial hemorrhage up to 14 days after thrombolysis was 6 out of 312 (1.9%), with two deaths. A larger analysis evaluated the data from 896 patients in 18 studies and determined the risk of ICH was approximately 1.2%, with a mortality rate of nearly 50%. Although the risk of ICH is low, it is associated with a very large probability of morbidity and mortality. Studies have suggested that the risk of ICH is further increased in patients with an elevated diastolic blood pressure, recent central nervous system surgery, trauma, recent stroke, intracerebral neoplasm, or aneurysm.

The risk of bleeding with the use of thrombolytics is much greater compared to the bleeding risk with the use of heparin alone. Various studies have reported different incidences of bleeding. This is due to differences in the definition of "major hemorrhage" in the studies as well as the use of venous cutdowns in the earlier literature. When studies are reviewed comparing thrombolysis with heparin therapy, the average incidence of bleeding is 6.3% and 1.8%, respectively. The risk of hemorrhage with the use of recombinant tissue plasminogen activator and streptokinase appears to be similar.

Anaphylactic reactions to thrombolytic agents are rare but may be increased in patients who are rechallenged with streptokinase. Other minor reactions may include fever, flushing, urticaria, and hypotension. These may be treated with acetaminophen, antihistamines, and corticosteroids such as Solu-Medrol.

Kanter DS, Mikkola KM, Patel SR, et al: Thrombolytic therapy for pulmonary embolism: Frequency of intracranial hemorrhage and associated risk factors. Chest 111:1241–1245, 1997.

Meyer G, Gisselbrecht M, Eieht JL, et al: Incidence and predictors of major hemorrhagic complications from thrombolytic therapy in patients with massive pulmonary embolism. Am J Med 105:472–477, 1998.

26. **What are the long-term results for patients treated with thrombolytics?**
Thrombolysis is advocated to reduce the acute morbidity and mortality from PE, to reduce the recurrence rate of pulmonary emboli, to preserve pulmonary microvasculature, and to decrease the risk of chronic pulmonary hypertension from persistent pulmonary arterial clots. Over a decade, it was shown that patients treated with thrombolytic therapy had better preservation of measurable carbon monoxide diffusion in the lung (DLCO) than those treated with heparin. The investigators proposed that the pulmonary capillary blood volume (i.e., the pulmonary microcirculation) is better preserved after thrombolytic therapy than after standard heparin anticoagulation. A preliminary report of follow-up hemodynamic evaluations of these patients 7 years later found that patients treated with thrombolytic agents had lower mean arterial pressures and pulmonary vascular resistance at rest and during exercise than patients who had been treated with heparin. However, the clinical and functional significance of these findings remains uncertain.

Schwarz F, Stehr H, Zimmerman R, et al: Sustained improvements of pulmonary hemodynamics in patients at rest and during exercise after thrombolytic treatment of massive pulmonary embolism. Circulation 71:117–123, 1985.

Sharma GVRK, Burleson VA, Sasahara AA: Effect of thrombolytic therapy on pulmonary capillary blood volume in patients with pulmonary embolism. N Engl J Med 303:842–845, 1980.

27. **Is there a difference between local and systemic thrombolytic therapy for PE?**
There is no difference in efficacy or side effects when full-dose thrombolysis administered through an intrapulmonary catheter is compared with similar doses of thrombolytic agents administered peripherally (i.e., systemically). However, patients, even those with contraindications to thrombolysis therapy, may be able to be treated using catheter-directed intraembolic infusions of the thrombolytic agents. Doses ranging from 10–20% of usual systemic doses have been given through a catheter embedded within the massive PE with evidence of neither systemic fibrinogenolysis nor bleeding complications.

Tapson VF, Davidson CJ, Bauman R, et al: Rapid thrombolysis of massive pulmonary emboli without systemic fibrinogenolysis: Intra-embolic infusion of thrombolytic therapy. Am Rev Respir Dis 145:A719, 1992.

Sharma GVRK, Folland ED, McIntyre KM, et al: Long-term hemodynamic benefit of thrombolytic therapy in pulmonary embolic disease. J Am Coll Cardiol 15:65A, 1990.

Verstraete MI, Miller GAH, Bounameaux H, et al: Intravenous and intrapulmonary recombinant tissue type plasminogen activity in the treatment of acute massive pulmonary embolism. Circulation 77:353–360, 1988.

28. Is consideration of aggressive therapeutic intervention (i.e., thrombolysis or surgical embolectomy) warranted in patients with upper-extremity DVT?

An aggressive approach to the treatment of upper-extremity DVT, particularly primary or spontaneous DVT, clearly appears warranted, especially in younger patients. Upper-extremity DVT can result in post-thrombotic syndrome with chronic arm pain, swelling, impaired arm function, and compromised quality of life; the consequences of these were particularly pronounced when the affected arm was the dominant arm.

Kahn SR, Elman EA, Bornais C, et al: Post-thrombotic syndrome, functional disability and quality of life after upper extremity deep venous thrombosis in adults. Thromb Haemost 93:499–502, 2005.

Thomas IH, Zierler BK: An integrative review of outcomes in patients with acute primary upper extremity deep venous thrombosis following no treatment or treatment with anticoagulation. Vasc Endovascular Surg 39:163–174, 2005.

29. What is the therapeutic role of an inferior vena cava filter in patients with PE?

The inferior vena cava (IVC) filter was introduced more than 30 years ago as a means of reducing the incidence of recurrent pulmonary emboli. These devices are placed angiographically in the IVC and trap thromboemboli from the lower extremity. The primary indication for placement of an IVC filter is the presence of DVT in a patient who cannot undergo systemic anticoagulation. A 20-year review of experience with the stainless steel Greenfield filter showed a 4% incidence of recurrence of PE in patients with contraindications to anticoagulation. In comparison, the incidence of recurrence of PE in anticoagulated patients is approximately 5.7% with heparin and 1.9% with Coumadin.

A recent study in France randomized 400 patients with proximal DVT to receive an IVC filter (200 patients) or no IVC filter (200 patients). All patients received either enoxaparin (195 patients) or heparin (205 patients). By day 12, 1.1% in the filter group, compared with 4.8% of the no-filter group, had suffered asymptomatic or symptomatic PE. At 2 years of follow-up, 6 patients (with 1 death) had symptomatic PE in the filter group, and 12 patients (with 5 deaths) had symptomatic PE in the no-IVC-filter group. Although not statistically significant, a trend toward lower rates of recurrent PE was noted in the enoxaparin group by day 12 (4.2%, compared with 1.6%). No difference was found between these groups at 3 months, nor by 2 years of follow-up. This study suggests that IVC filters prevent PE in high-risk patients at risk for PE. LMWH appears to be as safe as unfractionated heparin in the initial treatment of DVT.

Decousus H, Leigorovicz A, Parent F, et al: A clinical trial of vena cava filters in the prevention of pulmonary embolism in patients with proximal deep-vein thrombosis. N Engl J Med 338:409–415, 1998.

Greenfield LJ, McCurdy JR, Brown PP, et al: A new intracaval filter permitting continued flow and resolution of emboli. Surgery 73:599–606, 1973.

Greenfield LJ, Proctor M: Twenty-year clinical experience with the Greenfield filter. Cardiovasc Surg 3:199–205, 1995.

30. What is the factor V Leiden mutation? How does it relate to venous thromboembolism and PE?

The factor V Leiden mutation is a point mutation in the gene that codes for coagulation factor V. This is now known to be the cause of the most common heritable hypercoagulable state. In the mutated gene, glutamine replaces arginine at position 506, causing the activated factor V product to be resistant to degradation by activated protein C (APC). APC is a potent anticoagulant; thus, APC resistance causes thrombophilia. Heterozygosity for factor V Leiden is associated with a fivefold to 10-fold increased risk of thrombosis, and homozygous patients have up to a 50-fold to 100-fold increased risk of thrombosis. It was shown in the Physicians' Health Study that the relative risk of venous thrombosis in men with the mutation was 2.7. The factor V Leiden mutation also appears to increase the risk of recurrent PE after the discontinuation of anticoagulation treatment by a factor of 2–4. Interestingly, although the mutation greatly increases the risk for DVT, the risk for PE is not as large. The reason for this apparent discrepancy is not understood at the present time.

Other factors are also known to greatly increase the risk of venous thromboembolism. It has been estimated that women with the factor V Leiden mutation who take oral contraceptives may have a 35-fold increase in risk for venous thromboembolism compared to women without the mutation. Hyperhomocysteinemia, often caused by deficiency in folate, vitamin B_6, or vitamin B_{12}, may increase the risk of venous thromboembolism twofold to threefold over patients without hyperhomocysteinemia. However, hyperhomocysteinemia in patients with the factor V Leiden mutation may have a 10-fold to 20-fold increase in the risk for thrombosis.

Bertina RM: Genetic approaches to thrombophilia. Thromb Haemost 86:92–103, 2001.

Ridker PM, Hennekens CH, Lindpaintner K, et al: Mutation in the gene coding for coagulation Factor V and the risk of myocardial infarction, stroke and venous thrombosis in apparently healthy men. N Engl J Med 332:912–917, 1995.

31. **What is the relationship between PE and pregnancy?**

Pulmonary embolism is five to six times more common in pregnant women than in nonpregnant women. Over a 5-year period of review in Australia, PE–associated mortality in pregnant women equaled the mortality caused by hypertensive complications of pregnancy. Pregnancy is associated with variations in the clotting cascade protein levels, which may contribute to a relatively hypercoagulable state. Although the risk of PE is increased prenatally (particularly in the third trimester), the greatest risk occurs postpartum, when the relative risk is approximately 20%. Other factors that contribute to the risk of PE during pregnancy are as follows:

- Previous PE (5–15% recurrence rate)
- Immobilization
- Age more than 40 years
- Cesarean section
- Gravida more than 4
- African American race
- Hormonal therapy to promote fertility

Rutherford SE, Phelan JP: Deep venous thrombosis and pulmonary embolism in pregnancy. Obstet Gynecol Clin North Am 18:345–370, 1991.

32. **Should pregnant patients with suspected PE undergo a conventional diagnostic evaluation?**

Diagnosis of PE in pregnant women presents concerns about fetal radiation exposure. Undiagnosed and untreated PE represents a greater risk, however, to the well-being of the fetus. Current recommendations, therefore, encourage physicians to perform conventional diagnostic tests in pregnant patients with suspected PE. Some special precautions, however, should be initiated. Abdominal shields should be used during any radiographic procedure. Because the technetium used as the radiolabel in perfusion scans is excreted through the kidneys, we recommend hydration and placement of a Foley catheter (with the drainage bag as far from the patient as possible) to decrease the length of time that radionucleotide is in the bladder. Using this methodology, lung scanning may represent less radiation exposure to a fetus than helical CT scanning.

33. **Can pregnant patients with PE be treated with systemic anticoagulation?**
Coumadin is contraindicated in pregnant patients because of risk to the fetus. Heparin is the standard of care for use during the acute event and during long-term anticoagulation. Heparin therapy for longer than 5 months or at doses greater than 20,000 units per day, however, may be associated with the development of osteoporosis.

Ginsberg JS, Greer I, Hirsh J: Use of antithrombotic agents during pregnancy. Chest 119:122S–131S, 2001.

Jeffries WS, Bochner F: Thromboembolism and its management in pregnancy. Med J Aust 155:253–258, 1991.

Rutherford SE, Phelan JP: Deep venous thrombosis and pulmonary embolism in pregnancy. Obstet Gynecol Clin North Am 18:345–370, 1991.

34. **Do you need to think of PE when seeing a patient with an acute stroke?**
Paradoxical embolism (i.e., thrombotic material embolizing into the systemic circulation) through an atrial septal defect or a patent foramen ovale (PFO) can cause strokes, myocardial infarction, or organ or limb compromise. Paradoxical embolus should be considered when seeing a young patient with an otherwise unexplained acute neurologic event. When thrombus has been identified trapped in a PFO (an impending paradoxical embolus), emergent surgical intervention may be required.

Chow BJ, Johnson CB, Turek M, Burwash IG: Impending paradoxical embolus: A case report and review of the literature. Can J Cardiol 19:1426–1432, 2003.

Deeik RK, Thomas RM, Sakiyalak P, et al: Minimal access closure of patent foramen ovale: Is it also recommended for patients with paradoxical emboli? Ann Thoracic Surg 74:1326–1329, 2002.

Travis JA, Fuller SB, Ligush J Jr, et al: Diagnosis and treatment of paradoxical embolus. J Vasc Surg 34:860–865, 2001.

BIBLIOGRAPHY

1. Hirsh J: Advances and contemporary issues in prophylaxis for deep vein thrombosis. Chest 124(6 suppl): 347S–396S, 2003.
2. Schunemann HJ, Cook D, Grinshaw J, et al: Seventh ACCP Conference on Antithrombotic and Thrombotic Therapy. Chest 126(Suppl 3):163S–696S, 2004.

CHAPTER 38

NONTHROMBOTIC PULMONARY EMBOLI

Michael P. Gruber, MD, and Mark W. Geraci, MD

1. What is fat embolism syndrome (FES)?

FES is a poorly understood complication of skeletal trauma. Although rare, FES most often occurs after fractures of long bones or other conditions resulting in bone marrow disruption. FES is characterized by the appearance of free fat and fatty acids in the blood, lungs, brain, kidneys, and other organs. The classic triad of respiratory insufficiency, neurologic abnormalities, and petechial rash occurs in 0.5–2% of solitary long bone fractures. The incidence increases to 5–10% in multiple fractures with pelvic involvement. In addition, FES has been associated with numerous nontraumatic etiologies. FES should be distinguished from isolated fat embolism, which may or may not be associated with clinically significant embolization.

KEY POINTS: CLASSIC TRIAD OF FAT EMBOLISM SYNDROME

1. Respiratory insufficiency

2. Neurologic abnormalities

3. Petechial rash

2. Who is at risk for FES?

Fat embolism to the lungs and peripheral microcirculation occurs in over 90% of long bone fractures, yet only 2–5% of patients develop the clinical syndrome. FES most commonly occurs after femoral or pelvic fractures but has been reported after fractures of the humerus. The incidence in children is 100 times less frequent than in adults with comparable injuries. This finding is secondary to differences in either the content or the composition of marrow fat. Certain clinical conditions cause increased liquid marrow fat content and medullary cavity enlargement, which can predispose to FES.

Traumatic	Nontraumatic
▪ Fractures (more than 90% of all cases)	▪ Osteomyelitis
Long bones (femur, tibia, and humerus)	▪ Diabetes mellitus
Pelvis	▪ Pancreatitis
▪ Orthopedic procedures (e.g., joint reconstruction)	▪ Sickle cell disease
▪ Soft tissue injuries	▪ Alcoholic liver disease
▪ Burns	▪ Total parenteral nutrition (i.e., lipids)
▪ Liposuction	▪ Decompression sickness
▪ Bone marrow harvesting and transplantation	▪ Cardiopulmonary bypass
	▪ Propofol infusions

Fabian TC: Unraveling the fat embolism syndrome. N Engl J Med 329:961–963, 1993.

King MB, Harmon KR: Unusual forms of pulmonary embolism. Clin Chest Med 15:561–580, 1994.

Mellor A, Soni N: Fat embolism. Anaesthesia 56:145–154, 2001.

3. **Describe the pathogenesis of FES.**

   The pathogenesis is controversial. Two major theories have been proposed, and both probably contribute.

   - The **mechanical theory** postulates that bone marrow contents enter the venous system and lodge in the lungs as emboli. Smaller fat droplets (7–10 μm in diameter) may travel through the pulmonary capillaries into the systemic circulation with resulting multiorgan dysfunction. Systemic embolization may also occur through a patent foramen ovale, a defect found in 20–34% of the population, but more it likely occurs through intrapulmonary shunts.

   - The **biochemical theory** suggests that embolized circulating free fatty acids are concentrated in the pulmonary bed and serve to activate the clotting cascade, to increase platelet function, to induce fibrinolysis, and to further catecholamine-mediated mobilization of free fatty acids. These free fatty acids directly stimulate the release of inflammatory mediators, resulting in increased capillary permeability, leading to critical impairment of gas exchange and clinical findings of acute respiratory distress syndrome (ARDS).

   A more recent theory argues that fat embolism may be derived in part from chylomicrons and very-low-density lipoproteins agglutinating in the plasma. Acute-phase reactant proteins, particularly C-reactive proteins (CRPs), have been involved in the process of causing agglutination of intravenous fat emulsions in trauma victims and other critically ill patients.

   Hulman G: The pathogenesis of fat embolism. J Pathol 76:3–9, 1995.

   Nixon J, Brock-Utne J: Free fatty acid and arterial oxygen changes following major injury: A correlation between hypoxemia and increased free fatty acid levels. J Trauma 18:23–26, 1978.

   Pell ACH, Hughes D, Keating J, et al: Fulminating fat embolism syndrome caused by paradoxical embolism through a patent foramen ovale. N Engl J Med 329:926–929, 1993.

   Sulek CA, Davies LK, Enneking FK, et al: Cerebral microembolism diagnosed by transcranial Doppler during total knee arthroplasty: Correlation with transesophageal echocardiography. Anesthesiology 91:672–676, 1999.

4. **Describe the clinical presentation of FES.**

   FES typically manifests as respiratory insufficiency, neurologic abnormalities, and petechial rash within 12–72 hours of initial injury. Respiratory impairment leads to hypoxemia in up to 30% of patients and, on occasion, respiratory failure and the need for mechanical ventilation. The chest radiograph often shows diffuse infiltrates but can appear normal. Cerebral symptoms may occur in 60% of patients and tend to follow the pulmonary symptoms. Neurologic findings may range from restlessness, confusion, and altered sensorium to focal deficits, seizures, and coma. The characteristic petechial rash is observed in 50% of patients and is usually found on the neck, axilla, trunk, or conjunctiva. The rash is often the last of the triad to develop and resolves within a range of hours to days.

5. **How is the diagnosis of FES made?**

   FES is a clinical diagnosis. The two most widely accepted clinical criteria for the diagnosis of FES are presented. Gurd's (1970) criteria are grouped into major and minor features (Table 38-1). Schonfeld (1983) advocates a fat embolism index score (Table 38-2).

6. **Are there specific tests to aid in the diagnosis of FES?**

   There is no single test to diagnose FES, but a pattern of biochemical abnormalities may be seen. Hematologic studies may reveal decreased hematocrit and platelets, whereas fibrin degradation products, prothrombin time, erythrocyte sedimentation rate, and C5a levels are often elevated.

TABLE 38-1. DIAGNOSIS OF FAT EMBOLISM SYNDROME ACCORDING TO GURD'S (1970) CRITERIA

Major Features	Minor Features	Laboratory Features
Respiratory insufficiency	Fever	Anemia
Cerebral involvement	Tachycardia	Thrombocytopenia
Petechial rash	Retinal changes	Elevated erythrocyte sedimentation rate
	Jaundice	Fat macroglobulinemia
	Renal changes	

A positive diagnosis requires the presence of one major feature plus four minor features plus fat macroglobulinemia in the appropriate clinical setting.
Adapted from Gurd AR: Fat embolism: An aid to diagnosis. J Bone Joint Surg 52:732–737, 1970.

TABLE 38-2. DIAGNOSIS OF FAT EMBOLISM SYNDROME ACCORDING TO SCHONFELD'S (1983) CRITERIA

Symptom	Score
Petechiae	5
Diffuse alveolar infiltrates	4
Hypoxemia (PaO$_2$ ≤ 70 torr)	3
Confusion	1
Fever > 38°C	1
Heart rate ≥ 120 beats/min	1
Respiratory rate ≥ 30 breaths/min	1

FES is diagnosed when the cumulative score is 5 or more in the appropriate clinical setting.
Adapted from Schonfeld SA, Ploysongsang Y, DiLisio R, et al: Fat embolism prophylaxis with corticosteroids: A prospective study in high-risk patients. Ann Intern Med 99:438–443, 1983.

Biochemical abnormalities include hypocalcemia and the presence of fat microaggregates in samples of clotted blood. In a large prospective series, the commonly held tenet of fat globules presenting in the urine was not found in patients with FES. Both bronchoalveolar lavage (BAL) (looking for lipid-laden alveolar macrophages) and pulmonary arterial catheter blood sampling for cytology have been proposed as methods of early diagnosis of FES. Unfortunately, both lack specificity. Radiographic studies are particularly useful in cases of suspected cerebral involvement. Although computed tomography (CT) of the brain may be normal, magnetic resonance imaging (MRI) characteristically reveals multiple high-density lesions on T2-weighted images and low-density lesions on T1-weighted images. Common areas of involvement include basal ganglia, the corpus callosum, cerebral deep white matter, and the cerebral hemispheres. Radiographic findings tend to resolve in association with clinical improvement.

Chastre J, Fagon JY, Soler P, et al: Bronchoalveolar lavage for rapid diagnosis of the fat embolism syndrome in trauma patients. Ann Intern Med 113:583–588, 1990.
Gurd AR: Fat embolism: An aid to diagnosis. J Bone Joint Surg 52:732–737, 1970.

Parizel PM, Demey HE, Veeckmans G, et al: Early diagnosis of cerebral fat embolism syndrome by diffusion-weighted MRI (starfield pattern). Stroke 32:2942–2944, 2001.

Roger N, Xambet A, Agusti C, et al: Role of bronchoalveolar lavage in the diagnosis of fat embolism syndrome. Eur Respir J 8:1275–1280, 1995.

Vedrinne JM, Guillaume C, Gagnieu MC, et al: Bronchoalveolar lavage in trauma patients for the diagnosis of fat embolism. Chest 102:1323–1327, 1992.

7. How is FES treated?

A number of treatment modalities have been studied. The uses of ethanol, heparin, low-molecular-weight dextran, and hypertonic glucose have shown inconsistent results and are not currently recommended. The first successful treatment of FES with corticosteroids was reported by Ashbaugh and Petty in 1966. Schonfeld and colleagues, in a well-designed, prospective, randomized, double-blind study of patients at high risk for FES, demonstrated that prophylactic use of methylprednisolone (7.5 mg/kg IV every 6 hours for 12 doses) significantly reduced the incidence of FES. Lindeque and colleagues found similar results with even less stringent diagnostic criteria, using a dose of methylprednisolone of 30 mg/kg IV on admission and a single repeat dose after 4 hours.

In both studies, the use of steroids had no adverse effects on fracture healing. The mechanism of steroid effectiveness likely involves membrane stabilization, limitation in the rise of plasma free fatty acids, and inhibition of complement-mediated leukocyte aggregation. The effectiveness of steroids other than for prophylaxis remains to be demonstrated. In short, FES treatment includes aggressive supportive care, early ventilatory support, and early steroid use.

Ashbaugh DG, Petty TL: The use of corticosteroids in the treatment of respiratory failure associated with massive fat embolism. Surg Gynecol Obstet 123:493–500, 1966.

Lindeque BGP, Schoeman HS, Dommisse GF, et al: Fat embolism and the fat embolism syndrome: A double-blind therapeutic study. J Bone Joint Surg 69B:128–131, 1987.

Schonfeld SA, Ploysongsang Y, DiLisio R, et al: Fat embolism prophylaxis with corticosteroids: A prospective study in high-risk patients. Ann Intern Med 99:438–443, 1983.

8. How do you decrease the risk of FES?

Early immobilization and operative stabilization of long bone fractures reduces the incidence of FES. As mentioned above, the use of corticosteroids has been shown in prospective randomized trials to decreased both the incidence and the severity of FES when administered prophylactically to high-risk groups. Other strategies include intraoperative techniques to limit the elevations in intraosseous pressure in order to reduce the intravasation of intramedullary fat and other debris.

Pitto RP, Koessler M, Kuehle JW: Comparison of fixation of the femoral component without cement and fixation with use of a bone-vacuum cementing technique for the prevention of fat embolism during total hip arthroplasty. A prospective randomized clinical trial. J Bone Joint Surg 81A:39–48, 2002.

Riska R, Myllynen P: Fat embolism in patients with multiple injuries. J Trauma 22:891–894, 1982.

9. What is the prognosis in FES?

Mortality from FES often depends on the underlying extent of injury and preexisting comorbidities. For uncomplicated FES, the mortality is 5–15%. FES is self-limited. With appropriate supportive care, including maintenance of adequate oxygenation, pulmonary function can be expected to return to normal. Long-term morbidity is most often associated with neurologic complications, particularly focal neurologic deficits.

Mellor A, Soni N: Fat Embolism. Anaesthesia 56:145–54, 2001.

10. Define air embolism.

Air embolism is a consequence of air entry into the vascular system resulting in mechanical obstruction, end-organ ischemia, or hemodynamic compromise, or a combination thereof. A venous air embolism (VAE) results from the introduction of air into the venous system, where it travels into the right ventricle or pulmonary vasculature, causing mechanical obstruction and vasospasm, leading to hemodynamic compromise. Arterial air embolism (AAE) can also occur, typically leading to distal end-organ ischemia.

11. **In which clinical settings has VAE been described?**

Air can enter the venous system when two simultaneous conditions coexist: first, a direct communication between the source of air and the venous system, and second, a pressure gradient favoring the passage of air into the venous system. Under high pressure, gas may be forced into the venous system, such as with laparoscopic procedures, pressurized infusion sets, or mechanical ventilation. Conversely, generating high negative intrathoracic pressures (as in hyperventilation, exacerbation of underlying lung disease, hypovolemia, or upright positioning) may predispose patients to VAE by increasing the pressure gradient between the atmosphere and the thorax. The causes of VAE are summarized in Table 38-3.

Dudney TM, Elliott CG: Pulmonary embolism from amniotic fluid, fat and air. Prog Cardiovasc Dis 36:447–474, 1994.

Unusual forms of pulmonary embolism. Clin Chest Med 15:561–580, 1994.

TABLE 38-3. CAUSES OF VENOUS AIR EMBOLISM	
Surgical Procedures	**Trauma-Related Causes**
Laparoscopic or video-assisted procedures	Head and cervical spine injuries
Neurosurgery	Penetrating or blunt injuries
Intravascular catheter insertion	Positive pressure ventilation
Central lines	Invasive mechanical ventilation
Dialysis catheters	Noninvasive ventilation
Coronary artery bypass grafting or angioplasty	Decompression sickness
Pacemaker or defibrillator placement	Radiologic procedures
Removal of intravascular catheters	Intravenous contrast injections

12. **How does VAE result in hemodynamic collapse?**

Rapid entry of air into the venous system migrates to the pulmonary circulation, causing acute right heart strain. As the pulmonary arterial pressure increases, right ventricular outflow decreases and venous return is impaired. The impairment in venous return leads to decreased left ventricular preload with resulting decreased cardiac output, systemic hypotension, and, ultimately, hemodynamic collapse. Increased resistance to flow within the pulmonary vasculature results in greater ventilation-perfusion (V/Q) mismatch with increased intrapulmonary right-to-left shunting, increased dead-space ventilation, and resulting hypoxemia and hypercarbia. Air may enter the arterial system from a right-to-left shunt, either from an open patent foramen ovale as a result of the acute right heart strain or through microvascular intrapulmonary shunts. In addition, a complex interaction occurs when air and blood mix in the right heart, causing a network of air bubbles, fibrin strands, platelet aggregates, erythrocytes, and fat globules. Factors other than simple mechanical obstruction may contribute to acute lung injury, including the recruitment of inflammatory mediators such as neutrophils, with resulting endothelial injury and microvascular disruption, causing an increase in capillary permeability and clinical ARDS.

Muth CM, Shank ES: Gas embolism. New Engl J Med 342:476–482, 2000.

13. **How much air does it take to cause VAE?**

    The factors that determine the severity of VAE were identified by Durant in 1947. The volume of air, the speed of entry, and the body position are all important factors. A volume of 3–8 mL of air per kilogram of body weight is necessary to produce death. Most VAE occurs in relation to central venous catheters (0–2% incidence). Mortality for VAE associated with central venous catheters has been reported to be as high as 32%. In humans, the lethal volume of air is estimated to be 300–500 mL. With a pressure gradient of only 5 cm of water (as with normal tidal breathing), air can pass through a 14-gauge catheter at a rate of 100 mL/sec.

    Durant TM, Long J, Oppenheimer MJ: Pulmonary (venous) air embolism. Am Heart J 33:269–281, 1947.

    Orebaugh SL: Venous air emboli: Clinical and experimental considerations. Crit Care Med 20:1169–1177, 1992.

14. **What are the clinical features of VAE?**

    The clinical symptoms of VAE are nonspecific. Care providers must maintain a high index of suspicion to consider the diagnosis of VAE in patients who develop sudden cardiopulmonary or neurologic decompensation in the appropriate clinical setting. Patients may experience a gasping reflex, lightheadedness, dizziness, chest pain, or sudden-onset dyspnea. If venous gas reaches the arterial circulation, evidence of myocardial or central nervous system injury may occur. Physical examination may reveal tachycardia, tachypnea, and elevated jugular venous pressure. A mill-wheel murmur produced by movement of air bubbles in the right ventricle is considered the only specific sign, but it is a rare, transient, late finding. Wheezing or rales may occur secondary to induced bronchospasm.

15. **How is VAE diagnosed?**

    VAE is typically a clinical diagnosis made under the appropriate setting. Confirming the diagnosis of VAE can be challenging as air may be rapidly absorbed from the circulation prior to diagnostic testing. Transthoracic or transesophageal echocardiography is the most sensitive method for detection of venous air and may show evidence of both acute right ventricular dilatation and pulmonary hypertension. Decreased end-tidal carbon dioxide suggests increased V/Q mismatch and increased dead-space ventilation. Indwelling pulmonary artery (PA) catheters will show an acute increase in PA pressure. Although this finding has a sensitivity of only 45%, the presence of a PA catheter at the time of VAE can result in early therapeutic intervention.

    Bedford RF, Marshall WK, Butler A, et al: Cardiac catheters for diagnosis and treatment of venous air embolism: A prospective study in man. J Neurosurg 55:610–614, 1981.

16. **How is VAE treated?**

    Treatment of VAE is aimed at restoring flow within the cardiopulmonary circulation and promoting the reabsorption of intravascular air. If VAE is suspected, the patient should be placed left side down in Trendelenburg's position, allowing air to migrate toward the right apex of the heart, thus diminishing pulmonary outflow obstruction. Manual removal of air from an indwelling central line or a PA catheter may be attempted and is most effective at or above the right atrial junction, not in the right ventricle or the PA outflow tract. Closed-chest cardiac massage improves survival to the same extent as proper positioning, presumably by mechanically forcing air out of the right ventricle and the pulmonary outflow tract. Patients should be administered 100% FiO_2 to increase the rate of bubble absorption. For patients with persistent cardiopulmonary or cerebrovascular deficits despite these modalities, hyperbaric oxygen therapy should be initiated. If the patient needs to travel over a great distance, an aircraft pressurized to 1.0 atmospheres should be used. High altitude (more than 300–500 feet) may increase bubble size.

    Hanna PG, Gravenstein N, Pashayan AG: In vitro comparison of central venous catheters for aspiration of venous air embolism: Effect of catheter type, catheter tip position, and cardiac inclination. J Clin Anesth 3:290–294, 1991.

KEY POINTS: TREATMENT OF VENOUS AIR EMBOLISM

1. Place patient left side down in Trendelenburg's position.

2. Administer supplement oxygen at 100% FiO$_2$.

3. Attempt catheter-directed aspiration of air if an indwelling central line or a pulmonary artery catheter is present.

4. Consider hyperbaric oxygen therapy if persistent hemodynamic instability or cerebrovascular deficits exist.

17. **How do you minimize the risk of VAE when inserting or discontinuing a central line?**

Several important routine measures should be followed during central catheter insertion and removal to reduce the risk of VAE. First, the patient should be placed in Trendelenburg's position, which serves to increase central venous pressure, thus decreasing the pressure gradient, favoring the passage of air into the circulation. Second, when possible, ask the patient to breath-hold or to perform a Valsalva maneuver at the time of insertion or removal to minimize existing pressure gradient. Last, occlude the hubs of the central venous catheter during insertion and maintain all access ports closed and locked when not in use.

McGee DC, Gould MK: Preventing complication of central venous catheterization. N Engl J Med 348:1123–1133, 2003.

18. **What is the amniotic fluid embolism syndrome?**

Amniotic fluid embolism syndrome (AFES) is a rare complication of pregnancy with variable manifestations and high morbidity and mortality. The reported incidence of this catastrophic syndrome ranges from 1 in 8000 to 1 in 80,000 pregnancies, with a maternal mortality rate of 30–90%. Amniotic fluid is a complex mixture of both maternal and fetal components including particulate matter such as fetal squamous cells, lanugo hairs, and, variably, meconium. Amniotic fluid is postulated to enter the maternal circulation through endocervical veins, the site of placental insertion, or through uterine trauma. Once in the circulation, amniotic fluid triggers an immunologically mediated systemic inflammatory response leading to cardiovascular compromise, respiratory failure, coagulopathy, and disseminated intravascular coagulation.

Aurangzeb I, Liziamma G, Raoof S: Amniotic fluid embolism. Crit Care Clin 20:643–650, 2004.

19. **When can AFES occur?**

Analysis of a national registry revealed that AFES occurred during labor but before delivery in 70% of cases, after vaginal delivery in 11%, and during cesarean section in 19%. In the patients who developed AFES following delivery, 69% occurred within the first 5 minutes postpartum. AFES has also been reported to occur as early as the second trimester and as late as 36 hours postpartum.

Clark SL, Hankins GDV, Dudley DA, et al: Amniotic fluid embolism: Analysis of the national registry. Am J Obstet Gynecol 172:1158–1169, 1995.

20. **Who is at risk for AFES?**

AFES may occur during therapeutic abortion, abdominal trauma, amniocentesis, and labor and delivery. Factors historically associated with increased risk for AFES include advanced maternal age, multiparity, large fetal size, premature placental separation, fetal death, fetal male sex, meconium staining, and a history of allergy or atopy in the mother.

21. **What are the clinical manifestations of AFES?**
The clinical presentation of AFES is often dramatic, with sudden-onset respiratory distress, cyanosis, convulsions, and cardiovascular collapse classically occurring during labor and delivery. Patients may rapidly progress to asystole or pulseless electrical activity. Patients who survive the initial event later go on to develop a major coagulopathy in 40% of cases.

22. **Are there any tests available to diagnose AFES?**
AFES remains a clinical diagnosis. The identification of amniotic fluid debris from samples obtained from the distal port of a PA catheter lacks specificity and is not advocated for diagnostic purposes. Several serologic tests and immunohistochemistry stains to detect the presence of fetal antigens in maternal serum have been shown to be highly sensitive methods to diagnose AFES. However, further validation is needed, and these tests are not routinely available in clinical practice.

Oi H, Kobayashi H, Hirashima Y, et al: Serologic and immunohistochemical diagnosis of amniotic fluid embolism. Semin Thromb Hemost 24:479–484, 1998.

23. **How is AFES treated?**
AFES is a life-threatening condition that requires prompt resuscitation, including airway and hemodynamic support, in an intensive-care setting. Early aggressive support is imperative as most maternal deaths occur within 1 hour of symptom onset. Hemodynamic monitoring with a pulmonary artery catheter (PAC) typically shows elevated wedge pressures and left ventricular dysfunction. The use of a PAC may be beneficial in fluid management due to dynamic changes in left and right ventricular function. Hematologic abnormalities are best treated by serial laboratory assessment and the judicious use of blood products. Approximately 70% of cases of AFES occur during labor but before delivery; in these circumstances, immediate delivery of the fetus should be considered.

24. **What is the prognosis for patients treated with AFES?**
Maternal mortality for AFES ranges from 30–90%. The fetal survival is 40% when the fetus is *in utero* at the time of AFES onset. Furthermore, FES is associated with significant morbidity. Clark and colleagues reported neurologically intact survival in only 15% of maternal survivors.

Clark SL, Hankins GDV, Dudley DA, et al: Amniotic fluid embolism: Analysis of the national registry. Am J Obstet Gynecol 172:1158–1169, 1995.

25. **Describe the pathogenesis of pulmonary tumor embolism.**
Pulmonary tumor embolism occurs when solid tumors seed the systemic circulation with individual cells, clusters of cells, or large tumor fragments. Emboli travel to the pulmonary vasculature, causing microvasculature obstruction. Furthermore, tumor emboli may activate the coagulation system, resulting in concomitant thrombotic obstruction. The pathologic spectrum of tumor embolism varies from large tumor masses that may mimic pulmonary embolism to the more common microvessel embolism in small arterioles and capillaries, which causes a subacute clinical syndrome.

Roberts KE, Hamele-Bena D, Saqi A, et al: Pulmonary tumor embolism: A review of the literature. Am J Med 115:228–232, 2003.

26. **Are pulmonary emboli considered metastases?**
Pulmonary emboli should not be considered metastases. For metastases to develop, malignant cells must adhere to the endothelium and proliferate, initiating invasive and angiogenic processes. Intraluminal tumor emboli have not been observed to proliferate or spread locally. Some authors propose that microvascular emboli are ultimately the source of lymphangitic carcinomatosis; however, this remains disputed.

Bassiri AG, Haghighi B, Doyle RL, et al: Pulmonary tumor embolism. Am J Resp Crit Care Med 155:2089–2095, 1997.

27. **What tumors are associated with pulmonary tumor embolism?**

The incidence of tumor embolism is estimated by autopsy series to be between 3% and 26% of patients with solid tumors. Tumor embolism appears to be more common in patients with mucin-producing adenocarcinomas such as breast, gastric, and lung carcinoma; however, this observation may be explained by the higher prevalence of these tumors within the population. The following tumors have been reported to be associated with microvascular tumor emboli:

Hepatocellular	Stomach	Choriocarcinoma
Gynecologic	Pancreas	Breast
Gallbladder	Parotid	Skin
Renal	Prostate	Colon
Atrial myxoma	Bladder	Esophagus
Thyroid	Lung	

Roberts KE, Hamele-Bena D, Saqi A, et al: Pulmonary tumor embolism: A review of the literature. Am J Med 115:228–232, 2003.

28. **Describe the clinical presentation of tumor embolism.**

Most cases of pulmonary tumor embolism occur in patients with known malignancy. No clinical presentation is specific for the diagnosis. The clinical course is usually subacute, with dyspnea developing over the course of weeks. Patients may also complain of pleuritic chest pain. Cough and hemoptysis are less frequent. On physical exam, patients typically are tachypneic and tachycardic, and they may show signs of pulmonary hypertension including elevated jugular venous pressure, a loud pulmonic second sound (P_2), and a right-sided heave.

29. **How is tumor embolism diagnosed?**

Tumor embolism occurs in patients who are also at high risk for thromboembolic events. Findings of dyspnea, tachypnea, tachycardia, right heart strain, and clear chest radiography may suggest either diagnosis, making differentiation between the two challenging. A **confirmed diagnosis** requires surgical intervention to demonstrate tumor cells within the pulmonary vasculature. A **presumptive diagnosis** is based on a typical clinical presentation in conjunction with the exclusion of thromboembolic disease. A V/Q scan may be helpful in making this distinction. In tumor embolism, the V/Q scan may demonstrate peripheral subsegmental perfusion defects with a mottled appearance. This result is similar to that seen in primary pulmonary hypertension or fat embolism and is distinct in appearance from the focal mismatched defects seen in thromboembolic disease. Computed tomographic angiography (CTA) of the chest and pulmonary angiography are insensitive for tumor emboli. The major role for both these modalities is to rule out the presence of thromboembolic disease. Although they are rare findings, dilated and beaded peripheral pulmonary arteries by either CTA or pulmonary angiography may suggest tumor emboli.

Chan CK, Hutcheon MA, Hyland RH, et al: Pulmonary tumor embolism: A critical review of clinical, imaging, and hemodynamic features. J Thorac Imaging 2:4–14, 1987.

Shepard JA, Moore EH, Tempelton PA, et al: Pulmonary intravascular tumor emboli: Dilated and beaded peripheral pulmonary arteries at CT. Radiology 187:797–801, 1993.

30. **How is tumor embolism treated?**

Appropriate therapy for microvessel tumor embolism is poorly understood because diagnosis is rarely made before death. Controlling the source of the primary tumor with surgical resection affords some benefit. In patients with subdiaphragmatic tumors, placement of an inferior vena cava (IVC) filter may be beneficial. Embolectomy is generally reserved for patients with a large central embolic burden. Chemotherapy has a limited role in this disorder unless the tumor is highly chemoresponsive. Patients who exhibit cancer-related thrombosis need to be treated with anticoagulation unless this is contraindicated.

31. **Who is at highest risk for septic pulmonary emboli?**

Septic pulmonary emboli result from the embolization of a concomitant endovascular infection. Common predisposing factors include chronic alcohol abuse, periodontal disease, skin infections, immunologic deficiencies, malignancy, tricuspid valve endocarditis with or without intravenous drug abuse, and thrombophlebitis with or without associated intravascular catheter.

32. **What are the clinical manifestations and complications of septic pulmonary emboli?**

Clinical manifestations include fever, chills, rigor, dyspnea, pleuritic pain, cough, and hemoptysis. Physical examination reveals a cardiac murmur in only 20% of cases. Plain or computed radiography may be characteristic, showing multiple small, patchy, peripherally located densities with or without cavitation that can change rapidly on serial examinations. Complications include large abscess formation, pulmonary gangrene, empyema, and pneumonia.

Iwasaki Y, Nagata K, Nakanishi M, et al: Spiral CT findings in septic pulmonary emboli. Eur J Radiol 37:190–194, 2001.

33. **What is the treatment for septic pulmonary emboli?**

Treatment for septic pulmonary emboli centers on management of the primary infectious focus. Numerous organisms have been reported to cause septic pulmonary emboli, including aerobic and anaerobic bacteria, fungi, and parasites. Therefore, in selecting empirical therapy, one must consider the appropriate clinical circumstance. The mainstay of treatment is prolonged parenteral administration of high-dose antibiotics. Duration of treatment varies based on the underlying condition but is generally on the order of weeks. If the emboli are secondary to suspected catheter-related bloodstream infection, the catheter should be removed promptly and appropriate cultures should be obtained.

CHAPTER 39

PULMONARY HYPERTENSION

Richard N. Channick, MD

1. **What is required to establish a diagnosis of idiopathic pulmonary arterial hypertension (IPAH)?**

   The criteria developed by the National Institutes of Health (NIH) registry on IPAH (formerly primary pulmonary hypertension [PPH]) required the demonstration of a mean pulmonary artery pressure (PAP) at rest of more than 25 mmHg or more than 30 mmHg with exercise in the absence of an associated condition (e.g., connective tissue disease, human immunodeficiency virus [HIV], portal hypertension, congenital heart disease, or drug use; Table 39-1) or a known secondary cause of pulmonary hypertension (PH) (i.e., lung or respiratory disease, left-sided heart disease, or thromboembolic disease).

   D'Alonzo GE, Barst RJ, Ayers SM, et al: Survival in patients with primary pulmonary hypertension: Results form a national prospective registry. Ann Intern Med 115:343–349, 1991.

TABLE 39-1.   CAUSES OF PULMONARY ARTERIAL HYPERTENSION (CATEGORY 1 CAUSES IN THE VENICE CLASSIFICATION SYSTEM)

- Idiopathic pulmonary arterial hypertension (PAH)
- Familial PAH
  - Associated PAH
  - Connective tissue disease
  - Congenital systemic-to-pulmonary shunts
  - Portal hypertension
  - HIV infection
  - Drugs or toxins
- PAH with venous or capillary involvement
  - Pulmonary veno-occlusive disease (PVOD)
  - Pulmonary capillary hemangiomatosis (PCH)
- Persistent PH of the newborn

---

2. **What are the physical examination findings of PH?**

   Signs of PH include right ventricular heave, a loud pulmonic second sound (P_2), a murmur of tricuspid regurgitation (i.e., a systolic murmur, heard best at left lower sternal border), a pulmonic insufficiency murmur, and a wide splitting of the second heart sound. Another useful sign is the presence of pulmonary flow bruits, heard over the posterior lung fields and usually indicating chronic proximal thromboemboli. Signs of right ventricular failure include jugular venous distention, peripheral edema, and a right-sided third heart sound (S_3).

3. **Can patients with left heart disease develop severe PH?**
Patients with any left-sided cardiac disease, including systolic or diastolic dysfunction or valvular disease, can develop severe PH that is out of proportion to pulmonary venous hypertension. In fact, the signs of left heart dysfunction in these patients may be relatively mild (i.e., left atrial enlargement or left ventricular hypertrophy). Suspicion should be high for a left-heart cause of PH in older patients, in those with a history of hypertension or diabetes mellitus, and in patients with scleroderma. These patients are particularly challenging, as treating PH may actually unmask the left heart disease, leading to clinical worsening.

4. **How severe is the PH expected in patients with lung or respiratory disease?**
In general, PH seen in patients with underlying lung diseases (i.e., idiopathic pulmonary fibrosis [IPF], chronic obstructive pulmonary disease [COPD], or obstructive sleep apnea [OSA]) is mild (i.e., mean PAP < 30 mmHg). However, there appears to be a subgroup of patients with more severe PH, possibly due to genetic predisposition. Of course, in these patients, other causes must be excluded (e.g., concomitant left heart disease or thromboemboli). A challenge for the clinician is determining whether the pulmonary vascular disease or the lung or respiratory disease is contributing most to exercise intolerance.

5. **Should every patient with unexplained PH undergo polysomnography?**
Sleep-disordered breathing can produce a chronic pulmonary hypertensive state, although it is usually not as severe or progressive as PPH. Routine polysomnography in unexplained PH is not recommended. Polysomnography should be performed when clinical suspicion of sleep apnea exists, based on a history of nocturnal snoring or apnea, daytime somnolence, or chronic hypercapnia.

6. **What is the best screening test to rule out chronic thromboembolic PH?**
Ventilation-perfusion (V/Q) lung scanning is the recommended diagnostic technique and should be performed on all patients. Helical computed tomography (CT) may lack sensitivity when evaluating for chronic disease, especially at the segmental level. On V/Q scanning, most patients with chronic thromboembolic disease have multiple mismatched perfusion defects. Patients with an abnormal lung scan should undergo angiography in order to confirm the presence of thromboembolic disease and to determine if lesions are amenable to pulmonary thromboendarterectomy (PTE).

McGoon M, Gutterman D, Steen V, et al: Screening, early detection, and diagnosis of pulmonary arterial hypertension: ACCP evidence-based clinical practice guidelines. Chest 126:14S–34S, 2004.

7. **When should pulmonary veno-occlusive disease (PVOD) be suspected?**
PVOD should be suspected when PH is present and the chest radiograph shows pulmonary venous engorgement, often with Kerley's B lines. Clinically, these patients often have severe hypoxemia and a reduction in diffusing capacity. The pulmonary capillary wedge pressure in PVOD is usually normal because the disease affects small and medium-sized veins in a patchy manner, thereby allowing transmission of postcapillary pressure through the larger veins. A clinical diagnosis of PVOD can be confirmed by the development of acute, reversible pulmonary edema with acutely infused prostacyclin, caused by an increased pulmonary blood flow in the presence of downstream vascular obstruction. Although a definitive diagnosis of PVOD requires histologic examination, this is rarely necessary. Patients with PVOD are often less responsive to medical therapy and should be referred for lung transplantation as soon as possible.

8. **What is the incidence and cause of PAH in HIV patients?**
   Studies show that approximately 0.5% of HIV patients have PH. The cause of PH in HIV is not known; the presence of PAH is not related to CD4 count, activity of disease, or viral load. HIV is not present in pathologically examined vessels. One confounding factor is that many HIV-associated PAH patients have a concomitant history of stimulant drug use, another known risk factor for PAH. The clinical course in these patients is similar to that of IPAH patients, and the treatment approach is the same.

   Humbert M, Nunes H, Sitbon O, et al: Risk factors for pulmonary arterial hypertension. Clin Chest Med 22:459–475, 2001.

9. **How is echocardiography useful in the diagnosis of PH?**
   Echocardiographic findings in PH include tricuspid regurgitation (TR), enlarged right-sided chambers, paradoxical septal movement with compression of the left ventricle, and pulmonic insufficiency. Pulmonary artery systolic pressure (PASP) can be estimated by the equation

   $$PASP = (TR\ velocity)^2 \times 4 + (estimated\ central\ venous\ pressure)$$

   In addition, echocardiography can evaluate left-sided valvular disease and left ventricular function and can assess for congenital lesions associated with PAH.

KEY POINTS: RECOMMENDED TESTS IN THE EVALUATION OF PULMONARY HYPERTENSION

1. Echocardiography with a contrast bubble study

2. Ventilation/perfusion scanning

3. Pulmonary function tests

4. Laboratory tests: antinuclear antibody (ANA), HIV, and liver function tests

5. Right heart catheterization

10. **Is right heart catheterization required in all patients with PAH prior to initiating therapy?**
    Yes. It is the consensus of worldwide experts that, before making a firm diagnosis of PAH and initiating therapy, right heart catheterization is mandatory. The procedure serves three main purposes: (1) confirming the diagnosis and ruling out other causes of PH including left heart disease and congenital heart disease; (2) determining severity through precise measurements of cardiac output, right atrial pressure, and PAPs; and (3) evaluating acute vasoreactivity using a short-acting pulmonary vasodilator (i.e., inhaled nitric oxide, adenosine, or prostacyclin).

11. **Which patients with PH should be treated with anticoagulants?**
    Patients with chronic thromboembolic PH and IPAH should be treated with anticoagulants. The preferred approach is use of warfarin, adjusting the dose to achieve an international normalized ratio (INR) of 2.0–2.5. An adjusted dose of subcutaneous heparin is a suitable alternative for patients who cannot tolerate warfarin. In addition to the risks of chronic anticoagulation, which exist for all patients, those with PH are also at risk for pulmonary hemorrhage resulting from rupture of hypertensive pulmonary vessels. No data exist regarding the use of anticoagulants in other forms of PH such as connective tissue diseases and severe respiratory disease

(i.e., cor pulmonale). Patients with severe PH may benefit from anticoagulation as long as they have a low risk of complications.

Rich S, Kaufmann E, Levy PS: The effect of high doses of calcium-channel blockers on survival in primary pulmonary hypertension. N Engl J Med 327:76–81, 1992.

12. **What is the role of calcium channel blocker (CCB) therapy in the treatment of PH?**
Recent data have confirmed that only a very small number of patients (6%) benefit in the long term from these agents. Only highly vasoreactive patients seem to garner benefit from CCBs. These patients have been defined by hemodynamic parameters in response to a vasodilator test as a reduction in PAP_{mean} by at least 10 mmHg to a level less than 40 mmHg, with no change or with an increase in cardiac output. Importantly, patients should not be started empirically on CCBs in the absence of such testing as these agents have clear adverse effects and may worsen clinical status dramatically.

Sitbon O, Humbert M, Jais X, et al: Long-term response to calcium channel blockers in idiopathic pulmonary arterial hypertension. Circulation 111:3105–3111, 2005.

13. **Which patients with chronic thromboembolic PH are candidates for PTE?**
All patients with a suggestion of chronic thromboembolic disease (i.e., with multiple V/Q mismatches) and PH should be considered potential surgical candidates and should be referred to an experienced center for further work-up. The only absolute contraindication to PTE surgery is inaccessible disease. PTE surgery leads to marked improvement and, in some cases, normalization of pulmonary hemodynamics.

Jamieson SW, Kapelanski DP, Sakakibara N, et al: Pulmonary endarterectomy: Experience and lessons learned in 1500 cases. Ann Thorac Surg 76:1457–1462, 2003.

KEY POINTS: CURRENT CLASSIFICATION OF PULMONARY HYPERTENSION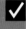

1. Pulmonary arterial hypertension

2. Pulmonary hypertension associated with left heart disease

3. Pulmonary hypertension associated with lung or respiratory disease or hypoxemia

4. Pulmonary hypertension due to thrombotic or other obstructive lesions of the pulmonary vasculature

14. **What are the best predictors of survival in patients with PAH?**
Parameters shown to be correlated with survival include hemodynamics (especially cardiac index and right atrial pressure), 6-minute-walk distance, and functional class. Improvement in these measures with therapy also correlates with improved survival.

McLaughlin VV, Presberg KW, Doyle RL, et al: Prognosis of pulmonary arterial hypertension: ACCP evidence-based clinical practice guidelines. Chest 126:78S–92S, 2004.

15. **What is the algorithm for initial therapy in patients with PAH?**
There is now an evidence-based algorithm for therapy based on vasoreactivity and initial functional class. Patients who meet criteria for acute vasoreactivity (see question 8) should be given

a trial of CCBs. For the remainder (the vast majority), Food and Drug Administration (FDA)-approved options include oral therapy with the endothelin receptor antagonist bosentan or with the phosphodiesterase type 5 inhibitor sildenafil; inhaled therapy with the prostacyclin (i.e., prostaglandin I_2 [PGI_2]) analogue iloprost; subcutaneous therapy with the PGI_2 analogue treprostinil; or IV therapy with another PGI_2 analogue, epoprostenol. In general, functional class III patients are begun on bosentan, whereas functional class IV patients are started on epoprostenol infusions. As sildenafil and inhaled iloprost have only recently become available, the role of these agents is still evolving.

Badesch DB, Abman SH, Ahearn GS, et al: Medical therapy for pulmonary arterial hypertension: ACCP evidence-based clinical practice guidelines. Chest 126:35S–62S, 2004.

Humbert M, Sitbon O, Simonneau G: Treatment of pulmonary arterial hypertension. N Engl J Med 351:1425–1436, 2004.

16. **What are the demonstrated benefits of bosentan in PAH patients?**
In two randomized, controlled trials, bosentan was shown to improve 6-minute-walk distance significantly. In addition, functional status was improved in patients on bosentan. Hemodynamic assessment, done in one of the trials, showed a significant improvement in pulmonary hemodynamics following 12 weeks of therapy. In the large bosentan randomized trial of endothelin receptor antagonist therapy (the BREATHE-1 trial), patients on bosentan had a reduced rate of clinical worsening (defined as withdrawal from the study with the need for more invasive therapy, hospitalization, or transplantation or because of death). In a recently published study, patients started on bosentan had a 2-year survival of 89%, compared to a predicted survival of 48%.

Channick RN, Simonneau G, Sitbon O, et al: Effects of the dual endothelin receptor antagonist bosentan in patients with pulmonary hypertension: A randomized placebo-controlled study. Lancet 358:1119–1123, 2001.

McLaughlin VV, Sitbon O, Badesch DB, et al: Survival with first-line bosentan in patients with primary pulmonary hypertension. Eur Respir J 25:244–249, 2005.

Rubin LJ, Badesch DB, Barst RJ, et al: Bosentan therapy for pulmonary arterial hypertension. N Engl J Med 346:896–903, 2002.

17. **What are the major adverse effects of bosentan?**
Liver function abnormalities constitute the side effect of bosentan requiring the most attention. Reversible transaminase elevations occur in 5–10% of patients, sometimes requiring discontinuation of the therapy. Monthly monitoring of liver function is required in all patients on bosentan. Other reported side effects include peripheral edema and nasal congestion.

18. **Should sildenafil be considered a first-line therapy in PAH patients?**
At this time, fewer data are available regarding the long-term safety and efficacy of oral sildenafil. A 12-week randomized clinical trial (RCT) demonstrated benefits on 6-minute-walk distance, functional class, and pulmonary hemodynamics. Based on this study, sildenafil was approved at a dose of 20 mg three times a day for patients with PAH who are class II–IV. There are no large head-to-head comparisons between the two approved oral therapies, bosentan and sildenafil; given that there are fewer long-term data for sildenafil, bosentan should probably be a first-line therapy in most patients.

19. **How effective is intravenous epoprostenol in PAH?**
Very effective. Numerous studies and reports confirm the potent, rapid benefit achieved when IV epoprostenol is instituted, even in gravely ill patients. Acute beneficial effects on cardiac output are seen and likely correspond to the rapid clinical benefit observed. Epoprostenol is typically begun at a low dose (1–2 ng/kg/min) and is titrated slowly. Side effects include flushing, headache, jaw claudication, leg pain, diarrhea, and catheter-related complications.

Barst RJ, Rubin LJ, Long WA, et al: A comparison of continuous intravenous epoprostenol with conventional therapy for primary pulmonary hypertension. The Primary Pulmonary Hypertension Study Group. N Engl J Med 334:296–302, 1996.

20. **What are the recommended studies for following PAH patients on therapy?**
The following tests have been demonstrated to predict more favorable prognosis in PAH patients on therapy:
- 6-minute-walk distance greater than 380 meters
- Functional class I or II
- Hemodynamic improvement with a decrease in PVR of at least 30% or an achievement of a mixed venous oxygen saturation of at least 63%
- Brain natriuretic peptide (BNP) level less than 180 μg/dL

KEY POINTS: APPROVED THERAPIES FOR PULMONARY ARTERIAL HYPERTENSION

1. Bosentan

2. Epoprostenol

3. Treprostinil

4. Iloprost

5. Sildenafil

21. **When should PAH patients be referred for lung transplantation?**
As lung transplantation carries a 5-year survival of only 50–60%, it should be reserved for patients failing medical therapy. Because of waiting times for transplantation, listing patients early has been the approach until now. A new allocation system may lead to a change in this approach because sicker patients will be given priority on the list, hopefully allowing more prompt transplantation in these patients. At present, it is still reasonable to refer patients for transplant evaluation at the time parenteral prostanoid therapy is initiated.

22. **Are there any restrictions in lifestyle that should be discussed with patients who have PH?**
Yes. Pregnancy is poorly tolerated in patients with PH because of dramatic hemodynamic stresses and hormonal changes that can affect the pulmonary circulation. Additionally, oral contraceptives can aggravate PH. Accordingly, safe and effective alternative methods of birth control should be practiced. Extremes in altitude should be avoided, but air travel is generally safe. Common over-the-counter decongestants should not be used because they frequently contain sympathomimetic drugs, which can produce tachycardia and vasoconstriction.

http://www.phassociation.org

GENERAL APPROACHES TO INTERSTITIAL LUNG DISEASE

Talmadge E. King, Jr., MD

CHAPTER 40

1. What are the causes of interstitial lung disease (ILD)?

The most common causes of ILD are related to occupational and environmental exposures, especially to inorganic or organic dusts. Sarcoidosis, idiopathic pulmonary fibrosis (IPF), and pulmonary fibrosis associated with connective tissue diseases (CTDs) are the most common ILDs of unknown etiology. Table 40-1 summarizes the etiologic classification of ILDs.

TABLE 40-1.   ETIOLOGIC CLASSIFICATION OF INTERSTITIAL LUNG DISEASES

Occupational and environmental exposures

Inorganic dust

    Silica, asbestos, hard metal dusts (e.g., cadmium or titanium oxide), beryllium

Organic dusts (causing hypersensitivity pneumonitis or extrinsic allergic alveolitis)

    Thermophilic bacteria (e.g., *Micropolyspora faeni, Thermoactinomyces vulgaris,* or *Thermoactinomyces sacchari*)

    Other bacteria (e.g., *Bacillus subtilis* or *Bacillus cereus*)

    True fungi (e.g., *Aspergillus* spp., *Cryptostroma corticale, Aureobasidium pullulans,* or *Penicillin* spp.)

    Animal proteins (e.g., bird fancier's disease)

    Bacterial products (byssinosis)

Chemical sources, gases, fumes, vapors, aerosols, paraquat, or radiation

Drugs and poisons

Chemotherapeutic agents (i.e., busulfan, bleomycin, or methotrexate)

Gold salts

Amiodarone

Antibiotics (i.e., nitrofurantoin or sulfasalazine)

Radiation

Drug-induced lupus (i.e., diphenylhydantoin and procainamide)

Connective tissue disease (CTD)

Systemic lupus erythematosus (SLE)

Polymyositis and dermatomyositis

Rheumatoid arthritis

Mixed collective tissue disease

Progressive systemic sclerosis

Ankylosing spondylitis

Sjögren's syndrome

TABLE 40-1.   ETIOLOGIC CLASSIFICATION OF INTERSTITIAL LUNG DISEASES—CONT'D

Other systemic diseases

Sarcoidosis

Vasculitides (i.e., Wegener's granulomatosis or Churg–Strauss syndrome)

Pulmonary Langerhans cell histiocytosis (i.e., pulmonary histiocytosis X or eosinophilic granuloma of the lung)

Hemorrhagic syndromes (i.e., Goodpasture's syndrome or idiopathic pulmonary hemosiderosis)

Alveolar proteinosis

Lymphangitic carcinomatosis

Chronic pulmonary edema

Chronic gastric aspiration

Chronic uremia

Idiopathic interstitial pneumonias

IPF

Nonspecific interstitial pneumonia (NSIP)

Respiratory bronchiolitis–associated interstitial lung disease (RB-ILD)

Desquamative interstitial pneumonia (DIP)

Lymphoid interstitial pneumonia (LIP)

Acute interstitial pneumonia (AIP), formerly Hamman–Rich syndrome

Infections (residue of active infection of any type)

American Thoracic Society/European Respiratory Society: International Multidisciplinary Consensus Classification of the Idiopathic Interstitial Pneumonias. Am J Respir Crit Care Med 165:277–304, 2002.
Collard HR, King TE Jr: Demystifying idiopathic interstitial pneumonias. Arch Intern Med 163:17–29, 2003.
Schwarz MI, King TE Jr: Interstitial Lung Diseases, 4th ed. Hamilton, Ontario, BC Decker, 2003.
Thomas KW, Hunninghake GW: Sarcoidosis. JAMA 289(24):3300–3303, 2003.

2. **Describe the modes of clinical presentation of patients with ILD.**
   Patients with ILD commonly come to clinical attention in one of the following ways:
   - Onset of progressive breathlessness with exertion (dyspnea) or persistent nonproductive cough. Other important symptoms and signs include hemoptysis, wheezing, and chest pain.
   - Identification of interstitial opacities on chest x-ray.
   - Pulmonary symptoms associated with another disease such as a CTD. Importantly, clinical findings suggestive of a CTD (i.e., musculoskeletal pain, weakness, fatigue, fever, joint pains or swelling, photosensitivity, Raynaud's phenomenon, pleuritis, dry eyes, or dry mouth) should be carefully elicited. The CTD may be difficult to rule out since the pulmonary manifestations occasionally precede the more typical systemic manifestations by months or years (particularly in rheumatoid arthritis, systemic lupus erythematosus (SLE), and polymyositis–dermatomyositis).

- Identification of lung function abnormalities on simple office spirometry, particularly a restrictive ventilatory pattern.

3. **What are the presenting clinical manifestations of ILD?**
   - **Dyspnea:** Shortness of breath is a common complaint of patients with cardiac or pulmonary disease. In most instances, the patient has attributed the insidious onset of breathlessness with exertion to aging, deconditioning, obesity, or a recent upper respiratory tract illness, and some patients deny the presence of dyspnea even when questioned. However, patients with sarcoidosis, silicosis, or pulmonary Langerhans cell histiocytosis may have extensive parenchymal lung disease without significant dyspnea, especially early in the course of their disease. Sudden worsening of dyspnea, especially if associated with pleural pain, may indicate a spontaneous pneumothorax.
   - **Cough:** A dry cough may be particularly disturbing for patients with processes that involve the airways such as sarcoidosis, organizing pneumonia, respiratory bronchiolitis, pulmonary Langerhans cell histiocytosis, hypersensitivity pneumonitis, lipoid pneumonia, or lymphangitic carcinomatosis.
   - **Hemoptysis:** Grossly bloody or blood-streaked sputum occurs in the diffuse alveolar hemorrhage syndromes, lymphangioleiomyomatosis, tuberous sclerosis, pulmonary veno-occlusive disease, long-standing mitral valve disease, and granulomatous vasculitides. Occasionally, diffuse alveolar bleeding may be present without hemoptysis; the clinical manifestations of dyspnea and an iron-deficiency anemia may be present. New onset of hemoptysis in a patient with known ILD should raise the possibility of a complicating malignancy.
   - **Wheezing:** Wheezing is an uncommon manifestation of ILD. It has been described in cases of lymphangitic carcinomatosis, chronic eosinophilic pneumonia, Churg-Strauss syndrome, and respiratory bronchiolitis.
   - **Inspiratory squeaks:** Scattered late inspiratory high-pitched rhonchi are frequently heard on chest examination in patients with bronchiolitis.
   - **Chest pain:** Clinically significant chest pain is uncommon in most ILDs, but pleuritic chest pain may occur in ILD associated with rheumatoid arthritis, SLE, mixed CTD, and some drug-induced disorders. Substernal chest pain or discomfort is common in sarcoidosis.

   American Thoracic Society. Dyspnea: Mechanisms, assessment, and management. A consensus statement. Am J Respir Crit Care Med 159:321–340, 1999.

4. **How long are clinical manifestations of ILD evident prior to presentation?**
   In the vast majority of ILDs, the symptoms and signs are chronic (i.e., having lasted months to years), as in IPF, sarcoidosis, and pulmonary histiocytosis X. In some, however, symptoms may be acute (i.e., days to weeks) or subacute (i.e., weeks to months). These latter processes are often confused with atypical pneumonias since many have diffuse radiographic opacities, fever, or relapses of disease activity; examples include acute idiopathic interstitial pneumonia, acute eosinophilic pneumonia, hypersensitivity pneumonitis, organizing pneumonia, some drug-induced ILDs, alveolar hemorrhage syndromes, and acute immunologic pneumonia that complicates either SLE or polymyositis.

5. **Describe an initial evaluation of a patient suspected of having ILD.**
   The initial evaluation should include a complete **history** and **physical examination**. The initial laboratory evaluation should include biochemical tests to evaluate **liver** and **renal function** and also **hematologic tests** to check for anemia, polycythemia, or leukocytosis. **Serologic studies** should be obtained if clinically indicated by features suggestive of a CTD or vasculitis: these tests should include sedimentation rate, antinuclear antibodies, rheumatoid factor, hypersensitivity panel, antineutrophil cytoplasmic antibodies, and antibasement membrane antibody. A recent **chest x-ray** should be obtained, and it also is important to review all old chest x-rays to

assess the rate of change in disease activity. **High-resolution computed tomography (HRCT)** is better than the chest x-ray for early detection and confirmation of suspected ILD. HRCT also allows better assessment of coexisting disease (e.g., emphysema, mediastinal adenopathy, or cancer). Complete **lung function testing** (i.e., spirometry, lung volumes, and diffusing capacity) and resting room air **arterial blood gases** (ABGs) should be obtained. Common diseases, such as chronic obstructive pulmonary disease (COPD), anemia, heart failure, and mycobacterial or fungal disease, can mimic ILD, so they must be ruled out. Most causes of ILD will be identified by this process.

6. **Why is the medical history so important in evaluating a patient with ILD?**
   Because the cause of the current illness is often recognized from the patient's history. Key areas of focus in the history include occupational and environmental exposures, smoking history, medication history, and family history.

7. **Describe the key features of the occupational history in a patient with ILD.**
   A strict chronologic listing of the patient's lifelong employment must be sought, including specific duties and known exposures to dusts, gases, and chemicals. The degree of exposure, the duration, the latency of exposure, and the use of protective devices should be elicited.

8. **What are the key environmental exposures to assess in a patient with ILD?**
   Review of the environment (home and work, including that of spouse and children) is valuable. It is especially important to determine if the patient has had exposures to pets (especially birds), air conditioners, humidifiers, hot tubs, evaporative cooling systems (e.g., swamp coolers), or water damage in the home or work environment. In hypersensitivity pneumonitis, respiratory symptoms, fever, chills, and an abnormal chest x-ray are often temporally related to the workplace (e.g., farmer's lung) or to a hobby (e.g., pigeon breeder's disease). Symptoms may diminish or disappear after the patient leaves the exposure for several days; similarly, symptoms reappear on returning to the exposure.

9. **Name the ILDs associated with a history of cigarette smoking.**
   Some ILDs occur largely among current or former smokers (e.g., pulmonary Langerhans' cell histiocytosis, desquamative interstitial pneumonitis, respiratory bronchiolitis, and IPF). Active smoking can lead to complications in some processes such as Goodpasture's syndrome, in which pulmonary hemorrhage is far more frequent in current smokers.

   Also, smoking was shown to have a significant impact on both histopathology and lung function in patients with ILDs. The quantity of cigarettes smoked may impact survival in some ILDs (e.g., in IPF, the higher the number of pack-years, the worse the prognosis).

   Sarcoidosis and hypersensitivity pneumonitis tend to be more common among never (or former) smokers.

   Hanley ME, King TE Jr, Schwarz MI, et al: The impact of smoking on mechanical properties of the lungs in idiopathic pulmonary fibrosis and sarcoidosis. Am Rev Respir Dis 144:1102–1106, 1991.
   Ryu JH, Colby TV, Hartman TE, Vassallo R: Smoking-related interstitial lung diseases: A concise review. Eur Respir J 17(1):122–132, 2001.

10. **What is the importance of prior medication use in defining ILD?**
    A detailed history of the medications taken by the patient, including over-the-counter medications, oily nose drops, and amino acid supplements, is needed to exclude the possibility of drug-induced disease. Lung diseases may occur weeks to years after the drug has been discontinued.

    Camus P: Drug-induced infiltrative lung disease. In Schwarz MI, King TE Jr (eds): Interstitial Lung Diseases, 4th ed. Hamilton, Ontario, BC Decker, 2003, pp 485–534.

11. **Are there any familial causes of ILD?**
The family history is occasionally helpful since familial associations (with an autosomal-dominant pattern) have been identified in cases of IPF, sarcoidosis, tuberous sclerosis, and neurofibromatosis. An autosomal-recessive pattern of inheritance occurs in Niemann–Pick disease, Gaucher's disease, and Hermansky–Pudlak syndrome.

   Loyd JE: Pulmonary fibrosis in families. Am J Respir Cell Mol Biol 29(3 Suppl):S47–S50, 2003.

12. **When are gender and age important in the evaluation of a patient with ILD?**
- **Gender** is important in lymphangioleiomyomatosis, which occurs almost exclusively in pre-menopausal women. Also, ILD in the CTDs is more common in women; the exception is ILD in rheumatoid arthritis, which is more common in men.
- **Age** is helpful given that the majority of patients with sarcoidosis and CTD present between the ages of 20 and 40 years. Conversely, most patients with IPF are over age 60 years.

13. **How useful is the physical examination in the diagnosis of ILD?**
The physical exam is commonly not specific but can be useful because it frequently reveals tachypnea, reduced chest expansion, bibasilar end-expiratory dry crackles, cyanosis, and digital clubbing.

   Crackles, or "Velcro rales," are common in most forms of ILD, although they are less common in the granulomatous lung diseases, especially sarcoidosis. Crackles may be present in the absence of radiographic abnormalities on the chest x-ray.

   Cyanosis is uncommon and is usually a late manifestation indicative of advanced disease.

14. **Describe clubbing.**
Clubbing of the digits (i.e., the distal part of the finger is enlarged compared with the proximal part; Fig. 40-1) is common in some patients (those with IPF or asbestosis) and rare in others (i.e., those with sarcoidosis, hypersensitivity pneumonitis, or histiocytosis X). In most patients, clubbing is a late manifestation suggesting advanced derangement of the lung.

   Myers KA, Farquhar DR: The rational clinical examination. Does this patient have clubbing? JAMA 286(3):341–347, 2001.
   Scharer L: Clinical description of nail clubbing. JAMA 286(16):1972–1973, 2001.

15. **What are the clinical implications of finding signs of cor pulmonale in patients with ILD?**
The cardiac examination is usually normal in patients with ILD except in the middle or late stages of the disease, when findings of pulmonary hypertension (PH) (i.e., an augmented pulmonic

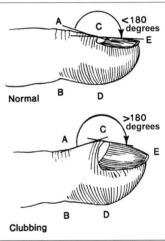

Figure 40-1. Clubbing of the fingers. In a normal finger, the length of a perpendicular dropped from point A to point B should be greater than a similar line from C to D. In clubbing, the relationships are reversed; that is, the distance from C to D is greater than the distance from A to B. The other important change is the angle described by A–C–E. In the normal finger, this angle is usually <180 degrees, whereas in clubbing it is >180 degrees. (From DeRemee RA: Facets of the algorithmic synthesis. In De Remee RA [ed]: Clinical Profiles of Diffuse Interstitial Pulmonary Disease. Mount Kisco, NY, Futura Publishing Company, 1990, pp 9–44, with permission.)

second sound [P_2], a right-sided lift, and a third-heart-sound [S_3] gallop) and cor pulmonale may become evident.

Signs of PH and cor pulmonale are generally secondary manifestations of advanced ILD, although they may be primary manifestations of a CTD (e.g., progressive systemic sclerosis).

16. **What extrapulmonary physical findings may be helpful in arriving at a diagnosis of ILD?**
See Table 40-2.

TABLE 40-2. EXTRAPULMONARY PHYSICAL FINDINGS HELPFUL IN THE DIAGNOSIS OF INTERSTITIAL LUNG DISEASE

Physical Findings	Associated Conditions
Skin changes	
Erythema nodosum	Sarcoidosis, CTD, Behçet's syndrome, histoplasmosis, coccidioidomycosis
Maculopapular rash	Drug-induced, amyloidosis, lipoidosis, CTD, Gaucher's disease
Heliotrope rash	Dermatomyositis
Telangiectasia	Scleroderma
Raynaud's phenomena	CTD
Cutaneous vasculitis	Systemic vasculitides, CTD
Subcutaneous nodules	Von Recklinghausen's disease, rheumatoid arthritis
Eye changes	
Uveitis	Sarcoidosis, Behçet's syndrome, ankylosing spondylitis
Scleritis	Systemic vasculitis, SLE, scleroderma, sarcoidosis
Keratoconjunctivitis sicca	Lymphocytic interstitial pneumonia (LIP)
Systemic arterial hypertension	CTD, neurofibromatosis, some diffuse alveolar hemorrhage syndromes
Calcinosis	Dermatomyositis, scleroderma
Salivary gland enlargement	Sarcoidosis, LIP
Peripheral lymphadenopathy	Sarcoidosis, lymphangitic carcinomatosis, LIP, lymphoma
Hepatosplenomegaly	Sarcoidosis, CTD, amyloidosis, LIP
Pericarditis	Radiation pneumonitis, CTD
Myositis	CTD, drugs
Muscle weakness	CTD

Adapted from King TE Jr, Schwarz MI: Approach to the diagnosis and management of the idiopathic interstitial pneumonias. In Mason RJ, Broaddus VC, Murray JF, Nadel JA (eds): Murray and Nadel's Textbook of Respiratory Medicine, 4th ed. Philadelphia, Elsevier, 2005, pp 1571–1608.

17. **What is the role of the routine laboratory evaluation in a patient suspected of having ILD?**

The routine laboratory evaluation is often not helpful because the findings are nonspecific. An elevated erythrocyte sedimentation rate and hypergammaglobulinemia are commonly observed but are nondiagnostic. Antinuclear antibodies and anti-immunoglobulin antibodies (i.e., rheumatoid factors) are identified in many of these patients, even in the absence of a defined CTD (especially in patients with idiopathic nonspecific interstitial pneumonia). Elevation of lactate dehydrogenase may be noted but is a nonspecific finding common to many pulmonary disorders. An increase in the angiotensin-converting enzyme (ACE) level may be observed in sarcoidosis but is nonspecific because elevated ACE levels have been noted in several interstitial diseases including hypersensitivity pneumonitis. Antibodies to organic antigens may be helpful in confirming exposure when hypersensitivity pneumonitis is suspected, although they, too, are nondiagnostic. The electrocardiogram (ECG) is usually normal in the absence of PH or concurrent cardiac disease.

18. **What is the role of the routine chest x-ray in a patient suspected of ILD?**

The diagnosis of ILD is often suspected initially on the basis of an abnormal chest roentgenogram. Unfortunately, the chest x-ray may be normal in as many as 10% of patients with some forms of ILD, particularly hypersensitivity pneumonitis. The physician should not ignore or incompletely evaluate a symptomatic patient with a normal chest x-ray or an asymptomatic patient with radiographic evidence of ILD. Failure to completely evaluate such patients often leads to progressive disease, which may be irreversible by the time the patient seeks additional medical attention.

19. **Describe the common chest radiographic patterns seen in a patient with ILD.**

The most common radiographic abnormality is a **reticular** or **nodular** pattern; however, mixed patterns of alveolar filling and increased interstitial markings are not unusual. Most ILDs have a predilection for the lower lung zones. As the disease progresses, the opacities become more widespread and associated with reductions in lung volume and the appearance of PH. A subgroup of ILDs have predilection for the upper lung zones and often produce nodular infiltrates that result in upward contraction of the pulmonary hilus. With progression of the disease, small cystic structures appear, representing fibrous replacement of the normal alveolar architecture and radiographic **honeycombing**. Figure 40-2 shows the radiograph of a patient with sarcoidosis.

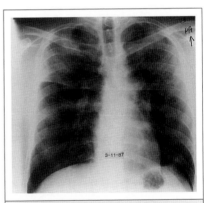

Figure 40-2. Sarcoidosis. This chest roentgenogram from a patient with sarcoidosis shows predominantly nodular and hazy opacities in the upper lung zones. The chest x-ray normalized following treatment with corticosteroids.

20. **How useful is the routine chest roentgenogram in the staging and follow-up of a patient with ILD?**

The correlation between the x-ray pattern and the stage of disease (i.e., clinical or histopathologic) is generally poor. Only the radiographic finding of **honeycombing** (i.e., small cystic spaces) correlates with pathologic findings; it portends a poor prognosis.

21. **What is the role of CT scanning of the chest in the evaluation of ILD?**

    HRCT is well suited for evaluation of diffuse pulmonary parenchymal disease. Pattern recognition in diffuse lung disease is enhanced because HRCT avoids the problem of superimposition of structures and is exposure independent. HRCT offers the following:

    - More accuracy than conventional chest x-ray in distinguishing air space from ILD.
    - Earlier detection and confirmation of suspected diffuse lung disease, especially in the investigation of a symptomatic patient with a normal chest radiograph.
    - Better assessment of the extent and distribution of disease.
    - Ability to disclose coexisting disease (e.g., occult mediastinal adenopathy, carcinoma, or emphysema).
    - Utility in more specifically selecting the appropriate type of and site for biopsy.

    In the appropriate clinical setting, HRCT may be sufficient to preclude the need for surgical lung biopsy (e.g., IPF, sarcoidosis, hypersensitivity pneumonitis, asbestosis, lymphangitic carcinoma, lymphangioleiomyomatosis, or pulmonary Langerhans cell histiocytosis). A predominant ground-glass pattern on HRCT is representative of a more active and potentially reversible process, particularly in hypersensitivity pneumonitis (Fig. 40-3), DIP, and nonspecific interstitial pneumonia. When the ground glass pattern is associated with traction bronchiectasis, the underlying pathologic finding is most likely fibrosis rather than cellular inflammation.

    Wittram C, Mark EJ, McLoud TC: CT-histologic correlation of the ATS/ERS 2002 classification of idiopathic interstitial pneumonias. Radiographics 23(5):1057–1071, 2003.

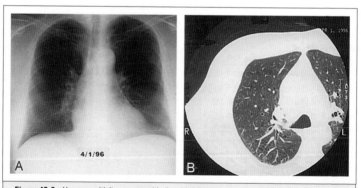

Figure 40-3. Hypersensitivity pneumonitis (i.e., bird fancier's disease). **A,** Chest roentgenogram is normal. **B,** HRCT scan of right lung reveals diffuse hazy or ground-glass increase in lung density (*i.e.,* an increase in CT lung density that does not obscure the underlying lung parenchyma). Lung biopsy confirmed the presence of a granulomatous pneumonitis.

22. **What is the role of pulmonary function testing (PFT) in the evaluation of a patient with ILD?**

    Measurement of lung volumes and spirometry function testing are important in assessing the severity of lung involvement. Also, the finding of an obstructive or restrictive pattern is useful in narrowing the possible diagnoses.

    Erbes R, Schaberg T, Loddenkemper R: Lung function tests in patients with idiopathic pulmonary fibrosis. Are they helpful for predicting outcome? Chest 111:51–57, 1997.

Flaherty KR, Mumford JA, Murray S, et al: Prognostic implications of physiologic and radiographic changes in idiopathic interstitial pneumonia. Am J Respir Crit Care Med 168(5):543–548, 2003.

Martinez FJ, Lynch JP III: Role of physiological assessment in usual interstitial pneumonia. In Lynch JP III (ed): Idiopathic Pulmonary Fibrosis. New York, Marcel Dekker, 2004, pp 137–165.

23. **What is the most common pattern of lung function abnormality in patients with ILD?**

    Most of the interstitial disorders have a **restrictive defect** with reduced total lung capacity (TLC), functional residual capacity (FRC), and residual volume (RV). Flow rates (the forced expiratory volume in 1 second [FEV_1] and the forced vital capacity [FVC]) are decreased, but this is related to the decreased lung volumes. The FEV_1-to-FVC ratio is usually normal or increased (Fig. 40-4). Smoking history must be assessed.

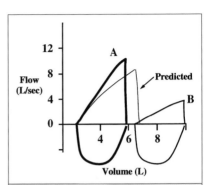

Figure 40-4. Maximal expiratory flow volume (MEFV) curve in IPF. **A,** MEFV curves at presentation in a 42-year-old nonsmoking man with a normal chest x-ray and lung biopsy-proven IPF. The ratio of the forced expiratory volume in 1 second (FEV_1) and forced vital capacity (FVC) values are low relative to the predicted values, but the FEV_1 to the FVC are increased. However, at any given lung volume, the flow rates are higher than expected because of elevated driving pressure due to an increased elastic recoil. **B,** MEFV curve for a patient with COPD. FEV_1 and FVC are low relative to the predicted values, and the lung volumes are increased.

24. **Does the presence of airflow obstruction on PFT rule out ILD as a major cause of the patient's illness?**

    No. A few disorders produce interstitial opacities on chest x-ray and obstructive airflow limitation on PFT (e.g., sarcoidosis, lymphangioleiomyomatosis, hypersensitivity pneumonitis, tuberous sclerosis, and COPD with superimposed ILD).

25. **Is there a role for measurement of lung elastic recoil?**

    Yes. In symptomatic patients with a normal chest radiograph and minimal or no restrictive disease, measurement of elastic recoil (i.e., the pressure-volume curve) may be helpful by identifying lung stiffness. Pressure-volume studies often yield a curve that is shifted downward and to the right, consistent with a stiff noncompliant lung. In general, as the disease progresses, lung compliance decreases and lung volumes fall.

26. **What is the relationship between the static deflation volume and pressure in a patient with IPF?**

    See Figure 40-5. The percent predicted TLC is plotted against the static transpulmonary pressure (in cmH_2O) for a patient with ILD. In general, the compliance, the maximum static transpulmonary pressure, and the coefficient of retraction (the maximum transpulmonary pressure to TLC) tend to correlate with the extent of parenchymal lung involvement observed on lung biopsy.

27. **Are there changes in the carbon monoxide diffusion in the lung (DLCO) in ILD?**

    Yes. A reduction in the DLCO is commonly found, but it is not specific for a particular type of ILD. The decrease in DLCO is due in part to effacement of the alveolar capillary units and, more importantly, to the extent of ventilation-perfusion (V/Q) mismatching of the alveoli. Lung regions with reduced compliance due either to fibrosis or to excessive cellularity may be poorly ventilated but still well perfused.

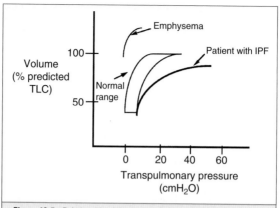

Figure 40-5. Relationship of the static deflation volume and pressure in a patient with IPF. The percent predicted total lung capacity (TLC) is plotted against the static transpulmonary pressure (cmH_2O) for a patient with ILD. In general, the compliance, the maximum static transpulmonary pressure, and the coefficient of retraction (i.e., maximum transpulmonary pressure to TLC) tend to correlate with the extent of parenchymal and lung involvement observed on lung biopsy.

28. **Do changes in DLCO correlate with disease stage in ILD?**
    No. The severity of the DLCO reduction does not correlate well with disease stage. In some ILDs, there can be considerable reduction in lung volumes or severe hypoxemia but normal or only slightly reduced DLCO, especially in sarcoidosis. The presence of moderate to severe reductions of DLCO in the presence of normal lung volumes should suggest ILD with associated emphysema, pulmonary vascular disease, pulmonary histiocytosis X, or lymphangioleiomyomatosis.

29. **Are there changes in the ABGs in ILD?**
    Yes. The resting ABGs may be normal or may reveal hypoxemia (secondary to V/Q mismatching) and respiratory alkalosis. Carbon dioxide retention is rare and is usually a manifestation of far-advanced end-stage disease.

30. **Does a normal resting ABG rule out the need for measurement of gas exchange with exercise?**
    A normal resting PaO_2 does *not* rule out significant hypoxemia during exercise or sleep. Furthermore, although hypoxemia with exercise and sleep is very common, secondary erythrocytosis is rarely observed in uncomplicated ILD.

31. **Why is the exercise gas exchange important in the evaluation of patients with ILD?**
    Because resting hypoxemia is not always evident and because severe exercise-induced hypoxemia may go undetected, it is important to perform exercise testing with serial measurement of ABGs. Arterial oxygen desaturation, a failure to decrease dead space appropriately with exercise (i.e., a high ratio of dead space [V_D] to total ventilation [V_T]), and an excessive increase in respiratory rate with a lower-than-expected recruitment of tidal volume provide useful information about physiologic abnormalities and the extent of the disease. There is increasing evidence that

KEY POINTS: INDICATIONS FOR SPECIALIZED TESTING AND REFERRAL TO A PULMONOLOGIST

1. No specific cause of dyspnea or cough were found.

2. Symptoms exceed the physiologic or radiographic abnormalities identified.

3. Empirical management (e.g., bronchodilators, diuretics, and smoking cessation) resulted in atypical or unsatisfactory clinical outcome.

4. Patient needs impairment or disability evaluation for worker's compensation or another reason as here.

5. Specialized cardiopulmonary testing is needed, such as:
   - Fiberoptic bronchoscopy and bronchoalveolar lavage
   - Lung biopsy, required to confirm diagnosis
   - Exercise testing with ABGs, to determine if physiologic limitation exists and whether its cause is cardiac or pulmonary
   - Right heart catheterization
   - Pulmonary angiography
   - Studies of respiratory drive

6. Therapeutic immunosuppressive or cytotoxic drug trial is contemplated.

serial assessment of resting and exercise gas exchange is the best method to identify disease activity and responsiveness to treatment.

KEY POINTS: INDICATIONS FOR SURGICAL LUNG BIOPSY IN PATIENTS WITH SUSPECTED INTERSTITIAL LUNG DISEASE

1. It often provides a specific diagnosis, especially in idiopathic interstitial pneumonias, alveolar proteinosis, sarcoidosis, pulmonary Langerhans' cell histiocytosis, respiratory bronchiolitis, lymphangioleiomyomatosis, organizing pneumonia (OP), veno-occlusive disease, and vasculitis limited to the lung.

2. It excludes neoplastic and infectious processes that occasionally mimic chronic progressive interstitial disease.

3. It occasionally identifies a more treatable process than originally suspected (e.g., hypersensitivity pneumonitis, OP, respiratory bronchiolitis–associated ILD, or sarcoidosis).

4. It provides the best assessment of disease activity.

32. **Is bronchoalveolar lavage (BAL) analysis useful in the assessment of ILD?**
    In selected cases, BAL cellular analysis may be useful to (1) narrow the differential diagnostic possibilities between various types of ILD, (2) define the stage of disease, and (3) assess the progression of disease or response to therapy. However, the utility of BAL in the clinical assessment and management of ILD patients remains to be fully established (Table 40-3).

    Rottoli P, Bargagli E: Is bronchoalveolar lavage obsolete in the diagnosis of interstitial lung disease? Curr Opin Pulm Med 9(5):418–425, 2003.

TABLE 40-3. LAVAGE FINDINGS IN INTERSTITIAL LUNG DISEASE	
Condition	**Lavage Finding**
Lymphangitic carcinomatosis, alveolar cell carcinoma, or pulmonary lymphoma	Malignant cells
Diffuse alveolar bleeding	Hemosiderin-laden macrophages and red blood cells
Alveolar proteinosis	Lipoproteinaceous intra-alveolar material (periodic acid-Schiff stain)
Lipoid pneumonia	Fat globules in macrophages
Pulmonary Langerhans' cell histiocytosis	Monoclonal antibody (T6)–positive histiocytes and electron microscopy demonstrating Birbeck granules in lavaged macrophages
Asbestos-related pulmonary disease	Ferruginous bodies
Lipoidosis	Accumulation of specific lipopigment in alveolar macrophages
Berylliosis	Lymphoblast transformation test
Silicosis	Dust particles by polarized light microscopy

33. **When should fiberoptic bronchoscopy with transbronchial lung biopsy be performed?**
This is often the initial procedure of choice, especially when sarcoidosis, lymphangitic carcinomatosis, eosinophilic pneumonia, Goodpasture's syndrome, or infection is suspected. If a specific diagnosis is not made by transbronchial biopsy, then a surgical lung biopsy is indicated.

   Churg A: Transbronchial biopsy: Nothing to fear. Am J Surg Pathol 25(6):820–822, 2001.

34. **When should surgical lung biopsy be performed?**
Open-lung (or thoracoscopic, which is preferred) biopsy is the most definitive method to diagnose and stage the disease so that appropriate prognostic and therapeutic decisions can be made. Failure to secure a definitive diagnosis or to determine the stage of disease prior to the initiation of treatment can result in unnecessary anguish for the physician and the patient with ILD. Having a definite diagnosis makes the physician and patient more comfortable proceeding with therapies that may have serious side effects. Also, a definitive diagnosis avoids confusion (and anxiety) later if the patient is failing therapy or is suffering serious side effects of therapy.

   Open-lung biopsy by thoracotomy or video thoracoscopy is a relatively safe procedure with little morbidity and <1% mortality. Currently, video-assisted thoracoscopic lung biopsy is the preferred method for obtaining multiple lung tissue samples for analysis.

   Hunninghake G, Zimmerman MB, Schwartz DA, et al: Utility of lung biopsy for the diagnosis of idiopathic pulmonary fibrosis. Am J Respir Crit Care Med 164:193–196, 2001.

35. **When should a lung biopsy *not* be performed?**
Relative contraindications to lung biopsy include serious cardiovascular disease, roentgenographic evidence of diffuse end-stage disease (i.e., honeycombing), severe pulmonary dysfunction, or other major operative risks (especially in the elderly).

36. **Describe the two major histopathologic patterns found in patients with ILD.**
    1. A **granulomatous** process is characterized by an accumulation of T lymphocytes, macrophages, and epithelioid cells organized into discrete structures (i.e., granulomas) that result in derangement of normal tissue architecture.
    2. The **inflammatory or fibrotic** process is characterized by interstitial inflammation accompanied by varying degrees of fibrosis, either in the form of abnormal collagen deposition or a proliferation of fibroblasts capable of collagen synthesis.

37. **Name the major histopathologic patterns found in patients with ILD.**
    The major histopathologic patterns of ILD include:
    - Usual interstitial pneumonia (UIP)
    - DIP
    - Respiratory bronchiolitis–associated interstitial lung disease (RB-ILD)
    - Nonspecific interstitial pneumonia (NSIP)
    - Diffuse alveolar damage
    - Lymphoid interstitial pneumonia
    - Diffuse alveolar hemorrhage

    Katzenstein ALA, Myers JL: Idiopathic pulmonary fibrosis: Clinical relevance of pathologic classification. Am J Respir Crit Care Med 157:1301–1315, 1998.

38. **Describe the pathophysiology of UIP.**
    UIP is the most common pattern of idiopathic interstitial pneumonia. Recent insight into the pathophysiology of UIP suggests that it is a model of abnormal wound healing in the lung resulting from multiple microscopic sites of ongoing alveolar epithelial injury and activation, leading to the formation of patchy areas of fibroblast and myofibroblast foci. These foci (now considered a reticulum extending from the pleural surface) of injury and abnormal repair are characterized by fibroblast and myofibroblast migration and proliferation, decreased myofibroblast apoptosis, and increased activity of the fibrogenic cytokines. In addition, there appears to be an absence of appropriate reepithelialization and impaired extracellular matrix remodeling, leading to basement membrane disruption, angiogenesis, and fibrosis.

    Selman M, King TE, Jr, Pardo A: Idiopathic pulmonary fibrosis: Prevailing and evolving hypotheses about its pathogenesis and implications for therapy. Ann Intern Med 134:136–151, 2001.

39. **Do the different histologic patterns of lung injury portend different prognoses?**
    Yes, patients with a granulomatous lung disease can progress to clinically significant pulmonary fibrosis. However, many of these patients remain free of severe impairment of lung function or even improve after immunosuppressive treatment (e.g., those suffering from sarcoidosis or hypersensitivity pneumonitis). Conversely, patients with the UIP lesion often have a more devastating illness characterized by unrelenting progression to end-stage fibrosis and death, especially patients with IPF.

    Flaherty KR, Thwaite EL, Kazerooni EA, et al: Radiological versus histological diagnosis in UIP and NSIP: Survival implications. Thorax 58(2):143–148, 2003.
    Vassallo R, Ryu JH, Schroeder DR, et al: Clinical outcomes of pulmonary Langerhans'-cell histiocytosis in adults. N Engl J Med 346(7):484–490, 2002.

40. **Which patients require treatment, and when should it begin?**
    Management of most ILDs is difficult, and different approaches are taken depending on the specific entity. Regardless of etiology, end-stage fibrosis is irreversible and untreatable. An extensive and aggressive diagnostic evaluation early on, even in patients with relatively few symptoms, is recommended. Patients with evidence of lung function impairment, signs of progression, or evidence of active disease should be treated if no contraindications to therapy exist.

Pursuing a diagnosis and instituting appropriate therapy early in the disease course, prior to extensive fibrosis, is likely to improve responsiveness to therapy, hopefully delaying or preventing the functional limitation and disability that commonly occur in these patients.

Davies HR, Richeldi L, Walters EH: Immunomodulatory agents for idiopathic pulmonary fibrosis. Cochrane Database Syst Rev (3):CD003134, 2003.

41. **Which patients require oxygen treatment, and when should it be started?**
Patients with ILD, especially IPF, typically are sufficiently dyspneic with exertion that they have stopped regular exercise. These patients need encouragement to develop a routine conditioning program to improve muscle strength and cardiovascular efficiency. Daily walks and stationary bicycling can help in weight control and can improve the patient's sense of well-being. Supplemental oxygen is often required during exercise. Severe hypoxemia ($PaO_2 < 55$ mmHg) at rest or during exercise should be managed with supplemental oxygen.

Education in energy management techniques may provide patients with the means to do more of their daily activities, hence improving their quality of life. For example, using labor-saving devices to simplify work, planning daily priorities, pacing physical activity, and improving breathing and body mechanics can significantly contribute to energy conservation.

Crockett AJ, Cranston JM, Antic N: Domiciliary oxygen for interstitial lung disease. Cochrane Database Syst Rev (3)CD002883, 2001.

CHAPTER 41

SARCOIDOSIS

Marc A. Judson, MD

1. **What is sarcoidosis?**

   Sarcoidosis is a systemic granulomatous disease of unknown origin that can affect any organ in the body. The lungs, eyes, skin, liver, and lymphatic systems are most commonly involved. The diagnosis of sarcoidosis is excluded if a known cause of granulomatous inflammation (e.g., tuberculosis or fungal disease) is identified.

2. **How is sarcoidosis diagnosed?**

   The diagnosis of sarcoidosis is usually established when suggestive clinical or radiologic findings are supported by histologic evidence of noncaseating granulomatous inflammation. Ideally, noncaseating granulomatous inflammation should be demonstrated in at least two organs because sarcoidosis is a systemic disease. In clinical practice, however, once biopsy-confirmed granulomas have been demonstrated in a single organ, sarcoidosis can be assumed to be present in a second organ without biopsy confirmation if clinical features compatible with the diagnosis are present and if there are no other explanations for the clinical findings. Sarcoidosis can also be diagnosed without a biopsy if the clinical features are so typical for the diagnosis that alternative diagnoses are extremely unlikely. An example of such a presentation is Löfgren's syndrome, which presents with a tender erythematous skin rash over the extensor surfaces of the extremities, bilateral hilar adenopathy on chest radiograph, and, often, fever and ankle arthritis.

3. **What causes sarcoidosis?**

   The cause of sarcoidosis is unknown. Studies have suggested that sarcoidosis is associated with certain infectious agents such as mycobacterium tuberculosis, nontuberculous mycobacteria, *Chlamydia* species, mycoplasma, and propionibacter acnes. Other studies have found an association between sarcoidosis and certain occupational exposures such as insecticides, glass fibers, rock wool, titanium, aluminum, and photocopier dust, which contains silica, iron, and copper. Many studies have been conflicting, with some showing no associations with these exposures.

   There are numerous reports of familial clustering of sarcoidosis. In the United States, 19% of African Americans have an affected first-degree relative, compared with 5% of Caucasians. Evidence of significant family clustering has also been reported in Ireland and Japan.

   These data suggest that multiple causes of sarcoidosis may exist and that the condition results from exposure of genetically susceptible hosts to specific agents.

4. **What evidence exists that antigen exposure causes sarcoidosis?**

   Granulomatous inflammation in conditions with known causes, such as tuberculosis, develops when antigen-presenting cells (i.e., histiocytes or macrophages) engulf and process antigens and then present antigen protein through a Class II human leukocyte antigen (HLA) molecule to a T-cell receptor on a T lymphocyte. This interaction results in the release of various cytokines that include interleukin 12 (IL-12) and tumor necrosis factor alpha (TNF-α) from the antigen-presenting cells and interferon-gamma and interleukin 2 (IL-2) from the T lymphocytes. These and other cytokines are of the T-helper-1 type and result in T-cell proliferation, macrophage recruitment, and resultant granuloma formation.

Although the antigens that cause granulomatous inflammation in sarcoidosis are unknown, various HLA Class II molecule polymorphisms are known to occur. This finding suggests that different antigens may cause sarcoidosis in different patients, as determined by an individual's unique immune response to antigen exposure. An interplay between specific combinations of exposures and host responses in the pathogenesis of sarcoidosis would explain why so many studies have come to conflicting conclusions regarding the etiology of the disease.

5. **Who gets sarcoidosis?**
Sarcoidosis occurs worldwide and affects all races and ages. The disease shows a predilection for the third decade of life, although a smaller second peak occurs in people over 50. There is a slightly higher prevalence rate in women. Sarcoidosis has certain geographic distributions; it is more frequent farther away from the equator. The frequency and severity of the disease also vary among different ethnicities and races. The highest prevalence of sarcoidosis is found in Sweden, in Denmark, and in persons of African descent in the United States. In the United States, the lifetime risk of sarcoidosis for Caucasians is 0.85%, and it is 2.4% for African Americans. The age-adjusted annual incidence rate of sarcoidosis in the United States is 35.5/100,000 for African Americans and 10.9/100,000 for Caucasians. African Americans tend to have more severe disease, whereas Caucasians are more likely to present with asymptomatic disease. The disease is more common in life-long nonsmokers.

6. **What organs are involved with sarcoidosis?**
Sarcoidosis may affect any organ in the body. The lungs are most commonly involved. Other organs that are frequently affected include the skin, the eyes, the liver, and the lymphatic system. Heart and neurologic involvement are less common but may be life threatening. Sarcoidosis may also affect the muscles, bones, bone marrow, sinuses, breast, spleen, and salivary glands. Sarcoidosis can cause a disorder in calcium metabolism leading to hypercalcemia, hyperkaluria, and nephrolithiasis. The disease may also result in constitutional symptoms of fatigue, weight loss, fever, and night sweats, which may be the result of the cytokine release discussed in question 3.

KEY POINTS: SARCOIDOSIS ORGAN INVOLVEMENT

1. The lung is the most common organ involved with sarcoidosis.
2. Sarcoidosis is a systemic disease, and involvement of multiple organs is required for a definitive diagnosis.
3. The eyes, skin, liver, and lymphatic systems are also commonly involved.
4. The most common cause of death from sarcoidosis in the United States is from lung involvement, which manifests as the insidious onset of respiratory failure over several years.
5. Heart sarcoidosis and neurosarcoidosis account for the remainder of deaths attributable to sarcoidosis.

7. **What are the typical features of pulmonary sarcoidosis?**
Sarcoid granulomas develop throughout the lung parenchyma, but they present most prominently in the upper two-thirds of the lung. They are common along the bronchovascular bundles, subpleural locations, and intralobular septae and also in the airways. Sarcoidosis also commonly involves the intrathoracic lymph nodes, particularly the hilar and paratracheal nodes. Less-common areas of involvement include the pulmonary vasculature and the pleura.

Many patients with pulmonary sarcoidosis are asymptomatic, even if their chest radiograph is abnormal. Nonproductive cough and dyspnea are the most common symptoms. Substernal pleuritic chest pain is also common. Because sarcoidosis may involve the airways, wheezing can be a prominent symptom and is often underappreciated. In contrast to idiopathic pulmonary fibrosis (IPF), auscultation typically reveals a quiet chest without crackles. Finger clubbing is rare unless there is associated bronchiectasis.

8. How is the severity of sarcoidosis staged?

Chest roentgenographic abnormalities occur in 90–95% of patients with pulmonary sarcoidosis. Bilateral hilar adenopathy is present in 50–85% of patients at diagnosis, and parenchymal disease is seen in 25–50%. A radiographic staging system was developed in the 1960s, as follows:

- **Stage 0:** Normal chest radiograph
- **Stage 1:** Bilateral hilar adenopathy, normal lung parenchyma
- **Stage 2:** Bilateral hilar adenopathy, nonfibrotic infiltrates
- **Stage 3:** No adenopathy, nonfibrotic infiltrates
- **Stage 4:** Fibrotic infiltrates, irrespective of adenopathy

In general, as the radiographic stage increases, the pulmonary function worsens and the likelihood of spontaneous remission decreases. The clinical utility of this stage system has been challenged because there is a poor correlation between radiographic stage and subjective impairment in individual patients. Computed tomography (CT) scans are not necessary for the routine diagnostic evaluation or follow-up of most patients with sarcoidosis.

As mentioned previously, sarcoidosis may involve the airways. Therefore, unlike most interstitial lung diseases that demonstrate a restrictive ventilatory defect, pulmonary sarcoidosis may manifest as an obstructive lung disease or a restrictive lung disease, or obstruction and restriction may occur concomitantly. Diffusion capacity is often normal. Gas exchange remains normal until late in the disease course. Resting hypoxemia and reductions in carbon monoxide diffusion in the lung (DLCO) are not commonly seen except with fibrocystic (Stage 4) disease or pulmonary hypertension (PH), which may develop.

9. What are the typical features of skin sarcoidosis?

Sarcoidosis skin lesions may be specific, showing noncaseating granulomas on biopsy, or nonspecific, showing a nondiagnostic inflammatory reaction pattern.

- **Specific skin lesions** include maculopapular eruptions, subcutaneous nodular lesions, skin plaques, infiltration of old scars, and lupus pernio. Lupus pernio is the most specific skin lesion of sarcoidosis. It is an indolent, red-purple or violaceous disfiguring skin lesion that usually affects the nose, cheeks, ears, and forehead. It is associated with chronic fibrotic pulmonary sarcoidosis.
- **Nonspecific sarcoidosis skin lesions** include erythema nodosum. This lesion is not diagnostic of sarcoidosis as it can be seen with infections, neoplasms, vasculitides, and drug reactions. However, when erythema nodosum is associated with bilateral hilar adenopathy on chest radiograph, it is called Löfgren's syndrome and, as mentioned in Question 2, is often specific enough for sarcoidosis to be clinically diagnosed without tissue confirmation. Erythema nodosum usually suggests a good prognosis.

10. What are the typical features of eye sarcoidosis?

- **Acute anterior uveitis** is the most common form of eye sarcoidosis and may present with acute onset of pain, photophobia, blurred vision, and red eyes. Up to one-third of patients with anterior uveitis will be asymptomatic; hence, a screening eye examination is required for all diagnosed sarcoidosis patients regardless of symptoms.
- **Chronic anterior uveitis** occurs in older patients, and the eye complaints tend to be milder. Posterior segment involvement, including vitreitis, may be the only manifestation of eye disease. Optic nerve involvement may occur, but it is rare.

- **Lacrimal gland** involvement may occur with gland swelling and keratoconjunctivitis sicca.
- **Conjunctival nodules**
- **Glaucoma and cataracts** may develop from the inflammation of sarcoid uveitis or steroid use. Therefore, it may be problematic to determine if corticosteroids are beneficial or harmful when these complications develop.
- **Heerfordt's syndrome,** or **uveoparotid fever,** is a classic presentation of sarcoidosis that features uveitis, parotiditis, fever, and facial or other cranial nerve palsies. Löfgren's syndrome, as mentioned previously, presents with erythema nodosum and bilateral hilar adenopathy on chest radiography and may also be associated with arthritis and iritis.
- **Posterior segment involvement**

11. **What are the typical features of cardiac sarcoidosis?**
    The clinical manifestations of cardiac sarcoidosis depend on the location and extent of the myocardial involvement. Most clinical problems are related to cardiac arrhythmias or left ventricular dysfunction. Electrocardiographic abnormalities include ventricular ectopy, ventricular tachycardia, atrioventricular block (including complete heart block), and supraventricular arrhythmias. Sudden death may occur. Congestive heart failure occurs when the myocardium is massively infiltrated with granulomata. Cardiomegaly occurs in fewer than 5% of patients with myocardial sarcoidosis, but more subtle abnormalities may occur, such as localized or diffuse wall motion abnormalities, thickening or subsequent thinning of the left ventricular free wall, papillary muscle dysfunction causing mitral valve prolapse or regurgitation, and diastolic stiffening of the left ventricle. Clinical pericarditis may occur. A multivariate analysis showed that death from myocardial sarcoidosis was related to New York Heart Association (NYHA) class, the left ventricular end-diastolic diameter, and the presence of sustained ventricular tachycardia.

12. **How is cardiac sarcoidosis diagnosed?**
    The diagnosis of myocardial sarcoidosis can be made definitively by endomyocardial biopsy. Although this is a specific test, it is only positive in 25–50% of cases because of the patchy distribution of the disease. Echocardiography may suggest the diagnosis if thinning, fibrosis, or wall motion abnormalities are seen that do not correspond to the distribution of the coronary circulation. Thallium-201 imaging suggests the diagnosis of sarcoidosis if focal defects on the myocardial wall at rest are not evident during the exercise or dipyridamole phase, the so-called reverse-redistribution phenomenon. Myocardial sarcoidosis may also be detected on gallium-67 scanning, gadolinium-enhanced magnetic resonance imaging (MRI), and positron emission tomography (PET).
    An electrocardiogram (ECG) has been recommended for every patient diagnosed with sarcoidosis. Clearly, patients with palpitations, syncope, chest pain, or signs of congestive heart failure should undergo a detailed evaluation that should include testing for arrhythmias and conduction system abnormalities, evaluation of left ventricular function, and invasive or noninvasive testing for the presence and extent of myocardial disease from sarcoidosis.

13. **What are the typical features of neurosarcoidosis?**
    Any portion of the central nervous system (CNS) or peripheral nervous system may be affected by sarcoidosis.
    - **Cranial neuropathies** are the most common manifestation. The facial nerve is the most common cranial nerve involved, causing a **Bell's palsy**. Often, a Bell's palsy develops prior to the diagnosis of sarcoidosis and has completely resolved once other manifestations of sarcoidosis appear.
    - **Peripheral neuropathy**
    - **Mass lesions** may develop in the **brain** or **spinal cord.**
    - **Diffuse encephalopathy**
    - **Aseptic meningitis** may occur with sarcoidosis. The findings in the cerebrospinal fluid (CSF) include a pleocytosis, usually of lymphocytes, and elevated protein levels. One in five cases with sarcoid meningitis has a low glucose level in the CSF (i.e., hypoglycorrhachia).
    - **Hydrocephalus**

14. **What are the typical features of other organs that are involved with sarcoidosis?**

Disturbances in calcium metabolism occur in sarcoidosis patients. The primary defect involves excessive alpha$_1$ hydroxylation of 25-hydroxyvitamin D to 1,25-dihydroxyvitamin D. This may lead to increased gut absorption of calcium, hypercalciuria, and hypercalcemia. The reported incidence of hypercalcemia is approximately 10%, whereas hypercalciuria is more common. The most common clinically important consequence of abnormal calcium is nephrolithiasis.

Acute sarcoid arthritis is often seen with Löfgren's syndrome. The ankles are almost always affected, but the knees, elbows, and wrists are often involved too. Chronic sarcoid arthritis is rare. It is usually a nondestructive polyarticular, oligoarticular, or monoarticular arthropathy that may involve the shoulder joints, wrists, knees, ankles, and small joints of the hands and feet. Joint fluid reveals inflammatory features with mononuclear or polymorphonuclear cell predominance, and synovial biopsy usually shows noncaseating granulomas.

Diffuse nonspecific myalgias or joint and muscle stiffness may occur in sarcoidosis patients; these symptoms are often major complaints and are often accompanied by fatigue and depression. These symptoms resemble those of fibromyalgia rheumatica. It is unknown if these symptoms relate to general symptoms associated with a chronic disease or if they relate to specific cytokines or another mechanism directly related to sarcoidosis. Carpal tunnel syndrome has also been reported with increased frequency in sarcoidosis patients.

Sarcoidosis may present in muscles as palpable nodules, chronic myopathy, atrophy, or acute myositis. Osseous involvement of sarcoidosis most commonly occurs in the hands and the feet but may be detected in any bone. Lesions are usually asymptomatic but can be painful. Lace-like lesions are often seen on radiographs of involved fingers and toes.

Hematologic abnormalities are common in sarcoidosis but rarely are of clinical significance. Anemia occurs in 5–28% of sarcoidosis patients. Leukopenia, lymphopenia, and eosinophilia are quite common. Thrombocytopenia is the least-common abnormality of all the blood cell lines.

The frequency of splenic involvement in sarcoidosis has been reported to range from 10% to over 50%, depending on whether it is detected on physical examination, a radiographic test, or a tissue biopsy. Five to fourteen percent of sarcoidosis patients have a palpable spleen on physical examination, whereas splenic sarcoidosis can be found histologically on biopsy in more than half of all sarcoidosis patients. CT scans of splenic sarcoidosis reveal splenomegaly and multiple discrete low-attenuation nodules. Patients with histologic evidence of splenic sarcoidosis usually have no symptoms related to involvement of this organ. Constitutional symptoms such as malaise, fever, and night sweats may develop. Hypersplenism with pancytopenia seldom occurs, and splenic rupture has rarely been reported.

Enlargement of peripheral lymph nodes is often observed during the course of sarcoidosis. The cervical lymph nodes are most commonly affected, although any lymph node may be involved. Occasionally, peripheral lymphadenopathy from sarcoidosis can become massive, and this presentation can be confused with lymphoma.

Sarcoidosis may involve any portion of the upper respiratory tract. The epiglottis, false vocal cords, arytenoids, larynx, and subglottic area may be involved. Involvement of the sinuses may range from hypertrophy of sinus tissue to ulceration, cartilage destruction, intracranial invasion, and saddle-nose deformity.

Parotid and salivary gland involvement may occur in sarcoidosis. Parotid involvement is seen in approximately 6% of cases. Parotid sarcoidosis involvement may be part of Heerfordt's syndrome and additionally may include uveitis, fever, and cranial nerve palsies (especially of the facial nerve). Parotid and salivary gland involvement may cause dry mouth, which may become chronic.

15. **What should the initial work-up of a patient with sarcoidosis include?**

Patients with sarcoidosis should have:
- **Medical history:** This should include particular attention to occupation and environment exposures because metal exposures such as beryllium may cause granulomatous disease

and inhalation of bioaerosols may cause hypersensitivity pneumonitis. Risk factors for tuberculosis and fungal diseases should be explored. The medical history should also question the patient concerning symptoms of pulmonary and extrapulmonary sarcoidosis.

- **Physical examination:** Auscultation of the chest is usually normal in pulmonary sarcoidosis, but extrapulmonary findings may be detected.
- **Purified protein-derivative tuberculosis skin test**

  An assessment of pulmonary involvement and severity should include the following:
- **Posteroanterior chest radiograph**
- **Measurement of spirometry and diffusing capacity**

  Detection and assessment of extrapulmonary sarcoidosis should include the following:
- Peripheral blood and platelet count
- Serum chemistries
- Serum calcium
- Liver function tests
- Serum blood urea nitrogen
- Serum creatinine
- Urinalysis
- ECG
- Ophthalmologic exam, including slit-lamp and retinal examination

16. **Is sarcoidosis fatal?**

    Sarcoidosis is rarely fatal. It is estimated that 3–5% of sarcoidosis patients will die from the disease. In these United States, three-quarters of the sarcoidosis deaths are from pulmonary sarcoidosis. These deaths are, for the most part, from respiratory failure that develops over 5–25 years. These patients have stage 4 fibrocystic sarcoidosis exclusively. The remaining deaths result from cardiac sarcoidosis and neurosarcoidosis. Death from involvement of these two organs may be abrupt and unexpected. In Japan, cardiac sarcoidosis is much more common than in the United States, and it is the leading cause of death.

17. **What is the prognosis of sarcoidosis?**

    The prognosis of sarcoidosis depends on the extent and severity of organ involvement. Patients with a stage I chest radiograph undergo spontaneous remission 60–80% of the time, while patients with stage II and stage III radiographs remit in 50–60% and less than 30% of cases, respectively. Patients presenting with Löfgren's syndrome have an excellent prognosis, with a rate of resolution exceeding 80%. Factors associated with a chronic course of disease include chronic uveitis, lupus pernio, cystic bone lesions, and chronic hypercalcemia. African-American patients also tend to have a higher rate of extrapulmonary involvement and a more severe disease than Caucasians.

18. **Does sarcoidosis mandate treatment?**

    Sarcoidosis does not mandate treatment because the disease may undergo spontaneous remission and there are significant potential toxicities from therapy. Pulmonary sarcoidosis may be observed unless pulmonary symptoms are severe or there is severe pulmonary dysfunction. Other forms of sarcoidosis that do not mandate treatment are asymptomatic hepatic sarcoidosis with mild to moderate elevations of serum liver function tests, bone marrow involvement causing a mild reduction in cell lines, and mild hyperkalemia or hyperkaluria that can be diet controlled. Symptomatic cardiac sarcoidosis always requires treatment as the disease may be life threatening, causing sudden death. Neurosarcoidosis, other than a Bell's palsy, usually requires treatment as it too may be suddenly life threatening.

19. **What is the standard treatment of sarcoidosis?**

    Corticosteroids are the usual treatment of sarcoidosis. Topical corticosteroids can be used when the disease is localized (e.g., corticosteroid creams or injections for localized skin lesions or corticosteroid eye drops for anterior sarcoid uveitis). Systemic corticosteroids must be used for diffuse skin disease, for eye disease deeper than the anterior chamber, and for visceral organ involvement.

KEY POINTS: TREATMENT OF SARCOIDOSIS

1. Treatment of sarcoidosis is not mandated.

2. Corticosteroids are the drug of choice.

3. Topical steroids can be given in the form of corticosteroid creams and injections for localized skin lesions and corticosteroid eye drops for anterior sarcoid uveitis.

4. Cardiac sarcoidosis and neurosarcoidosis (with the exception of Bell's palsy) always require treatment as these forms of sarcoidosis may be suddenly life threatening.

The dose of corticosteroids has not been standardized, and the effective dose varies depending on the organ involved. Pulmonary sarcoidosis almost always responds to an initial dose of 20–40 mg of prednisone equivalent per day. This dose can rapidly be tapered to 0.05–0.2 mg/kg prednisone equivalent per day within 2–8 weeks. Usually, therapy should be continued for 3–9 months as shorter courses of therapy are associated with relapse.

There is evidence that treatment may promote relapse, possibly by impairing the granuloma formation that was described in question 3. This further supports the concept that sarcoidosis does not mandate treatment unless there is a clinical reason for therapy, as outlined in question 15. In general, skin sarcoidosis (especially lupus pernio), cardiac sarcoidosis, and neurosarcoidosis are relatively recalcitrant to corticosteroid therapy and often require high doses.

20. **What alternative pharmacotherapy may be used for sarcoidosis?**
Several alternative agents have been found useful in sarcoidosis, although none has been subjected to a controlled clinical trial. The efficacy of a particular drug depends on the organ being treated.

- **Methotrexate** is the most-studied medicine for sarcoidosis next to corticosteroids. It has been found to improve spirometry and to reduce bronchoalveolar lavage lymphocyte counts to the same degree as corticosteroids. It seems to be particularly useful for lung, skin, brain, eye, joint, and neurosarcoidosis. Despite the potential for methotrexate to cause hepatotoxicity, it is not contraindicated for treatment of hepatic sarcoidosis.

- **Hydroxychloroquine** and **chloroquine** are most useful for the treatment of skin and joint sarcoidosis and for the treatment of hypercalcemia and hyperkaluria from sarcoidosis. Although chloroquine is more potent than hydroxychloroquine, its potential for retinal toxicity is greater.

- **Azathioprine** is not a potent antisarcoidosis agent, but it may be useful for selected patients with pulmonary or eye sarcoidosis.

- **Cyclophosphamide** is an effective agent for sarcoidosis, but its toxicity (causing, e.g., hemorrhagic cystitis and bladder cancer) prohibit its routine use except for neurosarcoidosis, which is often life threatening.

- Tetracycline derivatives such as **minocycline** and **doxycycline** may be useful for skin sarcoidosis.

- Drugs with activity against tumor necrosis factor, such as **thalidomide** and **pentoxifylline,** have some antisarcoidosis activity.

- **Monoclonal antibodies,** versus **tumor necrosis factor,** have also been shown to be effective in several case series of sarcoidosis patients, especially infliximab.

21. **When should organ transplantation be considered for sarcoidosis?**
Organ transplantation has been performed for pulmonary, cardiac, and hepatic sarcoidosis. Organ transplantation should be considered when all alternative treatments for sarcoidosis have

been exhausted. This should include, at a minimum, a reasonable trial of corticosteroids and at least one alternative agent. In the cases of pulmonary and hepatic sarcoidosis, transplantation should be considered if the disease is not only severe but also progressive. In the case of cardiac sarcoidosis, transplantation should be considered if there are significant risk factors for sudden death (see Questions 9 and 14). Although sarcoidosis is a systemic disease, transplantation should only be considered if the disease is minimal in the organs not being transplanted. Sarcoidosis often recurs in the allograft, which suggests that the disease involves a transmissible agent or, possibly, permanent alteration of the host's immune response.

BIBLIOGRAPHY

1. Baughman RP, Teirstein AS, Judson MA, et al: Clinical characteristics of patients in a case control study of sarcoidosis. Am J Respir Crit Care Med 164:1885–1889, 2001.

2. Hunninghake GW, Costabel U, Ando M, et al: ATS/ERS/WASOG statement on sarcoidosis. Sarcoid Vasc Diff Lung Dis 16:149–173, 1999.

3. Judson MA: Clinical aspects of sarcoidosis. J S C Med Assoc 96:9–17, 2000.

4. Judson MA, Baughman RP, Teirstein AS, for the ACCESS Research Group: Defining organ involvement in sarcoidosis: The ACCESS proposed instrument. Sarcoidosis Vasc Diffuse Lung Dis 16:75–86, 1999.

5. Judson MA, Baughman RP: Sarcoidosis. In Baughman RP, DuBois RM (eds): Diffuse Lung Disease: A Practical Approach. London, Arnold, 2004, pp 109–129.

6. Lynch JP, Kazerooni EA, Gay SE: Pulmonary sarcoidosis. Clin Chest Med 755–785, 1997.

7. Newman LS, Rose CS, Maier LA: Sarcoidosis. N Engl J Med 1224–1234, 1997.

CHAPTER 42

IDIOPATHIC PULMONARY FIBROSIS

John E. Heffner, MD

1. **What is idiopathic interstitial pneumonia?**

   Idiopathic interstitial pneumonia is a relentlessly progressive chronic fibrosing interstitial pneumonia of unknown etiology that is characterized by the histopathologic presence of usual interstitial pneumonia (UIP). The hallmark of UIP is a heterogeneous distribution of normal lung interspersed among regions of interstitial inflammation, fibroblast foci, and honeycombing. Fibroblast foci are collections of proliferating fibroblasts and myoblasts adjacent to damaged epithelial cells and basement membranes. These abnormalities occur most prominently in the peripheral subpleural regions of the lung. Idiopathic pulmonary fibrosis (IPF) is one form of the several different types of idiopathic interstitial pneumonia, which are subtypes of the broader category of diffuse interstitial lung disease (ILD).

   American Thoracic Society/European Respiratory Society: Idiopathic pulmonary fibrosis: Diagnosis and treatment. International consensus statement. Am J Respir Crit Care Med 161:646, 2000.

2. **Why do patients get IPF?**

   The pathogenesis and etiology of IPF remain unknown despite extensive investigation. Present theories center on the occurrence of one or more nonspecific microinjuries to airway epithelial cells that initiate an influx of fibroblasts and aberrant wound healing. The source of this injury is unknown, although infections, cigarette smoking, recurrent aspiration, drugs, and environmental pollutants have been proposed. These exogenous factors may require a genetic predisposition to cause the fibrotic response, although no underlying genetic or other host factors have been identified. Once initiated, the fibrosing process of IPF is self perpetuating and unremitting. Abnormal production of cytokines and growth factors in the lung may underlie progressive fibrosis. Although inflammation has been previously considered to be the initial pathophysiologic event in IPF, little histologic evidence of inflammation exists in lung biopsies when patients first present with symptoms.

   Noble PW, Homer RJ: Idiopathic pulmonary fibrosis: New insights into pathogenesis. Clin Chest Med 25:749–758, 2004.

   Thannickal VJ, Flaherty KR, Martinez FJ, Lynch JP 3rd: Idiopathic pulmonary fibrosis: Emerging concepts on pharmacotherapy. Expert Opin Pharmacother 5:1671–1686, 2004.

3. **What are the histopathologic features of IPF and UIP?**

   UIP has a specific histopathologic appearance with fibrotic zones characterized by scattered areas of fibroblastic proliferation (i.e., fibroblastic foci) with dense depositions of disorganized collagen. Other areas of the lung have honeycomb changes that comprise mucin-filled cystic fibrotic airspaces, often those lined by bronchiolar epithelium. Patchy interstitial inflammation involves alveolar septae, which have abnormal infiltrates of plasma cells, lymphocytes, and histiocytes. Evidence of hyperplasia of type 2 pneumocytes is also present. Smooth muscle hyperplasia is often found in regions of fibrosis and honeycombing. An identical histopathologic appearance occurs in patients with pulmonary fibrosis due to collagen vascular disease and several other conditions. The term UIP, however, is reserved for those biopsies in which the etiology of pulmonary fibrosis is unknown. When lung biopsy samples are taken during periods of rapid deterioration of lung function, histologic features of diffuse alveolar damage often coexist with findings of UIP.

KEY POINTS: HISTOPATHOLOGIC DIAGNOSES TO BE EXCLUDED ✓ IN EVALUATING LUNG BIOPSY SPECIMENS FOR IDIOPATHIC PULMONARY FIBROSIS

1. Desquamative interstitial pneumonia
2. Respiratory bronchiolitis–associated ILD
3. Nonspecific interstitial pneumonias
4. Acute interstitial pneumonia
5. Cryptogenic organizing pneumonia
6. Lymphocytic interstitial pneumonitis
7. Langerhans cell histiocytosis
8. Asbestosis
9. Connective tissue disease
10. Chronic hypersensitivity pneumonitis
11. Drug-induced lung diseases

4. **Who gets IPF?**
Men are affected more commonly than women. Most patients are middle-aged (i.e., 40–70 years old), with two-thirds of patients being over the age of 60 at the time of initial presentation. IPF does not occur more commonly in any geographic region and does not have a predilection for race or ethnicity. Although most cases of IPF are sporadic, a familial form of the disease occurs.

5. **How do patients with IPF present?**
Most patients present with an insidious onset of dyspnea with exertion and a nonproductive cough. Patients may have noted dyspnea for 6 months before seeking medical attention. Crackles are audible at the lung bases in more than 80% of patients and have been described to have a "Velcro" quality. Crackles are heard throughout all lung fields as the disease progresses. Digital clubbing is noted in 25–50% of patients. Pulmonary hypertension (PH) with clinical features of cor pulmonale may be apparent during the middle or late stages of the disease. Systemic signs or symptoms, other than generalized fatigue and weight loss, do not occur.

6. **What does IPF look like on a standard chest radiograph?**
Almost all patients with IPF have an abnormal chest radiograph at initial presentation. A normal chest radiograph, however, does not exclude the disease in patients with suggestive clinical manifestations. The standard chest radiograph demonstrates peripheral reticular opacities that are most prominent at the lung bases. These opacities are bilateral and usually asymmetric. The radiographic estimates of lung volumes are usually decreased. Confluent airspace opacities, pleural effusions, or mediastinal lymphadenopathy do not occur in IPF and suggest alternative diagnoses. Smokers with combined emphysema and IPF may demonstrate preserved or increased lung volumes with upper lobe oligemia. Even when radiologists using high-resolution computed tomography (HRCT) scanning are highly confident that an abnormal radiograph is diagnostic of IPF, they are correct in only 48–87% of instances.

7. **Does HRCT scanning assist the diagnosis?**

The radiographic pattern of IPF on HRCT scanning consists of patchy, primarily peripheral, subpleural, bibasal reticular abnormalities. Some ground-glass changes may also be noted, but involvement of more than 30% of the lung with this finding suggests an alternative diagnosis. Traction bronchiectasis and bronchiolectasis with subpleural honeycombing occur in more severely affected lung regions. Experienced radiologists can make a confident diagnosis of IPF by HRCT alone in only two-thirds of patients with the disease. The diagnostic accuracy of a "confident" HRCT reading for IPF is 90%. Similar HRCT findings occur in patients with scleroderma, rheumatoid arthritis, and asbestosis. Because physiologic testing is more sensitive than HRCT in detecting minimal manifestations of the disease, a normal HRCT does not exclude IPF.

Orens JB, Kazerooni EA, Martinez FJ, et al: The sensitivity of high-resolution CT in detecting idiopathic pulmonary fibrosis proved by open lung biopsy. A prospective study. Chest 108:109–115, 1995.

8. **What are the typical abnormalities noted on pulmonary function testing?**

Patients with IPF demonstrate a restrictive pattern on physiologic testing with decreased vital capacity (VC), residual volume (RV), total lung capacity (TLC) and thoracic gas volume. Smokers with emphysema may demonstrate normal lung volumes because the obstructive findings of airway obstruction and the restrictive findings of IPF counterbalance. Lung diffusion is usually decreased, and abnormalities in carbon monoxide diffusion in the lung (DLCO) often precede measured decreases in lung volumes.

Some patients with early IPF may have normal physiologic test results at rest. The presence of unexplained dyspnea in a patient with normal resting pulmonary function studies represents a need for exercise testing. Patients with IPF have stiff lungs and ventilation-perfusion (V/Q) mismatching that cause rapid shallow breathing and hypoxia during exercise.

9. **How can patients with IPF be diagnosed?**

The diagnosis of IPF begins with a careful history, physical, and laboratory evaluation. Although no clinical findings or tests short of lung biopsy can confirm the diagnosis, alternate explanations for dyspnea may be detected by a comprehensive examination. Most patients undergo fiberoptic bronchoscopy with bronchoalveolar lavage (BAL) and transbronchial biopsy in order to identify other diagnoses such as malignancy or sarcoidosis. No bronchoscopic findings, however, are diagnostic of IPF. IPF is diagnosed with certainty only by demonstrating the presence of UIP in a biopsied lung specimen obtained by thoracoscopy or a limited thoracotomy in patients without clinical evidence of known causes of UIP, which include asbestosis, connective tissue diseases, chronic hypersensitivity pneumonitis, and drug-induced lung diseases.

KEY POINTS: CRITERIA THAT MUST BE FULFILLED TO ✔ CONFIRM A DIAGNOSIS OF IDIOPATHIC PULMONARY FIBROSIS

1. Exclusion of known causes of ILD

2. Compatible pulmonary function test abnormalities that include a reduced VC, often with an increased ratio of the forced expiratory volume in 1 second (FEV_1) to forced vital capacity (FVC) or with impaired gas exchange (i.e., an increased alveolar-to-arterial pressure difference for O_2 at rest or exercise or a decreased DLCO)

3. Compatible findings on conventional chest radiographs or HRCT

10. **What if the patient cannot undergo a lung biopsy?**

Elderly patients, patients with severely compromised lung function, or patients with extensive honeycombing findings on radiographic studies may not tolerate lung biopsy. In the absence of histopathologic confirmation of UIP, a presumptive diagnosis of IPF may be made if patients fulfill all of the following major diagnostic criteria and at least three of the four minor criteria:

Major criteria

- Exclusion of other known causes of ILD
- Evidence of restriction and impaired gas exchange on pulmonary testing
- Bibasilar reticular abnormalities with minimal ground-glass features on HRCT scanning
- Absence of features suggestive of alternative diagnoses on transbronchial lung biopsy specimens or bronchoalveolar lavage samples

Minor criteria

- Age older than 50 years
- Insidious onset of unexplained dyspnea on exertion
- Duration of illness greater than 3 months
- Bibasilar, inspiratory crackles of a "Velcro" quality

It should be noted that some patients will be misclassified in the absence of a surgical lung biopsy, and the number misclassified will depend on the experience and skills of the evaluating clinicians and radiologists.

Peckham RM, Shorr AF, Helman DL Jr: Potential limitations of clinical criteria for the diagnosis of idiopathic pulmonary fibrosis/cryptogenic fibrosing alveolitis. Respiration 71:165–169, 2004.

Raghu G, Mageto YN, Lockhart D, et al: The accuracy of the clinical diagnosis of new-onset idiopathic pulmonary fibrosis and other interstitial lung disease: A prospective study. Chest. 116:1168–1174, 1999.

11. **What are the therapeutic options available for patients with IPF?**

Current therapies are of unproven benefit for IPF. Based on the rationale that lung inflammation precedes the fibrotic response, patients have been treated with various anti-inflammatory drugs that include corticosteroids and immunosuppressive agents such as cyclophosphamide and azathioprine. The poor response with these drugs, however, corresponds to the paucity of inflammation as compared with fibrosis found in lung biopsy specimens of patients who present with early symptoms of IPF. Emerging concepts of the pathogenesis of IPF that emphasize an initial epithelial injury followed by exaggerated fibroblast proliferation with excessive deposition of collagen suggest the value of newer drugs. These newer drugs, such as interferon gamma-1b, bosentan, zileuton, etanercept, pirfenidone, and N-acetylcysteine, focus on enhancing re-epithelialization and modulating fibroblastic and myofibroblastic foci. To date, however, no evidence demonstrates an improvement in mortality for interferon gamma-1b, which is the only newer drug that has undergone a large-scale clinical trial.

Collard HR, Ryu JH, Douglas WW, et al: Corticosteroid and cyclophosphamide therapy does not alter survival in idiopathic pulmonary fibrosis. Chest 125:2169–2174, 2004.

Raghu G, Chang J: Idiopathic pulmonary fibrosis: Current trends in management. Clin Chest Med 25:621–636, 2004.

Richeldi L, Davies HR, Ferrara G, Franco F: Corticosteroids for idiopathic pulmonary fibrosis. Cochrane Database Syst Rev (3):CD002880, 2003.

Thannickal VJ, Flaherty KR, Martinez FJ, Lynch JP III: Idiopathic pulmonary fibrosis: Emerging concepts in pharmacotherapy. Expert Opin Pharmacother 5:1671–1686, 2004.

12. **How are the effects of therapy monitored?**

In the absence of demonstrated effective therapy, most patients with IPF undergo a therapeutic trial with corticosteroids, immunosuppressive drugs, or both because of the poor prognosis associated with the disease. Markers of a therapeutic effect include decreased respiratory symptoms of cough and dyspnea with improved exercise tolerance, complete or partial resolution of radiographic abnormalities, a 25% increase in measured TLC or VC, a 40% increase in single-breath DLCO, or diminution of any oxygen desaturations during exercise. Stability of any of these clinical findings is also considered a therapeutic response.

13. **What can be done for patients who progress despite aggressive therapy?**

Otherwise healthy patients can be considered for lung transplantation. Single lung transplantation is most commonly performed for patients with IPF. Some centers limit transplantation for patients younger than 60 years of age. Ideal timing for transplantation has not been established, but patients with progressive disease should be referred for evaluation for transplantation early because of long waiting lists. The 5-year survival after transplantation is only 50–60%. Pulmonary rehabilitation can improve patients' perceived quality of life. Palliative interventions can relieve dyspnea for patients near the terminal stages of their disease. Some patients rapidly deteriorate with an acute exacerbation of their IPF. Such patients require careful evaluation to exclude pulmonary emboli, respiratory infections, and other reversible conditions. Those patients who require intubation for an acute exacerbation of IPF rarely survive to hospital discharge.

Al-Hameed FM, Sharma S: Outcome of patients admitted to the intensive care unit for acute exacerbation of idiopathic pulmonary fibrosis. Can Respir J 11:117–122, 2004.

CHAPTER 43

COLLAGEN VASCULAR DISEASE

Marvin I. Schwarz, MD

1. **Which components of the respiratory system are affected by the collagen vascular diseases (CVDs)?**

   Essentially, the CVDs can affect all components of the thorax including the lung parenchyma (i.e., the interstitium and pulmonary vessels), airways, pleura, and respiratory muscles. Treatments can also cause lung toxicity, such as the use of methotrexate in rheumatoid arthritis and polymyositis, resulting in parenchymal lung disease. Diffuse parenchymal lung disease, or interstitial lung disease (ILD), is most often caused by the CVD itself. Moreover, unusual infections can result from the use of immunosuppressive drugs such as cyclophosphamide and azathioprine (for pneumocystis pneumonia) or tumor necrosis factor-alpha (TFN-α)-blocking agents (for reactivation of tuberculosis).

   Schlesinger PA, Leatherman JW: Update in non-pulmonary critical care: Rheumatology. Am J Resp Crit Care Med 16:1161–1165, 1998.

2. **Can any of the CVDs initially present with pulmonary manifestations?**

   Although infrequent, ILD-complicating rheumatoid arthritis and polymyositis–dermatomyositis and, to a lesser extent, scleroderma may precede the more typical manifestations of these disorders by months to several years. The onset of lupus erythematosus is occasionally heralded by an acute immunologic pneumonia known as acute lupus pneumonitis. Pleuritis with or without pleural effusion can be the initiating event in rheumatoid arthritis, lupus erythematosus, and mixed connective tissue disease. An acute ILD also may be the presenting manifestation of polymyositis.

   Schwarz MI, Albert RK: Imitators of the ARDS. Chest 125:1530–1535, 2004.

3. **Are there any unique characteristics of the pleural effusions associated with the CVDs?**

   In lupus erythematosus, pleurisy and pleural effusion, which occur at some time during the course of the disease in up to 60% of patients, represent the most frequent noninfectious thoracic

---

KEY POINTS: COLLAGEN VASCULAR DISEASES

1. The pulmonary complication may be the presenting manifestation.

2. All CVDs may cause pleuritis except polymyositis–dermatomyositis.

3. Thromboembolism is most likely in patients with systemic lupus erythematosus.

4. Nonspecific interstitial pneumonitis is the most common interstitial lung disease histology present in the CVDs.

5. Scleroderma is associated with the highest incidence of interstitial lung disease when compared to other CVDs.

complication of this condition. Lupus-related effusions are exudates that contain both acute and chronic inflammatory cells. These effusions are characterized by high titers of antinuclear factor and low pleural fluid complement levels. Pleural effusions are also the most common noninfectious thoracic complication of rheumatoid arthritis. Rheumatoid effusions are exudates with mixed inflammatory cell populations and, occasionally, low pleural fluid complement levels. Typically, a low pleural fluid glucose concentration (i.e., less than 30 mg/dL) with rheumatoid factor titers exceeding 1:320 is present in rheumatoid effusions. Empyema, occurring spontaneously and thought to be the result of a ruptured necrobiotic nodule, complicates rheumatoid arthritis.

Sahn SA, Kaplan RL, Maulitz RM, et al: Rheumatoid pleurisy: Observations on the development of low pleural fluid pH and glucose. Arch Intern Med 140:1237–1238, 1980.

4. **What is the fate of a pleural effusion in either lupus erythematosus or rheumatoid arthritis?**
The majority of these effusions are self-limiting and require no more than treatment of symptoms. In some instances, however, persistent pain or increasing pleural effusions may require corticosteroid therapy, which is usually effective. In both disorders, pleural effusions tend to recur, and occasional patients may experience extensive pleural inflammation leading to fibrosis and pleural scarring. This, in turn, may lead to a trapped lung, in which a fibrotic pleural peel prevents adequate lung expansion.

5. **In which CVD is primary pleural involvement not a concern?**
In the CVDs, pleuritis and effusions occur most commonly in lupus erythematosus, mixed connective tissue disease, and rheumatoid arthritis. Pleural disorders occasionally develop in patients with systemic sclerosis (i.e., scleroderma) and Sjögren's syndrome. In systemic sclerosis, clinically apparent pleural disease occurs in only a few patients, but pleural fibrosis is common at postmortem examination. Primary pleural involvement does not occur in patients with polymyositis–dermatomyositis.

Tazelaar HD, Viggiano RW, Pickersgill J, et al: Interstitial lung disease in polymyositis and dermatomyositis: Clinical features and prognosis as correlated with histopathologic findings. Am Rev Respir Dis 144:727–733, 1990.

6. **Which pulmonary problem is most common in patients with the CVDs?**
Community-acquired pneumonia (CAP)—either from bacterial, viral, or mycoplasmal pathogens—or opportunistic organisms resulting from the immunosuppressive therapy used to treat the underlying disease are the most commonly experienced pulmonary problems. In immunosuppressed patients, *Pneumocystis jiroveci*, cytomegalovirus, *Nocardia* species, *Aspergillus* species, herpes simplex pneumonias, tuberculosis, and fungal pneumonitis must be considered when new infiltrates develop with fever. Additionally, patients with scleroderma or polymyositis–dermatomyositis frequently develop recurrent aspiration pneumonia. Aspiration occurs in patients with scleroderma because of esophageal dysmotility and dilatation with resultant gastroesophageal reflux. In polymyositis, inflammation of the upper-esophageal and pharyngeal musculature leads to degeneration of the muscle bundles and resultant dysphagia and aspiration.

Lee JH, Slipman, RL, Gershon SK, et al: Life-threatening histoplasmosis complicating immunotherapy with tumor necrosis antagonists infliximab and etanercept: Arthritis Rheum 4B:2565–2570, 2002.

7. **What causes pulmonary hypertension (PH) in patients with CVDs?**
Patients with CVDs may develop a primary form of PH that is not associated with other abnormalities of the lungs. The vessels undergo plexogenic changes characterized by endothelial proliferation, medial thickening, luminal obliteration, and, eventually, recanalization. This form of PH most commonly occurs in patients with scleroderma and develops, to a lesser extent, in those

with systemic lupus erythematosus, rheumatoid arthritis, and mixed connective tissue disease. A form of PH secondary to fibrotic ILD, occurs in any of the CVDs. The fibrosis results in hypoxemia, which in turn causes vasoconstriction.

8. **Which CVD is most likely to be complicated by pulmonary thromboembolism, and why?**

Patients with lupus erythematosus and, to a lesser extent, those with mixed connective tissue disease have a higher risk for pulmonary embolism (PE) compared to other CVDs. Patients with lupus often have a circulatory anticoagulant with procoagulant activity that predisposes them to deep venous thrombosis (DVT) and subsequent PE. The circulating anticoagulant is an antiphospholipid antibody. There is also a primary antiphospholipid antibody syndrome not associated with lupus.

Petri M, Rheinschmidt M, Whiting-O'Keefe Q, et al: The frequency of lupus anticoagulant in systemic lupus erythematosus study of sixty connective tissue disease patients by activated partial thromboplastin time, Russel viper venom time, and anticardiolipin antibody. Ann Intern Med 106:524–531, 1987.

9. **Can ILD be present in a patient with CVD who has a normal chest radiograph?**

Symptomatic ILD with a normal chest radiograph can occasionally occur in patients with any of the CVDs. In this setting, pulmonary vascular disease (i.e., primary PH or PE) is the first diagnostic consideration. After vascular disease is excluded, evaluation of these patients with a high-resolution computed tomography (HRCT) scan often shows parenchymal abnormalities even if the standard chest radiograph is normal. Moreover, physiologic testing, particularly rest and exercise arterial blood gas levels with measurement of alveolar-to-arterial oxygen gradients and dead space ventilation, may demonstrate abnormalities before any radiographic changes are present.

Petri M, Rheinschmidt M, Whiting-O'Keefe Q, et al: The frequency of lupus anticoagulant in systemic lupus erythematosus: A study of sixty connective tissue disease patients by activated partial thromboplastin time, Russel viper venom time, and anticardiolipin antibody. Ann Intern Med 106: 524–531, 1987.

Tazelaar HD, Viggiano RW, Pickersgill J, et al: Interstitial lung disease in polymyositis and dermatomyositis: Clinical features and prognosis as correlated with histopathologic findings. Am Rev Respir Dis 144:727–733, 1990.

10. **What is a necrobiotic nodule?**

Necrobiotic nodules occur in patients with rheumatoid arthritis, appearing on standard chest radiographs as either multiple bilateral or solitary rounded lesions of varying sizes. They are histologically identical to subcutaneous rheumatoid nodules but can undergo cavitation when they occur in the lung. Necrobiotic nodules are more likely to occur in men with high titers of rheumatoid factor and often appear during an active articular phase of the disease. They must be differentiated from other causes of lung nodules such as tuberculosis and peripheral bronchogenic carcinomas.

11. **What is Caplan's syndrome?**

Caplan's syndrome was first reported in coal miners who developed rheumatoid arthritis and rapidly appearing lung nodules. The nodules are often confined to the upper lobes and may undergo cavitation. Patients with rheumatoid arthritis who inhale other inorganic dusts, such as silica and asbestos, may also develop this syndrome. The nodules themselves have been termed "pneumoconiotic nodules."

Caplan A: Certain unusual radiographic appearances in the chest of coal miners suffering from rheumatoid arthritis. Thorax 8:29–37, 1953.

KEY POINTS: PULMONARY COMPLICATIONS OF COLLAGEN VASCULAR DISEASE

1. Infections, particularly in patients treated with immunosuppressive agents, often complicate the diagnosis of lung disease.

2. A normal chest radiograph does not exclude lung disease; therefore, high-resolution computed tomography (HRCT) of the chest and pulmonary function testing are often indicated.

3. Obstructive physiology, most often seen in patients with rheumatoid arthritis and Sjögren's syndrome, is the result of obliterative bronchiolitis or follicular bronchiolitis.

4. The acute presentation of diffuse pulmonary infiltrates may represent an infection, diffuse alveolar hemorrhage, diffuse alveolar damage, or organizing pneumonitis.

---

12. **What types of ILD complicate the CVD?**

Several histologic patterns of ILD occur in patients with underlying CVD. Usual interstitial pneumonia (UIP), characterized by a heterogeneous fibrotic process of the alveolar walls and by the presence of fibroblastic foci, is the same histologic pattern that occurs in the lung disease known as IPF. The most common histologic expression of ILD in CVD is nonspecific interstitial pneumonia (NSIP). This is a homogenous inflammatory fibrotic process that is more responsive to treatment than UIP. Other histologic appearances include:

- Bronchiolitis obliterans-organizing pneumonia (BOOP)
- Lymphoid interstitial pneumonitis (LIP)
- Diffuse alveolar damage (DAD)
- Diffuse alveolar hemorrhage (DAH) caused by either bland hemorrhage or pulmonary capillaritis

The ILDs listed above are much more responsive to anti-inflammatory therapy (i.e., corticosteroid drugs) and cytotoxic therapy (i.e., cyclophosphamide, azathioprine, and methotrexate) than UIP.

Myers JL, Katzenstein AL: Microangitis in lupus-induced pulmonary hemorrhage. Am J Clin Pathol 85:552–56, 1986.

Schuurawitzki H, Stiglbaver R, Graninger W, et al: Interstitial lung disease in progressive systemic sclerosis: High resolution CT vs. radiography. Radiology 176:755–759, 1990.

Tazelaar HD, Viggiano RW, Pickersgill J, et al: Interstitial lung disease in polymyositis and dermatomyositis: Clinical features and prognosis as correlated with histopathologic findings. Am Rev Respir Dis 144:727–733, 1990.

13. **What is the relative frequency of the various types of ILDs that occur in patients with CVD?**

Scleroderma has the highest incidence of ILD, which has been reported to be 75% in some patient series. The most common interstitial lesion in systemic sclerosis is NSIP, which usually leads to end-stage fibrosis in these patients. NSIP appears next in frequency in patients with rheumatoid arthritis, followed by those with polymyositis–dermatomyositis. LIP is the most common histologic pattern in patients with Sjögren's syndrome. DAD occurs as an acute immunologic pneumonia in lupus erythematosus (i.e., acute lupus pneumonitis) in mixed connective tissue disease and polymyositis–dermatomyositis. DAH, with or without pulmonary capillaritis, is most often seen in patients with established lupus erythematosus and, to a lesser extent, in the other collagen vascular disorders.

Cottin V, Thivolet-Bejic F, Reynaud-Guibert M, et al: Interstitial lung disease in polymyositis and dermato-myositis. Eur Resp J 22:245–250, 2003.

Matthay RA, Schwarz MI, Petty JL, et al: Pulmonary manifestations of systemic lupus erythematosus: Review of 12 cases of acute lupus pneumonitis. Medicine (Baltimore) 54:397–409, 1975.

Schuurawitzki H, Stiglbaver R, Graninger W, et al: Interstitial lung disease in progressive systemic sclero-sis: High resolution CT vs. radiography. Radiology 176:755–759, 1990.

Tazelaar HD, Viggiano RW, Pickersgill J, et al: Interstitial lung disease in polymyositis and dermatomyosi-tis: Clinical features and prognosis as correlated with histopathologic findings. Am Rev Respir Dis 144:727–733, 1990.

14. **Most ILDs and pleural diseases cause a restrictive defect as measured by pulmonary function testing. In which CVD can an obstructive lung disease appear, and why?**

In rheumatoid arthritis, bronchiolitis obliterans (BO) or bronchiectasis, and follicular bronchioli-tis can lead to progressive severe obstructive lung disease. Histologically, BO is a recurring process involving the terminal and respiratory bronchioles, represented by a concentric fibrotic obliteration of the bronchiolar lumen. Follicular bronchiolitis is characterized by lymphocytic infiltration of the walls of bronchioles. These conditions rarely occur with the other CVDs with the exception of Sjögren's syndrome.

Geddes DM, Corrin B, Brewerton DA, et al: Progressive airway obliteration in adults and its association with rheumatoid disease. Q J Med 46:427–44, 1977.

15. **What is a possible explanation for hypercarbic respiratory failure in a patient with polymyositis–dermatomyositis who does not have parenchymal lung involvement?**

Polymyositis–dermatomyositis is an inflammatory myopathy that can lead to generalized mus-cle weakness. If the respiratory muscles are extensively involved, respiratory failure resulting in hypoventilation and, in turn, hypoxemia will ensue. Respiratory failure occurs in up to 10% of patients and often requires mechanical ventilation. Subclinical involvement of the respiratory muscles does not cause overt respiratory failure but can cause tachypnea, dyspnea on exertion, and interference with cough generation, leading to development of hypostatic pneumonia.

Martin L, Chalmers IM, Dhingra S, et al: Measurements of maximum respiratory pressures in polymyositis and dermatomyositis. J Rheumatol 12:104–107, 1985.

16. **What laboratory value predicts the development of ILD in patients with polymyositis-dermatomyositis?**

ILD is more likely to occur in those patients who have positive titers to anti-Jo-1, an antibody to a cytoplasmic nuclear antigen. More than 60% of patients with polymyositis–dermatomyositis and ILD have this antibody in their serum.

Hochberg MC, Feldman D, Stevens MB, et al: Antibody to Jo-1 in polymyositis/dermatomyositis: Association with interstitial pulmonary disease. J Rheumatol 11:663–665, 1984.

CHAPTER 44

BRONCHIOLITIS, BRONCHIOLITIS OBLITERANS, AND SMALL AIRWAY DISEASE

Richard A. Helmers, MD

1. **What is bronchiolitis?**

   The small airways without cartilage in their walls and with a diameter of less than 2–3 mm are called bronchioles. These airways consist of membranous and terminal bronchioles that are purely air conducting and respiratory bronchioles that contain alveoli in their walls. These small airways account for approximately 25% of all airway resistance since the total cross-sectional area of small airways is much greater than that of the central airways. Consequently, these small airways are severely involved, often with considerable destruction pathologically, before a patient is symptomatic or airflow abnormalities are detected on pulmonary function testing (PFT). Bronchiolitis is a group of diseases affecting primarily the bronchioles and characterized by an inflammatory process in which inflammatory cells and mesenchymal tissue (including fibrosis) are both present. The concept of bronchiolitis can be difficult because the term has been utilized both as a morphologic description and as a clinicopathologic syndrome and also because the conditions with bronchiolar pathology are heterogeneous; understanding and characterization of them requires a multidisciplinary (i.e., clinical, pathologic, and radiologic) approach.

   Cordier JF: Organizing pneumonia. Thorax 55:318–328, 2000.

   Epler GR: Bronchiolitis obliterans organizing pneumonia. Arch Intern Med 161:158–164, 2001.

   Epler GR, Colby TV, McLoud TC, et al: Bronchiolitis obliterans organizing pneumonia. N Engl J Med 312:152–158, 1985.

   Wells AU: Cryptogenic organizing pneumonia. Semin Respir Crit Care Med (22):449–459, 2001.

2. **What is the clinical classification of the various forms of bronchiolitis?**

   There are several ways to clarify this fascinating group of disorders: bronchiolitis of known etiology versus idiopathic forms; clinical syndromes associated with constrictive bronchiolitis versus clinical syndromes associated with organizing pneumonia (descriptive pathologic terms are discussed below); or bronchiolar disorders with airflow obstruction versus interstitial bronchiolar disorders. The last classification has the advantage of being based on clinical and pulmonary function information, which is of most use to the respiratory practitioner and is most helpful in developing a differential diagnosis and a diagnostic and therapeutic plan.

KEY POINTS: CLINICAL CLASSIFICATION OF BRONCHIOLAR DISORDERS

1. Bronchiolitis of known etiology versus idiopathic forms

2. Clinical syndromes associated with constrictive bronchodilator versus clinical syndromes associated with organizing pneumonia

3. Bronchiolar syndromes associated with airflow obstruction versus interstitial bronchiolar disorders

3. **What are the key bronchiolar disorders associated with airflow obstruction, also associated usually with constrictive bronchiolitis and sometimes with cellular bronchiolitis, on pathologic examination?**
    These include bronchiolitis obliterans (also called constrictive bronchiolitis), which may be idiopathic, postinfectious, fume related, associated with connective tissue diseases, caused by drug reaction, or post-transplant (namely, bone marrow, heart-lung, or lung transplant). Smoker's respiratory bronchiolitis, mineral dust bronchiolitis, follicular bronchiolitis, and diffuse panbronchiolitis are the other disorders in this group.

    Moon J, duBois RM, Colby TV, et al: Clinical significance of respiratory bronchiolitis on open lung biopsy and its relationship to smoking related interstitial lung disease. Thorax 54:1009–1014, 1999.
    Schlesinger C, Meyer CA, Veeraraghavan S, Koss MN: Constrictive (obliterative) bronchiolitis: Diagnosis, etiology, and a critical review of the literature. Ann Diagn Pathol 2:321–334, 1999.

4. **What are the key bronchiolar disorders associated with interstitial lung disease (ILD) and, usually, organizing pneumonia (OP) or intraluminal polyps on pathologic examination?**
    These include respiratory bronchiolitis–interstitial lung disease (RB-ILD) and bronchiolitis obliterans-organizing pneumonia (BOOP). Bronchiolitis with inflammatory or intraluminal polyps (BWIP) is another term used to describe BOOP. When idiopathic, BOOP is also termed cryptogenic organizing pneumonitis (COP). COP is preferred to idiopathic BOOP because it covers the essential features of the syndrome and avoids confusion with airway diseases such as constrictive bronchiolitis obliterans (BO). BOOP may also be seen with connective tissue disorders, postinfection, and as a drug-related reaction.

    American Thoracic Society/European Respiratory Society: International Multidisciplinary Consensus Classification of the Idiopathic Interstitial Pneumonias. Am J Resp Crit Care Med 165:277–304, 2002.
    Turton CW, Williams G, Green M: Cryptogenic obliterative bronchiolitis in adults. Thorax 35:805–810, 1981.

5. **What are the pathologic manifestations of constrictive or obliterative bronchiolitis?**
    This lesion is characterized by alterations in the walls of membranous and respiratory bronchioles, often without extensive changes in the alveolar walls and ducts. There is a spectrum of changes, ranging from bronchiolar inflammation to peribronchiolar fibrosis and, ultimately, to concentric narrowing and obliteration of the bronchiolar lumen. Pathologic changes may often be subtle when clinical and radiographic findings are quite dramatic. Areas of fibrosis may be patchy and subtle, and the diagnosis may be missed if lesions are not adequately sampled. Bronchoscopic lung biopsy is relatively insensitive, and surgical lung biopsy is necessary in patients for whom histologic confirmation is necessary. The pathologic manifestation of constrictive or obliterative bronchiolitis may be termed "autoimmune airways disease."

6. **What are the pathologic manifestations of BOOP, BWIP, and COP?**
    The histologic hallmark is the presence of an organizing intraluminal exudate resulting in patchy intraluminal fibrosis, consisting of polypoid plugs of immature fibroblastic tissue that resembles granulation tissue. The characteristic intraluminal fibrotic buds or polyps are seen in respiratory bronchioles, alveolar ducts, and alveoli but do not completely occlude them. Chronic inflammatory cells can be seen within the granulation tissue plugs. The lumens in these lesions appear to be occluded from within, in contrast to the concentric narrowing seen in constrictive bronchiolitis. The fibroblastic plugs are eventually incorporated back into the interstitium and are broken down by unclear mechanisms.

7. **What are the radiographic manifestations of the bronchiolar disorders?**
    Nearly any radiographic pattern can be attributed to bronchiolitis. Dramatic clinical or functional findings may be present with minor radiographic changes; the chest x-ray may even be normal

in patients with documented advanced bronchiolitis, and its sensitivity to detect small airways disease is low. In constrictive or obliterative bronchiolitis, the chest x-ray may be normal, or it may show nonspecific patterns, ranging from normal lung volumes to hyperinflation with diminished vascular markings to vague reticulonodular opacities.

High-resolution computed tomography (HRCT) scanning is currently the best imaging technique for assessment of bronchiolar disease and evaluation of patients suspected of having bronchiolitis. Additional images acquired at residual volume (i.e., full expiration) are an invaluable adjunct in the detection of small airway disease and should be routinely performed when airway disease is suspected or documented clinically. Visibility on HRCT is limited to airways more than 2 mm in diameter, so normal bronchioles cannot be seen. Diseased bronchioles with lumen dilated to > 2 mm in diameter or with thickened walls can be visualized. Centrilobular tubular branching or nodular opacities usually represent abnormal bronchioles filled with fluid, mucus, or pus. Poorly defined centrilobular nodular opacities resulting from peribronchiolar inflammation or fibrosis also occur. Ground-glass attenuation or consolidation is mainly due to alveolar filling that can occur in RB-ILD or COP. Unilateral or bilateral areas of consolidation, usually patchy in distribution, are a characteristic finding in COP. The consolidation may be predominantly peribronchiolar or subpleural in distribution.

Air trapping due to small airway disease often results in the mosaic pattern of lung attenuation. Mosaic perfusion or mosaic attenuation consists of areas of reduced and increased lung density in a patchy distribution. This is due to decreased vascular perfusion associated with bronchiolar obstruction (with subsequent hypoventilation of alveoli distal to obstruction) and flow redistribution to normal areas; partial airway obstruction or collateral air drift into the alveoli past the obstructed bronchiole leads to air trapping, best seen on expiratory scans; the relative contributions of reduced airflow and reduced perfusion have yet to be quantified. These findings can be seen on HRCT when the radiograph is still normal.

Wells AU: Computed tomographic imaging of bronchiolar disorders. Curr Opin Pulmon Med 4:85–92, 1998.

8. **What is follicular bronchiolitis?**
In some chronic inflammatory conditions, lymphoid follicles form part of the mucosa-associated lymphoid tissue (MALT). When lymphoid hyperplasia occurs with subsequent hyperplastic lymphoid follicles with germinal cell hyperplasia and reactive germinal center formation distributed along bronchiolar bundles, the term "follicular bronchiolitis" is appropriate. Most cases are associated with collagen vascular diseases, immunodeficiencies, or hypersensitivity reactions. The major features of follicular bronchiolitis on HRCT consist of centrilobular nodules measuring 1–12 mm in diameter. In patients with no identifiable underlying cause, treatment is generally with bronchodilators and corticosteroids.

9. **Describe the important features of toxic fume-related bronchiolitis.**
Inhalation of toxic gases and fumes is an uncommon cause of bronchiolitis. The nitrogen oxides are the most common cause. The gases are poorly soluble in water and are able to reach the smaller airways before they become hydrolyzed. Fume-related bronchiolitis may be associated either with classical bronchiolitis obliterans with intraluminal polyps or with constrictive bronchiolitis. Inhaled gases and fumes can produce severe bronchiolitis with acute ulceration and inflammation, followed by occlusion of the airways by loose connective tissue and, finally, by complete stenosis. Once exposure has occurred, prevention of bronchiolitis obliterans may be possible by the administration of a short course of corticosteroids.

Nitrogen dioxide, sulfur dioxide, chlorine gas, ammonia, phosgene, smoke inhalation, and hydrogen chloride all can produce a disease with similar clinical, physiologic, and radiographic manifestations.

10. **Describe the important clinical characteristics of postinfection bronchiolitis.**
After either bacterial or viral infection, the lung may develop bronchiolitis. Respiratory tract infection in childhood may have long-term sequelae, including bronchiolitis and an increased

risk of developing chronic obstructive pulmonary disease (COPD) in adulthood. Compared to the pediatric population, there is relatively little information pertaining to the infectious agents of acute bronchiolitis in adults, but similar outcomes may be expected to result occasionally from respiratory tract infections acquired in adulthood. Only a limited number of agents have been reported to be causes of constrictive bronchiolitis: it is most commonly seen with infection with adenovirus or influenza in children or in adults infected with *Mycoplasma pneumoniae*. Sporadic cases in adults have been associated with *Nocardia* species, cytomegalovirus (CMV), *Serratia* species, *Legionella* species, *Cryptococcus* species, *Haemophilus* species, and *Klebsiella* species.

Adults present with nonproductive cough and dyspnea for days to weeks. On exam, inspiratory crackles are a prominent finding, with wheezing less common. Chest radiographs demonstrate heterogeneity of lung disease and also may demonstrate bronchiectasis.

KEY POINTS: MAJOR CATEGORIES OF BRONCHIOLAR DISORDERS

1. Constrictive bronchiolitis

2. Respiratory bronchiolitis

3. Follicular bronchiolitis

4. Occupational bronchiolitis

5. Cryptogenic organizing pneumonia

11. **What is respiratory bronchiolitis? Can smoking cause bronchiolitis?**
    Bronchiolitis, in some cases, may be induced by cigarette smoking. Several studies have demonstrated inflammation and fibrosis in the membranous and respiratory bronchioles associated with cigarette smoking. Respiratory bronchiolitis is defined by the presence of pigmented macrophages within the lumen of the respiratory bronchioles, alveolar ducts, and peribronchiolar alveolar spaces. Patchy submucosal infiltrates of lymphocytes and other chronic inflammatory cells and fibrosis of the bronchial wall are also present. Respiratory bronchiolitis has been found in nearly 90% of smokers operated on for spontaneous pneumothorax. Respiratory bronchiolitis usually occurs without symptoms, and pulmonary function may not be affected.

    The term "small airway disease" has also been used in several different ways to refer to chronic inflammation of distal bronchioles with physiologic evidence of airflow limitation, usually in cigarette smokers. This bronchiolar lesion may be important in the subsequent pathogenesis of centrilobular emphysema. The physiologic abnormalities in the small airways, however, do not predict the 15–20% of smokers who progress to chronic airflow limitation. Some radiologic studies have also suggested a relationship between duration and degree of cigarette smoking and the presence of small irregular opacities (so-called dirty lungs) on chest radiographs. Since smoking appears to cause bronchiolitis, smoking cessation appears to be very important in these patients.

    Meyers JL, Veal CF, Shin MS, Katzenstein AA: Respiratory bronchiolitis causing interstitial lung disease: A clinicopathologic study of six cases. Am Rev Respir Dis 135:880–884, 1987.

    Niewoehner DE, Kleinerman J, Rice DB: Pathologic changes in the peripheral airways of young cigarette smokers. N Engl J Med 291:755–758, 1974.

12. **What is RB-ILD?**

RB-ILD is a syndrome with features consistent with ILD found among current or former ciga-rette smokers. This may be confused with other diffuse parenchymal lung diseases, especially IPF. These patients probably represent a subset with a more severe stage on the spectrum of respiratory bronchiolitis and small airway disease of cigarette smokers. Lung biopsy is required for diagnosis because it is difficult to distinguish these patients from those with other causes of chronic ILD. There has been shown to be significant overlap in histologic and computed tomog-raphy (CT) findings of respiratory bronchiolitis, RB-ILD, and desquamative interstitial pneumo-nia (DIP). This is consistent with the concept that these entities represent different degrees of severity of small airway disease and parenchymal reaction to cigarette smoke.

Patients with RB-ILD present with cough and dyspnea, diffuse fine reticulonodular interstitial infiltrates on chest radiograph, and a restrictive or mixed restrictive–obstructive pattern on PFTs. Coarse crackles are often heard throughout inspiration and sometimes continue into expiration. Finger clubbing has not been reported. CT scans show diffuse or patchy ground-glass density or fine nodules. Histopathologically, respiratory bronchiolitis is characterized by an inflammatory process involving the membranous and respiratory bronchioles. The clinical course and prognosis of RB-ILD is unknown as there has not been a longitudinal study of a large group of patients. Smoking cessation appears quite important in the resolution of these lesions; patients may improve with smoking cessation only. A favorable response to corticosteroids, both functionally and radiographically, has also been reported.

13. **What are BOOP, BWIP, and COP?**

COP, or idiopathic BOOP, is a distinct clinicopathologic syndrome consisting of an idiopathic ill-ness responsive to corticosteroid therapy with distinctive histopathologic findings. The disease occurs, usually, in the fifth and sixth decade and affects men and women equally. A persistent nonproductive cough is the most common presenting symptom. Patients often have dyspnea on exertion and may note the onset of the disorder as a flu-like illness with cough, malaise, fatigue, fever, and weight loss. Less common symptoms are chest pain, hemoptysis, bronchorrhea, and night sweats. Most patients have had symptoms for less than 2–3 months. Cigarette smoking is not a precipitating factor. The symptoms often date to an acute upper respiratory tract infection of presumed viral etiology. Physical exam reveals bilateral crackles and, much less commonly, wheezes. In contrast to invasive pulmonary aspergillosis (IPA), clubbing is not found. However, in one series, one-fourth of patients had no pulmonary physical findings. There are no other extrathoracic clinical physical findings.

A mild-to-moderate restrictive defect is the most common PFT finding. The diffusing capacity is reduced in the majority of patients. Resting and exercise arterial hypoxemia is common. An increased erythrocyte sedimentation rate (ESR) is frequently found and is often greater than 100 mm/hr. The C-reactive protein level is increased. A moderate leukocytosis with, at most, only a minor rise in eosinophils is seen. Autoantibodies are negative or slightly positive. Bronchioalveolar lavage (BAL) reveals increased numbers of lymphocytes, but increased neu-trophils and eosinophils may be found as well. The lymphocytic alveolitis is associated with an expansion of $CD8^+$ cells and increased levels of Th1-related cytokines.

Forlain S, Retta L, Bulghoroni A, et al: Cytokine profile of broncho-alveolar lavage in BOOP and UP. Sarcoidosis Vasc Diffuse Lung Dis 19:47–53, 2002.

14. **Describe the radiographic features of COP.**

The characteristic radiographic finding is bilateral, symmetric, patchy airspace opacities ranging from 3–5 cm to the size of an entire lobe, often peripheral and pleura based, and most profuse in the lower lobes. The opacities may migrate spontaneously. A subgroup presents with focal lung lesions, sometimes manifesting as solitary pulmonary nodules. Cavitary nodules have also been described in some cases. Small pleural effusions are not uncommon. The lung volumes may be normal or decreased. Interstitial opacities, irregular linear infiltrates, or nodular interstitial infiltrates, however, may be the dominant or only abnormalities in a substantial minority of cases. These may be difficult to distinguish from those of IPF. Rarely is the radiograph normal. The severity of radiographic abnormalities correlates with the extent of histologic involvement of the respiratory bronchioles and the alveolar ducts.

HRCT may reveal much more extensive disease than is expected by the plain chest radiograph. The predominant findings are bilateral areas of consolidation associated with a predominantly subpleural or peribronchial distribution in a majority of patients. The consolidation usually involves all lung zones. Less-common findings include areas of ground-glass attenuation; small, ill-defined nodules; and irregular linear areas of increased attenuation. The consolidation tends to migrate, coming and going even without therapy. Bronchial wall thickening and dilation are often seen as well. Moderate mediastinal adenopathy may occur.

15. **How is COP diagnosed and treated?**
The diagnosis of COP depends on both the clinical setting and finding the characteristic pathology of the disease. An open-lung biopsy is recommended to confirm the diagnosis. A transbronchial biopsy should only be considered acceptable for diagnosis in a patient with classical clinical-radiologic features.

It is important to remember that a wide variety of clinical disorders are associated with the histologic finding of proliferative bronchiolitis besides COP, and a thorough search must be performed to rule out these other possibilities; the clinicopathologic syndrome of COP is a diagnosis of exclusion. These other disorders include hypersensitivity pneumonitis, chronic eosinophilic pneumonia, connective tissue disease, acute respiratory distress syndrome (ARDS), inhalation injury, vasculitides (especially Wegener's granulomatosis), ulcerative colitis, and drug-induced reactions.

In connective tissue disease, COP may be seen prior to any other active rheumatologic symptoms. The list of drugs that can cause COP is quite long. There have also been reports of a variant of COP with a rapidly progressive fulminating and life-threatening course, presenting as ARDS and respiratory failure.

A characteristic COP syndrome with lung infiltrates outside the radiation port (including the contralateral lung) may occur after radiation therapy to the breast, including tangential radiation to the lung. This suggests radiation therapy may prime the development of COP. There can be dramatic improvement with corticosteroids, but relapses may occur.

Corticosteroid therapy is the most common treatment. It results in clinical recovery, usually with complete physiologic improvement and normalization of the chest radiograph, in two-thirds of patients. Clinical improvement is usually within days to weeks. The treatment course is usually months. Often, patients will relapse when corticosteroids are tapered but will improve when retreated with corticosteroids. Cyclophosphamide has been successfully utilized in steroid-resistant cases. Focal nodular COP does not progress in a majority of cases, and resection results in cure.

Lohr RH, Boland BJ, Douglas WW, et al: Organizing pneumonia: Features and prognosis of cryptogenic, secondary and focal variants. Arch Intern Med 157:1323–1329, 1997.

Purcell IF, Bourke SJ, Marshall SM: Cyclophosphamide in severe steroid-resistant bronchiolitis obliterans organizing pneumonia. Respir Med 91:175–177, 1997.

Yousem SA, Lohr RH, Colby TV: Idiopathic bronchiolitis obliterans organizing pneumonia/cryptogenic organizing pneumonia with unfavorable outcome: Pathologic predictors. Mod Pathol 10:864–871, 1997.

16. **What is cryptogenic bronchiolitis? Is it a separate disorder from COP?**
Cryptogenic bronchiolitis (CB) is an uncommon clinicopathologic syndrome in adults, but it is a distinctly separate clinicopathologic entity from COP. It is an idiopathic syndrome of airflow obstruction, probably representing a heterogenous group of patients with bronchiolar injury with no specific etiology. In these patients, there is no evidence of underlying emphysema, chronic bronchitis, asthma, or bronchiectasis. CB has been estimated to cause approximately 4% of all obstructive lung diseases, and its true incidence may be higher. The disease usually

occurs in middle age, and the most common symptoms are exertional dyspnea and nonproductive cough of 6–24 months in duration. The most important clinical feature is that most chronic obstructive lung disorders develop over many years, whereas CB develops much more rapidly. Fifty percent of patients are current or prior smokers. Chest radiographs may be normal but typically demonstrate hyperinflation.

CT findings may be nearly diagnostic: there is marked heterogeneity of lung density, with lobules of increased and decreased lung density that create a "mosaic" appearance. This heterogeneity of lung density is exaggerated on expiration.

PFTs generally reveal airflow obstruction, often severe. The diffusing capacity may be normal or decreased. BAL reveals a marked increase in the number of neutrophils.

The cornerstone to the diagnosis of CB is a high index of clinical suspicion. Because treatment generally requires prolonged, high-dose corticosteroid therapy, open-lung biopsy should always be considered, especially if the diagnosis is in question or if the risks of steroid therapy are substantial. Cyclophosphamide has also been used in those who fail to respond to corticosteroid therapy. In contrast to COP, the course of CB can, in some cases, be rapidly progressive and severe.

Kindt GC, Weiland JE, Davis WB, et al: Bronchiolitis in adults: A reversible cause of airway obstruction associated with airway neutrophils and neutrophil products. Am Rev Respir Dis 140:483–492, 1989.

17. **Is bronchiolitis associated with connective tissue disease?**

Patients with connective tissue disease can have small airway narrowing as a result either of the distinct clinicopathological syndromes of bronchiolitis obliterans (i.e., constrictive bronchiolitis) or of BOOP.

The obstructive bronchiolitis seen in rheumatoid arthritis (RA) is the most common of the connective-tissue-disease-related bronchiolopathies. This is an increasingly recognized complication of RA and may be the most common form of lung involvement in this disorder. The majority of patients are middle-aged women with moderate-to-severe classic RA, high titers of rheumatoid factor, and at least 10 years of disease prior to symptom onset. Many also have evidence of advanced autoimmune exocrinopathy (i.e., Sjögren's syndrome). The condition may be advanced by the time symptoms are noticeable. Symptoms usually consist of either the abrupt or the insidious onset of dyspnea and dry cough.

The chest radiograph is normal or hyperinflated. Progressive airway obstruction is seen on PFT. The diffusing capacity is usually normal. The CT scan reveals widespread patchy increases in attenuation that are accentuated by expiration (i.e., a mosaic pattern).

The prognosis in this disorder is often poor. Treatment with bronchodilators is ineffective. Corticosteroid therapy appears to be effective in some patients; the use of either cyclophosphamide or azathioprine has been suggested as well.

Airflow or airway obstruction associated with constrictive bronchiolitis is a significant complication in both bone marrow transplant and lung transplant recipients. In these instances, the pathogenesis appears immune-mediated; there is an association with graft-versus-host disease (GVHD) in bone marrow recipients and with transplant rejection in lung transplant recipients. These patients may develop constrictive bronchiolitis as a chronic rejection phenomenon, which is a major threat to long-term survival.

18. **What is diffuse panbronchiolitis?**

Diffuse panbronchiolitis (DP) is a disease of chronic inflammation confined mainly to the respiratory bronchioles. DP presents almost exclusively in subjects of Japanese descent. In DP, the chest radiograph reveals diffusely disseminated small nodular shadows up to 2 mm in diameter, most prominent in the lung bases, sometimes accompanied by lung hyperinflation caused by air trapping. The natural history of DP is progressive respiratory dysfunction with episodic bacterial superinfection, often with *Pseudomonas* species. Untreated, the 10-year survival is as low as 25%. Long-term, low-dose (i.e., 600 mg/day) erythromycin has been shown to be efficacious; some positive experience has also been reported with the fluoroquinolones. The therapeutic efficacy of macrolides may be due to the ability of these antibiotics to impair production of proinflammatory cytokines rather than just their antibacterial properties.

Aubert JD, Pare PD, Hogg JC, Hayashi S: Platelet-derived growth factor in bronchiolitis obliterans organizing pneumonia. Am J Respir Crit Care Med 155:676–681, 1997.

Ichikawa Y, Hottam, Sumita S, et al: Reversible airway lesions in diffuse panbronchiolitis: Detection by high-resolution computed tomography. Chest 107:120–125, 1995.

19. Can mineral dust exposure result in bronchiolitis?

Airflow obstruction is being increasingly recognized in subjects with inorganic mineral dust exposure. Epidemiologic studies reveal that exposure to asbestos and other mineral dusts may cause obstructive pulmonary function in nonsmokers; animal exposure to asbestos or silica also produces airflow obstruction. A synergistic role with smoking appears likely.

Pathologic studies show fibrosis of the walls of respiratory and membranous bronchioles with minimal chronic inflammatory response. This lesion is morphologically recognizable and is specific for dust exposure. The degree of fibrosis in the bronchiole wall appears to be limited to local dust burden.

Terms used to describe the above include mineral dust–induced bronchiolitis or mineral dust–induced small airways disease. This has been found secondary to exposure to asbestos, silica, iron oxide, aluminum oxide, talc, silicates, and coal. The pathogenesis is unclear but probably involves the inflammatory response that follows the deposition of mineral particles or fibers in small airway walls. Two important factors in pathogenesis are local dust accumulation and the individual's inflammatory response to the dust (determined by the individual's ability to clear these particles). The inflammatory response likely leads to production of fibrogenic factors and the development of fibrotic lesions.

Chung A: Mineral dust induced bronchiolitis. In Epler GR (ed): Diseases of the Bronchioles. New York, Rowan Press, 1994.

20. Are there other known occupational causes of bronchiolitis?

In an outbreak of ILD in nylon flocking industry workers, lung biopsies demonstrated a characteristic pattern of lymphocytic bronchiolitis and peribronchiolitis with lymphoid hyperplasia. BO was also recently reported in workers in a microwave popcorn plant associated with exposure to diacetyl, an organic compound used in artificial butter flavoring.

Boag AH, Colby TV, Fraise AE, et al: The pathology of interstitial lung disease in nylon flock workers. Am J Surg Pathol 23(12):1539–1545, 1999.

Kreiss K, Gomea A, Kullman G, et al: Clinical bronchiolitis obliterans in workers at a microwave popcorn plant. N Engl J Med 347:330–338, 2002.

21. What is bronchocentric ILD?

Recently there have been two published series (with a total of 22 patients) of a distinct form of aggressive idiopathic diffuse lung disease. Lung biopsies from these cases show a distinctive pattern of interstitial fibrosis extending around the bronchioles. Chart radiographs demonstrate diffuse reticulonodular infiltrates. Idiopathic bronchiolocentric interstitial pneumonia appears thus far to be associated, with a relatively poor prognosis.

Chung A, Myers J, Suarez T, et al: Airway-centered interstitial fibrosis: A distant form of aggressive diffuse lung disease. Am J Surg Pathol 28:62–68, 2004.

Yousen SA, Dacic S: Idiopathic bronchiolocentric interstitial pneumonia. Mod Pathol 15:1148–1153, 2002.

WEBSITE

http://www.epler.com/whatsb.html

SMALL VESSEL VASCULITIS: WEGENER'S GRANULOMATOSIS, MICROSCOPIC POLYANGIITIS, AND CHURG–STRAUSS SYNDROME

Stephen K. Frankel, MD, and Kevin K. Brown, MD

CHAPTER 45

1. **What is vasculitis?**

   Vasculitis, or the vasculitides, refers to a number of distinct clinicopathologic syndromes characterized by histopathologic evidence of inflammation of the blood vessels. These diseases are systemic disorders that present with a wide variety of clinical manifestations.

   > Jennette JC, Falk RJ, Andrassy K, et al: Nomenclature of systemic vasculitides. Proposal of an international consensus conference. Arthritis Rheum 37:187–192, 1994.

2. **Which specific disease entities constitute the idiopathic small vessel vasculitides? (Hint: Look at the chapter heading.)**
   - Wegener's granulomatosis
   - Microscopic polyangiitis (MPA)
   - Churg–Strauss syndrome
   - Idiopathic pauci-immune glomerulonephritis
   - Idiopathic pauci-immune pulmonary capillaritis

3. **How common are the small vessel vasculitides?**

   The small vessel vasculitides have an incidence of 20–100 cases/million and a prevalence of 150–450 cases/million. Of these, Wegener's granulomatosis is the most common.

4. **List clinical scenarios that should make you think about the possibility of vasculitis.**
   - Rapidly progressive glomerulonephritis
   - Alveolar hemorrhage
   - Atypical pulmonary disease with multiple lung nodules or cavities
   - Chronic destructive upper airway or sinus disease
   - Mononeuritis multiplex
   - Palpable purpura (i.e., cutaneous vasculitis)
   - Retro-orbital mass
   - Multisystem illness with unusual constellations of signs or symptoms

5. **What other diseases can mimic small vessel vasculitis?**
   - Collagen vascular diseases (CVDs) (i.e., systemic lupus erythematosus, rheumatoid arthritis [RA], dermatomyositis or polymyositis, scleroderma, antiphospholipid antibody syndrome, and inflammatory bowel disease)
   - Malignancies
   - Infections (particularly atypical organisms such as *Mycobacterium* species, fungi, *Nocardia* species, *Actinomyces* species, and pulmonary abscess)
   - Subacute bacterial endocarditis (or other embolic phenomena)
   - Drug toxicity

- Sarcoidosis
- Immune-complex-mediated vasculitis (i.e., Goodpasture's syndrome, Behçet's syndrome, Henoch–Schönlein purpura, and cryoglobulinemia)
- Eosinophilic pneumonia or eosinophilic lung disease
- Interstitial lung disease (ILD)

6. **Name the clinical triad associated with Wegener's granulomatosis.**
   Wegener's granulomatosis is a necrotizing granulomatous vasculitis characterized by involvement of the (1) upper airways, (2) lower respiratory tract, and (3) kidneys.

KEY POINTS: SIGNS AND SYMPTOMS ASSOCIATED WITH WEGENER'S GRANULOMATOSIS

1. **Pulmonary:** Cough, chest pain, shortness of breath, hemoptysis, endobronchial lesions, and abnormal chest radiograph

2. **Ear, nose, and throat:** Rhinorrhea, epistaxis, ear or sinus pain or congestion, and ulcerative or destructive lesions of the upper airway

3. **Renal:** Glomerulonephritis, proteinuria, hematuria, red cell casts, and renal insufficiency

4. **Constitutional:** Fever, fatigue, malaise, anorexia, and weight loss

5. **Skin:** Palpable purpura, ulcers, vesicles, and nodules

6. **Eye:** Uveitis, eye pain, foreign body sensation, and retro-orbital mass

---

7. **Describe the pathologic triad of Wegener's granulomatosis.**
   Wegener's granulomatosis is characterized by (1) small and medium vessel vasculitis, (2) necrotizing granulomatous inflammation, and (3) a lymphocyte-predominant inflammatory infiltrate.

   Leavitt RY, Fauci AS, Bloch DA, et al: The American College of Rheumatology 1990 criteria for the classification of Wegener's granulomatosis. Arthritis Rheum 33:1101–1107, 1990.

   Lie JT: Illustrated histopathologic classification criteria for selected vasculitic syndromes. Arthritis Rheum 33:1074–1087, 1993.

8. **What signs and symptoms are commonly associated with MPA?**
   Rapidly progressive glomerulonephritis occurs in 95–100% of patients with MPA, and over 80% will have marked constitutional or musculoskeletal symptoms including fatigue, malaise, fevers, arthralgias, and myalgias. Alveolar hemorrhage occurs in 10–30% of patients (Fig. 45-1). Although less common, dermatologic, nervous system, gastrointestinal, ocular, and cardiac manifestations may also be seen with MPA.

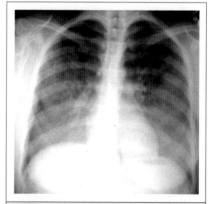

Figure 45-1. Chest radiograph of a patient with diffuse alveolar hemorrhage from MPA

9. **How are classic polyarteritis nodosa (PAN) and MPA, or microscopic PAN, different?**
   Classic PAN is a medium vessel vasculitis with a specific constellation of clinical findings that has historically been linked with the small vessel vasculitis MPA. However, they are now recognized as separate entities within the family of primary idiopathic vasculitis. Although constitutional symptoms, arthralgias, myalgias, peripheral nervous system involvement, and cutaneous involvement occur in both, classic PAN is associated with visceral aneurysms, hypertension, and, in up to one-third of cases, hepatitis B virus infection. Conversely, only about one-third of PAN patients have renal involvement, whereas it is near universal in MPA patients.

10. **What is the differential diagnosis for a patient with pulmonary–renal syndrome?**
    Pulmonary–renal syndrome refers to patients with diffuse alveolar hemorrhage (i.e., pulmonary capillaritis) and a rapidly progressive glomerulonephritis. The differential diagnosis includes Wegener's granulomatosis, MPA, Goodpasture's syndrome, and systemic lupus erythematosus.

    Niles JL, Bottinger EP, Saurina GR, et al: The syndrome of lung hemorrhage and nephritis is usually an ANCA-associated condition. Arch Intern Med 156:440–445, 1996.

11. **What is the clinical triad associated with Churg–Strauss syndrome?**
    (1) Asthma, (2) hypereosinophilia, and (3) necrotizing vasculitis.

12. **Name Lanham's three phases of Churg–Strauss syndrome.**
    - Prodromal phase of atopic disease, characterized by asthma, allergic rhinitis, rhinosinusitis, or a combination thereof, lasting years.
    - Eosinophilic phase, characterized by peripheral eosinophilia (>1500 cells/mm^3). Patients may also present with chronic eosinophilic pneumonia or other eosinophilic tissue infiltrates.
    - Vasculitic phase, with systemic disease.

    Lanham J, Elkon K, Pusey C, Hughes G: Systemic vasculitis with asthma and eosinophilia: A clinical approach to the Churg-Strauss syndrome. Medicine 63:65–81, 1984.

KEY POINTS: DIFFERENTIAL DIAGNOSIS FOR EOSINOPHILIC LUNG DISEASE

1. Churg–Strauss syndrome
2. Chronic eosinophilic pneumonia
3. Asthma
4. Allergic bronchopulmonary mycosis or aspergillosis
5. Hypereosinophilic syndrome
6. Parasitic infections
7. Drug reactions

13. **What clinical clues should suggest the possibility of Churg–Strauss syndrome?**
    Severe or refractory or steroid-dependent asthma, peripheral eosinophilia, elevated immunoglobulin E (IgE), pulmonary infiltrates, and positive perinuclear antineutrophilic cytoplasmic antibodies (P-ANCAs) or antimyeloperoxidase antibodies. Patients with severe

asthma who develop significant gastrointestinal disease (e.g., perforation, bleeding, or bowel ischemia) or cardiac disease (e.g., systolic or diastolic dysfunction, pericarditis, electrocardiogram [ECG] abnormalities, or cardiomyopathy) should raise suspicion for Churg–Strauss syndrome.

Cordier J-F: Eosinophilic pneumonias. In Schwarz MI, King TE Jr (eds): Interstitial Lung Disease, 4th ed. Hamilton, BC Decker, 2003, pp 657–700.

14. **Do leukotriene inhibitors cause Churg–Strauss syndrome?**
There have been several case reports associating Churg–Strauss syndrome with leukotriene inhibitors; however, to date there is no causal link between the two. Two competing theories hold that either (1) the leukotriene inhibitors improve asthma control and permit the withdrawal of systemic corticosteroids, which then unmasks the thus-far-treated underlying Churg–Strauss syndrome, or (2) the leukotriene inhibitors directly facilitate a progression from severe asthma to Churg–Strauss syndrome. Currently, there are no data to confirm the second theory.

Wechsler ME, Finn D, Gunawardena D, et al: Churg-Strauss syndrome in patients receiving montelukast as treatment for asthma. Chest 117:708–713, 2000.

15. **What are ANCAs?**
Antineutrophil cytoplasmic antibodies. The presence of these antibodies is associated with and may assist in the diagnosis of small vessel vasculitis. The role of these antibodies in the pathogenesis of small vessel vasculitis remains unclear but suggestive.

Hoffman GS, Specks U: Antineutrophil cytoplasmic antibodies. Arthritis Rheum 41:1521–1537, 1998.

16. **What is the difference between C-ANCAs and P-ANCAs?**
ANCA may further be divided into cytoplasmic ANCA (C-ANCA) and perinuclear ANCA (P-ANCA) staining patterns. C-ANCAs are primarily directed against the enzyme proteinase-3 (PR3), and specific enzyme-linked immunosorbent assay (ELISA) tests can look for anti-PR3 antibodies. P-ANCAs may be directed against a number of antigens, although myeloperoxidase (MPO) is the most common of these and can be identified with a specific ELISA of its own. C-ANCA or anti-PR3 is most commonly associated with Wegener's granulomatosis, whereas P-ANCA is commonly associated with Churg–Strauss syndrome and MPA. However, P-ANCA is much less specific and has also been associated with the immune-complex-mediated vasculitides, CVDs, and inflammatory bowel disease, among other disease entities.

17. **What are the sensitivity and specificity of ANCA and anti-PR3 antibodies for Wegener's granulomatosis?**
The sensitivity of ANCA testing in Wegener's granulomatosis depends upon the extent and severity of disease activity. In patients with generalized active disease, >90% will be ANCA-positive (and >90% of these will be C-ANCA- or anti-PR3-positive). However, in patients with limited Wegener's (i.e., without renal involvement) only 60% of patients will be ANCA-positive. In patients in whom the disease is in remission, only 40% will be ANCA-positive. Specificity is 85–90%; only rarely will cases of MPA, Churg–Strauss syndrome, inflammatory bowel disease, or other autoimmune diseases be C-ANCA-positive.

Hagen EC, Daha MR, Hermans J, et al: Diagnostic value of standardized assays for anti-neutrophil cytoplasmic antibodies in idiopathic systemic vasculitis. EC/BCR Project for ANCA Assay Standardization. Kidney Int 53:743–753, 1998.

Mandl LA, Solomon DH, Smith EL, et al: Using antineutrophil cytoplasmic antibody testing to diagnose vasculitis. Arch Intern Med 162:1509–1514, 2002.

18. **Can ANCA be used to predict disease relapse?**
Given the clinical usefulness of ANCA testing in diagnosing small vessel vasculitis, ANCA titers have been proposed as a surrogate marker for predicting impending relapse. However, clinical

trials evaluating ANCA titers as a predictor of disease relapse found them to be insufficiently sensitive or specific to be used as such and added little to the clinical assessment.

Girard T, Mahr A, Noel LH, et al: Are antineutrophil cytoplasmic antibodies a marker predictive of relapse in Wegener's granulomatosis? A prospective study. Rheumatology (Oxford) 40:147–151, 2001.

Kerr GS, Fleisher TA, Hallahan CW, et al: Limited prognostic value of changes in antineutrophil cytoplasmic antibody titre in patients with Wegener's granulomatosis. Arthritis Rheum 36:365–371, 1993.

19. **What are the broad principles that govern the treatment of the small vessel vasculitides?**

Therapy for Wegener's granulomatosis and the other small vessel vasculitides relies upon immunosuppression with corticosteroids and cytotoxic agents. Given that complications of such therapies may be life threatening, the therapy is carefully titrated to disease severity, with more aggressive immunosuppression being reserved for more severely affected patients. Moreover, as with cancer therapy, vasculitis therapy may be divided into an induction phase, in which more-intensive therapy is administered to induce a disease remission, and a maintenance phase, in which less-aggressive therapy is used to minimize side effects or complications while maintaining disease remission.

http://www.vasculitis.org

Jayne DN, Rasmussen K, Andrassy P, et al: A randomized trial of maintenance therapy for vasculitis associated with antineutrophil cytoplasmic autoantibodies. N Engl J Med 349:36–44, 2003.

20. **What is the differential diagnosis (broadly) for a patient with known vasculitis with new or worsening signs or symptoms?**

Disease flare versus infection versus drug toxicity. Approximately 50% of patients with small vessel vasculitis will have one or more recurrences of their disease, and these disease flares may manifest with either familiar or novel signs and symptoms compared with the initial presentation. However, it should also be remembered that vasculitis patients are often maintained on cytotoxic or immunosuppressive medications with serious complications and side effects of their own and that drug toxicity can mimic a disease flare. In addition, these patients are immunocompromised as a result of both their disease and their therapy, and because of their immunocompromised state, infections may present with atypical features. Infections, and especially unrecognized infections, represent a major cause of morbidity and mortality in vasculitis patients.

Frankel SK, Sullivan EJ, Brown KK: Vasculitis: Wegener granulomatosis, Churg-Strauss syndrome, microscopic polyangiitis, polyarteritis nodosa, and Takayasu arteritis. Crit Care Clin 18:855–879, 2002.

21. **What is the prognosis for patients with vasculitis?**

Prior to the use of corticosteroids and immunosuppressive agents, the majority of small vessel vasculitis patients died within 1 year. Currently available therapies are able to induce disease remission in 85–95% of patients, but 5-year mortality remains 15–30%.

Abdou NI, Kullman GJ, Hoffman GS, et al: Wegener's granulomatosis: Survey of 701 patients in North America. Changes in outcome in the 1990s. J Rheumatol 29:309–316, 2002.

22. **What factors are associated with a poor prognosis in patients with small vessel vasculitis?**

- Severe renal involvement (e.g., renal failure)
- Alveolar hemorrhage
- Advanced age
- Greater numbers of organ systems involved
- Anti-PR3/C-ANCA positive disease
- Elevated measures of disease severity (e.g., Birmingham Vasculitis Activity Score)

Guillevin L, Lhote F, Gayraud M, et. al: Prognostic factors in polyarteritis nodosa and Churg-Strauss syndrome. A prospective study of 342 patients. Medicine 75:17–28, 1996.

Koldingsnes W, Nossent H: Predictors of survival and organ damage in Wegener's granulomatosis. Rheumatology 41:572–581, 2002.

Mahr A, Girard T, Agher R, Guillevin L: Analysis of factors predictive of survival based on 49 patients with systemic Wegener's granulomatosis and prospective follow-up. Rheumatology 40:492–498, 2001.

ACKNOWLEDGMENTS

The authors thank Eugene Sullivan, MD, who wrote the previous edition of this chapter; Carlyne Cool, MD, who provided the photomicrographs in this chapter; and Gregory P. Cosgrove, MD, for his thoughtful review of this chapter.

CHAPTER 46

DIFFUSE ALVEOLAR HEMORRHAGE

Steve Yang, MBBS, MRCP, FAMS, and Ganesh Raghu, MD, FACP, FCCP

1. What is diffuse alveolar hemorrhage (DAH)?

DAH is a rare and potentially life-threatening syndrome of dyspnea and diffuse lung infiltrates caused by bleeding into the alveoli. The histopathologic features of microscopic alveolar hemorrhage (Table 46-1) can occur as a result of systemic disease, coagulopathy, inflammation, or local insults to pulmonary vasculature.

The most common histopathologic lesion found in patients with DAH is pulmonary capillaritis, in which there is neutrophilic infiltration of pulmonary capillaries and alveolar septae with resultant hemorrhage and nonspecific fibrosis of the alveolar wall. Pulmonary capillaritis may be associated with systemic vasculitis or connective tissue disease including systemic lupus erythematosus (SLE), Wegener's granulomatosis, microscopic polyangiitis (MPA) (the small-vessel variant of polyarteritis nodosa [PAN]), antiglomerular basement membrane (anti-GBM) disease, or Goodpasture's syndrome. Pulmonary capillaritis may also be isolated, without clinical or serologic evidence of an underlying systemic disorder.

A second, less-frequent histopathology in patients with DAH is bland alveolar hemorrhage, with blood in the alveoli but no abnormality of pulmonary architecture. Platelet dysfunction, coagulopathy, cardiac disease, inhaled toxins, and idiopathic pulmonary hemosiderosis (IPH) cause DAH with normal pulmonary capillaries.

A third histopathologic finding in patients with DAH is diffuse alveolar damage with hemorrhage. Crack cocaine use, bone marrow transplantation, drugs or toxins (rarely), and radiation (rarely) are associated with this finding.

Collard HE, Schwarz MI: Diffuse alveolar hemorrhage. Clin Chest Med 25:583–592, 2004.

Leatherman JW, Davies SF, Hoidal JR: Alveolar hemorrhage syndromes: Diffuse microvascular lung hemorrhage in immune and idiopathic disorders. Medicine 63:343–361, 1984.

Schwarz MI, Cherniak RM, King TE Jr: Diffuse alveolar hemorrhage and other rare infiltrative disorders. In Murray JF, Nadel JA (eds): Textbook of Respiratory Medicine, 3rd ed. Philadelphia, W.B. Saunders, 2000, pp 1733–1755.

http://www.chestnet.org

TABLE 46-1. DIFFUSE ALVEOLAR HEMORRHAGE AND HISTOPATHOLOGY

Pulmonary Capillaritis	Bland Alveolar Hemorrhage	Diffuse Alveolar Damage
MPA	Platelet dysfunction	Crack cocaine use
Wegener's granulomatosis	Coagulopathy	Bone marrow transplantation
Systemic lupus erythematosus	Cardiac disease	Drugs or toxins (rare)
Antiglomerular basement membrane disease	Inhaled toxins	Radiation (rare)
Other connective tissue diseases	IPH	
Isolated pulmonary capillaritis		

2. **How does DAH present?**

   Patients with DAH may present with acute or chronic symptoms. Acute symptoms include cough, sudden dyspnea, chest pain, and hemoptysis (which may not always be present, even in severe disease). Patients with more-chronic DAH may have fatigue, due to profound iron deficiency anemia, or dyspnea, due to interstitial fibrosis from repeated bouts of hemorrhage.

   On physical examination, patients with DAH may have rales and signs of anemia. Other evidence of systemic vasculitis such as skin rash, alopecia, arthritis, and abnormalities of the upper respiratory tract may be present.

   Chest radiography shows patchy alveolar infiltrates with air space filling. The differential diagnosis of the infiltrates includes pulmonary edema and pneumonia. Anemia is typical in patients with DAH, and, in patients with chronic alveolar hemorrhage, severe iron deficiency can occur.

   In acute alveolar hemorrhage, pulmonary function testing may show a transiently elevated carbon monoxide diffusion in the lungs (DLCO) as intra-alveolar red blood cells take up carbon monoxide. DAH causes ventilation/perfusion (V/Q) mismatch with hypoxemia. Chronic hemorrhage results in interstitial fibrosis with restrictive physiology and decreased DLCO.

3. **What is the connection between antineutrophilic cytoplasmic antibodies (ANCAs) and DAH?**

   ANCAs are antibodies directed at antigens in the cytoplasm of neutrophils. They show two distinct patterns of immunofluorescence: cytoplasmic ANCA (C-ANCA) and perinuclear ANCA (P-ANCA). The ANCA-associated small vessel vasculitides (i.e., Wegener's granulomatosis, MPA, and Churg–Strauss syndrome) can all cause pulmonary capillaritis and DAH. Immune complex deposition is not seen in these diseases.

4. **How frequently does Wegener's granulomatosis cause DAH?**

   DAH occurs in 10–15% of patients with Wegener's granulomatosis, a necrotizing vasculitis of small and medium vessels with associated granulomas. It can occur in established cases of Wegener's granulomatosis, or it can be the first manifestation of the illness. Clinical features of Wegener's granulomatosis include otorhinolaryngeal disease (i.e., sinusitis, otitis, hearing loss, and subglottic stenosis), pulmonary disease (i.e., nodular or cavitary infiltrates or hemoptysis), and renal disease. C-ANCA is found in 80–90% of patients with active Wegener's granulomatosis. DAH is the most immediately life-threatening complication of Wegener's granulomatosis and is treated with aggressive immunosuppression with cyclophosphamide and high-dose corticosteroids and, sometimes, with intravenous immunoglobulins.

5. **What is MPA?**

   MPA is a necrotizing small vessel vasculitis *without* the granulomatous changes seen in Wegener's granulomatosis. MPA can affect any organ system, but the most frequently involved is the kidney, with glomerulonephritis in over 90% of cases. Pulmonary capillaritis with DAH occurs in 10–30% of patients with MPA and can (rarely) occur in the absence of kidney disease. Treatment for DAH associated with MPA is the same as for Wegener's granulomatosis: cyclophosphamide and high-dose steroids, with plasmapheresis and intravenous immunoglobulins showing some benefit in resistant cases.

   Churg–Strauss syndrome is an even rarer small vessel vasculitis characterized by asthma, eosinophilia, and pulmonary infiltrates. ANCAs, usually P-ANCA, are present in 30–60% of patients with Churg–Strauss syndrome. DAH is uncommon in patients with Churg–Strauss syndrome, occurring in <3%.

6. **What connective tissue diseases are associated with DAH?**

   DAH is an uncommon complication of SLE, accounting for 4% of all SLE-related hospital admissions in one series, and must be distinguished from acute lupus pneumonitis, which has a similar presentation. It is caused by immune complex deposition, and histology usually shows pulmonary capillaritis. DAH is usually seen in patients with active extrapulmonary disease and can be catastrophic, with mortality rates exceeding 50%. High-dose corticosteroids alone have not been effective in treatment, and standard therapy includes adjunct cyclophosphamide with corticosteroids and plasmapheresis. Newer agents such as rituximab, a monoclonal antibody against CD20 that reduces B-cell function, are also potentially beneficial.

Antiphospholipid antibody syndrome may cause DAH, with histopathology showing microvascular thrombosis, with or without capillaritis. Cases of pulmonary capillaritis have also been reported in association with polymyositis, mixed connective tissue disease, scleroderma, and rheumatoid arthritis (RA).

Orens JB, Martinez FJ, Lynch JP III: Pleuropulmonary manifestations of systemic lupus erythematosus. Rheum Dis Clin North Am 20:159–193, 1994.

7. **What are the pulmonary–renal syndromes?**
The pulmonary–renal syndromes are a group of diseases characterized by alveolar hemorrhage and glomerulonephritis. Goodpasture described the first of these syndromes in 1919. Goodpasture's syndrome has since been found to be caused by antibodies (anti-GBM) directed against Type IV collagen in the basement membranes of the lungs and the kidney; it is most common in young male smokers. Almost all patients with Goodpasture's syndrome have involvement of the kidney, ranging from microscopic hematuria to crescentic, rapidly progressing glomerulonephritis with renal failure. Pulmonary involvement, which occurs in 60–80%, is more common in smokers and in those exposed to volatile hydrocarbons because alveolar permeability is increased in these individuals.

Circulating anti-GBM antibodies are found in almost all patients with Goodpasture's syndrome. Immunofluorescent staining of kidney and lung biopsies shows characteristic linear deposits of anti-GBM antibodies along alveolar and glomerular basement membranes. Goodpasture's syndrome is treated with immunosuppressive therapy and plasmapheresis. In cases refractory to conventional therapy, mycophenolate mofetil or anti-CD20 monoclonal antibodies may be helpful.

MPA is the most common cause of the pulmonary–renal syndrome. Other causes of DAH associated with glomerulonephritis are Wegener's granulomatosis, SLE, Henoch–Schönlein purpura, mixed cryoglobulinemia, and Behçet's syndrome.

8. **What is isolated pulmonary capillaritis?**
Isolated pulmonary capillaritis is a small vessel vasculitis confined solely to the lung. It is often be associated with a positive P-ANCA. Most cases arise sporadically, although it has been described to follow treatment with all-trans retinoic acid. Patients may present with respiratory failure and may require mechanical ventilation during the initial stages of clinical manifestations. However, the response to immunosuppressive therapy is good.

9. **What cardiac disease should be considered in patients with DAH?**
Occult mitral stenosis should be considered in any patient with DAH and no renal or other systemic manifestations of vasculitis. Mitral stenosis causes elevated pulmonary venous pressures, resulting in rupture of pulmonary capillaries with alveolar hemorrhage and hemoptysis. Elevated left atrial pressures can also cause varices of the bronchial circulation, with rupture leading to massive hemoptysis. Repeated episodes of hemorrhage can result in interstitial fibrosis.

Mitral stenosis should be strongly suspected in pregnant patients presenting with DAH because occult mitral stenosis may become clinically apparent with the increased intravascular volume associated with pregnancy.

10. **Which drugs can cause DAH?**
D-penicillamine, phenytoin, retinoic acid, hydralazine, minocycline, propylthiouracil, and drugs that affect coagulation (e.g., warfarin, heparin, thrombolytic agents, and antiplatelet agents) have all been associated with pulmonary capillaritis and DAH.

Camus P, Fanton A, Bonniaud P, et al: Interstitial lung disease induced by drugs and radiation. Respiration 71:301–326, 2004.

KEY POINTS: DIFFUSE ALVEOLAR HEMORRHAGE

1. A potentially life-threatening syndrome of dyspnea and diffuse lung infiltrates caused by bleeding into the alveoli.

2. Occurs as a result of systemic disease, coagulopathy, inflammation, or local insults to pulmonary vasculature.

3. Diagnosis is based on clinical evaluation, serologies (e.g., anti-GBM antibodies, ANCA panel, antinuclear antibody [ANA], and double-stranded DNA [dsDNA]), and bronchoscopy showing progressive or persistent bloody returns on lavage.

4. Treatment is dictated by the cause and includes correction of coagulopathy (if present), immunosuppressants, plasmapheresis, and intravenous immunoglobulins in addition to supportive measures like oxygen and mechanical ventilation.

11. **What occupational exposures are associated with DAH?**
Workers exposed to trimellitic anhydride (TMA) can develop DAH. TMA is used in the manufacture of plastics, paints, and epoxy resins. Illness can occur up to 3 months following exposure, and therapy is primarily supportive, with elimination of exposure. TMA exposure can also cause rhinitis and asthma. Isocyanate exposure has also been reported to cause DAH.

> Blanc PD, Golden JA: Unusual occupationally related disorders of the lung: Case reports and a literature review. Occup Med 7:403–422, 1992.

12. **What is IPH?**
Historically, the term "idiopathic pulmonary hemosiderosis" referred to patients with alveolar hemorrhage without an underlying cause or other known disorder associated with DAH. This is a very rare disease that affects mainly young children. Patients often present with dyspnea and interstitial fibrosis, without active hemorrhage. However, hemosiderin-laden macrophages are present in the alveoli, indicating prior hemorrhage.
Currently, IPH is a diagnosis of exclusion and is made only when no pulmonary capillaritis or other cause of DAH is found. It can be speculated that several patients with IPH may well have had recurrent or occult pulmonary capillaritis.

13. **What laboratory tests should be performed in a suspected case of DAH?**
An assessment of the severity of anemia, platelet count, and coagulopathy (prothrombin time and activated partial thromboplastin time [APTT]) is essential. A complete blood cell count (CBC) might reveal anemia in almost all patients with DAH. Creatinine, urinalysis, and microscopic examination of the urine should be obtained immediately to assess for red cell casts or dysmorphic red blood cells indicating glomerulonephritis. Serologic testing should include anti-GBM antibodies, an ANCA panel, antinuclear antibodies (ANAs), double-stranded DNA (dsDNA), and antiphospholipid antibodies.

14. **What is the role of bronchoscopy in cases of suspected DAH?**
Flexible fiberoptic bronchoscopy is indicated to inspect all bronchopulmonary segments to identify local source and extent of bleeding. Bronchoscopy can confirm the diagnosis of DAH if bleeding is noted from multiple bronchopulmonary segments, with bronchoalveolar lavage (BAL) fluid demonstrating gross evidence of increasing bloody returns on suctioning (i.e., progressive bloody returns). These hemorrhagic returns can be expected to be retrieved from any or all bronchopulmonary segments when the abnormality is diffuse. Bronchoscopy can also localize an alternative source of hemorrhage, such as a tumor, and can exclude infection as a cause of diffuse infiltrates and dyspnea. In subacute cases, methods such as quantitative

scoring of the hemosiderin-laden macrophages from a single BAL or increasing red blood cell counts in sequential aliquots of BAL fluid may be useful. However, these tests are not validated.

15. **What is the role of biopsy in the evaluation of DAH?**
Because therapy for many causes of DAH is long term and is associated with significant side effects, tissue biopsy should be obtained when the cause of DAH is not confirmed by clinical evaluation, serologies, and bronchoscopy. The site of the biopsy depends on the clinical situation. If there is evidence of glomerulonephritis, a renal biopsy typically is performed first. A sinus biopsy may confirm a diagnosis of Wegener's granulomatosis.

Surgical lung biopsy should be considered if diagnosis is not evident in tissue obtained from another site. Transbronchial lung biopsies are rarely helpful in identifying a cause of DAH but may show linear immune complex deposition in cases of Goodpasture's syndrome if adequate tissue is obtained. Surgical lung biopsy provides a better tissue sample. As described above, histopathology may show capillaritis, bland hemorrhage, or diffuse alveolar damage (DAD) with hemorrhage. Immunofluorescent staining should also be performed on lung biopsy specimens.

16. **What is the treatment of DAH?**
The treatment of DAH is dictated by the cause. Coagulopathy should be corrected if present. DAH associated with Wegener's granulomatosis, MPA, connective tissue diseases, and anti-GBM disease is typically treated with aggressive immunosuppression (i.e., combined corticosteroids plus cyclophosphamide or azathioprine) and, in some cases, plasmapheresis and intravenous immunoglobulins. Newer methods of treatment include specific agents to reduce B-cell function such as rituximab (a monoclonal antibody against CD20) and mycophenolate mofetil. Supportive measures include oxygen, mechanical ventilation, and transfusion (when necessary).

SLEEP APNEA SYNDROMES

Lee K. Brown, MD

CHAPTER 47

1. **What is meant by a sleep apnea syndrome?**
   Sleep apnea is a laboratory diagnosis, defined as the presence of abnormal numbers of breathing cessations (apneas) or reductions in ventilation (hypopneas) during sleep. Although often used synonymously with sleep apnea, a sleep apnea syndrome is characterized more precisely as sleep apnea associated with either nocturnal or daytime symptoms.

   Strollo PJ Jr., Rogers RM: Obstructive sleep apnea. N Engl J Med 334:99–104, 1996.

2. **How many types of respiratory events have been described?**
   Three types of apneas or hypopneas are recognized:
   - **Central:** Characterized by reduced or absent respiratory effort resulting in reduced or absent ventilation.
   - **Obstructive:** In which respiratory effort is maintained while ventilation decreases or disappears due to partial or total occlusion of the upper airway.
   - **Mixed:** Starts with one type of event (usually central) and concludes with the other. (Since it is believed that mixed and obstructive apneas are clinically the same disorder, they will not be discussed separately, and both will be referred to as obstructive sleep apnea [OSA].)

3. **By how much must ventilation decrease in order to diagnose hypopnea?**
   Hypopneas can be defined as a reduction in ventilation below a fixed percentage of baseline (70% of baseline is a common figure). However, many clinicians will count a hypopnea only if the required reduction in ventilation is followed by significant oxyhemoglobin desaturation or evidence that the patient aroused out of sleep. This excludes events that seem to be of no pathologic consequence.

4. **What is a respiratory effort–related arousal?**
   A third type of obstructive phenomenon has been described in which ventilation does not decrease at all. These events are the hallmark of **upper airway resistance syndrome** and consist of repeated partial obstructions of the upper airway associated with sufficiently increased respiratory effort such that normal levels of ventilation are maintained. The increases in respiratory effort, however, are not without consequence: they cause arousal out of sleep, resulting in many of the same symptoms that are associated with frank obstructive apneas and hypopneas. Such events are called **respiratory effort–related arousals** (RERAs).

   Guilleminault C, Stoohs R, Clerk A: A cause of excessive daytime sleepiness. The upper airway resistance syndrome. Chest 104:781–787, 1993.

5. **How long must ventilation decrease or stop during sleep to be considered hypopnea or apnea?**
   The standard definition for hypopnea or apnea in adults requires decreased or absent ventilation for 10 seconds or longer. In children, most clinicians require a duration of two previous respiratory cycles or greater.

6. **How many apneas or hypopneas must occur during sleep to be considered abnormal?**
   Severity of sleep-disordered breathing is commonly assessed in terms of the apnea, hypopnea, and apnea-plus-hypopnea indices (AI, HI, and AHI, respectively), calculated as the number of each event occurring per hour of actual sleep (not just time in bed). Based on currently available

data, many clinicians consider an AHI of greater than 5 to be abnormal in adults. Data from the Sleep Heart Health Study and other reports suggest that even in asymptomatic patients, an AHI of 15 or more is associated with elevated cardiovascular risk and should be treated. In children, an AHI as low as 1 may be abnormal.

Guilleminault C: Sleep and breathing. In Guilleminault C (ed): Sleeping and Waking Disorders: Indications and Techniques. Menlo Park, Addison-Wesley, 1982, pp 155–182.

7. **Where does the obstruction occur in OSA?**
   The obstruction most commonly occurs in the oropharynx, the hypopharynx, or both. In the oropharynx, there is posterior prolapse of the tongue and uvula and invagination of lateral and posterior pharyngeal tissues. In the hypopharynx, there is posterior prolapse of the root of the tongue and the epiglottis. In certain rare neurologic disorders (e.g., Shy–Drager syndrome), obstruction can occur at the laryngeal level from vocal cord paresis accentuated during sleep.

8. **Do patients with OSA have reduced upper airway caliber when awake?**
   Many, if not most, patients with OSA have some degree of upper airway abnormality while awake. These abnormalities most commonly include:
   - **Obesity:** Significantly overweight individuals are more likely to exhibit OSA, and changes have been demonstrated in the caliber and shape of the upper airway related to collections of adipose tissue.
   - **Adenotonsillar hypertrophy:** More commonly a factor in children.
   - **Macroglossia:** Most frequently attributed to hypothyroidism and myxedema.
   - **Mandibular deficiency:** Micrognathia or retrognathia can result in posterior displacement of the tongue and compromise of the upper airway lumen.

9. **Is an abnormal upper airway all that is necessary to cause OSA?**
   Usually not. A narrow upper airway is most likely a necessary but not sufficient factor in causing OSA. An abnormality in the control of upper airway muscle tone is almost always necessary as well. This situation stems from the multiplicity of roles that the upper airway must assume. It must alternately serve as a rigid conduit for airflow, a compliant waypoint for the passage of food to the esophagus, or a shape-shifting resonance chamber for phonation. Various muscles associated with the upper airway act to change its compliance and shape depending on the function *du jour*; it has been demonstrated that obstructive apneas during sleep are accompanied by failure of these muscles to maintain the degree of tone necessary to keep the airway patent. It is not known for certain why this occurs, but it most likely involves, at least in part, the normal decrease in muscle tone that accompanies sleep.

10. **Are there any other factors that promote upper airway obstruction?**
    The upper airway may tend to collapse if excessive pressure is generated during inhalation. Most often, this is attributed to the force necessary to overcome nasal obstruction (e.g., from allergic rhinitis or septal deviation).

11. **What causes the symptoms of OSA syndrome?**
    An obstructive apnea or hypopnea consists of an episode of asphyxia during sleep due to upper airway occlusion. During each episode there is increasing hypoxia, hypercapnia, acidosis, and progressively greater inspiratory effort against an occluded upper airway, finally leading to arousal from sleep. Upper airway muscle tone is restored during the arousal, allowing effective ventilation to resume; this in turn allows a return to sleep. This sequence of events occurs repeatedly throughout the night, modulated to some extent by body position (events are usually worse when supine) and sleep state (worse during rapid eye movement [REM] sleep). Many of the symptoms can be predicted based upon this known sequence of events.

12. **List the symptoms of OSA that occur during sleep.**
    - **Snoring:** Snoring is almost universal and may be intermittent (only occurring in the interval between apneas, when large tidal volumes are drawn through an upper airway that is just

beginning to achieve patency) or may be continuous if many events are hypopneas. It may also be described as resuscitative, a quality implying respiratory distress.

- **Abnormal motor activity:** The patient may flail about, kick, or even sit up during respiratory events. Patients predisposed to somnambulism or other arousal disorders may experience an increase in these behaviors.
- **Nocturia:** Nocturnal diuresis and natriuresis are frequently associated with OSA syndrome, at times leading to enuresis.
- **Night sweats:** Presumably, these are due to alternating increases in parasympathetic and sympathetic tone.
- **Nocturnal acid brash:** The large negative intrapleural pressures generated during obstructed inspirations promote gastroesophageal reflux.
- **Nocturnal awakenings:** Although each respiratory event typically is terminated by an arousal, the brevity of the arousal usually ensures that the patient does not remember awakening. A minority of patients report awakenings, sometimes associated with air hunger or choking.

13. **List the symptoms that may occur during wakefulness.**
    - **Excessive sleepiness:** The recurrent arousals disrupt sleep architecture, with a resultant shift to lighter stages of sleep and less restorative sleep. Some studies have suggested that the severity of nocturnal hypoxemia may contribute to daytime sleepiness as well.
    - **Cognitive impairment:** Difficulties with tasks involving memory or executive functions may occur, and personality changes are sometimes reported. These may be largely related to the nocturnal hypoxemia.
    - **Nocturnal or morning headache or nausea:** Recurrent hypercapnia from the nocturnal respiratory events may cause cerebrovascular dilatation and a "vascular" headache or related symptoms.

14. **Are any physical findings typical of OSA syndrome?**
    There are no physical findings *specific* to the disorder; that is, none can predict that any given patient will have the syndrome. However, the physical examination may reveal some of the following:
    - Obesity (common)
    - Enlarged uvula, which may be edematous or erythematous
    - "Crowded" oropharynx, which may be edematous or erythematous
    - Adenotonsillar enlargement (especially in children)
    - Retrognathia or micrognathia
    - Systemic hypertension
    - Signs of pulmonary hypertension (PH) or *cor pulmonale* (usually confined to patients with daytime hypoxemia as well, i.e., those with obesity-hypoventilation [Pickwickian] syndrome or coexisting chronic obstructive lung disease)
    - Plethora (from secondary polycythemia)

15. **Which laboratory studies should be performed when OSA syndrome is suspected?**
    - Arterial blood gas analysis (if obesity-hypoventilation [i.e., Pickwickian] syndrome is suspected)
    - Chest roentgenogram, electrocardiogram (ECG), and echocardiogram (consider if physical findings suggest PH or *cor pulmonale*)
    - Hematocrit (to aid in confirming a suspicion of secondary polycythemia)
    - Thyroid-stimulating hormone (in any adult who has not yet had this screening test performed)

    Lin C-C, Tsan K-W, Chen P-J: The relationship between sleep apnea syndrome and hypothyroidism. Chest 102:1663–1667, 1992.

16. **How is OSA syndrome diagnosed?**
    The gold standard test for diagnosing OSA syndrome is the polysomnogram. This test is performed in a sleep laboratory with a technologist in attendance while the patient sleeps for at least 6–8 hours during his or her customary sleep period. The following signals are recorded on a paper or computerized polygraph:

- **Electroencephalogram, submental electromyogram, bilateral electro-oculograms:** Sleep is divided into five different stages (I–IV and REM); these signals allow for the detection and staging of sleep.
- **Respiratory effort** (usually as a reflection of chest and abdominal movement) and **ventilation** (typically measured as airflow at the nose and mouth): These allow for the detection of apnea and hypopneas and their classification as obstructive or central. A microphone to detect snoring may also be included.
- **Oxyhemoglobin saturation by pulse oximetry**
- **ECG** (usually a single limb lead for assessment of cardiac rhythm)
- **Body position** (may be detected automatically or recorded manually by the technologist)

Figure 47-1 demonstrates the polysomnographic appearance of an obstructive apnea.

Keenan SA: Polysomnography: Technical aspects in adolescents and adults. J Clin Neurophysiol 9:21–31, 1992.

Sleep-related breathing disorders in adults: Recommendations for syndrome definition and measurement techniques in clinical research. The Report of an American Academy of Sleep Medicine Task Force. Sleep 22:667–689, 1999.

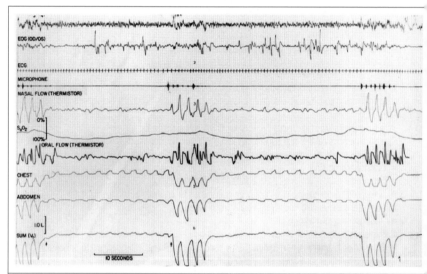

Figure 47-1. Polysomnogram showing an OSA lasting just over 10 seconds *(arrows)*. The electroencephalograms (EEGs), electro-oculograms (EOGs), and submentalis electromyogram (EMG) are consistent with Stage I sleep. The absence of nasal/oral airflow while respiratory efforts continue identifies the apnea as obstructive. Snoring resumes *(microphone)* when the apnea terminates. Note the ventricular premature contraction on the ECG channel toward the end of the respiratory event. (From Guido PS, Brown LK. A 45-year-old man with sleepiness, snoring, and disturbed nocturnal sleep. In Sahn SA, Heffner JE [eds]: Internal Medicine Pearls II. Philadelphia, Hanley & Belfus, 2001, pp 75–78.)

17. **What about portable recording in the patient's home?**

A number of devices are available that will record some of the signals used in standard polysomnography while the patient sleeps at home. Although there may be advantages to this technique from the standpoints of reduced cost and increased comfort and convenience for the patient, there are drawbacks as well: the quality of the data recorded may be suboptimal since a technologist is not available to replace electrodes and such that have malfunctioned, most systems record only a subset of the signals collected in the laboratory, therapeutic interventions cannot be made, and direct visual observations of nocturnal events by the technologist are not available. These drawbacks have recently led the Centers for Medicare and Medicaid Services to reaffirm that reimbursement will not be approved for these studies.

Chesson AL Jr, Berry RB, Pack A: Practice parameters for the use of portable monitoring devices in the investigation of suspected obstructive sleep apnea in adults. Sleep 26:907–913, 2003.

Flemons WW, Littner MR, Rowley JA, et al: Home diagnosis of sleep apnea: A systematic review of the literature. Chest 124:1543–1579, 2003.

18. **Is there any utility to screening with overnight pulse oximetry?**

Most studies have found oximetry to be relatively specific when the pretest probability of OSA is high, but sensitivity varies widely depending upon what level of AHI is used to define the presence of the disorder. For instance, one group of investigators recorded a sensitivity for pulse oximetry alone of only 75% when sleep apnea was defined as an AHI > 15, and it was only 60% using AHI > 5. In addition, pulse oximetry will not distinguish obstructive from central sleep apnea.

Cooper BG, Veale D, Griffiths CJ, Gibson GJ: Value of nocturnal oxygen saturation as a screening test for sleep apnoea. Thorax 46:586–588, 1991.

19. **Does OSA result in cardiac arrhythmias?**

Inspiratory effort against an occluded upper airway (i.e., Müller's maneuver) increases vagal tone and can result in bradyarrhythmias during the obstructive apnea itself, most commonly sinus bradycardia or sinus pauses. Various degrees of atrioventricular (A-V) block are also reported. Arousals from apnea are accompanied by sympathetic discharge and inhibition of parasympathetic tone, leading to sinus tachycardia. The combination of sinus bradycardia during an apnea and sinus tachycardia in between apneas leads to the phenomenon known as cyclic variation in heart rate (CVHR), and, when detected serendipitously during 24-hour ambulatory ECG monitoring, clinical evidence suggesting OSA syndrome should be sought. The sympathetic discharge at apnea termination promotes ventricular ectopy, more commonly when oxyhemoglobin saturation falls below 60%. Hypoxemia may also lead to atrial tachyarrhythmias such as atrial fibrillation or flutter or paroxysmal atrial tachycardia. See Figure 47-2 for a summary of the mechanisms for these and other complications of OSA.

Flemons WW, Remmers JE, Gillis AM: Sleep apnea and cardiac arrhythmias. Is there a relationship? Am Rev Respir Dis 148:618–621, 1993.

Shepard JW Jr., Garrison MW, Grither DA, Dolan GF: Relationship of ventricular ectopy to oxyhemoglobin desaturation in patients with obstructive sleep apnea. Chest 88:335–340, 1985.

20. **Will systemic hypertension worsen in patients with OSA?**

Hypertension is often seen in patients with OSA syndrome, and data from several cross-sectional studies made allowances for confounding factors such as obesity and still demonstrated a significant association, including a dose-response effect. Obstructive apneas are frequently associated with transient elevations of systemic blood pressure; among the mechanisms implicated are hypoxemia and increased sympathetic tone. The factors involved in converting this transient phenomenon in sleep to sustained diurnal hypertension are not known.

Hla KM, Young TB, Bidwell T, et al: Sleep apnea and hypertension. A population-based study. Ann Intern Med 120:382–388, 1994.

Nieto FJ, Young TB, Lind BK, et al: Association of sleep-disordered breathing, sleep apnea, and hypertension in a large community-based study. JAMA 283:1829–1836, 2000.

21. **Is there an increased risk of cardiovascular disease?**

An association between myocardial infarction and OSA has been demonstrated in several studies including the ongoing Sleep Heart Health Study, although causality has not necessarily been established: sleep apnea may predispose to arteriosclerotic and hypertensive heart disease, or these cardiac disorders may increase the likelihood of sleep-disordered breathing by leading to Cheyne–Stokes respiration. Snoring and OSA have been associated with increased risk of stroke in several studies, independent of the presence of hypertension and obesity. A wealth of data is accumulating that OSA promotes the development of the metabolic syndrome (i.e., insulin

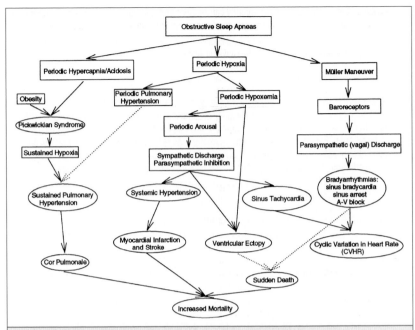

Figure 47-2. Pathogenesis of the complications of OSA syndrome. Postulated mechanisms are shown as dotted lines, and solid lines indicate mechanisms where supporting data exist.

resistance, plus two or more of the following: dyslipidemia, hypertension, central obesity, microalbuminuria, and hyperuricemia), probably through the promotion of inflammatory and other metabolic mediators such as leptin and tumor necrosis factor alpha (TNF-α). Furthermore, these markers of cardiovascular risk improve after effective treatment of sleep apnea. Thus, both an association and a plausible mechanism exist to suggest causality.

Punjab NM, Shahar E, Redline S, et al: Sleep-disordered breathing, glucose intolerance, and insulin resistance. The Sleep Heart Health Study. Am J Epidemiol 160:521–530, 2004.

Shahar E, Whitney CW, Redline S, et al: Sleep-disordered breathing and cardiovascular disease. Am J Respir Crit Care Med 163:19–25, 2001.

22. **Do OSA patients develop obesity-hypoventilation (pickwickian) syndrome?**
    A small percentage of morbidly obese patients with OSA are found to hypoventilate during wakefulness and thus carry the additional diagnosis of obesity-hypoventilation, or pickwickian syndrome (named after Dickens' character Joe the Fat Boy). Although the pathogenesis of this syndrome is not known, intriguing evidence exists suggesting that OSA syndrome may be an important factor in some of these patients: in one study, eight patients with both disorders were identified, and awake hypoventilation resolved in four after effective therapy for sleep apnea was instituted.

Kessler R, Chaouat A, Schinkewitch P, et al: The obesity-hypoventilation syndrome revisited. A prospective study of 34 consecutive cases. Chest 120:369–376, 2001.

Rapoport DM, Garay SM, Epstein H, Goldring RM: Hypercapnia in the obstructive sleep apnea syndrome. A reevaluation of the "Pickwickian syndrome." Chest 89:627–635, 1986.

23. **In view of the nocturnal hypoxemia that occurs in sleep apnea, are PH and cor pulmonale commonly seen?**
    Transient elevation in pulmonary artery pressure (PAP) occurs toward the end of an obstructive apnea and peaks shortly after termination of the event. This phenomenon is attributed largely to

hypoxic pulmonary vasoconstriction and can lead to mild-to-moderate degrees of fixed PH. However, severe PH and cor pulmonale rarely occur unless awake hypoxia is also present. Thus, sleep apnea patients with PH and right heart failure generally have coexistent chronic obstructive lung disease or obesity-hypoventilation syndrome.

24. **Does all of this morbidity result in increased mortality?**
Given the known associations between OSA and cardiovascular disease, it is not surprising that increased mortality has been demonstrated in this disorder. One study suggested that patients with an apnea index > 20 were more likely to suffer excess mortality, and this value has been widely used as a guideline for determining when treatment should be mandatory. Most studies have emphasized the cardiovascular origin of much of this excess mortality, although increasing evidence suggests that vehicular and work accidents attributable to hypersomnolence from the disorder also play an important role.

Marin JM, Carrizo SJ, Vicente E, et al: Long-term cardiovascular outcomes in men with obstructive sleep apnoea-hypopnoea with or without treatment with continuous positive airway pressure: An observational study. Lancet 365:1046–1053, 2005.

Stoohs RA, Guilleminault C, Itoi A, Dement WC: Traffic accidents in commercial long-haul truck drivers: The influence of sleep-disordered breathing and obesity. Sleep 17:619–623, 1994.

25. **When should a patient with OSA syndrome be treated?**
In making treatment decisions, it is important to take into account both disease severity (as assessed during polysomnography) and the presence of daytime or nocturnal symptoms. In view of the increase in hypertension and cardiovascular disease demonstrated in patients with an AHI ≥ 15, most clinicians treat patients in this group regardless of symptoms. Patients with milder degrees of sleep-disordered breathing (respiratory disturbance index ≥ 5 and < 15) are generally treated if significant symptoms (e.g., daytime sleepiness or recurrent nocturnal awakenings) are present.

26. **What is the treatment of choice at present for OSA?**
Currently, continuous positive airway pressure (CPAP) continues to represent the best treatment modality for most patients. This is applied using a nasal or oronasal mask with a soft plastic cushion to provide an airtight seal, held in place by headgear incorporating Velcro straps fastened around the back of the head. Nasal pillows, consisting of soft plastic cushions inserted

KEY POINTS: OBSTRUCTIVE SLEEP APNEA

1. Sleep apnea is a laboratory diagnosis; sleep apnea syndrome is sleep apnea plus symptoms attributable to the disorder.

2. Polysomnography for 6–8 hours in the sleep laboratory remains the gold standard for diagnosis.

3. CPAP remains the most reliable and effective treatment, although oral appliances or upper airway surgery may be reasonable alternatives, particularly in mild-to-moderate disease or when the patient cannot comply with CPAP treatment.

4. Close follow-up of the patient starting on CPAP treatment is essential in order to address factors that might affect compliance.

5. Treatment is recommended for any patient with AHI ≥ 15 and for any symptomatic patient with AHI ≥ 5 and < 15.

6. Adjunctive behavioral modifications are important, including weight loss and avoidance of alcohol, respiratory depressant drugs, and tobacco near to bedtime.

into the nares and also held in place by headgear, may be used instead. A swivel connection and suitably long tubing connect the patient interface to a blower unit, so the patient is free to move about in bed and change position at will. The blower unit incorporates either a pressure valve or another pressure regulatory apparatus so as to maintain a relatively constant system pressure regardless of the phase of respiration at any given time. CPAP acts as a pneumatic splint, such that the positive pressure maintained in the upper airway by the CPAP apparatus physically holds the airway open despite insufficient dilator muscle tone. The efficacy of CPAP has now been proven in randomized, controlled trials and has also been shown to reduce future medical expenditures in patients compliant with its use.

Bahammam A, Delaive K, Ronald J, et al: Health care utilization in males with obstructive sleep apnea syndrome two years after diagnosis and treatment. Sleep 22:740–747, 1999.

Engleman HM, Kingshott RN, Wraith PK, et al: Randomized placebo-controlled crossover trial of continuous positive airway pressure for mild sleep apnea/hypopnea syndrome. Am J Respir Crit Care Med 159:461–467, 1999.

Jenkinson C, Davies RJO, Mullins R, Stradling JR: Comparison of therapeutic and subtherapeutic nasal continuous positive airway pressure for obstructive sleep apnoea: A randomised prospective parallel trial. Lancet 353:2100–2105, 1999.

27. How is treatment with nasal CPAP initiated?

CPAP treatment is most commonly initiated by performing a titration study. The purpose of this study is threefold:

1. To determine the best interface (i.e., nasal mask, nasal pillows, or oronasal mask).
2. To determine the optimal CPAP pressure as evidenced by maximal elimination of apneas, hypopneas, snoring, and arousals, and to verify efficacy during REM sleep and in the supine position.
3. To educate the patient about the device.

CPAP titration may be performed during a second night of polysomnography or as part of a split-night polysomnogram, in which a diagnostic study during the first part of the night is followed by CPAP titration, thus combining two studies into one. It is likely that split-night protocols underestimate the severity of sleep apnea since the respiratory disturbance typically worsens during REM sleep, a stage that occurs more commonly toward the end of a night's sleep, when the titration has already commenced. There may also be insufficient time during one night to successfully titrate CPAP. However, when sleep apnea is sufficiently severe, these considerations often do not prevent successful consummation of a split-night protocol.

Finally, automatically titrating CPAP apparati are now available that, in some cases, may allow successful titration in the home.

Yamashiro Y, Kryger MH: CPAP titration for sleep apnea using a split-night protocol. Chest 107:62–66, 1995.

28. Will patients really wear this apparatus and use it regularly?

Compliance with CPAP therapy varies depending upon how you measure it. One can determine compliance using a patient questionnaire, by electrically timing how long the device is on each night, or by electronically recording how long the patient is actually breathing through it each night. Each method yields a progressively lower estimate of compliance. One study indicated that patients reported an average of 6 hours of CPAP use per night, and 60% said they used it every night. An electronic recorder indicated they actually used it an average of 5 hours per night, and usage patterns varied widely, with just under one-half of the patients using the device ≥ 4 hours/night for ≥ 70% of the nights. Usage did not decline significantly over the course of the 3-month study.

Kribbs NB, Pack AI, Kline LR, et al: Objective measurement of patterns of nasal CPAP use by patients with obstructive sleep apnea. Am Rev Respir Dis 147:887–895, 1993.

29. What factors affect nasal CPAP compliance, and what can be done about them?

Various studies have reported the following user complaints, all of which presumably affect compliance (Table 47-1).

TABLE 47-1. CONTINUOUS POSITIVE AIRWAY PRESSURE MACHINE–USER COMPLAINTS

Complaint	Solution
Claustrophobia	Try different interface (e.g., nasal pillows) Allow patient to become habituated to the mask during the day
Discomfort from interface including pain, air leaks, or contact allergy	Try different brands of mask or mask material or a different interface (e.g., nasal pillows) Change headgear or mask spacer size
Nasal Irritation	
Sneezing, rhinorrhea, or epistaxis	Humidification (heated is best) Topical intranasal steroids Topical intranasal disodium cromoglycate Antihistamines (nonsedating types)
Obstruction	See above, plus the following: Topical nasal decongestants Oral decongestants (e.g., pseudoephedrine)
Discomfort from airflow or pressure	Use ramp setting Convert to bilevel positive airway pressure Consider use of an adaptive CPAP device[*]
Leakage from mouth	Chin strap Full face (oronasal) mask

[*]These devices are designed to adjust the CPAP level periodically, maintaining just enough pressure to prevent respiratory events. They may result in lower average CPAP levels and therefore may be better tolerated.

30. **What about surgical therapy?**

The most common surgical technique advocated for treating sleep apnea is uvulopalatopharyngoplasty (UPPP), which involves resection of redundant lateral pharyngeal tissue, the margin of the soft palate, the palatine tonsils, and the uvula. This procedure increases the caliber of the oropharynx and may also reduce its compliance so that it is less likely to collapse. The success rate of UPPP depends upon how success is defined. Almost all patients will report that snoring is reduced or eliminated and will record a decline in AHI. However, only 40–60% of patients will experience a reduction in AHI of 50% or more, and as few as one-quarter of patients will record a fall in this index to below 20. The UPPP failures are related to the persistence of obstruction in the hypopharynx, an area not treated by this procedure. Although numerous attempts have been made to identify a preoperative strategy capable of distinguishing hypopharyngeal from oropharyngeal obstructors, thus far no practical techniques are available. An additional hazard to treatment failure after UPPP relates to the fact that snoring may be alleviated while, at the same time, a serious degree of sleep apnea remains; therefore, repeat polysomnography is mandatory following UPPP.

31. **Is surgical treatment of nasal obstruction recommended?**

In the presence of clinically important nasal obstruction refractory to medical treatment, consideration should be given to appropriate nasal surgery. This may also be necessary if CPAP cannot be properly administered due to nasal obstruction.

32. **Are there any other surgical treatments available?**

A variety of more-aggressive procedures have been developed if UPPP fails and the patient still cannot use CPAP. These are designed to address hypopharyngeal obstruction and range from techniques that put anterior tension on the base of the tongue to prevent posterior displacement during sleep (i.e., anterior sagittal mandibular osteotomy and genioglossus-hyoid advancement) to procedures that also increase the size of the bony skeleton enclosing the tongue (i.e., maxillary and mandibular osteotomies with advancement).

Maisel RH, Antonelli PJ, Iber C, et al: Uvulopalatopharyngoplasty for obstructive sleep apnea: A community's experience. Laryngoscope 102:604–607, 1992.

Shepard JW Jr., Olsen KD: Uvulopalatopharyngoplasty for treatment of obstructive sleep apnea. Mayo Clin Proc 65:1260–1267, 1990.

KEY POINTS: CENTRAL SLEEP APNEA

1. Determine which category of central sleep apnea (i.e., hypercapnic or eucapnic/hypocapnic) you are dealing with by reviewing history, physical examination, and laboratory tests.

2. Treat the underlying disease (e.g., congestive heart failure [CHF] or neurologic or neuromuscular disease).

3. Therapy for hypercapnic central sleep apnea requires ventilatory support modalities such as bilevel positive airway pressure.

4. Therapy for eucapnic/hypocapnic central sleep apnea has been most successful using oxygen or CPAP.

33. **What should I tell patients who ask about laser surgery, Somnoplasty, or the Pillar procedure for snoring and sleep apnea?**

Laser surgery for treatment of sleep apnea most commonly consists of a staged uvulopalatoplasty, in which the CO_2 laser is used to vaporize the uvula and part of the soft palate over the course of multiple sessions. A single-session technique has also been described. Laser surgery frequently relieves snoring by removing the vibrating tissues of the uvula and soft palate, but usually it does not include the excision of lateral pharyngeal tissues (a component of conventional UPPP) and may therefore be less effective for OSA than conventional UPPP.

Somnoplasty uses a proprietary device to introduce alternating-current electricity through a needle electrode into the tissues of the oropharynx or the base of the tongue (other similar, somewhat less sophisticated devices are also available), leading to protein degradation and shrinkage of the tissue.

The **Pillar procedure** involves insertion of prosthetic devices into the palate in order to reduce compliance and collapsibility.

None of these procedures has shown improved efficacy over UPPP in OSA (although they do frequently work for snoring alone), and, in some cases, they seem to be less effective. If performed for sleep apnea, postoperative polysomnography is mandatory, and when the indication is ostensibly snoring alone, screening polysomnography should be done first.

Powell N, Riley R, Troell R, et al: Radiofrequency volumetric tissue reduction of the palate in subjects with sleep-disordered breathing. Chest 113:1163–1174, 1998.

Standards of Practice Committee of the American Sleep Disorders Association: Practice parameters for the use of laser-assisted uvulopalatoplasty. Sleep 17:744–748, 1994.

34. **What other treatments are available?**

The following treatments may play a role in certain patients:

- **Weight loss:** Many studies have documented the salutary effect of weight loss in obese patients with sleep apnea. Adequate weight loss is often difficult to achieve and should not be the only modality employed, especially in more severe degrees of disease. In patients with morbid obesity, bariatric surgery may be indicated, particularly now that laparoscopic methods are available.

- **Sleep position training:** Certain individuals exhibit sleep-disordered breathing almost exclusively in the supine position. Such patients can sometimes be trained to remain in the lateral decubitus position by inserting tennis balls into a pocket sewn into the back of their pajama top.
- **Avoidance of alcoholic beverages, respiratory depressant medications (e.g., sedative hypnotics or opiates), and tobacco use within 4 hours of bedtime.**
- **Oxygen:** Oxygen is usually to be avoided as a single agent because it frequently prolongs episodes of apnea by delaying hypoxemia and subsequent arousal. Oxygen may be used in combination with other modalities if hypoxemia remains despite suppression of discrete respiratory events.
- **Oral appliances:** A variety of devices are available that either advance the mandible, hold the tongue anteriorly, or lift the palate. The mandibular advancement and tongue-retaining devices all have demonstrated efficacy, but the former are usually better tolerated. Up to 60% of patients will achieve an AHI of < 20 when wearing these appliances, and they may represent a useful alternative for some patients.

Schmidt-Nowara W, Lowe A, Wiegand L, et al: Oral appliances for the treatment of snoring and obstructive sleep apnea: A review. Sleep 18:501–510, 1995.

35. How should I advise my patients with sleep apnea about driving and using heavy machinery?

OSA syndrome is a cause of hypersomnolence, and sleepy individuals are less vigilant and less skillful—and may even fall asleep—while driving. One study demonstrated a seven-fold increase in the rate of automobile accidents in patients with OSA syndrome (AHI > 5) compared to a normal control group. Laws concerning the reporting of impaired drivers to licensing authorities vary from state to state, and physicians involved in the treatment of patients with sleep apnea would be well advised to become familiar with local regulations and to follow any reporting requirements. In the absence of a statutory duty to notify authorities about a pathologically sleepy driver, the physician is, at the very least, obligated in terms of good medical practice to warn such patients to refrain from driving or operating heavy machinery until their disorder is properly diagnosed and treated.

Findley LJ, Unverzagt ME, Suratt PM: Automobile accidents involving patients with obstructive sleep apnea. Am Rev Respir Dis 138:337–340, 1988.

36. What causes central sleep apnea syndrome?

The term "central sleep apnea syndrome" is a misnomer in that there is not one such disorder but rather a group of disorders that all manifest as central apneas during sleep. The first major distinction involves separating hypercapnic from eucapnic or hypocapnic central sleep apnea.

37. Describe hypercapnic central sleep apnea.

These patients have alveolar hypoventilation due to either defective central ventilatory control or respiratory muscle weakness. Disorders that affect brainstem respiratory centers include infarcts, encephalitis (including poliomyelitis), degenerative diseases, demyelinating diseases, congenital abnormalities, and iatrogenic injury (e.g., following cervical cordotomy). A host of disorders can impair respiratory muscle strength including primary muscle diseases (most commonly, muscular dystrophies), diseases of the neuromuscular junction, neuropathies, motor neuron diseases, and spinal cord disorders.

38. Describe eucapnic or hypocapnic central sleep apnea.

These syndromes are most often related to Cheyne–Stokes respiration, the waxing and waning respiratory pattern commonly associated with CHF and stroke. Periodic breathing at high-altitude represents another Cheyne–Stokes type of ventilatory instability induced by hypoxemia. The latter condition has proven to be a paradigm for the central sleep apnea of CHF: the hypoxemia and hypocapnia attendant to CHF cause instability in ventilatory control due to breathing near the CO_2 threshold for apnea. Central sleep apnea without the Cheyne–Stokes pattern may also occur.

Central sleep apnea without a Cheyne–Stokes pattern may be seen in the absence of known heart or central nervous system (CNS) disease. This idiopathic form of central sleep apnea implies an abnormality of medullary respiratory control, but the cause is generally unknown. Some of these patients have been found to demonstrate upper airway obstruction coincident with the loss of respiratory effort, and reflex inhibition of ventilatory drive due to airway occlusion (i.e., diving reflex) has been suggested as a possible mechanism. These patients often respond to CPAP treatment.

Bradley TD, Phillipson EA: Central sleep apnea. Clin Chest Med 13:493–505, 1992.
Brown LK: Sleep-disordered breathing in neurologic disease. Clin Pulm Med 3:22–35, 1996.

39. What are the symptoms and signs of the central sleep apnea syndromes?

The symptoms and signs depend upon whether the syndrome is hypocapnic or eucapnic/hypocapnic. Patients with hypercapnic central sleep apnea frequently snore and complain of daytime sleepiness, nocturnal or morning headache, and restless sleep. They are often hypoxemic during wakefulness, and thus are subject to developing PH, cor pulmonale, and polycythemia. Eucapnic/hypocapnic central sleep apnea more commonly results in complaints of insomnia and nocturnal choking and dyspnea; these patients may also experience daytime somnolence but rarely develop cor pulmonale.

Bradley TD, McNicholas WT, Rutherford R, et al: Clinical and physiologic heterogeneity of the central sleep apnea syndrome. Am Rev Respir Dis 134:217–221, 1986.

40. What treatments are available for the hypercapnic central sleep apnea syndromes?

In addition to effective treatment of the primary disease, hypercapnic central sleep apnea is most often managed with ventilatory support modalities. These are now most commonly "noninvasive"; that is, they do not require tracheotomy or endotracheal intubation. Available techniques include positive pressure ventilation through a nasal or oronasal mask or negative-pressure ventilation administered through a cuirasse (i.e., a shell), a body wrap, or a poncho. Nasal or oronasal bilevel positive airway pressure has become the most common technique due to the ready availability of masks (the same as used for CPAP) and pressure-generating equipment. This equipment supplies a higher level of pressure during inspiration compared to expiration; the expiratory pressure helps maintain upper airway patency, analogous to CPAP, while the higher inspiratory pressure augments or generates tidal volume. When used to treat central sleep apnea, a timed mode is used, enabling the apparatus to switch to its inspiratory pressure if no inspiratory effort is detected after a given length of time.

Other available treatments include diaphragmatic pacing and pharmacologic approaches. The former is of limited utility since an intact phrenic nerve and neuromuscular junction and normal diaphragmatic function are all necessary. The latter approach includes ventilatory stimulants such as progesterone or acetazolamide, REM-sleep-suppressant medication such as the tricyclic antidepressants, or oxygen. Oxygen must be used with care because it may potentiate hypercapnia.

41. Are the eucapnic/hypocapnic central sleep apnea syndromes treated differently?

CHF, if present, should be treated aggressively since most central sleep apnea (especially of the Cheyne–Stokes type) is caused by this disorder. Nocturnal oxygen therapy has been useful, especially in CHF, but may also be tried when hemispheric stroke is implicated. CPAP can be beneficial through mechanisms that include increasing pCO_2 due to rebreathing or ventilatory loading, reducing cardiac afterload leading to improvement in CHF, and relieving upper airway obstruction, if present. Periodic breathing of high altitude usually resolves with time, immediately upon returning to lower elevations, or with supplemental oxygen.

CHAPTER 48

ALVEOLAR HYPOVENTILATION

Robert D. Ballard, MD

1. **What is the definition of alveolar hypoventilation?**

   Alveolar hypoventilation arises when effective ventilation is inadequate to meet one's metabolic need. It is typically defined by an arterial pCO_2 ($PaCO_2$) greater than 45 mmHg. This condition can occur with decreased central ventilatory drive, respiratory muscle weakness, chest wall deformities, obstructive airway disease, and parenchymal lung disease, and many patients will have combinations of these processes.

2. **List disorders associated with alveolar hypoventilation.**

   Decreased central ventilatory drive
   - Primary alveolar hypoventilation (congenital central hypoventilation syndrome)
   - Drugs
   - Structural lesions (e.g., cerebrovascular accident, tumors, and hemorrhage)
   - Obesity-hypoventilation syndrome (may have mixed etiology)
   - Myxedema (may have mixed etiology)

   Neuromuscular and chest wall disorders
   Central nervous system (CNS) disorders
   - Poliomyelitis
   - Amyotrophic lateral sclerosis
   - Syringomyelia
   - Multiple sclerosis
   - Cervical cord injury

   Peripheral nervous system disorders
   - Polyneuropathy (Guillain–Barré syndrome)
   - Phrenic nerve injury

   Motor end plate disorders
   - Myasthenia gravis
   - Eaton–Lambert syndrome
   - Botulism

   Muscle dysfunction
   - Muscular dystrophy
   - Myopathy (inflammatory, metabolic, or hereditary)

   Chest wall disorders
   - Kyphoscoliosis (congenital or secondary)
   - Thoracoplasty
   - Obesity

   Airways or parenchymal disease
   - Upper airway obstruction (obstructive sleep apnea [OSA], which has a probable role in obesity-hypoventilation; tracheal stenosis; and tonsillar hypertrophy)
   - Chronic obstructive pulmonary disease (COPD)
   - Cystic fibrosis (CF)
   - Bronchiectasis
   - Interstitial lung disease (ILD)

3. **How is the work-up of hypoventilation approached?**
Work-up should begin with a careful **history and physical examination**. Because many forms of hypoventilation are initially asymptomatic and manifest only during sleep, detailed questioning of patients and family members about sleep patterns, snoring, daytime somnolence, orthopnea, fatigue, irritability, decreased mentation, and poor performance at work or school can be highly informative.

Laboratory tests include arterial blood gas (ABG) analysis, hematocrit (checking for secondary erythrocytosis), and levels of electrolytes, magnesium, phosphate, and thyroid-stimulating hormones.

Pulmonary function tests (PFTs) include spirometry, which can be used to characterize the nature and severity of a ventilatory disorder. Patients with neuromuscular disorders often have a forced vital capacity (FVC) below 50% of predicted before ventilatory insufficiency becomes apparent. The demonstration of a 25% or greater decrement in FVC from the upright to supine postures is an indicator of significant diaphragm weakness. Kyphoscoliosis is often severe (i.e., a Cobb angle > 100 degrees) with a FVC < 1.0 liter before onset of hypercapnia. In patients with obstructive airway disease, a forced expiratory volume in 1 second (FEV_1) > 1.0 liter suggests that a process other than the underlying airway disease is contributing to associated hypercapnia. Additional testing can include the measurement of lung volumes and respiratory muscle strength. If the diagnosis remains unclear at this point, nocturnal polysomnography may be useful. Finally, measurement of $PaCO_2$ during voluntary hyperventilation has traditionally been used to distinguish between those who cannot breathe and those who will not breathe, although there is often overlap between these disorders.

Cannot breathe	**Will not breathe**
Chest wall disorders	Impaired central ventilatory drive
Neuromuscular diseases	
Airways or parenchymal disease	

Chokroverty S: Sleep-disordered breathing in neuromuscular disorders: A condition in search of recognition. Muscle Nerve 24:451–455, 2001.

4. **Why should we treat hypoventilation?**
   Chronic hypoventilation and associated hypoxia lead to progressive pulmonary hypertension (PH). PH will lead to right heart strain and, eventually, failure. This will predispose the affected patient to edema formation and cardiac arrhythmia. Hypoventilation may worsen tissue hypoxia in the setting of underlying atherosclerotic disease, thereby increasing the risk of myocardial infarction. Hypoxia may also induce a secondary erythrocytosis that can create a hyperviscosity syndrome if the hematocrit exceeds 55%. Chronic hypercapnia can directly affect the CNS, triggering headache, altered mentation, and hypersomnolence. Thus, hypoventilation may lead to morbidity and even mortality by several different avenues.

5. **What changes occur during sleep that alter respiration and predispose one to hypoventilation?**
   During sleep, the reduced input from the behavioral control system results in reduced tidal volume and increased upper airway resistance (secondary to a decrease in upper airway muscular activity). This contributes to a reduction in ventilation. Hypoventilation is further promoted because the metabolic control system during sleep shifts its ventilatory hypercapnic response curve to the right, allowing a $PaCO_2$ that is typically 2–4 mmHg higher than that maintained in the awake state. These effects are most pronounced during rapid eye movement (REM) sleep, when activity in both upper airway dilator muscles and chest wall respiratory muscles is eliminated and breathing becomes dependent on the diaphragm. Thus, during REM sleep, individuals are predisposed to hypoventilation because upper airway patency is decreased and ventilation becomes dependent solely upon the diaphragm to meet the increased ventilatory demand.

   McNicholas WT: Impact of sleep on ventilation and gas exchange in chronic lung disease. Monaldi Arch Chest Dis 59:212–215, 2003.

6. **What is congenital central hypoventilation syndrome?**
   Congenital central hypoventilation syndrome (CCHS) is an uncommon disease usually characterized by adequate ventilation while awake, but with hypoventilation due to reduced tidal volume during sleep in the absence of other identifiable contributors. More-severely affected patients may also hypoventilate during wakefulness. Patients typically have absent or reduced ventilatory responsiveness to hypercarbia and hypoxia during both sleep and wakefulness, which also leads to reduced arousal responses to these stimuli during sleep. CCHS is associated with autonomic nervous system dysregulation and appears to have a genetic basis. Recent evidence suggests that *de novo* or inherited mutations in the PHOX2B gene (a key transcription factor for development of autonomic reflex pathways) are important determinants of CCHS.

   Weese-Mayer DE, Berry-Kravis EM: Genetics of congenital central hypoventilation syndrome. Am J Respir Crit Care Med 170:16–24, 2004.

7. **How does hypothyroidism cause hypoventilation?**
   Although the mechanisms are not completely understood, hypothyroidism is a known cause of central hypoventilation. In 1961, Wilson and Bedell described the pulmonary function of patients with myxedema, noting that most subjects had hypercapnia and hypoxia that improved with thyroid supplementation therapy. These investigators found such patients to have reduced hypercapnic ventilatory responsiveness that improved with subsequent therapy. Zwillich and colleagues subsequently reported reduced hypoxic ventilatory responsiveness in patients with both myxedema and hypothyroidism, but only the patients with true myxedema had reduced hypercapnic responses as well. After 3 weeks of thyroid supplementation therapy, only the hypoxic ventilatory response improved. It therefore appears that hypothyroidism alters the metabolic control of respiration. Hypothyroidism can also cause respiratory muscle weakness, as evidenced by reduced inspiratory and expiratory maximal pressures, which may also contribute to hypoventilation. Finally, many patients with hypothyroidism gain weight and

develop OSA, necessitating increased ventilatory work to overcome the elastic load of the chest wall and the obstructive load of the upper airway.

Wilson WR, Bedell GN: The pulmonary abnormalities in myxedema. J Clin Invest 12:42–55, 1960.
Zwillich CW: Ventilatory control in myxedema and hypothyroidism. N Engl J Med 292:662–665, 1975.

8. **How is central hypoventilation treated?**

The first approach to therapy is the identification of reversible causes such as space-occupying lesions, CNS infections, thyroid disease, and the use of sedating medications. Once reversible causes are addressed, patients may be offered many noninvasive and, in more difficult cases, invasive methods of treatment. Obese patients should aggressively pursue weight reduction, including bariatric surgery if indicated. Supplemental oxygen is effective in attenuating hypoxia induced by hypoventilation but may blunt hypoxic ventilatory drive and increase dead space within the lungs, further increasing hypercapnia. Consequently, oxygen should be administered and titrated in a monitored setting, both in the awake and asleep states.

Respiratory stimulants, such as theophylline and acetazolamide, augment ventilatory drive, but their effectiveness in long-term settings is poor. Medroxyprogesterone has been shown to increase central ventilatory drive, and some patients have demonstrated prolonged benefit from this agent. However, it is difficult to predict who will respond, and many patients develop side effects such as impotence.

An alternative therapy is the use of ventilatory assistance. Negative pressure ventilation, a technique first demonstrated by the iron lung used to treat polio patients, is cumbersome and tends to create or worsen upper airway obstruction secondary to increasingly negative pharyngeal pressures that are not coordinated with upper airway dilator muscle activity. Positive pressure ventilation administered through a tight-fitting nasal or facial mask during sleep can be effective in reversing both nocturnal and daytime hypercapnia and hypoxia and now has largely replaced negative pressure ventilation. Patient tolerance and compliance are primary determinants of treatment success.

Other treatment options include diaphragmatic pacing and tracheotomy for the maintenance of airway patency or the administration of positive pressure ventilation. Both of these strategies are invasive and should be used only when noninvasive treatment fails. Diaphragmatic pacing is ineffective in many patients with neuromuscular and chest wall disorders. In addition, because it creates negative pharyngeal pressure that is typically not coordinated with upper airway dilator muscle activity, when used alone it may trigger upper airway occlusion.

9. **What is the pickwickian syndrome?**

The pickwickian syndrome, or obesity hypoventilation syndrome, was first described by Burwell and associates in 1956 and named for a character described in Charles Dickens' *The Posthumous Papers of the Pickwick Club*. Marked obesity, somnolence, cyanosis, periodic breathing, secondary erythrocytosis, and right ventricular heart failure were the initially described clinical characteristics of this syndrome.

Morbid obesity decreases total lung capacity (TLC), functional residual capacity (FRC), and tidal volume because of increased adipose tissue in the chest wall and elevation of the diaphragm caused by increased intra-abdominal adipose tissue. The reduced lung volumes lead to atelectasis, which alters ventilation-perfusion (V/Q) matching and causes hypoxia. There is also evidence that respiratory muscles become less effective in morbid obesity. Most patients also have OSA, which further increases ventilatory work in a system already predisposed to hypoventilation. Finally, hypoxic and hypercapnic responses are diminished in most patients, either secondary to chronic hypoxia and hypercapnia or, perhaps, congenitally. Even though the exact sequence of events is not always clear, it is easy to conceptualize that affected patients with reduced lung volumes, atelectasis, noncompliant chest walls, ineffective respiratory muscles, upper airway obstruction, and altered metabolic control of breathing are prone to develop hypoventilation, especially during sleep.

10. **How common is the obesity hypoventilation syndrome?**

Recent findings suggest that obesity hypoventilation syndrome may be much more common than previously thought. Nowbar and colleagues evaluated 150 hospitalized obese (i.e., body mass index [BMI] > 35 kg/m^2) patients, finding unexplained elevation of $PaCO_2$ (52 + 7 mmHg) in 47 (31%) of these patients. Affected patients had more cognitive dysfunction, increased somnolence, and higher post-discharge mortality in comparison to hospitalized obese patients without hypoventilation. Only 6 (13%) of the obesity hypoventilation patients were discharged from the hospital on therapy for hypoventilation.

In another study of 57 obese residents of Mexico City, Valencia-Flores and associates found that 33 (58%) met their criteria for hypoventilation ($PaCO_2$ > 35 mmHg; PaO_2 < 65 mmHg). Fifty-five (96.5%) of the study population had echocardiographic evidence of pulmonary hypertension, and hypoventilation was clearly the major risk factor for elevation of pulmonary artery pressure. Both of these studies suggest a very high prevalence of hypoventilation in the obese population, with an associated increase in both morbidity and mortality.

Nowbar S, Burkhart KM, Gonzales R, et al: Obesity-associated hypoventilation in hospitalized patients: Prevalence, effects, and outcome. Am J Med 116:1–7, 2004.

Valencia-Flores M, Rebollar V, Santiago V, et al: Prevalence of pulmonary hypertension with respiratory disturbances in obese patients living at moderately high altitude. Internat J Obesity 28:1174–1180, 2004.

11. **How should patients with obesity hypoventilation syndrome be treated?**

Nasal continuous positive airway pressure (nCPAP) is now clearly established as the most effective therapy for OSA. nCPAP is also effective in the majority of patients with obesity hypoventilation, not only resolving upper airway obstruction during sleep, but also increasing the ventilatory response to CO_2 while awake and improving awake hypercapnia. However, there are many patients with severe OSA and hypercapnia who are only partially responsive to CPAP alone and continue to demonstrate sleep-associated hypoventilation and elevated $PaCO_2$ during wakefulness.

This is consistent with observations by Berger and colleagues, who studied 23 obesity hypoventilation patients and demonstrated upper airway obstruction alone in 11 patients during sleep (which therefore responded to nCPAP). The other 12 patients demonstrated hypoventilation during sleep that persisted after effective treatment of upper airway obstruction. A change to nocturnal ventilatory assistance (i.e., bilevel positive airway pressure) was found effective for these patients. Bilevel positive airway pressure will benefit the vast majority of obesity hypoventilation patients who fail nCPAP alone, and this role for nocturnal ventilatory assistance has been endorsed by a national consensus conference.

Berger KI, Ayappa I, Chatr-amontri B, et al: Obesity hypoventilation syndrome as a spectrum of respiratory disturbances during sleep. Chest 120: 1231–1238, 2001.

Berthon-Jones M, Sullivan CE: Time course of change in ventilatory response to CO_2 with long-term CPAP therapy for obstructive sleep apnea. Am Rev Respir Dis 135:144–147, 1987.

Consensus Conference Report: Clinical indications for noninvasive positive pressure ventilation in chronic respiratory failure due to restrictive lung disease, COPD, and nocturnal hypoventilation. Chest 116:521–534, 1999.

12. **Why does chest wall disease sometimes lead to hypoventilation? Which patients are susceptible?**

Chest wall diseases, such as kyphoscoliosis, reduce the efficiency of respiratory musculature. This is demonstrated by the lower inspiratory and expiratory maximal pressures that these patients generate. Chest wall deformity also contributes to reduced lung volumes. When lung volumes decrease, atelectasis can occur, causing V/Q mismatch and resultant hypoxia. Thus, patients with chest wall disorders have reduced lung volumes and poor respiratory muscle function leading to reduced alveolar ventilation and hypoxia.

Kyphoscoliosis is usually quite severe before significant respiratory impairment arises, with the angle of spinal deformity (Cobb angle) exceeding 100 degrees and the FVC falling below 1.0 liter. Respiratory failure is particularly likely when the inspiratory and expiratory maximum pressures fall below 30% of predicted. However, even in the absence of such indicators, the physician should always inquire about sleep-related complaints that could indicate sleep-associated hypoventilation.

13. **What is the treatment for hypoventilation in neuromuscular diseases and chest wall disorders?**

Because these patients have more severe hypoventilation during sleep due to decreased behavioral input, much of the focus has been on nocturnal therapy. Oxygen alone can allow unacceptable increases in $PaCO_2$, sometimes exceeding 95 mmHg. Masa and colleagues compared nocturnal oxygen therapy with nocturnal ventilatory assistance in 21 patients with chest wall disorders. They observed that, in comparison to the oxygen therapy, ventilatory assistance improved daytime oxygenation and symptoms (i.e., dyspnea, morning headaches, and morning alertness).

One recent review of the medical literature identified four randomized trials that assessed the efficacy of nocturnal ventilatory assistance in relieving hypoventilation in patients with neuromuscular or chest wall disorders. All studies confirmed that nocturnal ventilatory assistance decreased daytime $PaCO_2$ and improved oxygenation, and two of the studies suggested subsequent improvement in survival. It was concluded that mechanical ventilation should be offered to patients with chronic hypoventilation due to neuromuscular disease. As negative-pressure ventilation is cumbersome and may predispose such patients to upper airway collapse, positive-pressure devices (such as bilevel positive airway pressure) are now the therapy of choice. In the most severe cases, home ventilation through a tracheotomy can be considered.

Annane D, Chevrolet JC, Raphael JC: Nocturnal mechanical ventilation for chronic hypoventilation in patients with neuromuscular and chest wall disorders. Cochrane Database Syst Rev 2:CD001941, 2000.

Masa JF, Celli BR, Riesco JA, et al: Noninvasive positive pressure ventilation and not oxygen may prevent overt ventilatory failure in patients with chest wall diseases. Chest 112:207–213, 1997.

14. **Why does nocturnal ventilation often improve daytime hypercapnia in patients with chest wall disorders?**

Many theories exist to explain this effect, but none are well substantiated. It has been speculated that nocturnal ventilation rests chronically fatigued respiratory muscles, thereby making them more effective during the day. Alternatively, improvement of nocturnal hypoxia and hypercapnia may improve respiratory muscle endurance. Nocturnal reductions in hypercapnia may lower the body's bicarbonate pool, which may in turn reset chemosensors and augment metabolic control. Finally, nocturnal ventilation may raise lung volume and improve pulmonary compliance, thereby reducing dead space and ventilatory work. Thus, hypercapnia can be improved by several different mechanisms.

15. **What are clinical indicators of sleep-associated hypoventilation in Duchenne's muscular dystrophy?**

Duchenne's muscular dystrophy (DMD) will inevitably lead to respiratory failure, and, as in all neuromuscular disorders, hypoventilation during sleep is one of the first occurrences. Hukins and Hillman studied 19 patients with DMD in an attempt to identify what characteristics were predictive of sleep-associated hypoventilation and would therefore warrant a nocturnal polysomnogram. They reported that an FEV_1 < 40% predicted was sensitive to, but not specific for, sleep-associated hypoventilation. A $PaCO_2$ > 45 mmHg was also sensitive, but more specific to hypoventilation, whereas a base excess > 4 mmol/L was highly specific. These findings suggest that in addition to monitoring for clinical indicators of sleep-associated hypoventilation (i.e., restless sleep, daytime somnolence, and morning headaches), one should routinely monitor spirometry. When the FEV_1 falls below 40% predicted, ABGs should be checked. If the $PaCO_2$ is > 45 mmHg, and especially if base excess is > 4 mmHg, nocturnal polysomnography should be conducted.

Hukins CA, Hillman DR: Daytime predictors of sleep hypoventilation in Duchenne muscular dystrophy. Am J Respir Crit Care Med 161:166–170, 2000.

16. Why do some patients with COPD develop hypercapnia?

Hypoxia and hypercapnia initially develop in patients with COPD during sleep and ultimately progress to become daytime abnormalities. During sleep, patients with COPD, like normal individuals, have a generalized decrease in ventilatory drive. The resultant decrease in accessory inspiratory muscle activity (observed most markedly during REM sleep), upon which many COPD patients depend during wakefulness, leaves sleeping patients dependent solely upon the diaphragm, which may also be less effective because of hyperinflation-induced muscle shortening. Consequently, tidal volume is reduced and the amount of functional lung receiving adequate ventilation declines, increasing dead space. Hypoventilation and increased dead space result in hypercapnia. As the disease progresses, dead space increases further as a result of increasing tissue destruction. Despite accessory muscle use, the patient ultimately cannot meet ventilatory demands, and daytime hypercapnia ensues. Evidence exists that hereditary factors related to ventilatory control may play a role in determining who develops hypoventilation at a given level of disease, but these factors remain poorly understood.

Roussos C, Koutsouko A: Respiratory failure. Eur Respir J 22:Suppl.47, 3s–14s, 2003.

17. Should a sleep study be done for all patients with COPD?

Nocturnal oximetry is often conducted in COPD patients who have marginal oxygenation while awake in order to assess the adequacy of oxygenation during sleep. In a recent study of 54 stable hypercapnic COPD patients, O'Donoghue and colleagues found that the severity of hypoventilation during sleep was best predicted by a combination of baseline $PaCO_2$, body mass index, and percentage of sleep time spent in REM sleep. However, Connaughton and associates demonstrated that nocturnal measurements of hypercapnia and hypoxia were no more predictive of survival than awake measurements. Daytime hypoxia and hypercapnia indicate a poor prognosis, and nocturnal measurements do not provide additional prognostic data unless OSA is also present. When COPD patients do require supplemental oxygen during wakefulness, many physicians advocate the increase of their nocturnal oxygen flow rate by approximately 1 liter per minute.

Connaughton JJ, Catteral JR, Elton RA: Do sleep studies contribute to the management of patients with chronic pulmonary disease? Am Rev Respir Dis 138:341–345, 1988.

O'Donoghue FJ, Catcheside PG, Ellis EE, et al: Sleep hypoventilation in hypercapnic chronic obstructive pulmonary disease: Prevalence and associated factors. Eur Respir J 21:977–984, 2003.

18. What therapies are available for patients with COPD and hypoventilation?

Long-term oxygen therapy is the only treatment demonstrated to improve survival in patients with COPD. Because supplemental oxygen may diminish hypoxic ventilatory drive, it is tempting to perform sleep studies on all patients to ensure that hypercapnia does not increase during sleep, although this is infrequently done. The studies demonstrating that even nocturnal oxygen therapy alone improved survival in COPD patients titrated oxygen flow based on awake measurements, and whether patients should have nocturnal measurements remains unclear.

Other therapies, such as medroxyprogesterone, acetazolamide, theophylline, and negative pressure ventilation, have not been promising. Positive pressure ventilation, using methods such as bilevel positive airway pressure, may lower carbon dioxide acutely in patients with COPD and has been clearly established as an effective therapy for acute respiratory failure in these patients. However, this mode of therapy appears less effective for chronic, stable COPD, perhaps mostly due to poor patient tolerance and compliance. Multiple controlled, randomized trials assessing nocturnal positive pressure ventilation in stable, hypercapnic COPD patients demonstrated no consistent treatment effects upon PFTs, PaO_2, $PaCO_2$, survival, or number of days hospitalized, although there may be some improvement in quality-of-life indicators.

Casanova C, Celli BR, Tost L, et al: Long-term controlled trial of nocturnal nasal positive pressure ventilation in patients with severe COPD. Chest 118:1582–1590, 2000.

Clini E, Sturani C, Rossi C, et al: The Italian multicenter study on noninvasive ventilation in chronic obstructive pulmonary disease patients. Eur Respir Dis 20:529–538, 2002.

SILICOSIS, COAL WORKERS' PNEUMOCONIOSIS, AND CHRONIC BERYLLIUM DISEASE

Lisa A. Maier, MD, MSPH

CHAPTER 49

1. What is silicosis?

Silicosis is a major impairing chronic occupational disease that occurs throughout the world. Long-term exposure to free silica causes a nodular fibrotic lung disease in the interstitium. Disease presentation and severity depend on the intensity and duration of exposure, the nature of the silica inhaled, and poorly understood host susceptibility factors. The pathogenic mechanism remains obscure. The histologic hallmark of silicosis is the silicotic nodule, composed of weakly birefringent silica and a whorled hyalinized central collection of collagen surrounded by dust-laden macrophages. These nodules coalesce to form larger masses, and more diffuse interstitial fibrosis can occur over time, usually after 20–30 years of silica exposure.

American Thoracic Society Committee of the Scientific Assembly on Environmental and Occupational Health: Adverse effects of crystalline silica exposure. Am J Respir Crit Care Med 155:761–768, 1997.

Castranova V, Vallyathan V: Silicosis and coal workers' pneumoconiosis. Environ Health Perspect 108(Suppl 4):675–684, 2000.

Cohen R, Velho V: Update on respiratory disease from coal mine and silica dust. Clin Chest Med 23:811–826, 2002.

2. Who develops silicosis?

The element silicon is abundant and constitutes approximately 25% of the earth's crust. Exposure to silica occurs in numerous occupations (Table 49-1). The prevalence of silicosis increased after the industrial revolution with the introduction of mechanized tools, such as the

TABLE 49-1. OCCUPATIONS AND INDUSTRIES IN WHICH EXPOSURE TO SILICA OCCURS	
Occupation/Industry	**Examples of Specific Jobs**
Hard rock mining for metals, nonmetals, or coal; excavating or tunneling	Miner, driller, blaster, or crusher
Stonework	Sculptor, mason, or monument carver
Stone quarrying	Crusher, trucker, or laborer
Foundries	Casting, polishing, mold making, or sandblasting
Construction	Sandblaster
Abrasives	Manufacturer of sandpaper, silica flour, or sandblast grit
Tool grinding or sharpening	
Ceramics	Manufacturers of pottery, kilns, or refractory
Diatomaceous earth production	
Glass manufacture	

pneumatic drill, that amplified the amount of airborne silica dust in many industries. In this century, the prevalence of silicosis has declined in the United States because of tighter regulation of silica dust levels. However, silica-related lung disease is still found in this country. Throughout the developing world, many workers are exposed to levels of silica high enough to cause silicosis.

American Thoracic Society Committee of the Scientific Assembly on Environmental and Occupational Health: Adverse effects of crystalline silica exposure. Am J Respir Crit Care Med 155:761–768, 1997.

Cohen R, Velho V: Update on respiratory disease from coal mine and silica dust. Clin Chest Med 23:811–826, 2002.

Davis GS: Silicosis. In Harber P, Schenker MA, Balmes JR (eds): Occupational and Environmental Respiratory Disease. St. Louis, Mosby-Year Book, 1996, pp 379–399.

3. **Can silica exposure result in acute lung disease?**
Yes. Silica exposure results in a spectrum of diseases ranging from acute to chronic. Acute silicoproteinosis develops within days to months after high-level exposure such as can occur with sandblasting. This disease is clinically and histologically indistinguishable from pulmonary alveolar proteinosis; it presents with symptoms of dyspnea, radiographic findings of basilar alveolar infiltrates, and alveolar filling with protein-rich surfactant-like material. Individuals with this form of silicosis have a poor prognosis and may progress rapidly to respiratory insufficiency and death.

American Thoracic Society Committee of the Scientific Assembly on Environmental and Occupational Health: Adverse effects of crystalline silica exposure. Am J Respir Crit Care Med 155:761–768, 1997.

Centers for Disease Control and Prevention: Silicosis deaths among young adults—United States, 1968–1994. MMWR 47:331–335, 1998.

4. **What are the radiographic manifestations of silicosis?**
Silicosis can be diagnosed clinically in most individuals with a history of exposure and typical chest radiographic findings (Fig. 49-1). The classic chest radiographic abnormalities consist of rounded opacities, 1–5 mm in size, that are predominantly in the upper lung zones but sometimes are throughout all lung fields. Eggshell calcification of the hilar or mediastinal lymph nodes is almost pathognomonic of silicosis, although it is rarely seen. Computed tomography (CT) is more sensitive than plain radiography in detecting changes caused by silicosis. Over time, coalescence of fibrotic upper lobe nodules into large conglomerate masses that cause restrictive pulmonary physiology and impaired gas exchange may develop. This is known as progressive massive fibrosis (PMF). It is associated with high cumulative levels of silica exposure.

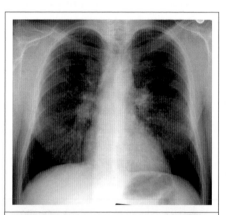

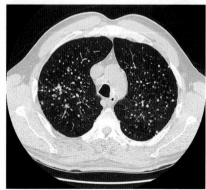

Figure 49-1. **A,** Posteroanterior chest radiograph of an individual with silicosis demonstrating diffuse parenchymal nodularity, with upper lobe predominance. **B,** High-resolution computed tomography scan revealing 2- to 5-mm nodules of silicosis with some coalescence of nodules.

Cohen R, Velho V: Update on respiratory disease from coal mine and silica dust. Clin Chest Med 23:811–826, 2002.

Davis GS: Silicosis. In Harber P, Schenker MA, Balmes JR (eds): Occupational and Environmental Respiratory Disease. St. Louis, Mosby-Year Book, 1996, pp 379–399.

5. Is there an increased risk of tuberculosis in silica-exposed workers?

An individual with silicosis or exposure to silica is at increased risk for tuberculosis and nontuberculous mycobacteria. Screening silicotics and possibly all workers exposed to silica with a skin test for tuberculosis has been recommended. Individuals with silicosis should be evaluated for mycobacterial infection if there are any signs, symptoms, or radiographic changes suggestive of the disease. Although the symptoms of tuberculosis and silicosis may be similar, typically they progress more quickly in silicotuberculosis than is expected in silicosis alone. Individuals with silicotuberculosis have an increased tuberculosis mortality than nonsilicotics. Tuberculosis or nontuberculous infections in silicotics should be treated according to standard protocols.

American Thoracic Society Committee of the Scientific Assembly on Environmental and Occupational Health: Adverse effects of crystalline silica exposure. Am J Respir Crit Care Med 155:761–768, 1997.

Cowie RL: The epidemiology of tuberculosis in gold miners with silicosis. Am J Respir Crit Care Med 150:1460–1462, 1994.

Snider DE: The relationship between tuberculosis and silicosis. Am Rev Respir Dis 118:455–459, 1978.

6. Does silica exposure result in other lung diseases?

Silica exposure may result in two other types of lung disease besides those discussed above. In numerous studies, workers exposed to silica dust have been found to have an increased frequency of symptoms of chronic bronchitis, including chronic sputum production, airflow obstruction, and even pathologic evidence of emphysema. The association between silica dust exposure, chronic bronchitis, and airflow obstruction has been confirmed even among nonsmokers. There may be an additive effect between smoking and silica exposure in the development of these diseases. The International Agency for Research on Cancer (IARC) recently classified silica as carcinogenic to humans, based on the weight of evidence from human and animal studies. A strong relationship between lung cancer and silicosis has been well established, and it may be further increased by tobacco smoke and exposure to other carcinogens in the workplace. Although the relationship is less robust, there is evidence to suggest that nonsilicotics with silica exposure may also be at higher risk for lung cancer. It is important to counsel workers with silicosis and silica exposure to stop smoking because tobacco use may further increase the risk of airway disease and lung cancer associated with silica exposure.

American Thoracic Society Committee of the Scientific Assembly on Environmental and Occupational Health: Adverse effects of crystalline silica exposure. Am J Respir Crit Care Med 155:761–768, 1997.

International Agency for Research on Cancer, World Health Organization: Silica, some silicates, coal dust and para-Aramid fibrils. IARC: Monographs on the Evaluation of Carcinogenic Risks to Humans. Lyon, IARC 68:21–242, 1997.

7. What is the therapy for silica-related lung disease?

There is no specific treatment for silica-related lung disease. Individuals with silicosis are treated symptomatically to prevent cor pulmonale. A high index of suspicion for mycobacterial infection should be maintained. Corticosteroids may produce short-term improvement in lung function, but long-term steroid therapy is not advocated because its long-term benefits are unknown. The airway disease should be treated with inhalers. Silica-related disease may be prevented by reducing exposure to silica, although the level that is safe remains the subject of debate. For 100% respirable quartz, in an average 8-hour work day, the time-weighted average of 0.1 mg per cubic meter of air is the recommended exposure limit. Even at this level, silicosis may develop. A diagnosis of silicosis should be reported to health authorities who can investigate whether the industry is in compliance with current exposure regulations. Removal from exposure is recommended once disease has developed.

Cohen R, Velho V: Update on respiratory disease from coal mine and silica dust. Clin Chest Med 23:811–826, 2002.

Davis GS: Silicosis. In Harber P, Schenker MA, Balmes JR (eds): Occupational and Environmental Respiratory Disease. St. Louis, Mosby-Year Book, 1996, pp 379–399.

KEY POINTS: SILICA-RELATED LUNG DISEASE

1. Exposure to silica can result in a number of pulmonary diseases including the fibrotic lung disease silicosis, pulmonary alveolar proteinosis, and lung cancer, and it increases the risk of developing tuberculosis for those exposed to mycobacteria tuberculosis.

2. Silica can cause airway diseases including chronic bronchitis, airflow obstruction, and emphysema.

3. A diagnosis of silicosis is based on a history of silica exposure and a chest radiograph or CT scan consistent with silicosis.

4. The radiographic manifestations of silicosis include simple silicosis with rounded opacities in the upper lung zones, with increasing profusion of opacities and coalescence of small opacities into conglomerate masses and PMF at later stages.

5. There is no specific therapy for silica-related lung diseases.

8. **What is black lung? What causes it?**
"Black lung" is a term usually applied to any respiratory disorder associated with work in the coal mines. Other terms have been applied to the lung diseases associated with coal dust including miner's asthma, anthracosis, and phthisis. Coal workers' pneumoconiosis (CWP) is the fibrotic lung disease that results from inhalation and deposition of coal dust. The pathologic lesion observed in CWP consists of focal collections of macrophages laden with coal dust and is known as a dust macule. With more progressive disease, these macules coalesce and form firm and palpable nodules.

9. **How does CWP present clinically and radiographically?**
Chest radiographs may reveal small rounded opacities in the upper lung zones, not unlike those seen in silicosis. Some individuals with radiographic evidence of CWP may be asymptomatic. Those with advanced disease may report symptoms of dyspnea, cough, sputum production, or melanoptysis, the production of black-pigmented sputum. As in silicosis, nodules of CWP may coalesce and form progressive massive fibrosis or PMF, usually bilaterally in the upper lobes. The development of PMF is related to more significant coal dust exposure. Symptoms and physiology generally correlate poorly with the severity of disease seen on radiographs in CWP.

Castranova V, Vallyathan V: Silicosis and coal workers' pneumoconiosis. Environ Health Perspect 108(Suppl 4):675–684, 2000.

Lapp NL, Parker JE: Coal workers' pneumoconiosis. Clin Chest Med 13:243–252, 1992.

10. **Does exposure to coal dust result in airway disease?**
Exposure to coal dust causes emphysema, chronic bronchitis, and airflow obstruction. Focal emphysema is found commonly around coal macules and nodules and is associated with the degree of fibrotic lung disease, the intensity of previous exposure, and the amount of retained coal dust. Pulmonary function tests (PFTs) may reveal reduced lung volumes, airway obstruction, or both and may be indistinguishable from those seen with tobacco abuse. This disease process occurs in both smoking and nonsmoking coal-exposed individuals. Symptoms of chronic cough, sputum production, and wheezing are common. The diagnosis is based on

a careful occupational history. These diseases are treated in the same way as other airway diseases. Coal miners with airway disease should be counseled to stop smoking.

Cohen R, Velho V: Update on respiratory disease from coal mine and silica dust. Clin Chest Med 23:811–286, 2002.

Seixas NS, Robins TG, Attfield MD, et al: Exposure-response relationships for coal mine dust and obstructive lung disease following enactment of the Federal Coal Mine Health and Safety Act of 1969. Am J Ind Med 21:715–734, 1992.

11. **Are some miners more likely to develop CWP than others?**
Not all coal miners are at equal risk for developing CWP. For example, miners working at the face of a mine, where higher exposure occurs, are more likely to develop CWP. Higher cumulative exposure levels are associated with higher rates of disease development. Anthracite coal found in the eastern United States is more likely to cause disease than bituminous coal found in the western part of the country. In general, miners working underground are at greater risk of developing disease than surface or strip miners because of dilution of exposures above ground. The prevalence of CWP has been decreasing in the United States, probably because of reduced exposure levels and decreasing numbers of workers employed in the industry. The current permissible exposure limit for coal is 2 mg/m^3.

Cohen R, Velho V: Update on respiratory disease from coal mine and silica dust. Clin Chest Med 23:811–826, 2002.

Lapp NL, Parker JE: Coal workers' pneumoconiosis. Clin Chest Med 13:243–252, 1992.

12. **What is Caplan's syndrome (rheumatoid pneumoconiosis)?**
Anthony Caplan described the constellation of CWP, rheumatoid arthritis, and large nodular lesions, initially mistaken for PMF on chest radiograph. The nodules tend to be well defined, in contrast to those seen in PMF, and occur with little or no fibrotic lung disease. These necrobiotic nodules may cavitate or calcify and sometimes disappear. Caplan's syndrome also has been noted in individuals with silicosis. Some individuals with CWP or silicosis may have an elevated rheumatoid factor level or antinuclear antibody titer level without having rheumatoid arthritis.

Caplan A: Certain unusual radiological appearances in the chest of coal-miners suffering from rheumatoid arthritis. Thorax 8:29–37, 1953.

Castranova V, Vallyathan V: Silicosis and coal workers' pneumoconiosis. Environ Health Perspect 108(Suppl 4):675–684, 2000.

KEY POINTS: COAL-RELATED LUNG DISEASE

1. Coal exposure can result in the fibrotic lung disease CWP, silicosis, emphysema, chronic bronchitis, and airflow obstruction.

2. The term "black lung" is used to indicate any lung disease due to coal exposure and may have medicolegal implications.

3. Risk of CWP is related to exposure: increased risk is associated with higher cumulative exposures, exposure to anthracite coal, and work underground and at the face of a mine.

4. Coal miners may develop an increased rheumatoid factor or rheumatoid arthritis and the large nodular lung disease known as Caplan's syndrome.

13. **What are the health effects related to beryllium exposure?**
The granulomatous lung disease, chronic beryllium disease (CBD), continues to occur in many industries, among family members exposed to second-hand dust, and in members of

communities surrounding beryllium industries. CBD rates in industry range from 1–16%, depending on the worker group studied. Beryllium is used in the aerospace, aircraft, nuclear weapons, electronics, ceramics, telecommunications, and automotive-parts industries and in dental alloy manufacture. Another health effect related to beryllium exposure is beryllium sensitization. These individuals demonstrate an immune response to beryllium but have no evidence of pathologic or physiologic defect. They can progress on to develop CBD at approximately 6–8% per year of follow-up and thus require long-term follow-up.

Maier LA: Genetic and exposure risks for chronic beryllium disease. Clin Chest Med 23:827–839, 2002.

Maier LA, Newman LS: Beryllium disease. In Rom WN (ed): Environmental and Occupational Medicine, 3rd ed. Boston, Little, Brown, 1998, pp 1021–1035.

14. **Is there an exposure–response relationship for beryllium sensitization and CBD?**
CBD can occur at very low levels, significantly below the existing federal standard of 2 $\mu g/m^3$. It has been observed in secretaries, office managers, and security guards; however, there is an exposure–response relationship. People who work in high-exposure jobs, such as machinists, are more likely to develop disease than low-exposure workers. A glutamic acid at amino acid position 69 (Glu69) in HLA-DPB1 is associated with disease, present at a rate of 75–95% of workers with sensitization and CBD, compared to 35–45% of nondiseased workers. Thus, both exposure and host susceptibility contribute to disease. Physicians should suspect CBD in any patient with granulomatous lung disease who has worked with metals, especially with beryllium, regardless of how low the reported exposure has been.

Maier LA: Genetic and exposure risks for chronic beryllium disease. Clin Chest Med 23:827–839, 2002.

Martyny JW, Hoover MD, Mroz MM, et al: Aerosols generated during beryllium machining. J Occup Environ Med 42:8–18, 2000.

Saltini C, Winestock K, Kirby M, et al: Maintenance of alveolitis in patients with chronic beryllium disease by beryllium-specific helper T cells. N Engl J Med 320:1103–1109, 1989.

15. **Can CBD be differentiated from other granulomatous lung diseases such as sarcoidosis?**
CBD is often misdiagnosed as sarcoidosis. A blood and bronchoalveolar lavage (BAL) test called the beryllium lymphocyte proliferation test (BeLPT) can differentiate between these diseases. Cells from an individual with suspected CBD are exposed to beryllium salts *in vitro*. Because CBD results from an antigen-specific cell-mediated immune response to beryllium, cells from individuals with CBD proliferate, whereas those from patients with other granulomatous lung diseases do not. Although 10–30% false-negative rates have been reported with the blood test, it is still more sensitive than chest radiograph or PFTs. In cases in which CBD is suspected but the blood BeLPT is normal, BAL BeLPT may improve the diagnostic yield.

Kreiss K, Wasserman S, Mroz MM, et al: Beryllium disease screening in the ceramics industry. J Occup Med 35:267–274, 1993.

Maier LA: Beryllium health effects in the era of the beryllium lymphocyte proliferation test. Appl Occup Environ Hyg 16:514–520, 2001.

16. **What is required to make a diagnosis of CBD and beryllium sensitization?**
The current diagnostic criteria for CBD and sensitization rely on the use of the BeLPT to demonstrate a beryllium-specific immune response and, thus, exposure to beryllium. This test indicates if an individual is sensitized to beryllium. To confirm that someone has CBD requires the demonstration of granulomatous inflammation on biopsy, usually by a bronchoscopy with transbronchial biopsies. The absence of granulomas on biopsy confirms the diagnosis of beryllium sensitization. In a situation in which an individual is unable to undergo bronchoscopy but has evidence of a chest radiograph (Fig. 49-2) or CT scan consistent with CBD and an abnormal BeLPT, a diagnosis of CBD may be provided.

17. What is the treatment for beryllium-related health effects?

There is no cure for beryllium sensitization or CBD. Treatment of CBD is aimed at suppressing the immune and inflammatory response with prednisone. Prednisone indications include evidence of significant impairing lung disease on PFT, evidence of gas exchange abnormalities at rest or with exertion, severe disabling symptoms such as cough, or evidence of cor pulmonale. As the name implies, this disease usually has a chronic course; individuals without current evidence of severe disease need to be followed for their lifetime for development of disease impairment. Inhalers may be used to treat symptoms in earlier or later stages of disease. Removal from exposure is recommended for individuals with sensitization and disease as this is an immune-mediated disease.

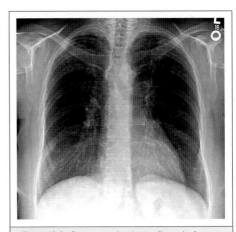

Figure 49-2. Posteroanterior chest radiograph of an individual with CBD, with hilar prominence and nodularity predominantly in the upper lobe.

Maier LA: Genetic and exposure risks for chronic beryllium disease. Clin Chest Med 23:827–839, 2002.

Maier LA, Newman LS: Beryllium disease. In Rom WN (ed): Environmental and Occupational Medicine, 3rd ed. Boston, Little, Brown, 1998, pp 1021–1035.

KEY POINTS: BERYLLIUM-RELATED HEALTH EFFECTS

1. Beryllium exposure in the workplace today still causes the granulomatous lung disease CBD and its precursor, beryllium sensitization.

2. A blood test, the beryllium lymphocyte proliferation test (BeLPT), is the cornerstone of the diagnosis of CBD and beryllium sensitization and differentiates CBD from other granulomatous lung diseases.

3. Individuals with beryllium sensitization demonstrate an immune response to beryllium but have no evidence of granulomatous lung disease; they do carry a risk of developing CBD at a rate of 6–8% per year.

4. The exposure–response relationship between beryllium and its health effects is not purely linear. This relationship is affected by a known genetic susceptibility factor, a glutamic acid at amino acid position 69 in HLA-DPB1 known as Glu69.

5. There is no cure for CBD; treatment is aimed at reducing the immune and inflammatory response in this disease using the nonspecific immunosuppressant prednisone. Removal from exposure is recommended for CBD and beryllium sensitization as these are immune-mediated processes.

CHAPTER 50

ASBESTOS-RELATED LUNG DISEASE

E. Brigitte Gottschall, MD, MSPH

1. What is asbestos?

Asbestos is the name given to a family of naturally occurring, fibrous, hydrated silicates present everywhere in the soil. The two major geologic types of asbestos fibers are **serpentine** (curly and long) and **amphibole** (rod-like and straight). Chrysotile, the only serpentine asbestos fiber, accounts for 95% of all asbestos used commercially worldwide. Of the amphibole fibers, crocidolite, amosite, and anthophyllite have been used commercially in small quantities, whereas tremolite and actinolite are mostly found as contaminants of other minerals such as chrysotile, talc, and vermiculite. All six asbestos fibers are resistant to the effects of heat, fire, acids, and alkali. They have great tensile strength and are flexible and weaveable. In addition, they are efficacious as insulators against heat, cold, and noise. These physical properties led to more than 3000 commercial applications of asbestos, most of which are banned in the United States and the western world now, but not in developing countries.

Bégin R, Samet JM, Shaikh RA: Asbestos. In Harber P, Schenker MB, Balmes JR (eds): Occupational and Environmental Respiratory Disease. St. Louis, Mosby, 1996, pp 293–329.

Burgess WA: Asbestos products. In Burgess WA (ed): Recognition of Health Hazards in Industry. New York, John Wiley & Sons, 1995, pp 443–451.

2. What determines the pathogenicity of asbestos fibers?

The toxicity of the various types of asbestos varies in part because of their distinct morphology and physicochemical properties. The width-to-length ratio (the aspect ratio) of asbestos fibers is one property that is critically important in determining their potential pathogenicity. An aspect ratio of 1:3 defines a fiber; an aspect ratio of ≥ 1:8 is associated with enhanced pathogenicity in asbestos fibers.

Dodson RF, Atkinson MA, Levin JL: Asbestos fiber length as related to potential pathogenicity: A critical review. Am J Indust Med 44(3):291–297, 2003.

Stanton MF, Layard M, Tegeris A, et al: Relation of particle dimension to carcinogenicity in amphibole asbestoses and other fibrous minerals. J Natl Cancer Inst 67(5): 965–975, 1981.

3. What occupations are associated with asbestos exposure?

Because there were more than 3000 commercial uses for asbestos, a listing of all occupations associated with potential exposure is not feasible. General industries in which exposure occurred range from asbestos mining and milling to the primary manufacturing of asbestos products including asbestos cement pipes, floor tiles, gaskets, thermal insulation, electrical insulation, friction products (e.g., brake and clutch pads), and textiles. The largest number of exposed workers is found in industries in which asbestos products are used, such as the construction industries, the automotive servicing industry, and the shipbuilding and repair industry. When taking a patient's occupational history, it is important to ask about job duties, work processes, and specifically whether asbestos exposure occurred. A job title is often uninformative. Some occupations associated with asbestos exposure are:

Asbestos miners	Gasket makers
Asbestos paper makers and users	Glass workers
Asbestos removal workers	Insulators
Automobile repair workers	Laborers
Boilermakers	Maintenance and custodial workers

Brake lining makers or repair workers	Petroleum refinery workers
Construction workers	Pipe fitters
Demolition workers	Plumbers
Electricians	Railroad workers
Roofers	Shipyard workers
Sheet metal workers	Textile workers

4. **Are people still exposed to asbestos?**

Yes. From the beginning of the 20th century until 1973, asbestos was used extensively in a large number of construction materials because of its physical properties (see question 1). In 1973, the U.S. Environmental Protection Agency banned its use in many, but not all, applications; however, large numbers of schools, public and commercial buildings, and even private homes continue to house asbestos-containing materials (e.g., acoustic ceiling tiles, vinyl floor tiles, paints, plasters, and insulation materials on pipes, boilers, and structural beams). Currently, exposure to asbestos may occur during the degradation of asbestos-containing materials in existing buildings. Occupational exposure to asbestos is also still of concern as asbestos removal workers, brake and clutch repair workers, construction workers involved in remodeling, and many others are still at risk of exposure to asbestos on their jobs.

Bates DV: Environmental Health Risks and Public Policy: Decision Making in Free Societies. Seattle, University of Washington Press, 1994, pp 27–35.

Oliver LC: Asbestos in public buildings. In Rom WN (ed): Environmental & Occupational Medicine, 3rd ed. Philadelphia, Lippincott-Raven, 1998, pp 387–395.

http://www.osha.gov/SLTC/asbestos/index.html

5. **What is paraoccupational exposure to asbestos?**

Paraoccupational exposure refers to exposure to a hazardous agent that is not directly associated with an individual's job or activity. Many construction workers who did not handle asbestos directly may have experienced significant exposure from use of asbestos by coworkers in their vicinity. For example, electricians and laborers were exposed as bystanders when insulators prepared asbestos mixtures to insulate steam pipes in shared working areas. Inadvertent domestic exposures occurred when asbestos workers carried large fiber burdens into the home on work clothing and hair. This "fouling of the nest" led to an increased incidence of mesothelioma and lung cancer in the families (including children) of asbestos workers.

Epler GR, Fitz Gerald MX, Gaensler EA, Carrington CB: Asbestos-related disease from household exposure. Respiration 39(4):229–240, 1980.

Schneider J, Woitowitz HJ: Pleural mesothelioma and household asbestos exposure. Rev EnvironHealth 11(1–2):65–70, 1996.

6. **What is a latency period?**

A latency period is the time between the first exposure and the clinical manifestations of disease. The latency period varies for the different manifestations of asbestos-related lung disease. Benign pleural effusions have the shortest latency at 5–20 years. Pleural plaques develop within 10–20 years. Asbestosis develops over 20–40 years. Lung cancer has a latency of > 15 years, and mesotheliomas often occur 15–40 years after exposure. These ranges are averages and may vary depending on exposure intensity and other factors. A manifestation of asbestos inhalation that develops outside these ranges may still be related to asbestos exposure.

7. **Describe the symptoms of asbestosis.**

Since asbestosis is defined as bilateral interstitial fibrosis of the lung parenchyma, the symptoms of asbestosis are similar to those of other interstitial lung fibroses and include slowly progressive dyspnea on exertion and dry cough. Chest pain, weight loss, and hemoptysis are not common and should raise the suspicion of asbestos-related malignancy.

KEY POINTS: RESPIRATORY DISEASES ASSOCIATED WITH ASBESTOS EXPOSURE

1. Pleural plaques (circumscribed, often partially calcified)

2. Diffuse pleural thickening

3. Benign pleural effusions

4. Rounded atelectasis

5. Asbestosis

6. Bronchogenic carcinoma

7. Mesothelioma

8. **How is asbestosis diagnosed?**
   The diagnosis of asbestosis usually can be based on clinical findings without histologic proof. A history of significant exposure (asbestosis has a well-established dose-response relationship), an appropriate interval between exposure and disease detection (i.e., 20- to 40-year latency), and radiographic evidence of interstitial fibrosis on chest radiograph or chest computed tomography (CT) scan are the primary means of establishing the diagnosis. Confirmatory but nonessential findings include other radiographic evidence of asbestos exposure such as pleural thickening or pleural calcification, pulmonary function tests (PFTs) with a restrictive pattern and decreased carbon monoxide diffusing capacity (DLCO), and bilateral inspiratory crackles on physical exam. Digital clubbing, cyanosis, and signs of cor pulmonale are seen in advanced stages of asbestosis. The main differential diagnoses are the other pneumoconioses and other causes of pulmonary fibrosis such as metal or organic dusts, drugs, infectious agents, collagen vascular disorders, and idiopathic pulmonary fibrosis (IPF).

   Although clinical assessment is usually sufficient to make a probable determination of asbestosis for medical and legal purposes, a more sensitive and specific method is the histologic and mineralogic evaluation of lung tissue. This, however, can be obtained only through an invasive procedure, with all of its associated risks. Transbronchial lung biopsy is generally inadequate to diagnose asbestosis. Video-assisted thoracic surgery (VATS) biopsy should be

KEY POINTS: CHEST COMPUTED TOMOGRAPHY FINDINGS TYPICAL FOR ASBESTOSIS

1. Pleural plaques or thickening (in almost all cases)

2. Thickened intralobular and interlobular lines (must be confirmed on prone imaging)

3. Parenchymal bands, often contiguous with the pleura

4. Honeycombing (in advanced cases)

5. Curvilinear subpleural lines of varying length, often parallel to the pleura (must also be confirmed on prone imaging)

obtained only if a thorough history and noninvasive testing yield no clues to the causes of pulmonary fibrosis. Even then, the risk-to-benefit ratio for biopsy must be weighed carefully.

Aberle DR, Balmes JR: Computed tomography of asbestos-related pulmonary parenchymal and pleural diseases. Clin Chest Med 12:115–131, 1991.

American Thoracic Society Documents: Diagnosis and initial management of nonmalignant diseases related to asbestos. Am J Respir Crit Care Med 170:691–715, 2004.

Asbestos, asbestosis, and cancer: The Helsinki criteria for diagnosis and attribution. Scand J Work Environ Health 23:311–316, 1997.

9. **What is a chest radiograph B-reading?**
The International Labor Organization (ILO) has assisted in designing a system of classifying chest radiographs of persons with pneumoconiosis to achieve better standardization for epidemiologic use. The strength of the ILO system lies in its systematic and more reproducible manner of assessing pneumoconiosis chest radiographs. The ILO classification, based on the posteroanterior chest radiograph, is a descriptive system consisting of a glossary of terms and a set of 22 standard radiographs illustrative of the pleural and parenchymal changes of the pneumoconioses. The classification grades the parenchymal, typically reticulonodular, pattern of the pneumoconioses based on size, shape, extent, and profusion (i.e., severity). Pleural abnormalities are also categorized and quantified. The National Institute for Occupational Safety and Health (NIOSH), in conjunction with the American College of Radiology (ACR), offers courses on the ILO classification. A physician who attends the course and passes a subsequent test is a NIOSH-certified B-reader. Of interest, 10–20% of symptomatic patients with asbestosis and gas exchange abnormalities have a normal chest radiograph. In such patients, high-resolution CT (HRCT) scan often shows early interstitial changes. HRCT has, therefore, become an essential tool in the diagnosis of asbestosis.

ILO: Guidelines for the use of the ILO international classification of radiographs of pneumoconioses. Geneva, International Labour Office, Occupational Safety and Health Series, No. 22 [REV], 2000.

10. **How does asbestosis appear histologically?**
Lung tissue taken from the lower lobes adjacent to the pleura is most likely to show histologic evidence of asbestosis. The development of end-stage asbestosis with severe lung fibrosis and honeycombing is a process that takes many years. The evolution of asbestosis lesions, from the early appearance of fibrosis surrounding only the respiratory bronchiole to honeycombing with destruction of alveoli, has been divided into four grades of severity by a panel from the College of American Pathologists:

- **Grade 1:** Discrete foci of fibrosis limited to the walls of first-order respiratory bronchioles
- **Grade 2:** Fibrosis extends into some adjacent alveolar ducts and septae
- **Grade 3:** Grade 2 fibrosis with more diffuse coalescent involvement of the respiratory bronchioles and the surrounding alveoli
- **Grade 4:** Obliteration of the parenchyma, with fibrous tissue and honeycombing

Occupational lung diseases and pneumoconioses. In King DW, Sobin LH, Stocker JT, et al (eds): Non-Neoplastic Disorders of the Lower Respiratory Tract, First Series, Fascicle 2. Washington, DC, American Registry of Pathology and the Armed Forces Institute of Pathology, 2002, pp 793–856.

Yamamoto S: Histopathological features of pulmonary asbestosis with particular emphasis on the comparison with those of usual interstitial pneumonia. Osaka City Med J 43:225–242, 1997.

11. **What is an asbestos body?**
Characteristically, two different types of asbestos are found in the lungs: (1) the uncoated, bare fiber and (2) the coated fiber, also called asbestos body. The bare fiber is an inhaled particle that may have undergone change due to fracture or digestion but has not accumulated a coating. The asbestos body is an asbestos fiber coated with proteins and iron compounds. It is a histologic marker of asbestos exposure and is associated more with amphibole than with chrysotile fibers.

Occasionally, the term "ferruginous body" is used in this context. Strictly speaking, a ferruginous body is any fiber coated by protein and iron compounds. Thus, the asbestos body is a specific kind of ferruginous body: a coated asbestos fiber. The asbestos body is the hallmark of asbestos exposure and an important feature of the histologic diagnosis of asbestosis. Asbestos bodies are best looked for on iron-stained tissue sections.

Occupational lung diseases and pneumoconioses. In King DW, Sobin LH, Stocker JT, et al (eds): Non-Neoplastic Disorders of the Lower Respiratory Tract, First Series, Fascicle 2. Washington, DC, American Registry of Pathology and the Armed Forces Institute of Pathology, 2002, pp 793–856.

12. **Is asbestosis treatable?**
There is no specific treatment for asbestosis. Corticosteroids and immunosuppressive agents have been tried without success and generally are not indicated. Treatment is supportive. Intercurrent respiratory infections may occur frequently and should be treated aggressively. Oxygen therapy is necessary for patients with hypoxemia at rest or during exercise. In the late stages of asbestosis, right heart failure (i.e., cor pulmonale) may develop; treatment consists of oxygen and diuretics. Influenza and pneumococcal vaccinations are warranted. Patients should be counseled to abstain from smoking to decrease the risk of developing lung cancer and to minimize the risks of other smoking-related diseases. The lack of viable treatment options for asbestosis emphasizes the critical need for primary prevention: reduction or elimination of asbestos exposure by using asbestos substitutes, engineering controls, or administrative controls.

Rom WD: Asbestos-related diseases. In Rom WN (ed): Environmental & Occupational Medicine, 3rd ed. Philadelphia, Lippincott-Raven, 1998, pp 349–375.

13. **Does everyone exposed to asbestos develop asbestosis?**
No. The most important factor in the development of asbestosis is the cumulative fiber dose to which a person is exposed. When exposure levels were very high in the early part of the century, the time from first asbestos exposure to clinical manifestations of asbestosis (i.e., the latency period) was reported to be around 5 years. With the introduction and implementation of exposure limits, latency periods have increased. Latency is inversely proportional to cumulative fiber dose. Some data suggest that the threshold fiber dose, below which asbestosis is not seen, is 25–100 fibers/mL/year. Although the cumulative fiber dose remains the strongest predictor of asbestosis, recent research suggests a possible component of individual susceptibility. What renders one person potentially susceptible at a lower cumulative dose than another is under intense investigation. Susceptibility probably is influenced by many factors including genetics, gender, ethnic origin, immune function, and fiber clearance.

14. **What is the significance of pleural plaques?**
Pleural plaques are focal, often partially calcified, irregular, fibrous tissue collections on the parietal pleura, diaphragm, or mediastinum (Fig. 50-1, *arrowheads*). They are the most frequent manifestation of

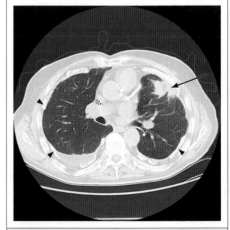

Figure 50-1. Chest CT image with multiple large, localized, partially calcified pleural plaques *(arrowheads)* and rounded atelectasis *(long arrow)*.

asbestos exposure and typically develop bilaterally, with a latency of 10–20 years. Often, they are noticed incidentally on a chest radiograph taken for a different reason. Pleural plaques alone rarely, if ever, lead to symptoms. A standard chest radiograph can identify 50–80% of pleural plaques actually present on chest CT scan. Over time, pleural plaques may calcify, making them more visible on plain chest radiograph. The greatest significance of pleural plaques lies in their recognition as markers of asbestos exposure.

Although the most common cause of pleural plaques is asbestos exposure, other diagnoses should be considered. Previous hemothorax, empyema, or repeated pneumothorax associated with tuberculosis may be implicated, especially if the pleural thickening or calcification is unilateral. Mesothelioma, lymphoma, multiple myeloma, and pleural metastasis may lead to localized pleural thickening. Occasionally, the callus of an old rib fracture may give the appearance of pleural thickening. Other exposures connected with pleural plaques are talc, mica, tin, barite, and silica; however, concomitant exposure to asbestos cannot be excluded.

Gottschall EB, Newman LS: Benign asbestos-related pleural disease. In Bouros D (ed): Pleural Disease. New York, Marcel Dekker, 2004, pp 545–569.

15. **What is diffuse pleural thickening?**

Diffuse pleural thickening (i.e., pachypleuritis) refers to more extensive fibrosis of the pleura (i.e., visceral pleura) than is seen with circumscribed pleural plaques. By definition, diffuse pleural thickening involves the costophrenic angles, which are not affected by circumscribed pleural plaques. The incidence of diffuse pleural thickening is much lower than that of pleural plaques. Diffuse pleural thickening is more likely to produce symptoms of dyspnea on exertion and restrictive physiology on PFT. Patients with pachypleuritis may die of hypercapnic respiratory failure as their lungs become encased by a thick pleural rind that prevents the lungs from expanding.

Kee ST, Gamsu G, Blanc P: Causes of pulmonary impairment in asbestos-exposed individuals with diffuse pleural thickening. Am J Respir Crit Care Med 154:789–793, 1996.

16. **What is rounded atelectasis?**

Rounded atelectasis is a form of partial collapse in the peripheral part of the lung. It is also called folded lung syndrome, Blesovsky's syndrome, shrinking pleuritis with atelectasis, atelectatic pseudotumor, and pleuroma. The pathogenesis is controversial. The most accepted theory postulates that a pleural inflammatory reaction is followed by pleural shrinkage, which causes atelectasis in the immediately adjacent lung parenchyma that assumes a rounded configuration. The principal cause is believed to be asbestos exposure; however, conditions such as parapneumonic effusions, congestive heart failure, Dressler's syndrome, pulmonary infarcts, chest trauma, and therapeutic pneumothoraces have been associated with rounded atelectasis.

Its clinical significance lies in its presentation as a pulmonary mass, which must be distinguished from a malignancy. It is often an incidental finding on chest radiograph, ranging from 2.5–7 cm in size. The angle between the pleura and the mass is usually sharp. The classic radiographic feature is a "comet tail" extending from the hilum toward the base of the lung and then sweeping into the inferior pole of the lesion (*see* Fig. 50-1, *long arrow*). In the past, the diagnosis often was made only at decortication, but CT of the chest permits recognition of this benign condition noninvasively.

Hillerdal G: Rounded atelectasis: Clinical experience with 74 patients. Chest 95:836–841, 1989.

17. **How do you diagnose an asbestos-related benign pleural effusion?**

Benign asbestos-related effusion is a diagnosis of exclusion. In patients with a significant history of asbestos exposure and an appropriate latency interval, in whom other causes (including bronchogenic carcinoma, mesothelioma, tuberculosis, and pulmonary embolism) have been considered, exudative, serosanguineous pleural effusions are probably due to asbestos exposure. These benign effusions may have white blood cell counts (WBCs) of up to 28,000/mm^3, and polymorphonuclear or mononuclear cells may predominate in the WBC differential. Some series have shown pleural fluid eosinophilia. Asbestos-related benign pleural effusions produce few symptoms and may be discovered incidentally on serial chest radiographs. The effusion, on average, lasts several months and eventually clears without residual effects.

Epler GR, McLoud TC, Gaensler EA: Prevalence and incidence of benign asbestos pleural effusions in a working population. JAMA 247:617–622, 1982.

18. **What are the important facts about lung cancer in asbestos-exposed workers?**
The association between occupational asbestos exposure and an increased risk for lung cancer is well established. Although the majority of these cancers occur in individuals with asbestosis, it is important to remember that underlying asbestosis is not a requirement to attribute lung cancer to asbestos exposure. Every patient diagnosed with a bronchogenic carcinoma should be asked about occupational exposure to lung carcinogens including asbestos. Cigarette smoke and asbestos exposure have a well-documented synergistic (i.e., multiplicative) effect on the risk of lung cancer. Asbestos-exposed smokers carry a 60-fold greater risk of developing lung cancer than people who have never smoked and who have not worked with asbestos. This emphasizes how critically important smoking cessation is in the care of asbestos-exposed workers. The clinical presentation, diagnostic evaluation, pathology, treatment, and prognosis of lung cancer due to asbestos do not differ from lung cancer due to tobacco use. However, the diagnosis of asbestos-related lung cancer may have legal implications, and patients should be guided to obtain further information to this effect.

Asbestos, asbestosis, and cancer: The Helsinki criteria for diagnosis and attribution. Scand J Work Environ Health 23:311–316, 1997.

19. **What is mesothelioma?**
Mesothelioma is an uncommon but increasingly recognized malignant neoplasm, typically of the pleura (80%) and rarely of other mesothelial surfaces (e.g., the peritoneum, pericardium, or tunica vaginalis testis). It is one of the few malignant tumors for which the specific etiologic agent has been identified. Of patients diagnosed with malignant mesothelioma, 80–85% have had occupational, paraoccupational, or environmental exposure to asbestos. The latent period between first exposure and clinical detection of the neoplasm is usually 15–40 years. Unlike bronchogenic carcinoma, cigarette smoking does not confer an increased risk of developing mesothelioma.

Dull, aching chest pain combined with slowly progressive dyspnea and weight loss are often the presenting symptoms. Pleural effusions occur in approximately 60% of patients. A biopsy with video-assisted thoracoscopy is usually needed to establish the diagnosis; only one-third of blind, closed pleural biopsies yield a diagnosis.

Pistolesi M, Rusthoven J: Malignant pleural mesothelioma: Update, current management, and newer therapeutic strategies. Chest 126:1318–1329, 2004.

20. **What is the medical management of mesothelioma?**
In general, treatment of mesotheliomas, either by surgery, radiotherapy, or chemotherapy, has extended survival by only a few months, if at all. New directions in therapy include aggressive combined modality treatment in potentially resectable patients and targeted chemotherapy with new-generation antifolates, antiangiogenesis agents, and agents directed at the epidermal growth factor receptor in unresectable cases. During such therapy regimens and if therapy fails, treatment is supportive, including pain management, nutritional support, treatment of infections, and counseling of patient and family. Death usually occurs 8 months to 2 years after diagnosis as a result of extensive local spread, infection, or respiratory failure.

Maziak DE, Gagliardi A, Haynes AE, et al: Surgical management of malignant pleural mesothelioma: A systematic review and evidence summary. Lung Cancer 48(2):157–169, 2005.

Steele JP, Klabatsa A: Chemotherapy options and new advances in malignant pleural mesothelioma. Ann Oncol 16(3):345–351, 2005.

21. **How do you counsel a patient with asbestos-related disease?**

The care of a patient with a work-related disorder does not stop with medical treatment and psychologic support. Each patient should be counseled that the diagnosis of an asbestos-related disorder may raise legal issues that can be further explored with a knowledgeable lawyer. Either written or verbal communication of a diagnosis of work-related disease may trigger the legal statute of limitations (i.e., the time frame in which the patient must file a legal claim for benefits). Thus, patients should be counseled to seek appropriate legal support.

CHAPTER 51

HYPERSENSITIVITY PNEUMONITIS AND OTHER DISORDERS CAUSED BY ORGANIC AGENTS

Cecile Rose, MD, MPH

1. **What is meant by the term *organic agent*?**

   Substances of animal and vegetable origin are generally referred to as *organic agents*. Airborne organic agents are called *bioaerosols*; these are airborne particles, large molecules, or volatile compounds that are living or were released from a living organism. Common bioaerosols capable of causing human diseases include bacteria, fungi, protozoa, viruses, algae, green plants, arthropods, and mammalian byproducts. For example, aerosols of cat saliva can cause asthma and rhinitis in cat-sensitive individuals.

   The conditions necessary to produce aerosolization of an organism or its parts are (1) a reservoir, (2) amplification (i.e., an increase in numbers or concentration), and (3) dissemination (by aerosolization). Human hosts are reservoirs for some organisms (e.g., *Mycobacterium tuberculosis*) disseminated through aerosols from coughing. Environmental reservoirs may act as amplifiers or disseminators (e.g., *Legionella* bioaerosol dissemination from cooling towers or respirable mycobacterial aerosols from hot tub sprays).

   Burge HA: Airborne allergenic fungi: Classification, nomenclature, and distribution. Immunol Allergy Clin North Am 92:307–319, 1989.

2. **Describe the spectrum of diseases caused by exposure to organic agents.**

   The spectrum of diseases associated with inhalation of organic agents includes:
   - Hypersensitivity pneumonitis (HP)
   - Rhinoconjunctivitis
   - Asthma
   - Inhalation fevers such as grain fever, organic dust toxic syndrome (ODTS), and humidifier fever
   - Infections such as *Legionella* pneumonia or unusual infections from outbreaks in laboratory workers
   - Chronic airflow limitation and accelerated decline in lung function such as the decline in the forced expiratory volume in 1 second (FEV_1) often found in workers exposed to cotton dust, grain workers, and animal confinement workers

3. **What pathophysiologic mechanisms occur in the diseases caused by organic agents?**

   Organic agents are capable of causing disease by both immune and nonimmune mechanisms.
   - Bronchoalveolar lavage (BAL) studies of HP show an acute neutrophilia followed by macrophage activations and thymus-dependent lymphocyte (T-L) alveolitis.
   - Rhinoconjunctivitis and allergic asthma from organic dust exposures involve an immunoglobulin E (IgE)-mediated, immediate-type hypersensitivity reaction.
   - Inhalation fevers are noninfectious, nonallergic, acute, self-limited febrile responses to inhalation of high concentrations of grain dusts and some microbial bioaerosols associated with increases in several cytokines including interleukin 6 (IL-6).
   - Chronic airflow limitation and chronic bronchitis are probably a combination of toxic and immune-mediated processes from exposure to a variety of organic dust contaminants includ-

ing endotoxins from the cell walls of gram-negative bacteria, glucans contained in fungal cell walls, and inhaled microorganisms that cause the immunologic effects.

4. **What industries or occupational groups are most likely to be affected by exposure to organic agents?**

Bioaerosol exposures have been described in a wide variety of environmental and occupational settings including home and recreational hot tubs, contaminated humidifiers in homes or office buildings, and particulates from decaying wood and damp walls in inner-city dwellings. Common occupational and environmental settings in which exposure to organic agents is likely to occur include the following:

- **Agriculture:** The classic form of HP, farmer's lung, is associated with inhalation of thermophilic bacteria and fungal contaminants in hay and grain. Mushroom workers, cheese workers, and wood workers are at risk for both HP and asthma from exposure to microbial bioaerosols.
- **Bird fanciers:** Proteins capable of causing HP are present in the serum and droppings of birds. Indirect exposures to avian antigens (e.g., from feather pillows and bed clothes) or to those laundering bird-dust-contaminated clothing have been associated with cases of HP.
- **Health care industries:** Potential workplace bioaerosols include a variety of infectious agents such as viruses and mycobacteria. Laboratory animal workers are at risk for unusual infections such as Q fever (caused by *Coxiella burnetii*) and for allergic rhinoconjunctivitis and occupational asthma (from exposure to aerosolized proteins in the urine of laboratory animals or from powdered latex gloves).

Rose CS, Martyny JW, Newman LS, et al: "Lifeguard lung": Endemic granulomatous pneumonitis in an indoor swimming pool. Am J Public Health 88:1795–1800, 1998.

5. **How many people are affected by diseases resulting from exposure to organic agents?**

The number is not known, but, probably, many more are affected than are clinically recognized. Our understanding of disease incidence and prevalence is hampered by the lack of a national database and reporting system, the nonspecificity of the symptoms associated with exposures to bioaerosols and other organic agents, and the lack of a gold standard for diagnosis of diseases such as HP.

Most of the population-based studies of HP focus on the prevalence of illness among agricultural workers. In Scotland, the prevalence of farmer's lung in three agricultural areas ranged from 2.3–8.6%. A questionnaire survey of western Wyoming dairy and cattle ranchers elicited a history typical of acute farmer's lung disease in 3% of those surveyed. The prevalence of HP among bird hobbyists is estimated to range from 0.5–21%.

Yoshizawa Y, Ohtani Y, Hayakawa H, et al: Chronic hypersensitivity pneumonitis in Japan: A nationwide epidemiologic survey. J Allergy Clin Immunol 103:315–320, 1999.

Zejda JE, McDuffie HH, Dosman JA: Epidemiology of health and safety risks in agriculture and related industries. Practical applications for rural physicians. West J Med 158:56–63, 1993.

6. **Describe the symptoms and signs of disease caused by exposure to organic agents.**

Hypersensitivity pneumonitis (i.e., allergic alveolitis) is characterized in its acute form by recurrent pneumonitis with fever, chills, cough, chest tightness, shortness of breath, and myalgias. The subacute and chronic forms of HP are manifested by insidious and progressive dyspnea, fatigue, cough, weight loss, and decreased appetite.

Asthma is characterized by complaints of wheezing, chest tightness, cough, and shortness of breath. Symptoms may occur immediately after exposure or 6–12 hours later. Diagnosis usually relies on the patient's history, wheezing on examination, and reversible airflow limitation on pulmonary function (PF) testing, including methacholine challenge testing.

Allergic rhinitis is diagnosed by history, physical examination, the finding of eosinophils on nasal smear, elevated total or specific IgE antibody levels, and immediate skin prick testing to relevant aeroallergens.

Inhalation fevers are characterized by fevers, chills, malaise, and muscle aches but have no prominent pulmonary symptoms or signs. Symptoms usually occur within 48 hours after exposure and subside within 24–48 hours, with no long-term sequelae.

Richerson HB, Bernstein IL, Fink JN, et al: Guidelines for the clinical evaluation of hypersensitivity pneumonitis. Report of the Subcommittee on Hypersensitivity Pneumonitis. J Allergy Clin Immunol 84:839–844, 1989.

7. **How is the diagnosis of HP established?**
   Since there is no single diagnostic test for HP, diagnosis relies on a constellation of historical, imaging, pulmonary function, and histologic findings (Table 51-1). The usual approach includes:
   - **Detailed clinical and exposure histories.**
   - **Physical examination:** It may be normal, but bibasilar inspiratory crackles and clubbing occur in more advanced HP.
   - **PF testing:** May be normal in early or mild disease, but typically shows restrictive, obstructive, or mixed abnormalities, sometimes with a decreased diffusion capacity for carbon monoxide. Gas exchange abnormalities are often present with exercise.
   - **Imaging:** Chest radiograph may be normal in early stages of disease but typically reveals small, discrete, scattered 1- to 3-mm nodules, often predominant in the lower lobe. Diffuse, patchy infiltrates or a ground-glass appearance may be present. Radiographic abnormalities in acute illness typically regress or resolve over 4–6 weeks if further exposure is avoided. In the subacute or chronic form of HP, linear interstitial markings become more distinct and are often associated with progressive loss of lung volume (Fig. 51-1). High-resolution computed tomography (HRCT) scanning may be normal if disease is diagnosed early. In subacute or chronic HP, the predominant HRCT pattern is poorly defined centrilobular micronodules, often with ground-glass attenuation. These findings probably reflect the histologic findings of cellular bronchiolitis, noncaseating granulomas, and active alveolitis (Fig. 51-2).
   - **Biopsy:** Fiberoptic bronchoscopy with BAL and transbronchial biopsies is often necessary to confirm the diagnosis of HP. If this is nondiagnostic and doubt remains, surgical lung biopsy

---

TABLE 51-1.   DIAGNOSTIC APPROACH TO PATIENTS WITH POSSIBLE HYPERSENSITIVITY PNEUMONITIS

1. Detailed history of occupational and environmental exposures, along with regular clinical history
2. Physical examination
3. Pulmonary function tests including spirometry, lung volumes, and carbon monoxide diffusion in the lung (DLCO)
4. Chest radiograph (posteroanterior and lateral)
5. HRCT if chest film is negative or nonspecific
6. Exercise ventilatory and gas exchange parameter assessment if exertion dyspnea is prominent
7. Consider serum precipitin analysis. Negative results do not rule out HP, but a positive precipitin result helps confirm relevant antigenic exposures.
8. Fiberoptic bronchoscopy (FOB) with bronchoalveolar lavage if diagnosis is in doubt. Surgical lung biopsy may be indicated if FOB is nondiagnostic.

is sometimes necessary. The classic histologic triad for HP includes airway-centered cellular bronchiolitis, mononuclear interstitial inflammation (often with organizing pneumonia), and noncaseating granulomas, although all three features are not always present.

Ando M, Arima K, Yoneda R, Tamura M: Japanese summer-type hypersensitivity pneumonitis. Geographic distribution, home environment, and clinical characteristics of 621 cases. Am Rev Respir Dis 144:765–769, 1991.

Coleman A, Colby TV: Histologic diagnosis of extrinsic allergic alveolitis. Am J Surg Pathol 12:514–518, 1988.

Lacasse Y, Selman M, Costabel U, et al: Clinical diagnosis of hypersensitivity pneumonitis. Am J Respir Crit Care Med 168:952–958, 2003.

Lynch DA, Rose CS, Way D, King TE Jr: Hypersensitivity pneumonitis: sensitivity of high-resolution CT in a population-based study. Am J Roentgenol 159:469–472, 1992.

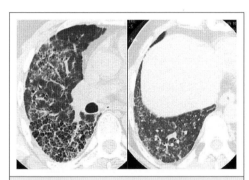

Figure 51-1. In the subacute or chronic form of HP, linear interstitial markings become more distinct and are often associated with progressive loss of lung volume.

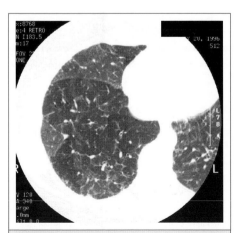

Figure 51-2. In subacute or chronic HP, the predominant CT pattern is poorly defined centrilobular micronodules, often with ground-glass attenuation.

8. **Are precipitating antibodies useful in the diagnosis of HP?**
Precipitin testing is neither sensitive nor specific in making a diagnosis of HP. The finding of specific precipitating antibodies in the serum of a patient with suspected HP indicates exposure sufficient to generate a humoral immunologic response; this may be a helpful diagnostic clue, particularly for avian precipitins. However, specific precipitating antibodies are frequently not demonstrable in patients with HP. Moreover, positive precipitins are often found in antigen-exposed individuals without clinically evident disease.

9. **What information should be included in the occupational and environmental histories of patients with suspected exposure to organic agents?**
The most important approach to diagnosis of diseases caused by organic agents is a high index of suspicion and careful occupation and environment history-taking. The occupation history should contain a chronology of current and previous occupations, a description of job processes and specific work practices (e.g., baling moldy hay), and a list of specific exposures.
Improvement in symptoms away from work or a worsening of symptoms with specific exposures can be a helpful diagnostic clue when present. Additionally, the presence of persistent respiratory or constitutional symptoms, or both, in exposed coworkers can be helpful in identifying exposure-related disease.
    The environmental and home history should include:
- A list of pets and other domestic animals
- Hobbies and recreational activities that may involve exposures to organic dusts
- Use of hot tubs, saunas, or indoor swimming pools
- Presence of leaking or flooding in a basement or occupied space
- Presence of humidifiers, dehumidifiers, swamp coolers, or cool mist vaporizers
- Water damage to carpets and furnishings
- Visible mold or mildew contamination in the occupied space
- Use of feathers in pillows, comforters, or clothing

Embil J, Warren P, Yakrus M, et al: Pulmonary illness associated with exposure to *Mycobacterium-avium* complex in hot tub water. Hypersensitivity pneumonitis or infection? Chest 111:813–816, 1997.

10. **What treatment options are available for diseases caused by exposure to organic agents?**
For the hypersensitivity diseases (i.e., rhinoconjunctivitis, asthma, and hypersensitivity pneumonitis), early recognition and removal from antigen exposure is important for disease management.

KEY POINTS: HYPERSENSITIVITY PNEUMONITIS

1. The three major categories of agents capable of causing HP are microbial agents (i.e., bacteria, fungi, and their byproducts), animal proteins (particularly those from birds), and a few low-molecular-weight chemicals (including isocyanates).

2. If a lung HRCT scan shows features of patchy ground-glass opacities or small centrilobular nodules, a diagnosis of HP should be considered.

3. Negative serum-precipitating antibodies does not rule out a diagnosis of HP. Positive precipitins do not confirm the diagnosis.

4. Lung biopsy in HP typically features the triad of bronchiolitis, lymphoplasmacytic interstitial infiltrates, and poorly formed nonnecrotizing granulomas (60–70%). Giant cells, airspace foam cells, and bronchiolitis obliterans may occur. A fibrotic pattern similar to usual interstitial pneumonitis may be seen in chronic HP.

Pharmacologic therapy for asthma and rhinoconjunctivitis using inhaled and topical antiinflammatories is similar to that for other causes of these diseases. In patients with HP who have more severe abnormalities at presentation or persistent symptoms despite removal from exposure, short-term (i.e., 2–6 months') treatment with oral corticosteroids may be helpful. Treatment is generally not required for the inhalation fevers as they are self limited. Prevention of recurrent episodes is recommended because little is known about risk from repeated attacks of inhalation fever.

Kokkarinen JI, Tukiainen HO, Terho EO: Effect of corticosteroid treatment on the recovery of pulmonary function in farmer's lung. Am Rev Respir Dis 145:3–5, 1992.

11. What is the prognosis for recovery from HP?

The clinical course of HP is variable, but permanent sequelae may include persistent airway hyperresponsiveness, emphysema, or interstitial fibrosis. An accelerated decline in lung function with continued antigen exposure has been demonstrated for most forms of HP, underscoring the importance of exposure cessation. Acute HP generally resolves without sequelae. The subacute and chronic forms are frequently recognized later in the disease course, resulting in a poorer prognosis. Factors that predict mortality from HP include age at diagnosis > 44 years, smoking, clubbing, male gender, honeycombing on HRCT, total lung capacity (TLC) < 65% predicted, and symptoms for 20 months or more before diagnosis.

Erkinjuntti-Pekkanen R, Rytkonen H, Kokkarinen JI, et al: Long-term risk of emphysema in patients with farmer's lung and matched control farmers. Am J Respir Crit Care Med 158:662–665, 1998.

Munakata M, Tanimura K, Ukuta H: Smoking promotes insidious and chronic farmer's lung disease, and deteriorates the clinical outcome. Intern Med 34:966–971, 1995.

12. For patients with immunologic lung diseases from organic agents, how are causal exposures effectively eliminated?

Eliminating antigen exposure is the most challenging part of the treatment. In some cases, an investigation aimed at assessing the bioaerosol status of the building or home can be undertaken. Although it is often difficult to prove the connection between specific exposures and disease, it may be possible to demonstrate bioaerosol reservoirs, amplifiers, and disseminators during an on-site inspection. The presence of potential bioaerosol sources may be sufficient for remedial action to be undertaken without further investigation.

If additional exposure documentation is required, quantitative bioaerosol sampling can be considered. The primary objective of air sampling is to identify the source of bioaerosol components so that effective corrective action can be undertaken. Dose-response information is not available. Positive results may document the presence of a specific source; however, negative results are usually inconclusive with respect to confirming the presence or absence of sources. An exposure may be considered potentially significant when indoor levels of the bioaerosol are at least an order of magnitude higher than those in outdoor air or when the types of bioaerosols differ between the control environment and the complaint environment. The mere presence of an unusual organism or antigen in an environment does not prove a causal relationship between the exposure and the illness.

For patients with bird-related HP, removal of the birds should be followed by efforts to eliminate reservoirs of their dust from the environment through methods such as wet wiping of surfaces; removal of carpets, mats, and other fleecy furnishings that harbor protein dusts; and cleaning of air-handling systems.

Bracker A, Storey E, Yang C, Hodgson MJ: An outbreak of hypersensitivity pneumonitis at a metalworking plant: a longitudinal assessment of intervention effectiveness. Appl Occup Environ Hygiene 18:96–108, 2003.

Craig TJ, Hershey J, Engler RJ, et al: Bird antigen persistence in the home environment after removal of the bird. Ann Allergy 69:510–512, 1992.

Yoshida K, Ando M, Sakata T, Araki S: Prevention of summer-type hypersensitivity pneumonitis: Effect of elimination of Trichosporon cutaneum from the patients' homes. Arch Environ Health 44:317–322, 1989.

13. **Are diseases caused by organic agents preventable?**

There is little research on prevention of these diseases. Complete elimination of indoor allergens is probably impossible, so it may be necessary to relocate immunologically sensitized individuals once hypersensitivity lung disease has occurred.

Appropriate design and maintenance of heating, ventilation, and air conditioning systems is important in limiting microbial amplification and dissemination. Contaminants can be diluted by an increase in the amount of outdoor air in a building, and high-efficiency filters can be added to the ventilation system to improve quality of recirculated air.

Indoor microbial contamination is often related to problems with moisture control. Source control includes preventing leaking and flooding; removing stagnant water sources; eliminating aerosol humidifiers, vaporizers, or hot tubs; and maintaining indoor relative humidity below 70%.

The efficacy of various types of respirators in preventing antigen sensitization and disease progression is unknown. Helmet-type powered air purifying respirators have been used to prevent episodic exposure in individuals with previous acute episodes of farmer's lung. Prolonged wearing of respiratory protection is limited by the fact that most respirators are hot and cumbersome. Dust respirators offer incomplete protection against organic particulates and are not recommended once sensitization has occurred.

Mauny F, Polio JC, Monnet E, et al: Longitudinal study of respiratory health in dairy farmers: Influence of artificial barn fodder drying. Eur Respir J 10:2522–2528, 1997.

CHAPTER 52

OCCUPATIONAL ASTHMA

Anne E. Dixon, MD, and Ronald Balkissoon, MD

1. **What is occupational asthma?**
   Occupational asthma refers to disorders characterized by variable airflow limitation, airway hyperresponsiveness, or both, attributable to specific exposures found in the workplace. Occupational asthma may be subclassified into two groups: occupational asthma with latency and occupational asthma without latency.

2. **How common is occupational asthma?**
   Over 300 different agents are recognized as potentially causing occupational asthma, and the list continues to grow. It is believed that approximately 10–20% of adult-onset asthma is work related. In many industrialized countries, the annual number of reported cases of occupational asthma has surpassed that of dust-related lung diseases such as silicosis and asbestosis.

3. **Define occupational asthma with latency.**
   Occupational asthma with latency generally implies an immune-mediated asthma caused by a workplace agent (i.e., a sensitizer). After variable periods of exposure, susceptible individuals develop an immune response (i.e., a sensitization) to a specific agent. Once an individual has become sensitized, he or she may report developing symptoms a few hours into the work shift, late in the work shift, after returning home, or sometimes even during sleeping hours. These latencies correspond to the well-recognized patterns of early, late, or dual asthmatic responses.

4. **What is a sensitizer?**
   The term *sensitizer* refers to an agent that appears to cause asthma through immune-mediated mechanisms. In other words, they cause characteristic patterns of early, late, or dual responses or else (or in addition) they demonstrate positive skin test, immunoglobulin response, or radioallergosorbent test (RAST) responses, or other evidence of immune system activation. Sensitizers have been divided into high-molecular-weight and low-molecular-weight compounds.

5. **Give some examples of high-molecular-weight compounds that can induce asthma.**
   See Table 52-1.

6. **Give some examples of low-molecular-weight compounds that can induce asthma.**
   See Table 52-2.

7. **What is occupational asthma without latency?**
   Occupational asthma without latency is considered to be nonimmunologically mediated. Common terms used to describe this phenomenon include irritant-induced asthma and reactive airways dysfunction syndrome (RADS). Individuals develop the clinical characteristics of asthma (i.e., variable airflow obstruction and airway hyper-responsiveness) immediately following high-level exposure to an agent that is recognized to have strong irritant properties.

TABLE 52-1. HIGH-MOLECULAR-WEIGHT COMPOUNDS THAT CAN INDUCE ASTHMA	
Products	**Occupation**
Animal products (proteins)	Lab workers, veterinarians
Bird proteins	Breeders, poultry workers
Insect proteins	Grain workers, researchers
Plant proteins	Bakers, food processors, latex workers
Biologic enzymes	Detergent and pharmaceutical industries
Vegetables (gums)	Printers
Fish proteins	Crab, shrimp, and oyster processing industries

TABLE 52-2. LOW-MOLECULAR-WEIGHT COMPOUNDS THAT CAN INDUCE ASTHMA	
Products	**Occupation**
Diisocyanates	Plastic, polyurethane, and paint workers
Anhydrides	Manufacturers of epoxy resins and plastics
Wood dust (e.g., plicatic acid in redwood cedar)	Carpenters and saw mill and construction workers
Fluxes, colophony	Soldering, welders
Drugs	Pharmaceutical and health care workers
Metals	Platers, welders, metal and chemical workers
Ethanolamines, ethylenediamines, aromatic amines, methacrylates	Workers in cosmetics, manufacturing, and rubber and fur industries
Biocides	Hospital workers
Reactive dyes	Reactive dyes manufacturers, wool dye house workers

8. **Does low-level chronic exposure to irritants cause asthma?**

   It remains controversial whether chronic occupational exposure to irritants such as acid mists or various types of dusts or smoke can lead to asthma or asthma-like conditions. Workers report the gradual onset of asthma-like symptoms following chronic exposure to irritants (i.e., a latency period), but these disorders do not appear to be immune mediated. The terms *irritant-induced bronchitis* and *industrial bronchitis* have been used to describe these patients.

   Irritant-induced asthma must be distinguished from preexisting asthma aggravated by workplace irritants.

9. **What are some common irritants?**

   Agents that are responsible for irritant-induced asthma are presumed to cause direct airway injury, although the precise mechanism remains unknown and likely varies with the agent in question. Some common irritants include

- Fire smoke
- Gases such as chlorine and ammonia
- Atmospheric pollutants such as ozone and sulfur dioxide
- Oil-based and certain acrylic-based paints
- Formaldehyde used in hospitals, embalming, and rubber and plastic industries (may be immune mediated)
- Aluminum smelter emissions containing gaseous fluorides, hydrofluoric acid, sulfur dioxide, and cold tar volatiles (causing pot room asthma)
- Machining lubricant and coolant fluids containing trace amounts of metals, additives, and bactericidal agents that are potential respiratory irritants
- Machining fluids with inadequate bactericide agents, allowing growth of bacteria and fungi

10. **Is there a difference between occupational asthma and work-related asthma?**
The term *work-related asthma* encompasses not only asthma caused by work (i.e., occupational asthma) but also preexisting asthma aggravated by workplace exposures. Work-related asthma has a much broader definition than occupational asthma and is used for medicolegal and work-ers' compensation purposes. Some jurisdictions recognize workplace aggravation of underlying asthma as compensable, but many jurisdictions do not.

KEY POINTS: CAUSES OF OCCUPATIONAL ASTHMA

1. Occupational asthma with latency: an immune response to a workplace antigen (e.g., flour or latex)

2. Occupational asthma without latency: a nonimmunologic response caused by high-level exposure to a strong irritant (e.g., chlorine gas)

3. Work-aggravated asthma: Preexisting asthma is aggravated by workplace exposures

4. Note that controversy exists over whether chronic low-level expose to irritants can induce asthma

11. **Are there any risk factors for developing occupational asthma?**
Level of exposure to an agent is an important determinant of whether asthma develops, with higher exposures associated with higher incidences of asthma. Certain human lymphocyte anti-gen (HLA) class II subtypes have been associated with an increased risk of occupational asthma in response to low-molecular-weight agents. Atopy may be a risk factor for sensitization to cer-tain high-molecular-weight compounds. Risks related to gender may be related to different job exposures. Cigarette smoking has been shown to be a risk factor for developing asthma in response to certain exposures.

12. **What conditions should be considered in the differential diagnosis of occupational asthma?**
The initial differential should include underlying asthma or chronic bronchitis irritated by work-place exposures. Hypersensitivity pneumonitis or other respiratory diseases that may have air-way involvement, such as sarcoidosis, may also be aggravated by workplace exposures.
    The remainder of the differential diagnosis is similar to that for nonoccupational asthma and includes such varied entities as gastroesophageal reflux disease, rhinosinusitis with postnasal drip, vocal cord and upper-airway dysfunction, irritant tracheobronchitis, and psychogenic or factitious conditions (e.g., malingering).

13. **What clinical criteria suggest RADS?**
    - There has been no prior history of asthma-like respiratory disease.
    - Onset follows high-level exposures, typically occurring with accidents or spills.
    - Toxicants are usually recognized irritant gases, vapors, fumes, aerosols, or dusts, present in very high concentrations.
    - The onset of symptoms is abrupt, occurring within minutes to hours, but always within the first 72 hours (original definition was 24 hours) of exposure.
    - Symptoms are identical to those of asthma (i.e., chest tightness, wheezing, dyspnea, and cough).
    - Spirometry may demonstrate reversible airflow obstruction (i.e., >12% improvement in the forced expiratory volume in 1 second [FEV_1] after administration of a bronchodilator).
    - Nonspecific bronchial provocation with methacholine or histamine reveals a positive response.
    - Other respiratory disorders that simulate asthma are ruled out.

14. **Is the clinical course of RADS distinct in any way from other asthmas?**
    The clinical course of RADS is very much like that of other asthmas, having a variable response to steroids and a variable long-term prognosis. Some patients have complete recovery within days to weeks, and others never completely recover. Some studies suggest that early treatment with steroids (inhaled and oral) may improve prognosis.

15. **What are the current methods used to evaluate patients for possible occupational asthma?**
    A thorough medical and exposure history documenting the temporal relationship between exposures and onset of symptoms is essential, followed by pulmonary function (PF) tests to assess airway obstruction, reversibility, and hyperresponsiveness. Once the presence of asthma is confirmed, the relationship to occupational exposure is determined based on reviewing history and objectively assessing symptoms and lung function over 2–4 weeks at work and 2–4 weeks away from work (if feasible). Lung function is evaluated using peak flow monitors, spirometry, or methacholine inhalation tests, or a combination thereof.

16. **What are the essential points in evaluating a history of occupational asthma?**
    - **Temporal relationship of symptoms:** Worse at work or better on weekends, holidays, and vacations.
    - **Duration of exposure (including current and previous jobs) before the onset of symptoms:** Will establish the latency period and whether it is more likely to be an immune versus an irritant effect.
    - **Symptoms during the work shift:** Individuals who report symptoms developing right away (within minutes) after starting the work shift are more likely to have irritant effects rather than immune-mediated effects.
    - **Progressive symptoms through a day or work week:** Suggest aggravation of preexisting asthma from a chronic irritant or, possibly, an unrecognized sensitivity.

17. **What is the usefulness of PF testing in evaluating occupational asthma?**
    - Serial peak-flow measurements are highly operator dependent, and recent studies suggest they are unreliable in diagnosing occupational asthma. They may be used as an adjunct in patients thought to be reliable and compliant or who are in supervised situations.
    - Serial spirometry comparisons are difficult to obtain during periods at and away from work because of the requirements for a technician and sophisticated equipment.
    - Serial methacholine challenge tests are fairly reliable measurements of nonspecific bronchial hyperresponsiveness and should show a significant improvement (i.e., a twofold to threefold increase in PC_{20}) during a period away from exposure lasting 4 or more weeks.

18. **Are tests of immunoreactivity useful in occupational asthma?**
    As a general rule, tests of immunoreactivity are supportive evidence but neither confirm or rule out the possibility of occupational asthma.

19. **Can skin testing be used to confirm sensitivity to a workplace irritant?**
    Skin tests are not very specific for asthma because some individuals may have positive skin tests and no objective evidence for asthma. Nor are they sensitive, because individuals may have negative skin tests and positive inhalation challenges.

20. **What is the role of RAST, enzyme-linked immunosorbent assay (ELISA), and serum immunoglobulins in the evaluation?**
    These tests may confirm exposure and immune sensitization but do not confirm a diagnosis of asthma. No prospective cohort studies have been performed to establish the proportion of individuals with positive immunoglobulin levels to a particular agent who go on to develop work-related asthma.

21. **What are specific inhalation challenges?**
    These tests are considered the gold standard for establishing whether a particular agent is the cause of a person's asthma. Specific inhalation challenges involve testing individuals by direct exposure to the potential workplace agent in a controlled lab environment (i.e., a challenge chamber). This typically requires observing a person during control (i.e., sham) exposures and increasing doses of the putative causative agent over several days. After the final exposure for a given day, subjects need to be observed for up to 8 or more hours in a hospital to ensure that they do not have a significant late reaction. Because there are few reliable, specialized centers that perform these tests, the reliability and reproducibility of these methods have not been thoroughly documented.

22. **What are appropriate clinical indications for specific inhalation challenges?**
    - Individuals who may have become sensitized to a specific agent and in whom confirming the diagnosis has significance for possible job modification or compensation purposes.
    - Individuals having a prior history of asthma or other respiratory conditions in whom there is a question of whether a specific workplace agent is causing a true immune (i.e., a sensitized) response. If the worker is truly sensitized, he or she may need to switch jobs; if it is only an irritant effect, then lowering exposure levels through relocation, substitution, engineering controls, or personal protective equipment may be sufficient.
    - Individuals who report a compelling history for work-related symptoms when exposed to a specific agent that has not been previously recognized as causing occupational asthma.

23. **Does a negative specific inhalation challenge test rule out occupational asthma?**
    A negative specific inhalation test does not rule out occupational asthma. It is possible that exposure to the agent in the workplace may be different or that another agent may be causing the asthma. Furthermore, if patients have been removed from work exposure for a prolonged period of time before being challenged, they may not demonstrate hyper-responsiveness.

24. **How should occupational asthma be managed?**
    The primary management of immune-mediated occupational asthma should be avoidance of exposure because this can result in a cure and continued exposure can lead to more severe asthma. Pharmacologic treatment is similar to that for nonoccupational asthma, involving the judicious use of systemic and inhaled steroids and bronchodilator medications. After a period of removal from the offending exposure, some individuals will be able to discontinue all asthma medication.

    In contrast, patients with irritant-induced asthma or RADS may be able to remain in their job with certain process modifications, such as substance substitution, process isolation (i.e.,

KEY POINTS: DIAGNOSIS OF OCCUPATIONAL ASTHMA

1. History of symptoms at workplace, with improvement during periods away from work

2. Peak-flow monitoring, ideally four times per day for 4 weeks (requires a reliable, compliant patient)

3. Decline of bronchial hyper-responsiveness to methacholine after a period (which may take up to 4 weeks) away from work

4. Specific inhalation challenge to a causative agent (only available at specialist centers, and sensitivity is not 100%)

enclosure), improved ventilation, or personal protective equipment (i.e., respirators), or a combination thereof. Pharmacologic treatment is the same as for immune-mediated occupational asthma.

25. **What is the prognosis for individuals with occupational asthma?**
Individuals who are identified early and are managed appropriately generally have a better prognosis than those who are identified after prolonged periods of symptoms with ongoing exposure. Certain persons simply require removal from exposure, whereas others may require steroid and bronchodilator medication temporarily or permanently. Some unfortunate patients develop steroid-dependent asthma despite removal from exposure. To date, we do not know if there are significant differences in prognosis among immune-mediated, RADS, and irritant-induced occupational asthma.

26. **How should impairment ratings be established?**
Occupational asthma is one of the occupational respiratory disorders that requires special evaluation when assessing impairment and disability. Strict adherence to the American Medical Association's guidelines for the basic evaluation of the respiratory system is inadequate. The guidelines actually allude to this fact and place occupational asthma in a special category.
Evaluation of individuals with occupational asthma should incorporate the degree of symptoms and medication requirements during periods of clinical stability with measurements of spirometry and nonspecific bronchial hyperresponsiveness (i.e., methacholine challenge PC_{20}). Determining maximum medical improvement for individuals with occupational asthma may take up to 2 years following the final exposure to the causative agent. Individuals requiring evaluation and impairment ratings of occupational asthma should generally be referred to pulmonary physicians or allergists with a particular interest and expertise in occupational asthma.

BIBLIOGRAPHY

1. American Thoracic Society: Guidelines for the evaluation of impairment/disability in patients with asthma. Am Rev Respir Dis 147:1056–1061, 1993.

2. Bernstein IL, Chan-Yeung M, Malo JL, Bernstein DI (eds): Asthma in the Workplace, 2nd ed. New York, Marcel Dekker, 1999.

3. Brooks SM, Weiss MA, Bernstein IL: Reactive airways dysfunction syndrome (RADS): Persistent asthma syndrome after high level irritant exposures. Chest 88:376–384, 1989.

4. Kennedy SM: Acquired airway hyperresponsiveness from nonimmunogenic irritant exposure. Occup Med State Art Rev 7:287–300, 1992.

5. Mapp CE, Boschetto P, Maestrelli P, Fabbri LM: Occupational asthma. Am J Respir Crit Care Med 172:380–305, 2005.

6. Nicholson PJ, Cullinan P, Taylor AJ, et al: Evidence based guidelines for the prevention, identification, and management of occupational asthma. Occup Environ Med 62(5):290–299, 2005.

7. Vigo PG, Grayson MH: Occupational exposures as triggers of asthma. Immunol Allergy Clin North Am 25(1):191–205, 2005.

CHAPTER 53

DRUG-INDUCED LUNG DISEASE

Andrew H. Limper, MD, and Edward C. Rosenow III, MD, MS

1. **Why are drug-induced diseases of any kind (e.g., pulmonary, renal, liver, and skin diseases) still such a problem? I thought all new drugs went through intensive screening before being released to the public.**

   Most drugs do go through a rather thorough process, namely animal and human phase trials, before they are released, but phase 3 trials may include only 1000 people and may last for no more than 1 year. The screened population may not have been followed long enough, or they may not be as sensitive to side effects as the general population that is to receive the drug.

   Some day, pharmacogenetics will help us determine the proper dose for each person. Some people will require a fraction of what the majority will require and thus will be less likely to develop side effects.

2. **How is the diagnosis of drug-induced lung disease made?**

   It is almost always a diagnosis of exclusion since, unfortunately, there are no diagnostic blood tests or characteristic chest imaging findings. Criteria used with most drug-induced diseases are as follows:
   - The patient is taking or recently has taken the drug.
   - Discontinuing the drug causes the symptoms to abate or improve, although a course of corticosteroids may be required.
   - Findings recur with rechallenge (*not* recommended).

   With rare exceptions, even sufficient tissue removal at open lung biopsy or autopsy is not diagnostic; it just helps the clinician exclude other diseases that will produce the symptoms and chest imaging changes seen in this particular patient.

   Morales JE, Diaz PT: How to determine when lung disease is drug-induced. J Resp Dis 25:519–526, 2004.

KEY POINTS: PROBLEMS ENCOUNTERED IN DIAGNOSING DRUG-INDUCED LUNG DISEASE

1. The true incidence is unknown.

2. We have almost no ideas regarding the characteristics of patients predisposed to an adverse reaction.

3. The majority of patients do not even know what drugs they are taking, and they rarely perceive over-the-counter drugs or eye drops as legitimate therapy.

4. No patient is taking only one drug, and we have very little concept of the role of synergism.

3. **What are the uncommon exceptions to characteristic histologic changes that might give me the diagnosis?**

   There are over 20 drugs, including radiation, that will produce bronchiolitis obliterans–organizing pneumonia (BOOP). This entity usually is associated with typical histologic findings and typical findings on a computed tomography (CT) scan of the lungs. Pulmonary eosinophilia from drugs, of course, has eosinophils in the lung tissue and usually in the bronchoscopic lung biopsy (BAL), but not always in the peripheral blood. ara-C, a chemotherapeutic agent, produces an intense proteinaceous pulmonary edema without interstitial changes; we know of no other condition that will produce this change.

Allen JN: Drug-induced eosinophilic lung disease. Clin Chest Med 25(1):77–88, 2004.
Epler GR: Drug-induced bronchiolitis obliterans organizing pneumonia. Clin Chest Med 25(1):89–94, 2004.
Flieder DB, Travis WD: Pathologic characteristics of drug-induced lung disease. Clin Chest Med 25(1): 37–46, 2004.

4. **What is the best way of knowing what drugs the patient is taking?**
   Unfortunately, asking the patient is not very helpful. Most patients do not know all the drugs they are taking and certainly do not know all the doses and frequencies. They will almost never volunteer or write down the over-the-counter (OTC) drugs that they take. The only sure way is to have the patient or family bring in *every* original bottle of pills or liquids, including eye drops and all OTC medications, in his or her medicine chest.

   Nitrofurantoin is classically one of the drugs that patients (almost always women, for urinary tract symptoms) do not mention because they think that, since it is taken on an as-needed basis, it does not count as a real medicine.

KEY POINTS: DIAGNOSIS OF DRUG-INDUCED LUNG DISEASE

1. It is almost always a condition of exclusion.

2. Animal studies are of no value in research.

3. Imaging studies are of little value in except in a few conditions (e.g., BOOP, dense lesions of amiodarone, and migratory infiltrates of pulmonary infiltration with eosinophilia [PIE]).

4. Blood and serum levels of the drug or metabolite are of no help.

5. **What are a few of the more serious drugs that patients may use but almost never list as medication?**
   - **Timoptic ophthalmic solution:** A beta-blocker prescribed for glaucoma. Patients assume that since an eye drop never gets into the systemic circulation and since the medication was not prescribed by their family physician, it cannot cause any trouble! There have been hundreds of fatalities (perhaps more) from ophthalmic beta-blockers that aggravate bronchospasm, namely in asthma and emphysema.
   - **Aspirin:** Over 200 medications contain acetylsalicylic acid (ASA). One, of which few physicians are aware, is Percodan, which contains 325 mg of ASA. Up to 10% of intensive care unit (ICU) admissions of asthmatics are caused by the inadvertent ingestion of aspirin by an asthmatic who is sensitive (but not necessarily allergic) to aspirin.

6. **List several drugs, both illicit and legitimate, that will cause an acute pulmonary insufficiency without venipuncture marks.**
   Heroin is notoriously given intravenously but can be overdosed by nasal insufflation. Aspirin, our friend from question 5, can acutely cause a noncardiac pulmonary edema. In two-thirds of the cases, edema is a result of a suicide attempt, but in the other third it is due to the gradual

accumulation of salicylate in the blood in patients with rheumatologic conditions. Their PaCO$_2$ is unusually low from brainstem hyperventilation (with heroin, the PaCO$_2$ will be high from central nervous system [CNS] suppression). Get a salicylate level—it should be above 40 mg/dL. Nitrofurantoin will produce an acute pulmonary insufficiency that usually clears within 48 hours of discontinuing the drug. Overdosing on tricyclics is a common form of suicide, producing an acute pulmonary reaction.

Heffner JE, Sahn SA: Salicylate-induced pulmonary edema: Clinical features and prognosis. Ann Intern Med 95:405–409, 1981.

Roy TM, Ossorio MA, Cipolla LM, et al: Pulmonary complications after tricyclic antidepressant overdose. Chest 96:852–856, 1989.

7. **If I suspect that the patient may be having an adverse reaction to a particular drug, what are the best methods of investigation?**
The Web site http://www.pneumotox.com is about the best single e-source, and it offers further references. The *Physicians' Desk Reference* (PDR) is also good, but it has to list any reaction ever reported to the Food and Drug Administration (FDA), even if the circumstances are very weak and are poorly documented. Calling the pharmaceutical manufacturer directly can be rewarding; phone numbers are listed in the front of the PDR.

Camus P, Rosenow EC III (eds): Iatrogenic Lung Disease. Clin Chest Med 25(1):XIII–XIX, 2004.
http://www.pneumotox.com

8. **Why are medications such a problem in the immunocompromised host (ICH)?**
There are a few dozen medications used by oncologists and hematologists in treating various malignant conditions that can mimic other complications of immunosuppression that occur in most, but not all, patients treated for a malignancy. The two major complications of these drugs are fever and diffuse pulmonary infiltrates. The most common complication that they mimic is opportunistic infection. Again, the diagnosis of drug-induced lung disease in this setting is one of exclusion. Some drugs produce an atypia of Type 2 pneumocytes seen histologically, but this finding can be present in the majority of those on the drugs without pulmonary disease. Its absence would help eliminate the possibility.

Limper AH: Chemotherapy-induced lung disease. Clin Chest Med 25(1):53–64, 2004.

9. **What is the best way of coming up with a differential diagnosis in the immunocompromised host who is receiving medication that can produce an adverse lung reaction?**
Table 53-1 can be of great help in narrowing your differential diagnosis of diffuse pulmonary infiltrate in immunocompromised hosts.

10. **Is there a reasonable noninvasive approach to determining whether the clinician is dealing with a possible drug-induced lung disease in an immunocompromised host?**
Several years ago, a group came up with a reasonable way of dealing with these patients, in whom you really do not want to do a lung biopsy. They used the following criteria, with weighted scores, with good results in bone marrow transplant patients:
1. **Velcro crackles at the bases:** 2 points
2. **Decrease in carbon monoxide diffusion in the lung (DLCO) >10%:** 3 points
3. **Decrease in oxygen saturation (SaO$_2$) >4% with a 2-minute walk test:** 3 points
4. **Abnormal chest x-ray (interstitial):** 3 points
Patients with scores of 6 or more points, after noninvasive exclusion of other diseases, were treated with prednisone on the assumption that the problem was drug-induced lung disease.

Chap L, Shpiner R, Levine M: Pulmonary toxicity of high-dose chemotherapy for breast cancer: A noninvasive approach to diagnosis and treatment. Bone Marrow Transplant 20:1063-1067, 1997.

TABLE 53-1. DIFFERENTIAL DIAGNOSIS OF DIFFUSE PULMONARY INFILTRATE IN IMMUNOCOMPROMISED HOSTS

Opportunistic infection	"Unrelated"
Recurrence of the underlying disease	Congestive heart failure
Hematologic	Pulmonary embolism
AIDS (e.g., Kaposi sarcoma)	Adult respiratory distress syndrome
Connective tissue disease (e.g., systemic lupus erythematosus)	Oxygen toxicity
	Community-acquired pneumonia
Transplant rejection (several)	Others
Neoplasm	Unusual complications
Drug effect	Pulmonary veno-occlusive disease
Opportunistic neoplasm	Alveolar proteinosis
Idiopathic "fibrosis" (likely due to drug and/or radiation)	Goodpasture's syndrome
Two or more of the above	

Adapted from Limper AH: Chemotherapy-induced lung disease. Clin Chest Med 25(1):53–64, 2004.

11. **Almost all patients treated by an oncologist are given two or more drugs, and sometimes they are given four or five, any of which could cause an adverse pulmonary reaction. In a patient with a diffuse pulmonary infiltrate that I suspect is due to one of the drugs, how can I decide which drug is the culprit so that I can drop it from the program?**
Sorry—you can't. Synergism may be present, but the evidence is weak because so many patients take the same various combinations without any problem. Animal studies have provided no help. We know that concomitant radiation (perhaps not even to the lungs) can be synergistic.

12. **Despite all the miracle drugs for the treatment of rheumatoid arthritis (RA), low-dose methotrexate (MTX) is still widely used. What should the clinician be looking for as a pulmonary complication of MTX?**
Low-dose MTX is also used for other conditions besides RA. The most common complication is diffuse interstitial lung disease (ILD), which, on biopsy, may show noncaseating granulomas. But a more serious complication (not commonly known) is opportunistic infection with all of the usual pathogens, most commonly *Pneumocystis jiroveci*. Keep in mind that these patients usually are not taking any other immunosuppressing agents.

   Saravanan V, Kelly CA: Reducing the risk of methotrexate pneumonitis in rheumatoid arthritis. Rheumatology 43:143–147, 2004.

13. **How can I separate rheumatoid lung disease from MTX-injured lung?**
This distinction is not always easy. A lung biopsy, such as a transbronchial lung biopsy, shows granulomas in the majority of cases of MTX-injured lung if adequate tissue is sampled and thus excludes rheumatoid lung disease. Peripheral blood eosinophilia can be found in one-third to one-half of MTX-injured lungs. Discontinuing MTX and perhaps adding corticosteroids will usually bring about a resolution of MTX pneumonitis. Corticosteroids are not usually very effective in rheumatoid lung disease. Finally, rheumatoid lung disease is more insidious in onset, but this may not be a good diagnostic criterion.

Saravanan V, Kelly CA: Reducing the risk of methotrexate pneumonitis in rheumatoid arthritis. Rheumatology 43:143–147, 2004.

14. **A well-to-do young businessman repeatedly presents to the emergency department (ED) with flare-ups of asthma. You finally get a clue as to what is going on when he also coughs up black sputum. What is the problem?**

With this evidence, he now admits to smoking cocaine. In many inner city EDs, the use of cocaine is one of the most common precipitators of an acute asthma attack. The black material is not old blood, but rather is a chemical reaction from smoking free-based cocaine; however, pulmonary hemorrhage is also another complication of cocaine use.

Wolff AJ, O'Donnell AE: Pulmonary effects of illicit drug use. Clin Chest Med 25(1):203–216, 2004.

15. **My patient had an intractable cough from using an angiotensin-converting enzyme (ACE) inhibitor. I switched her to another ACE inhibitor with no improvement. I then put her on losartan, and the cough cleared. Now, however, she is in the hospital with asthma, which she has never had before. Could the losartan be a contributing factor?**

You betcha. (She's from Minnesota.) But it is not asthma, although originally it was thought to be so. It is acute laryngeal edema, which losartan can cause. Many such patients have repeated ED visits for "asthma" until the diagnosis is reconsidered and the drug is stopped. Why the edema does not persist despite continued use of losartan between episodes is unknown. Many of these patients have been intubated or have undergone a tracheostomy, and some have died. A view with a fiberoptic laryngoscope is diagnostic. So would be a flow-volume study.

Jain M, Armstrong L, Hall J: Predisposition to and late onset of upper airway obstruction following angiotensin-converting enzyme inhibitor therapy. Chest 102:871–874, 1992.

16. **A 42-year-old woman is being treated for her lymphoma with chemotherapy and radiation therapy directed to the mediastinum. After about 6 weeks, she develops a low-grade fever and progressive dyspnea. Chest x-ray shows a unilateral infiltrate of a homogeneous pattern in the upper half of her right lung field. Transbronchoscopic lung biopsy and BAL from the right upper lobe show mostly lymphocytes. What drug will cause this predominantly lymphocytic pattern?**

You are seeing acute radiation pneumonitis. If you had done a BAL from the left lung, you would have also seen lymphocytes predominate, even though the chest x-ray from this side appeared normal. Because of the lymphocytes, some have believed that this is a hypersensitivity pneumonitis (HP)—but hypersensitivity to what? We do not know much more about this disorder than we did when it was first described over 10 years ago. It is usually treated with prednisone, with unpredictable results.

Roberts CM, Foulcher E, Zaunders JJ, et al: Radiation pneumonitis: A possible lymphocyte-mediated hypersensitivity reaction. Ann Intern Med 118:696–700, 1993.

17. **You are called in the middle of the night to see a 22-year-old woman in labor with acute pulmonary edema. She was admitted in premature labor that was treated with a tocolytic agent to inhibit uterine contractions, but it failed. Labor progressed, and the tocolytic agent was stopped. She was given hydrocortisone to accelerate fetal lung maturation. There was no evidence that she aspirated. Appropriate work-up ruled out cardiac disease and venous thromboembolism (VTE). What is the probable cause of her acute pulmonary edema?**

The tocolytic agent plus the aggravation of fluid retention from the steroid. Tocolytic drugs such as albuterol and terbutaline have been used for at least the past 2 decades, but the entity of tocolytic-induced pulmonary edema is not widely recognized by the nonobstetrician. The drug normally causes dilation of the peripheral vessels with an increase in the intravascular volume, as demonstrated by a diluted hematocrit and a drop in blood pressure. Discontinuing the tocolytic agent returns the tone of the vessels to normal, squeezing out a large volume of fluid into the tissues, including the lungs. Supportive treatment is all that is usually needed.

Pisani RJ, Rosenow EC III: Pulmonary edema associated with tocolytic therapy. Ann Intern Med. 110:714–718, 1989.

18. **What two drugs can cause acute respiratory failure when a patient taking either of them receives supplemental oxygen?**
Bleomycin and amiodarone. Patients who are taking either of these drugs and who then receive supplemental oxygen may develop acute respiratory distress syndrome (ARDS). But the oxygen is almost always administered during surgery, so you have to be suspicious of barotrauma as an aggravating factor. It is important that the anesthesiologist be aware of the drugs the patient is taking currently and also of those taken previously as a few of these events have occurred after the patient was off the drug for a while.

Ashrafian H, Davey P: Is amiodarone an underrecognized cause of acute respiratory failure in the ICU? Chest 120:275-82, 2001.
Ingrassia TS III, Ryu JH, Trastek VF, Rosenow EC III: Oxygen-exacerbated bleomycin pulmonary toxicity. Mayo Clin Proc 66:173–178, 1991.

19. **Can hexamethonium cause lung disease?**
Yes. This is a question of historic as well as educational value. In the 1950s and 1960s, ganglionic blockers were used in the treatment of malignant hypertension. There was a 5–8% incidence of "fibrinous pulmonary edema," with onset at weeks to months after receiving the drug and a 90% mortality rate. A few years ago, a widely publicized fatality occurred after an experimental study of the therapeutic use of inhaled hexamethonium in asthma. The newspaper descriptions of the death were very similar to those that occurred from orally or intravenously administered ganglionic blockers.

Heard BE: Fibrous healing of old iatrogenic pulmonary edema ("hexamethonium lung"). J Path Bact 83:159–164, 1962.

CHAPTER 54

RADIATION INJURY TO THE LUNG

Deborah Z. Rubin, MD, and Marie E. Wood, MD

1. **List the phases of radiation injury to the lung.**
   - **Acute phase:** Within 1–6 months of completing radiation treatments, *radiation pneumonitis* becomes apparent.
   - **Chronic phase:** *Radiation fibrosis* may ensue within 4–24 months of completion of radiation treatments.

2. **What are the clinical symptoms of radiation pneumonitis?**
   A clinical triad of dyspnea, nonproductive cough, and, occasionally, low-grade fever. Postradiation pneumonitis will occur in less than 10% of patients who have undergone thoracic irradiation.

KEY POINTS: CLINICAL TRIAD OF SYMPTOMS OF RADIATION PNEUMONITIS

1. Dyspnea

2. Nonproductive cough

3. Low-grade fever

---

3. **What are the clinical signs of radiation pneumonitis?**
   Occasionally, rales or pleural rub can be heard. Low-grade fever and elevated sedimentation rate are additional signs of radiation pneumonitis.

4. **Provide the radiographic findings of radiation pneumonitis.**
   - Infiltrate on plain radiograph
   - Computed tomography (CT) findings include a geometric infiltrate, often with a ground-glass appearance that commonly corresponds to the beam fields of treatment
   - Fluorodeoxyglucose–positron-emission-tomography and computed tomography (FDG–PET/CT) is very sensitive in detecting the inflammatory response and, therefore, is more sensitive and more specific than CT alone in defining the areas of pneumonitis corresponding to the beam fields

   http://radiographics.rsnajnls.org/cgi/content/full/20/1/83

5. **How is the diagnosis made?**
   To some degree, it is a diagnosis of exclusion. The differential includes infection (viral or bacterial), heart disease (i.e., congestive heart failure), exacerbation of preexisting lung disease, and (not uncommonly in this population of patients) lymphangitic spread of the tumor.

6. **What diagnostic tests can be done?**
   Measurement of pulmonary diffusing capacity for carbon monoxide (DLCO) is the most specific test. Because many of these patients have preexisting lung disease (e.g., emphysema, post-

KEY POINTS: DIFFERENTIAL DIAGNOSIS FOR RADIATION PNEUMONITIS AND FIBROSIS

1. Infection

2. Heart disease

3. Exacerbation of prior lung disease

4. Lymphangitic spread of cancer

obstructive pneumonia, atelectasis, or lobar collapse), other pulmonary function tests (PFTs) are likely to be abnormal and, therefore, not specific.

7. **How is radiation pneumonitis treated?**
Steroids are the mainstay of treatment. Prednisone at doses of 60–100 mg/day or methylpred-nisolone at doses of 16–24 mg/day can be used initially for 1–2 weeks. If the symptoms subside, then consideration can be given to switching to nonsteroidal anti-inflammatory drugs or cyclooxygenase-2 (COX-2) inhibitors to avoid complications of prolonged steroid use.
   A course of antibiotics can be used before starting steroids to confirm that the process is not infectious.

8. **How is radiation fibrosis treated?**
Although the fibrotic injury to the lung is irreversible, referral to a pulmonary rehabilitation program is likely to improve the patient's functional status and quality of life. By training the muscles to use oxygen more efficiently, the oxygen demand is lowered and exercise tolerance is increased. Steroids given concurrently with radiation treatments have not been shown to reduce the risk of pneumonitis or fibrosis.

9. **What clinical course can be expected with radiation pneumonitis?**
Radiation pneumonitis is self limited. Symptoms are likely to resolve within weeks to a few months. The DLCO is likely to drop 20–60% during the acute phase, but a partial recovery is generally expected 12–18 months after treatment.
   Some degree of **radiation fibrosis** will follow the resolution of the acute phase and may or may not cause further pulmonary symptoms.
   Marks LB, Lebesque JV: The challenge of predicting changes in pulmonary function tests after thoracic irradiation. Int J Radiol Oncol Biol Physiol 55(5):1331–1340, 2003.

10. **What is the clinical course with radiation fibrosis?**
Patients may note increased shortness of breath and increased dyspnea with exertion. Correspondingly, a decreased PaO_2 and a decreased lung compliance can be measured with pulmonary function studies.

11. **Describe the radiographic changes that are seen with radiation fibrosis.**
Plain radiographs may show increased density with volume loss, retraction of the mediastinum, tenting of the diaphragm, or a combination thereof, as the lung parenchyma continue to scar down, losing elasticity and vascular permeability, thereby becoming nonfunctioning.
   On PET or CT there will no longer be uptake by the FDG as this is no longer an inflammatory response; the CT, however, will show scarred lung tissue with geometric, and not anatomic, borders. Retraction of pleura, bronchus, and vessels may be noted.
   http://radiographics.rsnajnls.org/cgi/content/full/20/1/83

12. **What increases the risk of radiation injury to the lung?**
Combined radiation and chemotherapy may increase the incidence of radiation injury to as high as 20–30%. Drugs such as 5-fluorouracil, cyclophosphamide, cisplatin, and gemcitabine, when given before, during, or after radiation treatment, will potentiate the risk. The use of doxorubicin may initiate radiation recall, a condition in which previously irradiated lung is injured with the subsequent administration of the drug weeks or months after radiation therapy has been completed.

   Kwa SL, Lebesque JV, Theuws JC: Radiation pneumonitis as a function of mean lung dose: An analysis of pooled data of 540 patients. Int J Radiat Oncol Biol Physiol 42(1):1–9, 1998.

13. **How can the risk of radiation injury to the lung be reduced?**
Using three-dimensional radiation treatment planning, the volumes of tissue treated can be measured. Limiting the volume of lung treated to less than 20% of the total lung volume and keeping the daily dose fractions below 260 centi-Gray (cGy) will reduce the risk of lung injury to less than 10%, even in high-risk patients.

   Kim TH, Cho HR, Pyo JS, et al: Dose volumetric parameters for predicting severe radiation pneumonitis after three-dimensional conformal radiation therapy for lung cancer. Radiology 235:208–215, 2005.

14. **What does radiation injury look like under the microscope?**
In the later stages of injury, when the stroma is fibrosed, there may be fibrinous exudates, necrosis with minimal inflammatory cells, and atypical fibroblasts. The parenchymal cells may show atrophy, metaplasia, atypia, or dysplasia.

15. **What is the common vascular injury in radiation injury?**
The medium-sized venules and arterioles are most likely to be affected, with fibrinoid necrosis, thrombosis, arteritis, and neointimal proliferation. Vascular damage to the large vessels is least common and occurs more in the arteries than in the veins, with neointimal proliferation, atheromatosis, and thrombosis.

16. **Does amifostine lower the risk of developing radiation pneumonitis?**
The data are mixed. The largest study from the Radiation Therapy Oncology Group showed no benefit in risk reduction; however, smaller institutional studies have shown a benefit, as measured by DLCO.

   Antondau D: Radiotherapy or chemotherapy followed by radiotherapy with or without amigostine in locally advanced lung cancer. Sem Rad Oncol Jan 12(1):50–58, 2002.

17. **What is the risk of pulmonary injury associated with breast irradiation?**
When only the tangent fields are treated, the risk is less than 1%. When the treatment fields include the local-regional lymph nodes, the risk rises to 4%. The addition of chemotherapy increased the risk slightly in one study.

   Lind PA, Marks LB, Hardenbergh PH, et al: Technical factors associated with radiation pneumonitis after local ± regional radiation therapy for breast cancer. Int J Radiat Oncol Biol Physiol 52(1):137–143, 2002.

18. **What risk factors are associated with a higher incidence of radiation pneumonitis in patients with lung cancer who are receiving thoracic irradiation?**
   - Daily fraction of radiation dose greater than 2.67 cGy
   - Concurrent chemotherapy
   - Chronic obstructive pulmonary disease (COPD) (i.e., forced expiratory volume in 1 second [FEV_1] less than 2.0 liters)
   - Treatment of more than 30% of the total lung volume
   - Poor performance status

KEY POINTS: RISK FACTORS FOR RADIATION PNEUMONITIS

1. Volume and fraction size of radiation used

2. Underlying pulmonary disease

3. Specific concurrent or prior chemotherapy

4. Decreased function status of the patient

19. **What is three-dimensional treatment planning? How is it different from prior treatment planning?**

    Three-dimensional conformal planning utilizes CT imaging and computerized treatment planning, which allow the radiation oncologist to identify the critical anatomic structures (i.e., the heart, esophagus, spinal cord, lung, nodal drainage beds, and tumor mass) and to view these structures volumetrically. Computer planning allows optimization and tailoring of the doses of radiation throughout the treated area, limiting doses to normal structures and maximizing doses to the target volume. The ability to measure the volume of lung treated relative to the total lung volume is critical in minimizing the risk of injury to the lung.

CHAPTER 55

INHALATIONAL INJURIES

David A. Kaminsky, MD

1. **Describe the factors involved in determining the toxicity of inhalational agents.**
   In general, substances causing primarily upper airway injury tend to be larger (i.e., >5 μm) and more water-soluble (e.g., ammonia), whereas those causing lower airway and alveolar damage are smaller (i.e., < 1 μm) and less water soluble (e.g., phosgene). Substances may also be categorized as primarily irritating or asphyxiating. Irritating substances usually cause immediate symptoms, which allows the victim early warning of exposure. Less-irritating substances (e.g., phosgene) often result in more prolonged and intense exposure, and toxic effects may be delayed. Asphyxiating agents result in tissue hypoxia either due to displacement of oxygen, usually in confined spaces (as is the case with methane), or from chemical interference of cellular respiration (as happens with carbon monoxide, cyanide, and hydrogen sulfide).

   Kales, SN, Christiani DC: Acute chemical emergencies. N Engl J Med 350:800–808, 2004.
   Miller K, Chang A: Acute inhalational injury. Emerg Med Clin North Am 21:533–557, 2003.
   Rabinowitz PM, Siegel MD: Acute inhalation injury. Clin Chest Med 23:707–715, 2002.

2. **What are the consequences of exposure to toxic inhalational agents?**
   Severe upper airway irritation occurs within minutes following exposure to irritating gases. Pulmonary edema and pneumonia may also result following acute exposure to such substances as ammonia, chlorine, and oxides of nitrogen, phosgene, and sulfur dioxide. In addition, many substances have immediate systemic effects from cellular asphyxia (e.g., hydrogen cyanide), central nervous system (CNS) dysfunction, or bone marrow suppression (e.g., benzenes). Weeks later, some substances cause more-chronic respiratory problems, such as bronchitis (caused by ammonia), bronchiolitis obliterans (caused by oxides of nitrogen), and airway hyperreactivity (caused by sulfur dioxide).

   Valent F, McGwin G, Bovenzi M, Barbone F: Fatal work-related inhalation of harmful substances in the United States. Chest 121:969–975, 2002.

3. **List some common toxic inhalation agents and their characteristics.**
   - **Acrolein:** Clear yellow liquid with a pungent odor; found in manufacturing, sewage treatment, cigarette smoke, smog, and products of combustion of wood, paper, and cotton; upper airway irritant; causes mucosal irritation, lacrimation, and pulmonary edema.
   - **Ammonia:** Highly water soluble; clear and colorless; pungent odor; widely used as an industrial chemical in fertilizers, dyes, plastics, and pharmaceuticals; causes thermal and chemical airway burns, pulmonary edema, and pneumonia.
   - **Chlorine:** Dense, irritating gas; pungent odor; wide variety of sources; moderate water solubility allows exposure to the entire respiratory tract, resulting in airway injury and pulmonary edema.
   - **Formaldehyde:** Colorless gas with a pungent odor; commercial, medical, and industrial sources; component of smog; chronic in-home exposure may produce recurrent respiratory and systemic symptoms; causes upper airway irritation and airway hyperreactivity.
   - **Hydrofluoric acid:** Used in many commercial processes including semiconductor manufacturing; may cause severe local and systemic effects including mucosal burns; exposure may result in hypocalcemia and hypomagnesemia; calcium gluconate is a specific treatment.

- **Ozone:** Naturally occurring gas with chlorine-bleach-like odor; moderate water solubility; exposures can occur from welding, waste treatment, cold storage, and food preservation; component of smog; causes upper and lower respiratory tract inflammation; results in chest pain, cough, and dyspnea; may cause new or worsened airway hyperresponsiveness.
- **Phosgene:** Poorly water soluble; exposures occur from chemical plants, fires, dry cleaning, and welding; delayed (15–48 hours) symptoms from time of exposure due to slow hydrolysis to hydrochloric acid; causes small airway injury and pulmonary edema.
- **Sulfur dioxide:** Highly water soluble; clear, dense gas; byproduct of industry and a component of smog; upper airway irritant; may cause upper airway obstruction, cyanosis, and pulmonary edema; may cause new or worsened airway hyperresponsiveness.

4. **What is silo filler's disease?**
Silo filler's disease is a syndrome of respiratory failure following exposure to toxic levels of nitrogen dioxide that form during fermentation of grain within the first few days of its storage. Nitrogen dioxide is a dense, reddish-brown gas that has a characteristic sweet odor. It tends to accumulate in silos just above the grain surface. The pulmonary toxicity results from the formation of nitric acid when the oxides of nitrogen react with lower-respiratory-tract water. Potent oxidation products are released, causing local tissue inflammation and damage. Short-term (i.e., <24 hours) manifestations include bronchospasm and pulmonary edema; long-term (i.e., >5 weeks) sequelae may include bronchiolitis obliterans.

5. **A patient presents with headache, weakness, and confusion. She recently had a new gas furnace installed. Her arterial blood gas (ABG) shows a partial pressure of oxygen (PO_2) of 80 mmHg on room air, but her arterial saturation is 97% by pulse oximetry. What is the most likely diagnosis?**
Carbon monoxide (CO) poisoning. CO is a colorless, odorless gas produced by incomplete combustion of carbon-containing compounds such as wood, coal, and gasoline. Asphyxiation from CO is responsible for approximately 3000–6000 deaths per year in the United States, both accidental (especially in the winter months) and from suicide. CO does not directly injure the lung. Instead, it displaces oxygen from hemoglobin with a binding affinity for hemoglobin some 250 times higher than oxygen binding. In addition, CO shifts the oxyhemoglobin curve to the left, thereby reducing oxygen release at the tissue level, and binds to myoglobin in cardiac muscle, resulting in decreased oxygen availability to the heart. CO also causes tissue hypoxia by other mechanisms. Although the serum level of carboxyhemoglobin may not accurately reflect tissue levels of carboxyhemoglobin, there tends to be a correlation between blood levels and clinical signs, as seen in Table 55-1.

Ernst A, Zibrak JD: Carbon monoxide poisoning. N Engl J Med 339:1603–1608, 1998.

TABLE 55-1. SYMPTOMS RELATIVE TO CARBOXYHEMOGLOBIN LEVELS

Carboxyhemoglobin Level (% of total hemoglobin)	Symptoms
0–5	None
15–20	Headache, tinnitus
20–40	Disorientation, fatigue, nausea, weakness
40–60	Confusion, coma, respiratory failure
>60	Shock, death (the mortality rate is >50%)

6. **How is pulse oximetry affected by CO poisoning?**
   CO poisoning results in a discrepancy between the true arterial hemoglobin oxygen saturation and the saturation measured by pulse oximetry. The pulse oximeter interprets carboxyhemoglobin as oxyhemoglobin and will consistently overestimate the true arterial hemoglobin oxygen saturation by an amount somewhat less than the carboxyhemoglobin level. To overcome this problem, CO-oximetry should be used since this device utilizes four or more wavelengths, which are capable of differentiating among various hemoglobin species.

   Hampson NB: Pulse oximetry in severe carbon monoxide poisoning. Chest 114:1036–1041, 1998.

KEY POINTS: CLINICAL APPROACH TO PATIENTS WITH INHALATIONAL INJURY

1. Determine circumstances and type of exposure

2. Determine timing of onset of symptoms

3. Obtain past cardiopulmonary medical history and tobacco use

4. Administer a physical examination, focusing on the skin, hair, nares, upper airway, lungs, and nervous system

5. Administer laboratory tests including electrocardiogram, chest radiograph, spirometry, and evaluation of blood gases, toxin levels, and lactate levels

7. **What is the role of hyperbaric oxygenation (HBO) therapy in the treatment of CO poisoning?**
   The half-life for CO at room air is 240 minutes, but it decreases to approximately 75 minutes on 100% oxygen. The half-life of CO is even further reduced, to 20 minutes, with the use of HBO at 2 atmospheres. HBO may be useful in selected patients (see Table 55-2), but its use is controversial. Information on HBO chambers may be obtained from the Divers Alert Network

TABLE 55-2. SUGGESTED INDICATIONS FOR HYPERBARIC OXYGEN THERAPY IN PATIENTS WITH CARBON MONOXIDE POISONING

- Coma
- Any period of unconsciousness
- Any abnormal score on the Carbon Monoxide Neuropsychological Screening Battery
- Carboxyhemoglobin level > 40%
- Pregnancy and a carboxyhemoglobin level > 15%
- Signs of cardiac ischemia or arrhythmia
- History of ischemic heart disease and a carboxyhemoglobin level > 20%
- Recurrent symptoms for up to 3 weeks
- Symptoms that do not resolve with normobaric oxygen after 4–6 hours

Adapted from Ernst A, Zibrack JD: Carbon monoxide poisoning. N Engl J Med 339:1603–1608, 1998.

(http://www.diversalertnetwork.org) and from the Underwater Hyperbaric Medicine Society (http://www.uhms.org).

Juurlink DN, Stanbrook MB, McGuigan MA: Hyperbaric oxygen for carbon monoxide poisoning. Cochrane Database Syst Rev 2:CD002041, 2000.

Weaver LK, Hopkins RO, Chan KJ, et al: Hyperbaric oxygen for acute carbon monoxide poisoning. N Engl J Med 347:1057–1067, 2002.

8. **Which toxic inhalational agent has a characteristic smell of bitter almonds?**
    Hydrogen cyanide, a chemical asphyxiant that inhibits intracellular cytochrome oxidase activity and thus poisons cellular respiration. Hydrogen cyanide exposure may occur in electroplating, photographic development, and polishing of metals and from the burning of polyurethane, cellulose, nylon, wool, silk, and asphalt. Symptoms of headache, palpitations, giddiness, and dyspnea appear within seconds and may quickly progress to seizures, coma, and death. Clues to diagnosis are severe hypoxic symptoms without cyanosis, similar arterial and venous oxygen saturations, and an anion gap in lactic acidosis. The smell of bitter almonds, although pathognomonic, is only detectable by 20–40% of individuals.

9. **Why is it vitally important to diagnose cyanide toxicity?**
    Hydrogen cyanide toxicity must not be overlooked because, unlike most other causes of toxic inhalation, specific antidote therapy is available. The traditional regimen is detoxification with sodium nitrite and sodium thiosulfate. The nitrite converts hemoglobin to methemoglobin, which then competes with cytochrome oxidase for the cyanide ion. Thiosulfate further converts cyanide to the less-toxic thiocyanide, which is then excreted in the urine. One danger to this regimen is the excessive production of methemoglobin, so methemoglobin levels must be monitored carefully. Because of this potential toxicity, nitrite therapy is usually reserved for patients who are hypotensive, acidemic, or comatose.

10. **A rotten-egg odor is characteristic of which toxic inhalational agent?**
    Hydrogen sulfide, a dense gas. This odor rapidly becomes undetectable upon continued exposure because of olfactory fatigue. Exposures may occur in the petroleum industry as well as with sewage treatment and contact with volcanic gases, coal mines, and natural hot springs. Hydrogen sulfide is an even more potent inhibitor of cytochrome oxidase than cyanide. Unlike cyanide, however, hydrogen sulfide also causes upper airway irritation. Symptoms include rhinitis, bronchitis, and pulmonary edema, as well as significant CNS dysfunction including headache, seizures, and respiratory failure. In addition to supportive measures, treatment includes the use of sodium nitrite.

KEY POINTS: HIGH-RISK FACTORS RELATED TO FATAL INHALATION OF HARMFUL SUBSTANCES IN U.S. WORKPLACES ✓

1. Male sex

2. Age > 65 years

3. Employment in mining, firefighting, farming, forestry, fishing, or repair and maintenance work (e.g., construction, cleaning, painting, or inspecting)

4. Carbon monoxide exposure, especially in the winter

11. **What is meant by the term "inhalation fever"?**
    Inhalation fever refers to the febrile flu-like syndromes that occur following acute inhalation of fumes or dusts. Causes of inhalation fever include the following:

- **Metal fume fever:** Due to exposure to metallic oxides of zinc, copper, or magnesium
- **Polymer fever:** Due to exposure to heated polytetrafluoroethylene (i.e., Teflon)
- **Organic dust toxic syndrome:** Related to exposure to organic dusts, such as might occur in cleaning a grain storage bin or working in a swine confinement building

All three syndromes are characterized clinically by the acute onset of chills, fever, malaise, and myalgia approximately 4–8 hours following exposure. Respiratory complaints may include cough and mild dyspnea, but spirometry and chest radiographs are typically normal. Symptoms tend to resolve within 12–48 hours.

12. **True or False: The leading cause of death in fires is smoke inhalation, not burns.**
True. Smoke inhalation results in both direct lung injury and systemic effects. The heat from a fire usually causes thermal injury above the vocal cords because the upper airway is extremely efficient at dissipating heat. Thermal injury takes the form of burns to the face, oropharynx, and upper airway, and it may result in airway edema and obstruction. Lower airway injury is usually due to the chemical effects of smoke, which cause direct mucosal irritation and result in bronchorrhea, bronchoconstriction, and airway edema. Systemic effects of smoke inhalation are primarily due to cellular hypoxia and acidosis induced by the asphyxiants CO and hydrogen cyanide.

13. **Describe the three phases of injury following smoke inhalation.**
- **Phase 1 (0–36 hours):** During this phase, hypoxic injury may result from low inspired oxygen concentrations occurring during a fire or from the asphyxiant properties of CO and hydrogen cyanide; thermal and chemical airway injury occur.
- **Phase 2 (2–5 days):** This has been described as "the calm before the storm." During this phase, airway injury is resolving, but tracheobronchial sloughing continues.
- **Phase 3 (5+ days):** During this period, nosocomial pneumonia, respiratory fatigue, and acute respiratory distress syndrome (ARDS) may develop. Continued respiratory support and aggressive attention to fluid management and infection are crucial during this period until lung healing and burn wound healing take place.

14. **What are the best methods for determining whether inhalation injury has occurred in a burn patient?**
One of the most immediate concerns following smoke inhalation is adequate patency of the upper airway. History and clinical signs are important in this evaluation, but they do not reliably predict upper airway injury. Such signs include exposure in a closed space; steam, neck, or facial burns; singed nasal hairs; sooty sputum; bronchorrhea; hoarseness; and wheezing. Serial physiologic testing with spirometry and flow-volume loops may also be used to detect the earliest signs of upper airway narrowing. Upper airway endoscopy offers the most definitive assessment of airway injury.

Haponik EF, Meyers DA, Munster AM, et al: Acute upper airway injury in burn patients. Serial changes of flow-volume curves and nasopharyngoscopy. Am Rev Respir Dis 135:360–366, 1987.

15. **Name some important biological and chemical weapons and their characteristics.**
- **Anthrax:** Encapsulated, broad, gram-positive bacillus; biphasic illness; early phase, 1–6 hours following exposure, manifests as a nonspecific illness with fever, malaise, myalgia, cough, and chest and abdominal pain; later phase, 2–3 days following exposure, manifests as acute dyspnea, fever, cyanosis, and shock; chest imaging shows widened mediastinum, effusions, and adenopathy; meningitis occurs in 50% of cases; can be treated with ciprofloxacin or doxycycline.
- **Nerve agents:** Organophosphate compounds (e.g., sarin, tabun, soman, and VX) inhibit acetylcholinesterase, precipitating cholinergic crisis; increased muscarinic activity, causing

excessive secretions, miosis, bronchospasm, bradycardia, and intestinal hypermotility; increased nicotinic activity, resulting in fasciculations, weakness, and paralysis; death from respiratory failure may occur within minutes; treatment includes decontamination, atropine, pralidoxime (to restore acetylcholinesterase), and diazepam (to treat seizures).

- **Mustard gas:** Blistering, alkylating agent; inhibits cellular glycolysis; latent period of 4–12 hours following inhalation; causes chest pain, dyspnea, cough, sore throat, and (within 24–48 hours) hemorrhagic pulmonary edema.

- **Riot-control agents:**
  - Chlorobenzylidene (CS): Component of tear gas; causes intense lacrimation, coughing, sneezing, and (possibly) asphyxia.
  - Oleoresin capsicum (OC): Used in pepper spray; extract of Cheyenne peppers (i.e., capsaicin); causes upper airway irritation, bronchoconstriction, and pulmonary edema.

http://www.bt.cdc.gov/agent/vx/basics/facts.asp

XIII. LUNG NEOPLASMS

SOLITARY PULMONARY NODULES

Todd M. Bull, MD, and Elizabeth L. Aronsen, MD

CHAPTER 56

1. **Define solitary pulmonary nodule.**
   A solitary pulmonary nodule (SPN) is an isolated opacity seen on a plain chest radiograph. SPNs are located entirely within the lung parenchyma, are not associated with atelectasis or hilar adenopathy, and are generally <3.0–4.0 cm in diameter.

   Ost D, Fein AM, Feinsilver SH: Clinical practice. The solitary pulmonary nodule. N Engl J Med 348(25):2535–2542, 2003.

   Tang AW, Moss HA, Robertson RJ: The solitary pulmonary nodule. Eur J Radiol 45(1):69–77, 2003.

2. **How are SPNs usually discovered?**
   SPNs are usually asymptomatic and are found on routine chest radiographs obtained for other reasons such as preoperative evaluation. An estimated 1 in 500 chest radiographs will demonstrate a SPN. As the utility of screening for lung cancer is reevaluated, there likely will be an increase in the number of asymptomatic SPNs discovered. Less often, local (e.g., hemoptysis or cough) or systemic (e.g., fatigue or weight loss) symptoms may prompt the clinician to obtain the chest radiograph that detects the SPN.

   Toomes H, Delphendahl A, Manke HG, Vogt-Moykopf I: The coin lesion of the lung. A review of 955 resected coin lesions. Cancer 51(3):534–537, 1983.

3. **List the most common causes of benign SPNs.**
   From 75–85% of pathologically diagnosed SPNs are benign. Common causes include the following:
   1. **Granuloma:** More than half of all benign SPNs (and 40% of total SPNs) are granulomas, which are categorized as follows:
      - Infectious (i.e., histoplasmosis, coccidioidomycosis, or tuberculosis)
      - Noninfectious (i.e., sarcoidosis, rheumatoid arthritis, or vasculitides such as Wegener's granulomatosis)
   2. **Hamartoma:** Hamartomas represent the second-most-common benign cause, although they constitute less than 10% of all SPNs.
   3. **Other:** More than 100 benign causes of SPNs have been reported, including the following:
      - Bronchiolitis obliterans–organizing pneumonia (BOOP)
      - Parasitic infections
      - Arteriovenous malformations
      - Bronchogenic cysts
      - Pulmonary infarction
      - Eosinophilic granuloma
      - Nodular pulmonary amyloidosis
      - Anthrasilicotic intrapulmonary lymph nodes
      - "Round" pneumonia (a less-common presentation of acute pulmonary infection in which the alveolar-space-filling disease assumes a more rounded nodular appearance)
      - *Rhodococcus equi* pneumonia (may present as a cavitating SPN in an immunocompromised patient)

4. **List the most common causes of malignant SPNs.**
   1. **Primary bronchogenic**
      - Non–small cell lung cancer
      - Small cell lung cancer
      - Primary pulmonary lymphoma
   2. **Metastatic disease from nonpulmonary sources**
      - Kaposi sarcoma
      - Adenocarcinoma from any source
      - Angiosarcoma

5. **What patient characteristics make the diagnosis of malignant disease more likely?**
   - **Age:** In patients younger than 35 years, the vast majority of all SPNs are benign. The risk of malignant disease increases with age until age 65, at which point more than two-thirds of SPNs are malignant.
   - **History of prior malignancy:** Although primary bronchogenic carcinoma is the most frequent cause of resected malignant SPNs, metastatic disease, often originating from extrapulmonary adenocarcinomas of the breast, prostate, or colon, represent 30% of malignant SPNs. In one series, 50% of patients with SPN had a prior history of malignancy.
   - **Smoking history:** There is a well-known association between smoking and the development of primary bronchogenic carcinoma, although the effect of smoking on malignancy in the setting of SPNs has not been specifically determined. The risk diminishes after smoking cessation but never reaches that of a life-long nonsmoker.
   - **Obstructive lung disease:** There is growing evidence that the risk of lung cancer is significantly increased in patients with obstructive airways disease, as assessed by pulmonary function tests (forced expiratory volume in 1 second [FEV_1] < 0.7; FEV_1/[forced vital capacity (FVC)] < 0.7).

   Bechtel JJ, Kelley W, Coons T, et al: Lung cancer detection in asymptomatic patients with airflow obstruction. Chest 125(5 Suppl):163S, 2004.
   Bechtel JJ, Petty TL: Strategies in lung cancer detection: Achieving early identification in patients at high risk. Postgrad Med 114(2):20–26, 2003.
   Gurney JW: Determining the likelihood of malignancy in solitary pulmonary nodules with Bayesian analysis. Part I. Theory. Radiology 186(2):405–413, 1993.
   Petty TL: The early diagnosis of lung cancer. Dis Mon 47(6):204–264, 2001.

KEY POINTS: PATIENT CHARACTERISTICS THAT INCREASE THE LIKELIHOOD OF A MALIGNANT SOLITARY PULMONARY NODULE

1. Age of patient

2. History of prior malignancy

3. History of tobacco exposure

4. Diagnosis of chronic obstructive pulmonary disease (COPD)

---

6. **What imaging techniques can be used to evaluate an SPN?**
   - **Chest radiography:** Chest radiography is the imaging modality that is usually responsible for the initial diagnosis of an SPN. It is rarely relied upon, however, as the sole imaging technique in patients who appear to have an SPN because it often fails to detect additional parenchymal nodules.

- **Chest computed tomography (CT) scan:** Chest CT with contrast enhancement is almost always part of the work-up of the SPN for guiding the clinician in assessing the most likely diagnosis and determining the best approach for obtaining a tissue sample. A benign SPN is suggested by a lack of contrast enhancement. CT guidance is also used to localize the lesion with methylene blue or to hook wires before surgical resection.
- **Positron emission tomography (PET):** PET scanning is playing a more prominent role in the evaluation of the SPN, complementing chest x-ray and CT imaging. Positron-emitting radio-labeled isotopes of glucose (i.e., F-2-deoxy-D-glucose [FDG]) or amino acids are taken up by rapidly metabolizing cells that can then be imaged. The sensitivity of this modality for detecting malignancies is greater than 90%, but the specificity is much lower. A recent meta-analysis reported the sensitivity of PET for identifying a malignant process as 96.8% and its specificity as 77.8%. It is important to recognize that the sensitivity of PET may be significantly lower for lesions less than 1 cm in diameter.

Gould MK, Maclean CC, Kuschner WG, et al: Accuracy of positron emission tomography for diagnosis of pulmonary nodules and mass lesions: A meta-analysis. JAMA 285(7):914–924, 2001.

7. **Which lesions are often associated with false-negative or false-positive results on FDG–PET scan?**
   1. **False-negative results**
      - Bronchioloalveolar cell carcinoma
      - Typical carcinoids
      - Lesions less than 1 cm in diameter
   2. **False-positive results**
      - Infectious etiologies such as tuberculomas and fungal infection

Erasmus JJ, McAdams HP, Patz EF Jr, et al: Evaluation of primary pulmonary carcinoid tumors using FDG PET. Am J Roentgenol 170(5):1369–1373, 1998.

Higashi K, Ueda Y, Seki H, et al: Fluorine-18-FDG PET imaging is negative in bronchioloalveolar lung carcinoma. J Nucl Med 39(6):1016–1020, 1998.

8. **What CT characteristics make a diagnosis of malignant disease more likely?**
   - **Nodule size:** 20% or fewer of SPNs < 2.0 cm in diameter are malignant. In contrast, more than 80% of the SPNs > 3.0 cm in diameter are malignant.
   - **Presence and pattern of calcification:** Central, laminated, or diffuse patterns of calcification suggest a benign diagnosis such as granulomatous disease or hamartoma. Malignant disease only rarely shows evidence of calcification; when there is calcification, it usually exhibits an eccentric pattern.
   - **Nodular density and configuration:** Chest CT, with thin sections through the nodule, is very sensitive in defining the density and configuration of an SPN. The finding of a fat density within the nodule strongly suggests the diagnosis of hamartoma. A ground-glass appearance of the SPN is consistent with the diagnosis of bronchoalveolar carcinoma. A "halo sign" or ground-glass appearance surrounding an SPN is characteristic of hemorrhagic nodules, as seen in infectious processes (caused by fungus or virus) and, less frequently, noninfectious processes (i.e., Wegener's granulomatosis, Kaposi sarcoma, or metastatic angiosarcoma). The configuration of the SPN is less helpful in predicting malignancy because well-marginated spherical nodules can be either benign or malignant. Poorly marginated or spiculated nodules suggest malignancy 90% of the time.
   - **Adenopathy:** Both benign and malignant diseases may be associated with ipsilateral mediastinal or hilar adenopathy (defined as lymph nodes > 1.0 cm in diameter). Adenopathy involving the contralateral hemithorax, however, is highly suggestive of nonresectable malignant disease.
   - **Contrast enhancement:** Complete contrast enhancement by dynamic CT suggests malignancy, whereas capsular, peripheral, or no enhancement of the SPN is more consistent with benign causes such as hamartoma or tuberculoma. Pathologically, enhancement is thought to

be caused by the distribution of small vessels within the mass. Further study is needed to determine the characteristics of other benign SPNs and whether enhancement can be used to reduce the number of surgical procedures needed to obtain definitive diagnoses.

9. **How should the work-up of the SPN begin?**
   1. **Obtain an old chest radiograph or CT scan.** A nodule is very likely to be benign if previous radiographs confirm that it has been present and unchanged in size for at least 2 years. In this setting, no further work-up is necessary. Malignant lesions usually have a doubling time measured in weeks to months. In effect, a lesion that grows either very rapidly (days) or very slowly (years) is likely to be benign. In the event of rapid growth, the patient usually has additional symptoms suggesting a benign diagnosis such as infection or infarction. An SPN increasing very slowly in size may warrant only further observation for an additional period of time.
   2. **Obtain a chest CT.** Contrast-enhanced dynamic chest CT with thin sections through the nodule helps to characterize the nature of the SPN, to confirm its solitary nature, and to stage the disease should it prove to be malignant. Often, CT demonstrates several pulmonary nodules, suggesting the diagnosis of either granulomatous disease or pulmonary metastases. Less than 1% of primary bronchogenic cancers present as multiple synchronous lesions.
   3. **Assess clinical likelihood that the lesion is lung cancer.** By reviewing the patient's risk factors for lung cancer (e.g., age, tobacco history, and previous history of malignancy) and the characteristics of the lesion on radiograph (e.g., size and calcification pattern), the likelihood that a pulmonary lesion is benign or malignant can be assessed. The patient's risk of lung cancer will help determine the level of aggression employed in the work-up.

10. **What steps should be taken next in the work-up and diagnosis of the SPN?**
    - **Observation:** This is appropriate in many patients, particularly in those with a very low likelihood of malignancy based on clinical and radiologic features and in those for whom an invasive diagnostic procedure would carry an unacceptably high risk of morbidity and mortality. The course of the SPN can be monitored with serial chest radiographs or CT scans every 3 months for the first year, every 6 months for the second year, and on a yearly basis thereafter.
    - **Biopsy:** The alternative to observation is to obtain tissue for a definitive diagnosis. Biopsy can be performed using either CT- or fluoroscopy-guided transthoracic fine-needle aspiration (TTNA) or fiberoptic bronchoscopy with transbronchial biopsy (TBB). TTNA and TBB are often considered complementary procedures. The latter is associated with a lower diagnostic yield, particularly for small (i.e., <2 cm) peripheral SPNs. TTNA can be considered diagnostic for malignant and some benign lesions only when definitively positive. Nonspecific inflammation should not be construed as evidence of a benign lesion. Characteristic morphology seen after

Gomori methenamine silver stain of biopsy specimens includes extracytoplasmic spheroids and cytoplasmic inclusions in the case of histoplasmosis. If diagnosis is not definitive, more aggressive attempts to obtain tissue must be pursued in most clinical situations. Open lung biopsy (OLB) or video-assisted thoracoscopy (VATS) is performed in cases of high clinical suspicion with a nondiagnostic TTNA or TBB.

- **Resection:** Patients at high risk for malignant disease (e.g., an older patient with a large, noncalcified, enhancing SPN and a smoking history) without significant comorbid illnesses or contraindications for general anesthesia are frequently referred directly for surgical resection of the mass. Thoracotomy has the advantage of often being both a diagnostic and a therapeutic procedure. Unfortunately, however, it is also associated with higher morbidity. A peripheral SPN may be amenable to surgical resection by a VATS approach rather than by open thoracotomy, thus reducing operating room costs, duration of anesthesia, and the duration of the hospital stay.

11. **What percent increase in diameter represents a doubling of volume of an SPN?**
A common mistake is underestimating the rate of change of SPN over time on chest radiograph. If the lesion is considered spherical, a 30% increase in diameter represents a doubling of volume. Malignant lesions generally have doubling times of 20–400 days. Lesions with shorter doubling time are likely infectious in etiology, and a longer doubling time suggests a benign neoplasm. It is important to note, however, that typical carcinoid and bronchoalveolar cell carcinomas can have doubling times longer than 400 days.

Garland LH: The rate of growth and natural duration of primary bronchial cancer. Am J Roentgenol Radium Ther Nucl Med 96(3):604–611, 1996.

Yankelevitz DF, Gupta R, Zhao B, Henschke CI: Small pulmonary nodules: Evaluation with repeat CT—Preliminary experience. Radiology 212(2):561–566, 1999.

Yankelevitz DF, Reeves AP, Kostis WJ, et al: Small pulmonary nodules: Volumetrically determined growth rates based on CT evaluation. Radiology 217(1):251–256, 2000.

CHAPTER 57

LUNG CANCER

Marc A. Voelkel, MD, Teofilo L. Lee-Chiong, Jr., MD, and Richard A. Matthay, MD

1. **What are the prevalence, incidence, and risk of death from lung cancer in the United States?**

   The estimated cancer incidence for the United States in 2004 was 699,560 for men and 668,470 for women. The most common cancer was prostate cancer (33%) in men and breast cancer (32%) in women. Lung cancer is the second-most-common cancer in both men (13%) and women (12%).

   Lung cancer is the primary cause of cancer death in both men and women. In 2004, estimated cancer deaths totaled 563,700, of which 32% and 25% were attributable to lung and respiratory tract cancers, respectively. More people will die from lung cancer than from colon, breast, and prostate cancer combined.

   Nearly 60% of people diagnosed with lung cancer die within 1 year of their diagnosis, and nearly 75% die within 2 years. Although most other cancer death rates have declined since 1975, there has been little change in the median 1-year survival rate for lung cancer (15% in 1999).

   American Cancer Society: Surveillance, epidemiology, and end results program, 1975–2000. Washington, DC, Division of Cancer Control and Population Sciences, National Cancer Institute, 2004.

   Jemal A, Murray T, Ward E, et al: Cancer statistics, 2005. CA Cancer J Clin 55:10–30, 2005.

   http://caonline.amcancersoc.org

2. **What are the major risk factors?**

   Tobacco use is the primary risk factor for lung cancer and is estimated to account for 90% of all cases. Any source of smoking, including cigarette (unfiltered, filtered, and low-tar), pipe, cigar, and secondhand smoke, is associated with increased lung cancer risk. The duration of smoking appears to have a much greater effect than the amount smoked. It is estimated that tripling the amount smoked effectively triples the risk, whereas tripling the duration smoked increased the risk 100 times. In addition, there may be increased susceptibility to smoke-related lung cancer among women, as compared with men.

   Other risk factors include:
   - Radon and radon progeny from either uranium mining or household exposure
   - Arsenic; asbestos; chromates and chromium; chloromethyl ethers, vinyl chloride, and mustard gas; nickel; and polycyclic aromatic hydrocarbons (i.e., benzene and its related species)
   - Ionizing radiation
   - Air pollution from combustion engines and indoor pollution from cooking fires
   - Genetic factors
   - Infectious agents (e.g., *Mycobacterium tuberculosis*, human papilloma virus (HPV), and *Microsporidium canis*)

   Alberg AJ, Samet JM: Epidemiology of lung cancer. Chest 123(Suppl 1):21S–49S, 2003

3. **What are the major (known) occupational risk factors associated with lung cancer?**

   The worldwide occupational risk factor that is most related to lung cancer is asbestos exposure. It is estimated to increase the risk of cancer 50–60 times in smokers exposed to asbestos, as compared to those who have never smoked and have never been exposed to asbestos. Radon is another important cause of lung cancer in the United States. It is a decay product of uranium and is present in both uranium mines and indoor pollution from poorly ventilated cellars in areas of uranium-rich soil.

Alberg AJ, Samet JM: Epidemiology of lung cancer. Chest 123(1Suppl):21S–49S, 2003.

4. **Why was there a delay in the acceleration of lung-cancer–related mortality among women in the United States?**
Death rates from lung cancer in men have been declining since 1990; in contrast, death rates continue to rise in women. This disparity is believed to be related to differences in the timing, effect, and amount of smoking trends in the United States. The epidemic of smoking among men in the early part of the 20th century preceded that of women by about 15–20 years. Women historically started smoking in the 1930s, with greater numbers starting around World War II. The 15- to 20-year delay led to a rise in lung cancer deaths in women by the 1960s. The decrease in men's smoking following the Surgeon General's warning has resulted in the current peak fall in U.S. men's lung cancer rates. Lung cancer mortality in men peaked at about 1990, roughly the same time that U.S. women's lung cancer mortality surpassed that of breast cancer (1987).

Alberg AJ, Samet JM: Epidemiology of lung cancer. Chest 123(Suppl 1):21S–49S, 2003.

5. **What are the most common symptoms and presentations associated with lung cancer?**
A majority of patients are symptomatic at initial presentation. Symptoms associated with lung cancer are a result of the tumor itself, metastasis, or systemic paraneoplastic syndromes. Cough is the most common presentation (50–75%). Other symptoms include dyspnea (25–60%), chest discomfort (60%), hemoptysis (25–50%), hoarseness (due to recurrent laryngeal nerve involvement), bone pain (20%), superior vena cava syndrome (i.e., facial edema and dilated upper chest and neck veins), dysphagia, and neurologic symptoms (i.e., headache, seizures, cranial nerve defects, weakness, and sensory loss). Patients who present with symptoms at the time of diagnosis have a far worse outcome than those who do not. Approximately 5–23% of patients are asymptomatic at presentation.

Beckles MA, Spiro SG, Colice GL, Rudd RM: Initial evaluation of the patient with lung cancer: Symptoms, signs, laboratory tests, and paraneoplastic syndromes. Chest 123:97S–104S, 2003.

6. **What are the various paraneoplastic signs and symptoms of lung cancer?**
Approximately 10–20% of patients with lung cancer exhibit paraneoplastic syndromes. These clinical features do not result from the physical effects of tumors themselves. Rather, these phenomena are believed to arise from the excessive release of cellular products by tumors, ectopic production of hormones and other polypeptides, or neurovascular reflexes. The spectrum of clinical conditions includes the following:
- **Systemic disorders** such as anorexia, cachexia, fever, and malaise
- **Cutaneous and musculoskeletal disorders** including urticaria, acanthosis nigricans, erythema multiforme, digital clubbing, and hypertrophic pulmonary osteoarthropathy (HPOA) (i.e., painful arthropathy, periosteal elevation, and neurovascular involvement of the extremities, mostly related to non–small cell lung cancer (NSCLC), particularly adenocarcinoma and large cell carcinoma)
- **Rheumatologic disorders,** exemplified by polymyositis–dermatomyositis and systemic lupus erythematosus (SLE)
- **Renal disorders** such as membranous glomerulonephritis and nephrotic syndrome
- **Endocrine disorders** including Cushing's syndrome (most commonly caused by small cell lung cancer), hypercalcemia (most frequently associated with squamous cell carcinoma), carcinoid syndrome, and the syndrome of inappropriate secretion of antidiuretic hormone (SIADH) (seen most commonly with small cell lung cancer)

- **Hematologic disorders** such as anemia, polycythemia, leukocytosis, eosinophilia, thrombocytosis, thrombotic diseases, and hemorrhagic diathesis
- **Neurologic disorders** including Lambert–Eaton syndrome (encountered usually in small cell lung cancer), binocular visual loss, cerebellar degeneration, encephalomyelopathy, limbic encephalitis, necrotizing myelopathy, subacute peripheral neuropathy, psychosis, and dementia
- **Miscellaneous disorders,** consisting of nonbacterial thrombotic endocarditis and lactic acidosis

Several conditions may masquerade as paraneoplastic syndromes. Infection, fluid, and electrolyte abnormalities; vascular disorders; tumor metastasis; and drug reactions must be excluded before therapy is initiated for these various syndromes.

Management involves eradication of the underlying tumor by surgical resection, chemotherapy, or irradiation, or else by specific treatments for Cushing's syndrome, hypercalcemia, SIADH, or Lambert–Eaton syndrome.

Beckles MA, Spiro SG, Colice GL, Rudd RM: Initial evaluation of the patient with lung cancer: Symptoms, signs, laboratory tests, and paraneoplastic syndromes. Chest 123:97S–104S, 2003.

7. **What is a Pancoast's tumor?**

Pancoast's tumor, or superior sulcus tumor, was first described by Edwin Hare in 1838 and was named after the radiologist who described it in 1924. It produces a characteristic clinical syndrome that includes pain down the affected arm with eventual weakness and numbness along the eighth cervical nerve trunk (the ulnar nerve) and the first and second thoracic nerve trunks, Horner syndrome (ipsilateral ptosis, miosis, and anhidrosis), and radiographic evidence of destruction of the first thoracic rib or vertebral body.

It is caused by a benign or malignant tumor invading portions of the brachial plexus, subclavian vessels, vertebral bodies, parietal pleura, apical ribs, and stellate ganglion. The tumor represents less than 5% of all bronchogenic carcinomas and, on presentation, is usually at an advanced stage (i.e., stage T3 or T4, with invasion of the subclavian vessels or vertebral body). Of these tumors, 90–95% are NSCLC. They are usually difficult to diagnose with bronchoscopy, requiring percutaneous needle biopsy. A work-up for infectious processes (i.e., *Actinomyces, Staphylococcus,* and *Echinococcus* spp.), as well as for neurogenic thoracic outlet syndromes and pulmonary amyloidosis, should be done to rule out nonmalignant causes before treatment is initiated.

Pitz CC, de la Rieviere AB, van Swieten HA, et al: Surgical treatment of Pancoast tumours. Eur J Cardiothorac Surg 26(1):202–208, 2004.

8. **What are the most common lung cancer cell types?**

The four common cancer types are NSCLC, adenocarcinoma (including bronchoalveolar carcinoma), squamous cell and large cell carcinoma, and small cell lung cancer (SCLC). They account for over 90–95% of lung cancers discovered. Adenocarcinoma is the most frequent cell type, followed by squamous cell, small cell, and large cell carcinoma, in descending order.

Other lung cancer types include neuroendocrine (i.e., carcinoid, atypical carcinoid, and large-cell NSCLC with neuroendocrine differentiation), mesothelioma, mucoepidermoid, lymphoproliferative disorders (i.e., lymphoma and leukemia), Kaposi sarcoma, and benign neoplasms (i.e., tracheobronchial papillomas and hamartomas).

Franklin WA: Pathology of lung cancer. J Thorac Imag 15(1):3–12, 2000.

9. **What are the common histologic characteristics of the major lung cancer cells?**

Light microscopy (LM) is used to determine and differentiate lung cancer phenotype. Specimens can be obtained from either cytology (i.e., sputum, bronchial brushings or washings, alveolar lavage, transbronchial biopsies, transthoracic needle aspirates, or pleural fluid) or histologic biopsy specimens (from endobronchial or transbronchial biopsies or surgical resection).

- Under LM, squamous cell carcinoma is characterized by the presence of keratinization, squamous pearl formation, and desmosomes.
- Gland formation and intracytoplasmic mucin are often found in adenocarcinoma.
- Bronchoalveolar cell carcinoma is recognized by cell growth along alveolar septa (i.e., lepidic growth).
- Large cell carcinomas are not well differentiated and lack typical features of either adenocarcinoma or squamous cell carcinoma.
- Small cell carcinoma consists of small round or oval cells with variable amounts of cytoplasm and hyperchromatic nuclei.

Interobserver disagreement among pathologists is <5% for distinguishing between NSCLC and SCLC, but it can be as high as 25–40% for differentiating among the different types of NSCLC.

Franklin WA: Pathology of lung cancer. J Thorac Imag 15(1):3–12, 2000.

10. How does the histology of lung cancer predict difference in spread patterns?

- Squamous cell carcinomas characteristically develop in chronically damaged airway lining cells. Their tendency to extend centrally toward the mainstem bronchi is responsible for the frequent occurrence of atelectasis, hemoptysis, and postobstructive pneumonitis.
- Adenocarcinomas present commonly as a peripheral mass or nodule and metastasize early to the central nervous system (CNS), liver, adrenal glands, and bone.
- Large cell carcinomas also tend to present as a peripheral mass. The gastrointestinal tract is commonly involved in metastatic large cell cancers.
- Small cell carcinoma also tends to present as a central mass and is normally highly aggressive. It is usual to encounter extensive spread of cancer cells at the time of diagnosis. Bone, bone marrow, the liver, and the brain are the frequent sites of metastases. Of the different cancer cell types, SCLC has the greatest tendency to metastasize to the brain, bones, and liver.

Beckles MA, Spiro SG, Colice GL, Rudd RM: Initial evaluation of the patient with lung cancer: Symptoms, signs, laboratory tests, and paraneoplastic syndromes. Chest 123:97S–104S, 2003.

11. What are the current methods of staging NSCLC and SCLC?

NSCLC is staged by the tumor node metastasis (TNM) classification, first proposed by Denoix over 50 years ago. It was adopted by the American Joint Committee for Cancer Staging in 1974 and was revised in 1986 and 1997 by C.F. Mountain. It has undergone minor revisions in classification to group lesions with similar outcomes. SCLC is usually staged as limited stage (LS) or extensive stage (ES). LS is defined as SCLC confined to one radiation port, with disease that is limited to ipsilateral supraclavicular nodes and no pleural effusion (Table 57-1).

Passlick B: Initial surgical staging of lung cancer. Lung Cancer 42(Suppl 1):S21–S25, 2003.
Spira A, Ettinger DS: Multidisciplinary management of lung cancer. N Engl J Med 350(4):379–392, 2004.

12. Does staging affect the outcome and therapy available to patients with lung cancer?

Yes. Staging is required after making a diagnosis of lung cancer. Survival is based on available therapy. In NSCLC, a diagnosis of a locally advanced (IIIA resectable) tumor or a lower stage disease allows the possibility of resection and potential cure. Advanced (stages IIIA unresectable, IIIB, or IV) tumors can be treated only for palliation with chemotherapy and radiation therapy. LS SCLC should be treated with concurrent thoracic radiation therapy and chemotherapy. ES SCLC has a worse prognosis, and chemotherapy is indicated for these patients. Five-year survival in LS disease is 15–18% (with a median survival of 47–60 weeks) and is <3% in ES disease (with median survival of 36–28 weeks).

Passlick B: Initial surgical staging of lung cancer. Lung Cancer 42(Suppl1):S21–S25, 2003.
Spira A, Ettinger DS: Multidisciplinary management of lung cancer. N Engl J Med 350(4):379–392, 2004.

TABLE 57-1. TUMOR NODE METASTASIS STAGING FOR NON–SMALL CELL LUNG CANCER

Stage	Tumor	Node	Metastasis	Description	% Survival (1 year/5 year)
Local					
IA	T1	N0	M0	T1: tumor <3 cm, surrounded by lung or pleura; no tumor more proximal than lobe bronchus	94/67
IB	T2	N0	M0	T2: tumor >3 cm involving main bronchus >2 cm distal to carina, invading pleura; atelectasis or pneumonitis extending to hilum but not entire lung	87/57
IIA	T1	N1	M0	N1: involvement of ipsilateral peribronchial or hilar nodes by direct extension	89/55
Locally advanced					
IIB	T1	N2	M0		73/39
	T3	N0	M0	T3 tumor: invasion of chest wall, diaphragm, mediastinal pleura, pericardium; main bronchus <2 cm distal to carina; atelectasis or pneumonitis of entire lung	
IIIA	T1	N2	M0		64/23
	T2	N2	M0		
	T3	N1	M0	N2: involvement of ipsilateral mediastinal or supraclavicular nodes	
IIIB	Any	N3	M0	N3: involvement of contralateral lung or supraclavicular nodes	32/3
Advanced					
IIIB	T4	Any	M0	T4: Invasion of mediastinum, heart, great vessels, trachea, esophagus, vertebral body, carina; separate tumor nodules; malignant pleural effusion	7/7
IV	Any	Any	M1	M1: distant metastasis	20/1

Adapted from Spira A, Ettinger DS: Multidisciplinary management of lung cancer. N Engl J Med 350(4):379–392, 2004.

13. **What is the recommended method of evaluating someone with suspected lung cancer?**

The two most important features of the work-up for lung cancer are the determination of diagnosis and the tumor staging. Evaluation and management by a multidisciplinary team consisting of pulmonologists, cardiothoracic surgeons, pathologists, radiologists, and oncologists is highly recommended. An initial thorough history and physical examination, focused on features commonly encountered in lung cancer, is essential.

Recommended laboratory tests include a complete blood count and serum chemistry (including electrolytes, calcium, alkaline phosphatase, albumin, aspartate aminotransferase, alanine aminotransferase, total bilirubin, and creatinine). Hyponatremia secondary to SIADH may be detected. Liver enzymes are rarely disturbed unless there are extensive liver metastases. Serum albumin is prognostic in advanced disease. Initial radiographic studies should include a chest radiograph. Pathologic diagnosis by cytology (i.e., sputum, bronchial washings or brushings, transbronchial needle, BAL, or transthoracic needle) or biopsy (i.e., bronchoscopy or surgical resection) is paramount.

Initial staging consists of a high-resolution computed tomography (HRCT) scan that includes views of the lung apices, liver, and adrenal glands. Additional workup for distant metastases is recommended for patients (1) without evidence of distant metastases, (2) who have clinically operable disease (stage IIIa or less [including resectable Pancoast's tumor]), and (3) who are able to survive an operation. Further tests might include evaluation of mediastinal lymph nodes greater than 1 cm on chest computed tomography (CT) scans by fluorodeoxyglucose positron emission tomography (FDG-PET) scans or by mediastinoscopy. Alternatives to mediastinoscopy include fine-needle aspiration biopsies with a transthoracic approach, bronchoscopy, or endoscopic ultrasound. This is important as patients with T3N0 tumors are now therapeutically and prognostically similar to stage IIb NSCLC. Brain magnetic resonance imaging (MRI), liver scanning, and bone scanning are recommended for patients with N2 disease or when clinically indicated before aggressive local therapy is undertaken.

Passlick B: Initial surgical staging of lung cancer. Lung Cancer 42(Suppl 1):S21–S25, 2003
Sihoe AD, Yim AP: Lung cancer staging. J Surg Res 117(1):92–106, 2004.
http://www.chestjournal.org/content/vol123/1_suppl
http://www.chestnet.org/education/guidelines/currentGuidelines.php

14. **What is the role of sputum in the diagnosis of lung cancer?**

Sputum analysis alone has not been shown to be sensitive enough for screening of lung cancer. Data from the 1970s–1980s showed a sensitivity of 14% and a specificity of 99%. It is most reliable for diagnosing central, upper lobe, and large lesions. The diagnostic yield also varies with different cancer cell types. Sensitivity is greatest for squamous cell carcinoma, followed by adenocarcinoma and SCLC. A single sputum sample has a sensitivity of about 50%. The yield might be improved with multiple samples, by sputum induction using ultrasonic nebulizers, or by utilizing monoclonal antibodies, reverse transcriptase-polymerase chain reaction (RT-PCR), fluorescence *in situ* hybridization (FISH), and quantitative cytology. Newer techniques, including nuclear staining techniques, have a reported increased sensitivity and specificity of 75% and 98%, respectively.

Kennedy TC, Hirsch FR: Using molecular markers in sputum for early detection of lung cancer: A review. Lung Cancer 45(Suppl 2):S21–S27, 2004.

15. **What is the role of radiologic imaging in evaluation of lung cancer?**

Radiologic imaging (i.e., chest radiographs and chest CT scan) is useful in both diagnosis and staging of lung cancer. Nevertheless, a histologic confirmation of tumor is still necessary prior to initiation of therapy.

Serial imaging is recommended in any patient with a solitary pulmonary nodule (SPN). The likelihood that an SPN is malignant is influenced by several factors including

- **Size:** Likelihood of cancer is low for nodules < 1.5–2 cm and is rare in those <5 mm in size.
- **Change in size:** Cancer is less likely if doubling times are <1 month or >1 year.

- **Number of nodules:** The presence of >6 nodules often suggests an inflammatory disease.
- **Density on CT:** Cancer is more likely if the nodule is solid.
- **Calcification:** Cancer is less likely if calcifications are present.
- **Age:** Lung nodules in persons <40 years of age are less likely to be due to cancer.
- **Smoking history**
- **Spirometry:** Patients with reduced ratio of forced expiratory volume in 1 second (FEV_1) to forced vital capacity (FVC) have a higher risk of lung cancer.
- **Occupational history**
- **Risk of endemic granulomatous disease** (e.g., mycobacterial and fungal diseases such as histoplasmosis, blastomycosis, and coccidioidomycosis)

Additional assessments include FDG-PET scanning and bone scanning to look for metastasis. A quantitative ventilation/perfusion (V/Q) scan to assess lung perfusion may be useful in the perioperative setting. If the patient has evidence of neurologic dysfunction, SCLC, or advanced NSCLC, MRI of the brain, or a head CT scan with contrast is indicated. CT-guided fine-needle aspiration (FNA) may also be performed to obtain cytologic specimens of select lung nodules or lymph nodes.

Libby DM, Smith JP, Altorki NK, et al: Managing the small pulmonary nodule discovered by CT. Chest 125(4):1522–1529, 2004.

Toloza EM, Harpole L, McCrory DC: Noninvasive staging of non-small cell lung cancer: The guidelines. Chest 123 Suppl: 137S–146S, 2003.

KEY POINTS: EPIDEMIOLOGY OF LUNG CANCER

1. Lung cancer is the primary cause of cancer death in both men and women.

2. Tobacco use is the primary risk factor for lung cancer and is estimated to account for 90% of all cases.

3. Symptoms associated with lung cancer are a result of the tumor itself, its metastasis, or systemic paraneoplastic syndromes.

4. Cough is the most common presentation (50–75%).

5. Approximately 5–23% of patients are asymptomatic at presentation.

16. **What is "tumor growth doubling time"? How does it help in evaluation of lung cancer?**

    Tumor growth doubling time refers to the rate at which a lung mass increases in size (to double) over time. Mathematically, a tumor increases in size by a factor multiplied by the cube root of 2. A tumor doubles in size when it reaches 1.3 times its last linear dimension. Therefore, a 1-cm tumor has doubled when it measures 1.3 cm in width. Doubling times of malignant lesions range from 21–400 days. Benign processes usually have doubling times that are either faster or slower.

17. **Is there a role for PET imaging?**

    Due to the increased uptake of FDG by transformed cells, FDG–PET scanning has become useful in the diagnosis and staging of lung cancers. Uptake of FDG is also increased in granulomatous infections and other inflammatory processes. Several trials have suggested a specificity and sensitivity of 88% and 85%, respectively, for mediastinal staging of lymph nodes. PET imaging may be used to corroborate negative CT scan findings or to redirect biopsy to other sites of metastasis.

    http://www.asco.org

18. **Describe the role of bronchoscopy and transthoracic needle biopsy in lung cancer evaluation.**

Bronchoscopy can be used to provide pathologic diagnosis by transbronchial or endobronchial biopsy or by cytology using FNA of lymph nodes, BAL, bronchial brushings, or endobronchial washings. The diagnostic yield for central lesions is about 70%, and, for bronchoscopically visible endobronchial lesions, it is about 90%. The diagnostic yield is generally less for transbronchial biopsies, brushings, and washings of peripheral lesions, depending upon the size: it is about 30% for lesions < 2 cm; 60–70% for lesions > 2 cm; and 80% for lesions > 4 cm. Mediastinal lymph node biopsy and aspiration has a sensitivity of 50% and a specificity of 96%. Diagnostic yield of peripheral lesions < 3 cm in diameter is greater with fluoroscopic- or CT-guided transthoracic needle aspiration.

http://www.thoracic.org/statements
http://www.thoracic.org/adobe/statements/erj.pdf

19. **What is the role of mediastinoscopy and anterior mediastinotomy (Chamberlain procedure) in the evaluation of lung cancer?**

Mediastinoscopy is indicated to assess the mediastinum for tumor metastases if mediastinal lymph nodes are greater than 1 cm on CT scan in cases of potentially resectable NSCLC with no evidence of metastatic disease by FDG–PET. Due to a high potential for false positives, FDG-PET-positive mediastinal lymph nodes require tissue confirmation. Options for obtaining this tissue include mediastinoscopy, anterior mediastinotomy, FNA during bronchoscopy, or trans-esophageal ultrasound biopsy. These procedures are also recommended before resection if FDG–PET is not available.

Bunn PA Jr: Early stage non-small-cell lung cancer: Current perspectives in combined-modality therapy. Clin Lung Cancer 6(2):85–98, 2004.
Sihoe AD, Yim AP: Lung cancer staging. J Surg Res 117(1):92–106, 2004.
Spira A, Ettinger DS: Multidisciplinary management of lung cancer. N Engl J Med 350(4):379–392, 2004.

20. **What is the role of surgery in the treatment of lung cancer?**

Surgery is the mainstay of therapy in NSCLC (i.e., stage I disease, stage II disease, some stage IIIa disease, and T3 Pancoast's tumors, depending on the lesion). Surgery typically consists of lobectomy, bilobectomy or pneumonectomy, and mediastinal lymph node mapping.

Surgery for SCLC is not recommended outside of clinical trials since it has not been shown to alter survival in prospective randomized trials.

Bunn PA Jr: Early stage non-small-cell lung cancer: Current perspectives in combined-modality therapy. Clin Lung Cancer 6(2):85–98, 2004.
Sihoe AD, Yim AP: Lung cancer staging. J Surg Res 117(1):92–106, 2004.
Spira A, Ettinger DS: Multidisciplinary management of lung cancer. N Engl J Med 350(4):379–392, 2004.

21. **What is important in the preoperative evaluation of a patient with stage I–II operative lung cancer?**

Preoperative evaluation of NSCLC should focus on accurate staging. Patients with lung cancer might have compromised respiratory and cardiovascular function, and preoperative evaluation should include determination of cardiovascular risk from surgery, performance status, and likely postoperative FEV_1. Evaluation may include pulmonary function testing (PFT) and electrocardiography. Additional cardiovascular tests (e.g., exercise stress testing, echocardiography, or cardiac angiography) might be necessary in certain patients.

Martin J: Lung resection in the pulmonary compromised patient. Thorac Surg Clin 14(2):1571–1562, 2004.
Spira A, Ettinger DS: Multidisciplinary management of lung cancer. N Engl J Med 350(4):379–392, 2004.

22. **How do you predict postoperative FEV_1?**

Patients being evaluated for lung resection should have preoperative PFT. Patients with a significantly decreased FEV_1 (i.e., < 60–70%) should be evaluated for the amount of residual lung function after surgery (postoperative FEV_1 [$ppoFEV_1$]). Postoperative FEV_1 can be estimated by a quantitative V/Q scan. Patients should also be considered for exercise testing. Patients with a $ppoFEV_1$ < 1 liter or < 40% or with a preoperative maximum oxygen consumption (VO_2max) < 10 mL/kg/min are usually not deemed to be surgical candidates.

An estimate of FEV_1 lost can be calculated as follows:

- Right pneumonectomy = 60%
- Left pneumonectomy = 40%
- Upper lobectomy = 40% (of affected)
- Lower lobectomy = 60% (of affected)
- Lingula or middle lobectomy = 25%

23. Is there a role for operative therapy in stage III lung cancer?

Surgical therapy may be tried for Pancoast's tumors, locally advanced stage IIIA tumors (especially with neoadjuvant therapy), and, possibly, stage IIIB tumors that have responded to chemotherapy. A thorough evaluation of patients with stage III NSCLC is, therefore, recommended. T3 tumors have a 2-year survival rate of 50–70% with combined neoadjuvant chemoradiation therapy. N2 tumors may occasionally be resectable as well.

Martin J: Lung resection in the pulmonary compromised patient. Thorac Surg Clin 14(2):157–162, 2004.

Pfister DG, Johnson DH, Azzoli CG, et al, for the American Society of Clinical Oncology: American Society of Clinical Oncology treatment of unresectable non-small cell lung cancer guideline: Update 2003. J Clin Onc 22(2):330–353, 2004.

Spira A, Ettinger DS: Multidisciplinary management of lung cancer. N Engl J Med 350(4):379–392, 2004.

24. What is the role of bronchoscopy in the treatment of lung cancer?

Palliative therapeutic bronchoscopy, including use of brachytherapy, photodynamic therapy, and laser therapy (with neodymium/yttrium-aluminum-garnet [nd:YAG] laser), is evolving. All three modes of therapy have shown effective palliation of symptoms such as cough, hemoptysis, and dyspnea in patients with endobronchial disease. Palliative placement of Silastic or metallic stents into the airways to manage obstruction or tracheobronchial fistula is also an option.

http://www.thoracic.org/statements
http://www.thoracic.org/adobe/statements/erj.pdf

25. What is the role of radiation in the treatment of lung cancer?

Radiation therapy is considered in patients with stage III tumors and in patients with NSCLC who are deemed unresectable due to tumor location, poor lung function, or poor performance status. Treatment with radiation therapy, often in combination with chemotherapy, should be considered if patients have stage IIIa or IIIb disease, unresectable tumors, adequate pulmonary function, and disease confined to the thorax. Preoperative neoadjuvant combined chemotherapy and radiation therapy has been shown to increase survival in stages I–IIIa tumors. Postoperative adjuvant radiation therapy is not currently recommended. Palliative radiation in hypofractionated schedules may be tried to relieve patients with symptoms from local disease.

In summary, thoracic radiation is given as follows:

- Concurrently with chemotherapy in some neoadjuvant stage IIIa NSCLC protocols
- In combination with chemotherapy for locally advanced NSCLC
- For limited-stage SCLC
- For palliation treatment of hemoptysis
- For management of pain related to skeletal metastases
- For treatment of brain metastases

Toxic effects associated with radiation therapy include radiation pneumonitis, esophagitis, skin desquamation, myelopathies, and cardiac abnormalities; these side effects could be minimized using newer three-dimensional (3-D) CT-guided therapy.

Spira A, Ettinger DS: Multidisciplinary management of lung cancer. N Engl J Med 350(4):379–392, 2004.

26. **What is the role of chemotherapy in lung cancer?**

Neoadjuvant and adjuvant (post-surgery) chemotherapy, as well as chemotherapy for nonresectable tumors, continues to be a consideration in NSCLC due to the poor prognosis even with early-stage disease and despite apparently adequate resection. The poor survival rates are felt to be secondary to the presence of micrometastasis at the time of diagnosis and the likelihood of second primary tumors. Currently, the best outcomes have been achieved with platinum-containing agents (i.e., cisplatin or carboplatin). The addition of other agents (e.g., taxanes, etoposide, ifosfamide, irinotecan, or mitomycin) continues to be controversial, but trials have shown increased survival in stage I, II, and IIIa tumors.

In patients able to tolerate chemotherapy, it has been recommended to use a two-agent therapy, including platinum, for unresected stage III–IV NSCLC. In stage IV disease, two-drug, non-platinum-containing regimens may be substituted as alternatives. Neoadjuvant chemotherapy has been shown to have a small survival benefit for patients with stage I, II, or IIIa resectable NSCLC. Trials of adjuvant chemotherapy have so far shown little benefit.

Arrigada R, Bergman B, Dunant A, et al, for the Cisplatin-based International Adjuvant Lung Cancer Trial Collaborative Group: Cisplatin-based adjuvant chemotherapy in patients with completely resected non-small cell lung cancer. N Engl J Med 350(4):351–360, 2004.

Ramsey SD, Howlader N, Etzioni RD, Donato B: Chemotherapy use, outcomes, and costs for older persons with advanced non-small cell lung cancer: Evidence from surveillance, epidemiology, and end-results—Medicare. J Clin Oncol 22(24):4971–4978, 2004.

Spira A, Ettinger DS: Multidisciplinary management of lung cancer. N Engl J Med 350(4):379–392, 2004.

27. **What is the role of targeted chemotherapeutics in lung cancer?**

Studies of the biology of lung cancer in animal models have shown that inhibition of growth receptors and angiogenesis and intervention in the process of metastasis improves rates of progression, cure, outcomes, and survival. This finding has led to interest in molecular signaling pathways as novel targets for new chemotherapeutics. Agents being used in clinical trials include anti-epidermal growth factor receptor (anti-EGF-R) agents such as cetuximab (Erbitux) and gefitinib (Irressa).

Potential future directions include targeting other growth receptors such as insulin-like growth factor I receptor (IGFIR), platelet-derived growth factor receptor (PDGFR), vascular endothelial growth factor receptor (VEGFR), integrins, receptor-tyrosine kinase (RTK) signaling pathways (RAS, phosphatidylinositol 3-kinase [PI3K] and protein kinase C [PKC] pathways), and cell cycle pathways (cyclin-dependent kinases [CDKs], p53, and retinoblastoma gene and retinoid receptor pathways).

Reinmuth N, Mesters RM, Bieker R, et al: Signal transduction pathways as novel therapy targets in lung cancer. Lung Cancer 45(Suppl 2):S177–S186, 2004.

28. **What is the primary therapy in SCLC?**

SCLC has been shown to have an incidence of about 15–20% worldwide. SCLC is strongly associated with cigarette smoking and is far more malignant than NSCLC. Untreated, it is associated with a median life expectancy of 3 months. Being more sensitive to radiation therapy and chemotherapy than NSCLC, these modalities are used as the primary therapy.

Initial evaluation is similar to that of NSCLC. Brain imaging is important as metastases to the brain might be present. Isolated metastases may also involve the bone marrow and adrenals. Bone marrow aspiration detects tumor contamination in 10% of patients by light microscopy and in > 60% with molecular markers.

Only 20–25% of patients with SCLC have LS disease. LS disease is usually treated with a platinum-containing two-agent chemotherapy regimen along with radiation therapy to the tumor and ipsilateral lymph nodes. Often, prophylactic cranial irradiation should be considered, but its influence on outcome remains controversial.

ES disease is treated with at least a two-agent chemotherapy regimen. Platinum-containing regimens, because they are associated with a small but significant survival advantage, are preferred over older regimens (e.g., cyclophosphamide, adriamycin, and vincristin [CAV]). Newer agents such as irinotecan, topotecan, paclitaxel, and gemcitabine have been tried as well.

http://www.chestnet.org/education/guidelines/currentGuidelines.php

Spira A, Ettinger DS: Multidisciplinary management of lung cancer. N Engl J Med 350(4):379–392, 2004.

Stupp R, Monnerat C, Turrisi AT III, et al: Small cell lung cancer: State of the art and future perspectives. Lung Cancer 45(1):105–117, 2004.

29. What is the role of gene therapy in lung cancer?

Targeted gene therapy is currently not recommended outside of experimental and clinical trials. Use of genetic markers for molecular staging and for gene chip analysis has been shown to have prognostic significance but is thus far of no clinical significance. Chemotherapeutics are being developed for specifically targeting certain portions of the molecular biology of carcinogenesis, metastasis, and angiogenesis, and hopefully these will improve lung cancer survival.

Reinmuth N, Mesters RM, Bieker R, et al: Signal transduction pathways as novel therapy targets in lung cancer. Lung Cancer 45(Suppl 2):S177–S186, 2004.

30. What is the recommended follow-up for a patient treated for lung cancer?

There is a lack of evidence-based guidelines for follow-up of lung cancer. Consensus statements from the American Society of Clinical Oncology (ASCO) and the European Cancer Society agree that patients treated with curative intent should have a follow-up visit every 3 months for the first 2 years and then every 6 months for up to 5 years. A full history, physical examination, and screening chest radiograph are recommended. Patients are urged to quit smoking as there is a high chance of second primary cancers ($\geq$2.5% per year for at least 10 years in patients cured of an initial NSCLC). For patients treated with palliative intent, visits after initial acute reactions will depend on the adequacy of symptom control, generally every 1–2 months.

http://www.chestnet.org/education/guidelines/currentGuidelines.php

Saunders M, Sculier JP, Bali D, et al: Consensus: The follow-up of the treated lung cancer patient. Lung Cancer 42(Suppl 1):S17–S19, 2003.

KEY POINTS: MANAGEMENT OF LUNG CANCER

1. NSCLC is staged by the TNM classification. SCLC is usually staged as limited or extensive.

2. Surgery is the mainstay of therapy in NSCLC (i.e., stage I disease, stage II disease, some stage IIIa disease, and T3 Pancoast's tumors, depending on the lesion).

3. Radiation therapy is considered in patients with stage III tumors and in patients with NSCLC deemed unresectable due to tumor location, poor lung function, or poor performance status.

4. At this point, no conclusive evidence supports the routine use of chemopreventive agents for lung cancer.

31. What is the role of screening for lung cancer among the adult population?

Given that the majority of lung cancers are discovered in later stages (due to its being generally asymptomatic in early stages) and considering the better curative outcomes of surgical therapy in low-stage lung cancers (66%), the hope is that detecting and treating lung cancer early will have an impact on reducing lung cancer mortality. After prevention of smoking, the second-best strategy would be to detect and treat it as early as possible. However, trials in the 1970s and 1980s of chest radiograph and sputum cytology did not improve outcomes.

The purpose of screening at-risk persons (i.e., smokers and former smokers) is to detect lung cancers earlier and at a lower stage and thereby decrease mortality. Current trials of screening with low-dose high-resolution computed tomography (LDHRCT) in smokers and former smokers are underway. Trials adding sputum cytology with new markers to LDHRCT are also underway. Sputum cytology alone, although having a high specificity (90–99%) and frequent success at diagnosing central stage I lung cancers, has a low sensitivity (14–45%). New technologies to increase the sensitivity of sputum cytology using new monoclonal antibody (mAB) markers (e.g., heterogenous nuclear ribonucleoprotein [hnRNP] A2/B1), DNA-based assays with RT-PCR, gene chip analysis looking at DNA methylation, and FISH analysis for markers such as K-ras mutations and p53 mutations, are in progress.

The current recommendation for routine screening utilizing any modality is that interested high-risk individuals should sign up for a screening trial. Most investigators agree that screening of populations not at risk for lung cancer is not recommended.

Heyneman LE, Herndon JE, Goodman PC, Patz EF Jr: Stage distribution in patients with a small (≤ 3 cm) primary non-small cell lung carcinoma. Implications for lung cancer screening. Cancer 92(12):3051–3055, 2001.

32. **What is the role of chemoprevention in lung cancer?**

With chemoprevention, an agent is given to prevent lung cancer in susceptible individuals by interfering with the multistep model of carcinogenesis. In this model, a cell requires multiple genetic defects accumulated over time to become a malignant neoplasm. This process involves the following:

- Tumor initiation (mutation of the DNA, resulting in activation of oncogenes or loss of tumor suppressors)
- Tumor promotion (cellular proliferation through cellular selection, escape from immune surveillance, and clonal expansion)
- Tumor progression (conversion to malignancy by angiogenesis and invasion of nearby tissue)

Areas of research include anti-inflammatory agents (i.e., steroids and nonsteroidal anti-inflammatory agents including aspirin and cyclooxygenase-2 [COX-2] inhibitors such as celecoxib), antioxidants (i.e., vitamins D, C, and E, retinoids, green tea, resveritol, and selenium), and compounds that increase metabolism of carcinogens (i.e., D-glucaric acid salts). Thus far, the major antioxidant trials (the n-acetyl cysteine trial, the Alpha Tocopherol Beta Carotene Cancer Prevention Trial [ATBC], and the Beta Carotene and Retinol Efficacy Trial [CARET]) have shown either a lack of effect or a worsening of outcomes. Phase 1 trials with D-glucaric acid showed decreased K-ras mutations in peripheral blood monocytes. Data from the National Health and Nutrition Examination Surveys (NHANES) I and II have shown decreased incidence of lung cancer among aspirin users. There is no conclusive evidence at this point to support routine recommendation of chemopreventive agents.

Walaszek Z, Hanausek M, Slaga TJ: Mechanisms of chemoprevention. Chest 125(Suppl 5):128S–133S, 2004.

33. **What are the effects of diet on lung cancer, its risks, and its outcomes?**

An association between diets high in fruits and vegetables and lower lung cancer incidence has been reported. However, clinical trials that have supplemented specific nutrients (particularly natural antioxidants such as retinols [i.e., beta carotene] and vitamin C) to the diet were either ineffective in reducing cancer incidences or were inconclusive or potentially harmful. The Physician's Health Study (PHS), a trial of beta carotene and aspirin, showed no significant changes aside from a trend toward lower cancer rates. ATBC tested 29,133 male current smokers with beta carotene and alpha-tocopherol; CARET studied 18,314 current smokers and recent ex-smokers, as well as asbestos-exposed workers, treated with combined beta carotene and retinol versus a placebo. Both trials were stopped early because of increased lung cancer incidence in the treatment arm. Six-year follow-up on both trials has shown a persistent (but statistically insignificant) increase in lung cancer incidence in the intervention arms for all-cause and lung cancer mortality.

Alpha-Tocopherol, Beta Carotene Cancer Prevention Study Group: The effect of vitamin E and beta carotene on the incidence of lung cancer and other cancers in male smokers. N Engl J Med 330(15):1029–1035, 1994.

Goodman GE, Thornquist MD, Balmes J, et al: The Beta-Carotene and Retinol Efficacy Trial: Incidence of lung cancer and cardiovascular disease mortality during 6-year follow-up after stopping beta-carotene and retinal supplements. J Natl Cancer Inst 96(23):1743–1750, 2004.

Shekelle RB, Lepper M, Lius S, et al: Dietary vitamin A and the risk of cancer in the Western Electric study. Lancet 2(8257):1185–1190, 1981.

CHAPTER 58

MALIGNANT PLEURAL EFFUSIONS

Steven A. Sahn, MD

1. How is a malignant pleural effusion diagnosed?

The diagnosis is established by demonstrating exfoliated malignant cells in pleural fluid or by finding malignant cells in pleural tissue obtained by percutaneous pleural biopsy, thoracoscopy, or thoracotomy, or else malignant pleural effusion is discovered at autopsy.

2. What is a paramalignant effusion?

A paramalignant effusion is an effusion associated with a known malignancy but in which malignant cells cannot be demonstrated in pleural fluid or pleural tissue. Paramalignant effusions are caused by local effects of the tumor (i.e., lymphatic obstruction), systemic effects of the tumor (i.e., hypoalbuminemia), and complications of therapy (i.e., radiation pleuritis).

Sahn SA: Malignant pleural effusions. In Bouros D (ed): Pleural Disease. New York, Marcel Dekker, 2004, pp 411–438.

3. What is the most common cause of a malignant pleural effusion?

Lung cancer (causing approximately 40% of all malignant effusions) is the most common malignancy to metastasize to the pleura because of its close proximity to the pleural surface and its tendency to invade the pulmonary vasculature and to embolize to the visceral pleural surface. Breast cancer (25%), gastric carcinoma (3–5%), and ovarian carcinoma (3–5%) are the next most frequent carcinomas to metastasize to the pleura.

Chernow B, Sahn SA: Carcinomatous involvement of the pleura: An analysis of 96 patients. Am J Med 63:695–702, 1977.

Heffner JE, Nietert PJ, Barbieri C: Pleural fluid pH as a predictor of survival for patients with malignant pleural effusions. Chest 117:79–86, 2000.

KEY POINTS: CAUSES OF PARAMALIGNANT EFFUSIONS

1. Local effects of tumors

   - Lymphatic obstruction

   - Endobronchial obstruction (i.e., parapneumonic effusion or atelectasis)

2. Systemic effects of tumors

   - Hypoalbuminemia

   - Pulmonary embolism

3. Complications of therapy

   - Radiation pleuritis

   - Drug reaction

Sahn SA: Pleural effusion in lung cancer. Clin Chest Med 14:189–200, 1993.

Sahn SA: Malignant pleural effusions. In Bouros D (ed): Pleural Disease. New York, Marcel Dekker, 2004, pp 411–438.

4. **How often is the primary site unknown when a malignant pleural effusion is diagnosed?**
   In 5–10% of cases, the primary site is unknown at the time of diagnosis of a malignant pleural effusion. Work-up for the primary site should include an evaluation of the breasts in women and the prostate in men. Further work-up should be dictated by the patient's clinical presentation, by physical examination, and through ancillary laboratory tests.

Chernow B, Sahn SA: Carcinomatous involvement of the pleura: An analysis of 96 patients. Am J Med 63:695–702, 1977.

5. **What is the mechanism of formation of a malignant pleural effusion?**
   A blockage in lymphatic drainage of the pleural space at any point from the stoma of the parietal pleura to the mediastinal lymph nodes and increased pleural capillary permeability (particularly related to vascular endothelial growth factor [VEGF]) are the important mechanisms responsible for the development of a malignant effusion.

Myer PC: Metastatic carcinoma of the pleura. Thorax 21:437–443, 1966.

Sahn SA: Malignant pleural effusions. In Bouros D (ed): Pleural Disease. New York, Marcel Dekker, 2004, pp 411–438.

6. **What are the most common symptoms in patients with malignant pleural effusions?**
   Patients most commonly present with dyspnea on exertion and cough. The presence and degree of dyspnea depend on the volume of pleural fluid and the patient's underlying pulmonary function.

Chernow B, Sahn SA: Carcinomatous involvement of the pleura: An analysis of 96 patients. Am J Med 63:695–702, 1977.

7. **Are all patients with malignant pleural effusions symptomatic at the time of diagnosis?**
   No. In a large retrospective series of patients with metastatic carcinoma to the pleura, almost one in four patients was asymptomatic at presentation. One would suspect, however, that directed questions in a prospective study would elicit symptoms that the patient might not volunteer spontaneously. In contrast, patients with malignant mesothelioma are virtually always symptomatic at the time of diagnosis, with chest pain being the most common symptom.

Chernow B, Sahn SA: Carcinomatous involvement of the pleura: An analysis of 96 patients. Am J Med 63:695–702, 1977.

8. **List the radiologic features that suggest that a pleural effusion is caused by malignancy.**
   - Massive pleural effusion (opacification of the entire hemithorax)
   - Bilateral pleural effusions with a normal heart size (indicating nonlung primary cancer)
   - Interstitial lung disease, ipsilateral mediastinal adenopathy, and effusion (indicating lymphangitic carcinomatosis)
   - Absence of contralateral mediastinal shift with an apparent large effusion (indicating lung cancer of ipsilateral mainstem bronchus)
   - Multiple pulmonary nodules and effusions

Sahn SA: Malignant pleural effusions. In Bouros D (ed): Pleural Disease. New York, Marcel Dekker, 2004, pp 411–438.

9. **What diagnoses should be considered when there is no contralateral mediastinal shift with an apparent large effusion?**
   - Lung cancer of the ipsilateral mainstem bronchus, causing atelectasis
   - A fixed mediastinum caused by malignant lymph nodes
   - Malignant mesothelioma (the radiodensity represents predominantly tumor, with only a small effusion)
   - Extensive tumor infiltration of the ipsilateral lung radiographically mimicking a large effusion

   Sahn SA: Malignant pleural effusions. In Bouros D (ed): Pleural Disease. New York, Marcel Dekker, 2004, pp 411–438.

KEY POINTS: RADIOGRAPHIC FEATURES SUGGESTING A MALIGNANT PLEURAL EFFUSION

1. Massive effusion

2. Bilateral effusions with normal heart size

3. Absence of contralateral mediastinal shift with an apparent large effusion

4. Kerley's B lines with ipsilateral mediastinal adenopathy and pleural effusion

5. Multiple nodules and effusions

6. Unilateral effusion in a patient > 60 years of age

10. **Excluding cytologic examination, is pleural fluid analysis diagnostic for malignant pleural effusion?**
   No. Malignant pleural effusions may be serous, serosanguineous, or grossly bloody and are virtually always exudates. The nucleated cell count is modest (at approximately 1500–4000 cells/μL). The cell population generally consists of lymphocytes, macrophages, and mesothelial cells; lymphocytes often predominate (50–70%) in malignant effusions. In lymphoma, typically 80–100% of the nucleated cells are lymphocytes.

   Chernow B, Sahn SA: Carcinomatous involvement of the pleura: An analysis of 96 patients. Am J Med 63:695–702, 1977.
   Sahn SA: Malignant pleural effusions. In Bouros D (ed): Pleural Disease. New York, Marcel Dekker, 2004, pp 411–438.

11. **Does pleural fluid eosinophilia usually exclude a malignant pleural effusion?**
   No. The prevalence of malignancy is the same in eosinophilic and noneosinophilic effusions.

   Rubins JB, Rubins HB: Etiology and prognostic significance of eosinophilic pleural effusions: A prospective study. Chest 110:1271–1274, 1996.

12. **What is the significance of a low pleural fluid pH (i.e., <7.30) in malignant pleural effusions?**
   Patients whose malignant pleural effusion has a low pH have a high yield (95% positivity) on initial cytologic examination, tend to have a poorer survival from the time of thoracentesis, and tend to have a worse response to chemical pleurodesis than those with a pH > 7.30. However, the pH should not be used as the sole criterion for recommending pleurodesis.

   Heffner JE, Nietert PJ, Barbieri C: Pleural fluid pH as a predictor of pleurodesis failure: Analysis of primary data. Chest 117:87–95, 2000.

Heffner JE, Nietert PJ, Barbieri C: Pleural fluid pH as a predictor of survival for patients with malignant pleural effusions. Chest 117:79–86, 2000.

Sahn SA, Good JT Jr: Pleural fluid pH in malignant effusions: Diagnostic, prognostic, and therapeutic implications. Ann Intern Med 108:345–349, 1988.

KEY POINTS: MALIGNANT PLEURAL EFFUSIONS WITH pH < 7.30

1. Decreased survival

2. High diagnostic yield on pleural cytology

3. Less likely to have successful chemical pleurodesis

13. **Which is the more sensitive test for the diagnosis of malignant pleural effusion, pleural fluid cytology or percutaneous pleural biopsy?**

Cytology is a more sensitive test for diagnosis than percutaneous pleural biopsy because pleural metastases tend to be focal and the latter is a blind sampling procedure. Yield from percutaneous pleural biopsy averages 50%, whereas yield from exfoliated cytology may be as high as 95%. The yield of cytology and pleural biopsy increases as the disease progresses in the pleural space.

Chernow B, Sahn SA: Carcinomatous involvement of the pleura: An analysis of 96 patients. Am J Med 63:695–702, 1977.

Sahn SA: Malignant pleural effusions. In Bouros D (ed): Pleural Disease. New York, Marcel Dekker, 2004, pp 411–438.

14. **What are the options for the patient with suspected malignancy and negative pleural fluid cytology and pleural biopsy?**

The options include observation for a few weeks followed by repeat studies, thoracoscopy, or open pleural biopsy. If the patient wants an immediate diagnosis, thoracoscopy should be done because, in expert hands, it provides a yield of 95–100% in patients with malignant disease, with low morbidity.

Sahn SA: Malignant pleural effusions. In Bouros D (ed): Pleural Disease. New York, Marcel Dekker, 2004, pp 411–438.

15. **What is the prognosis for the patient with a malignant pleural effusion?**

Lung, gastric, and ovarian cancers tend to have a survival time of only a few months from the time of diagnosis of a malignant effusion. Patients with breast cancer may survive for several months to years, depending on the response to chemotherapy. Patients with lymphomatous pleural effusions tend to have survival times intermediate between those with breast cancer and other carcinomas.

Chernow B, Sahn SA: Carcinomatous involvement of the pleura: An analysis of 96 patients. Am J Med 63:695–702, 1977.

Heffner JE, Nietert PJ, Barbieri C: Pleural fluid pH as a predictor of survival for patients with malignant pleural effusions. Chest 117:79–86, 2000.

Sahn SA: Malignant pleural effusions. In Bouros D (ed): Pleural Disease. New York, Marcel Dekker, 2004, pp 411–438.

Sahn SA, Good JT Jr: Pleural fluid pH in malignant effusions: Diagnostic, prognostic, and therapeutic implications. Ann Intern Med 108:345–349, 1988.

16. **What are the usual clinical and physiologic responses to therapeutic thoracentesis?**
Therapeutic thoracentesis generally rapidly relieves dyspnea. However, the volume of pleural fluid removed at thoracentesis does not correlate closely with the improvement in lung volumes; in addition, PaO_2 may fall transiently in some patients despite relief of dyspnea.

> Sahn SA: Malignant pleural effusions. In Bouros D (ed): Pleural Disease. New York, Marcel Dekker, 2004, pp 411–438.

17. **What causes dyspnea in patients with large pleural effusions?**
Dyspnea appears to be caused by several factors including decrease in the compliance of the chest wall, a contralateral shift of the mediastinum, depression of the ipsilateral hemidiaphragm, and decrease in the ipsilateral lung volume. Reflex stimulation from the lungs and chest wall is also important.

> Sahn SA: Malignant pleural effusions. In Bouros D (ed): Pleural Disease. New York, Marcel Dekker, 2004, pp 411–438.

18. **Which patients are candidates for chemical pleurodesis?**
All patients who obtain relief following thoracentesis are potential candidates for pleurodesis. Decisions should be made on an individual basis, based upon general health status, expected survival, pleural fluid pH, primary tumor type, and evidence of lung entrapment.

> Heffner JE, Nietert PJ, Barbieri C: Pleural fluid pH as a predictor of pleurodesis failure: Analysis of primary data. Chest 117:87–95, 2000.
> Kennedy L, Sahn SA: Talc pleurodesis for the treatment of pneumothorax and pleural effusions. Chest 106:1215–1222, 1994.
> Sahn SA: Malignant pleural effusions. In Bouros D (ed): Pleural Disease. New York, Marcel Dekker, 2004, pp 411–438.
> Sahn SA, Good JT Jr: Pleural fluid pH in malignant effusions: Diagnostic, prognostic, and therapeutic implications. Ann Intern Med 108:345–349, 1988.
> Walker-Renard PB, Vaughan LM, Sahn SA: Chemical pleurodesis for malignant pleural effusions. Ann Intern Med 120:56–64, 1994.

19. **What are the complete success rates for the available chemical pleurodesis agents?**
Based on a retrospective literature review, the complete success rate (i.e., no recurrence of any fluid) for talc was 93%; the doxycycline, 72%; and bleomycin, 54%.

> Walker-Renard PB, Vaughan LM, Sahn SA: Chemical pleurodesis for malignant pleural effusions. Ann Intern Med 120:56–64, 1994.

20. **How should talc be administered?**
Talc given by poudrage through the thoracoscope or by slurry through a chest tube is equally effective in the control of malignant pleural effusions. Talc slurry is less expensive than poudrage because the latter requires thoracoscopy.

> Kennedy L, Sahn SA: Talc pleurodesis for the treatment of pneumothorax and pleural effusions. Chest 106:1215–1222, 1994.
> Sahn SA: Malignant pleural effusions. In Bouros D (ed): Pleural Disease. New York, Marcel Dekker, 2004, pp 411–438.

21. **How much talc should be used?**
The appropriate dose is probably 2–4 g of talc because this amount results in a high success rate with minimal adverse effects. Less than 1% of patients have been reported to have acute respiratory failure, of which possible causes include an inflammatory response to talc, sepsis, and reexpansion pulmonary edema.

> Sahn SA: Malignant pleural effusions. In Bouros D (ed): Pleural Disease. New York, Marcel Dekker, 2004, pp 411–438.

22. **When should the chemical agent be instilled into the pleural space for pleurodesis?**
Instillation should take place when the lung has reexpanded and minimal or no pleural fluid is observed on chest radiograph regardless of the volume of current drainage.

23. **Does the patient have to be rotated after instillation of the chemical agent?**
Not with soluble agents such as doxycycline. It has been shown with radiolabeled tetracycline that distribution is rapid and complete within seconds of pleural space instillation. However, patient rotation is recommended with talc slurry because the slurry may not spontaneously distribute well in the pleural space.

> Lorch DG, Gordon L, Wooten S, et al: The effect of patient positioning on the distribution of tetracycline in the pleural space during pleurodesis. Chest 93:527–529, 1988.

24. **When should the chest tube be removed during the pleurodesis procedure?**
Success rates tend to be higher when 24-hour chest tube drainage is less than 150 mL. However, successful pleurodesis can occur with larger volumes of drainage.

25. **What are the adverse effects of talc?**
Fever and chest pain are the most common adverse effects of talc and of most other chemical agents instilled into the pleural space. Other adverse effects that have been reported with talc include empyema, arrhythmias, and respiratory failure; the last may be related to high doses, very small talc crystals, simultaneous bilateral pleurodesis, or talc contaminated by bacteria and endotoxins.

> Kennedy L, Sahn SA: Talc pleurodesis for the treatment of pneumothorax and pleural effusions. Chest 106:1215–1222, 1994.
> Sahn SA: Malignant pleural effusions. In Bouros D (ed): Pleural Disease. New York, Marcel Dekker, 2004, pp 411–438.

26. **Which patients should not be treated with chemical pleurodesis?**
Patients whose disease appears to be terminal, those with severe comorbid disease, those with a very low pleural fluid pH, those with lung entrapment, and those with mainstem bronchial occlusion with tumor should not be treated with chemical pleurodesis.

> Heffner JE, Nietert PJ, Barbieri C: Pleural fluid pH as a predictor of pleurodesis failure: Analysis of primary data. Chest 117:87–95, 2000.
> Sahn SA: Malignant pleural effusions. In Bouros D (ed): Pleural Disease. New York, Marcel Dekker, 2004, pp 411–438.

CHAPTER 59

SYSTEMIC COMPLICATIONS OF LUNG CANCER

Peter Mazzone, MD, MPH, FRCPC, FCCP, and Alejandro Arroliga, MD, FCCP

1. **Define paraneoplastic syndrome.**

   Paraneoplastic syndromes are said to be present when symptoms or signs are caused by the presence of a cancer but are not the direct result of the physical effects of the tumor or its metastases. This may occur because the tumor produces and secretes peptide proteins that generate physiologic responses or because an immune response to the tumor affects other areas in the body. Paraneoplastic syndromes in lung cancer frequently lead to endocrine and neurologic disorders. Other organ systems that can be affected include the hematologic system, the skin, and the bones, as well as the kidneys.

2. **What are the most common paraneoplastic endocrine syndromes in lung cancer?**

   The most common paraneoplastic endocrine syndromes in lung cancer are the syndrome of inappropriate secretion of antidiuretic hormone (SIADH), humoral hypercalcemia of malignancy (HHM), and ectopic Cushing's syndrome (ECS).

3. **What criteria should be fulfilled to prove the existence of an endocrine paraneoplastic syndrome?**

   - Clinical or biochemical evidence of abnormal endocrine function should be present without metastatic tumor spread to the respective endocrine gland.
   - Removal of the tumor should eliminate the endocrine abnormality.
   - The endocrine abnormality should not be affected by physiologic feedback regulation.
   - The endocrine abnormality should persist after removal of the gland normally responsible for producing the hormone in question.
   - A hormone gradient should exist across the tumor bed.
   - The hormone should be shown to be present in tumor tissue.
   - Tumor cells should be shown to be capable of hormone synthesis.

   It is clearly not practical to meet all of these criteria in a given patient.

   Baylin SB, Mendelsohn G: Ectopic (inappropriate) hormone production by tumors: Mechanisms involved and the biological and clinical implications. Endocr Rev 1:45–77, 1980.

   Vorherr H: Para-endocrine tumor activity with emphasis on ectopic ADH secretion. Oncology 29:382–416, 1974.

4. **Describe the incidence and manifestations of SIADH in lung cancer.**

   Clinical SIADH occurs in 7–16% of patients, whereas elevated antidiuretic hormone (ADH) levels may occur in 30–70% of individuals tested. The incidence does not seem to vary with the stage of small cell carcinoma, nor has there been a difference in chemotherapy response or survival.

   Despite very low serum sodium levels (typically below 120 mEq/L), clinical manifestations are frequently absent. This is related to the prolonged period of time over which the syndrome develops during tumor growth. The most common symptoms found in lung cancer patients with SIADH are mental status changes, confusion, lethargy, and seizures.

   Bondy PK, Gilby ED: Endocrine function in small cell undifferentiated carcinoma of the lung. Cancer 50:2147–2153, 1982.

Hansen M, Hanse HH, Hirsch FR, et al: Hormonal polypeptides and amine metabolites in small cell carcinoma of the lung, with special reference to stage and subtypes. Cancer 45:1432–1437, 1980.

Lokich JJ: The frequency and clinical biology of the ectopic hormone syndromes of small cell carcinoma. Cancer 50:2111–2114, 1982.

KEY POINTS: DEFINITION OF SYNDROME OF INAPPROPRIATE SECRETION OF ANTIDIURETIC HORMONE

1. Hyponatremia

2. Plasma hypo-osmolality

3. Inappropriately concentrated urine

4. Absence of conditions that mimic this syndrome (including cardiac, renal, adrenal, and thyroid disorders)

---

5. **Name the treatments available for SIADH related to lung cancer.**
   Treatment of the tumor leads to resolution of over 80% of the cases of SIADH related to small cell carcinoma of the lung. While waiting for a response to chemotherapy, water restriction and medications may be needed. Demeclocycline, lithium, and phenytoin have been used; demeclocycline is the medication of choice as its effect on the concentrating abilities of the kidney is dose dependent and reversible, with minimal side effects. Isotonic or hypertonic saline may be needed in the worst cases. For an infusion of a saline solution to be of benefit, its tonicity must be greater than that of the urine. Serum sodium should rise no more than 0.5 mEq/L/hour to avoid the rare complications of osmotic demyelination syndrome.

   Hainsworth JD, Workman R, Greco A: Management of the syndrome of inappropriate antidiuretic hormone secretion in small cell lung cancer. Cancer 51:161–165, 1983.

   List AF, Hainsworth JD, Davis BW, et al: The syndrome of inappropriate secretion of antidiuretic hormone (SIADH) in small-cell lung cancer. J Clin Oncol 4:1191–1198, 1986.

6. **What other causes of hyponatremia need to be considered in lung cancer?**
   Medications (including chemotherapy) and end-organ dysfunction related to metastases or comorbidities can lead to hyponatremia. In addition, factors other than ADH have been looked for as contributors to hyponatremia. Plasma levels of atrial natriuretic peptide (ANP) have been found to be elevated in small cell carcinoma cell lines as well as in patients with a syndrome of inappropriate antidiuresis, with or without the concomitant elevation of ADH. Other natriuretic factors may also be present (e.g., brain natriuretic peptide).

   Campling BG, Sarda IR, Baer KA, et al: Secretion of atrial natriuretic peptide and vasopressin by small cell lung cancer. Cancer 75:2442–2451, 1995.

   Ohsaki Y, Gross A, Le PT, Johnson BE: Human small cell lung cancer cell (SCLC) lines produce brain natriuretic peptide (BNP). Proc Am Assoc Cancer Res 34:256, 1993.

   Vanhees SL, Paridaens R, Vansteenkiste JF: Syndrome of inappropriate antidiuretic hormone associated with chemotherapy-induced tumor lysis in small-cell lung cancer: Case report and literature review. Ann Oncol 11:1061–1065, 2000.

7. **Describe the cause of humoral hypercalcemia of malignancy (HHM).**
   Hypercalcemia is present in 2–6% of patients with lung cancer at presentation and is most commonly associated with squamous cell carcinoma. Most individuals with hypercalcemia and lung cancer are found to be free of bony metastases. A factor secreted by tumor cells has been found to lead to hypercalcemia. This factor, similar to but distinct from parathyroid hormone, is termed the parathyroid-hormone-related protein (PTHrP). It is the cause of HHM.

KEY POINTS: MANIFESTATIONS OF THE HUMORAL HYPERCALCEMIA OF MALIGNANCY

1. Weakness and fatigue

2. Mental status change

3. Polyuria

4. Gastrointestinal complaints (including pain, constipation, nausea, vomiting, and anorexia)

5. Electrocardiographic changes (i.e., prolongation of the P-R and QRS intervals, shortening of the Q-T interval, bradycardia, and heart block).

---

8. **How is the HHM treated?**

Infusion of isotonic saline helps to correct the dehydration and to enhance the renal excretion of calcium. A loop diuretic can be added once rehydration has occurred to further promote urinary excretion of calcium. Other therapies, designed to bind calcium or to inhibit bone resorption, have evolved. Treatments have included phosphate and sulfate, mithramycin, calcitonin, and gallium nitrate. All have been effective but carry significant side effects. More recently, bisphosphonates have become the most commonly used agent. They are effective, are relatively long lasting, and are well tolerated. Novel therapies are being investigated.

Gucalp R, Theriault R, Gill I, et al: Treatment of cancer-associated hypercalcemia. Double-blind comparison of rapid and slow intravenous infusion regimens of pamidronate disodium and saline alone. Arch Intern Med 154:1935–1944, 1994.

Onuma E, Sato K, Saito H, et al: Generation of a humanized monoclonal antibody against human parathyroid hormone-related protein and its efficacy against humoral hypercalcemia of malignancy. Anticancer Res 24:2665–2673, 2004.

Oyajobi BO, Anderson DM, Traianedes K, et al: Therapeutic efficacy of a soluble receptor activator of nuclear factor KB-IgG Fc fusion protein in suppressing bone resorption and hypercalcemia in a model of humoral hypercalcemia of malignancy. Cancer Res 61:2572–2578, 2001.

9. **Describe the hypercalcemia–leukocytosis syndrome.**

The presence of the HHM has been associated with an increased white blood cell count. Investigation of these individuals has revealed cases of squamous cell carcinoma of the lung that produces granulocyte colony–stimulating factor as well as PTHrP. This hypercalcemia–leukocytosis syndrome has been estimated to be present in 0.5% of lung cancer patients at presentation. It portends a worse prognosis than the presence of HHM alone.

Hiraki A, Ueoka H, Takata I, et al: Hypercalcemia-leukocytosis syndrome associated with lung cancer. Lung Cancer 43:301–307, 2004.

10. **List the main cell types of lung tumors associated with ECS.**

Approximately 27% of all individuals with ECS will be found to have small cell carcinoma of the lung, and another 21% will be found to have a bronchial carcinoid. Uncommonly, ECS may be seen in individuals with non–small cell carcinomas and pulmonary tumorlets.

Beuschlein F, Hammer GD: Ectopic pro-opiomelanocortin syndrome. Endocrinol Metab Clin North Am 31:191–234, 2002.

11. **What are the clinical differences between ECS in small cell carcinoma and in carcinoid tumors?**

ECS has different presentations in small cell carcinoma and in carcinoid tumors. In ECS due to small cell carcinoma, the classic signs of Cushing's syndrome are rarely present. The most common features of ECS in small cell carcinoma are proximal myopathy, moon facies, hypokalemia, and hyperglycemia. Infectious complications are not uncommon. In ECS due to carcinoid tumors, the classic appearance of Cushing's syndrome is more common. Cushingoid features are seen in most cases, hypertension is common, and hypokalemia is seen in 50% of patients. Cortisol levels may be suppressed by high-dose dexamethasone in carcinoids but not in small cell carcinoma.

Amer KMA, Ibrahim NBN, Forrester-Wood CP, et al: Lung carcinoid related Cushing's syndrome: Report of three cases and review of the literature. Postgrad Med J 77:464–467, 2001.

Delisle L, Boyer MJ, Warr D, et al: Ectopic corticotropin syndrome and small-cell carcinoma of the lung. Clinical features, outcome, and complications. Arch Intern Med 153:746–752, 1993.

12. **Explain the molecular differences between ECS in small cell carcinoma and ECS in carcinoid tumors.**

In addition to differences in the aggressiveness of small cell carcinoma versus carcinoid, molecular differences exist that help to explain the clinical differences. In ECS due to small cell carcinoma, there is aberrant processing of proopiomelanocortin (POMC). Secretion of adrenocorticotropic hormone (ACTH) and ACTH precursors occurs in a nonpulsatile fashion. In ECS due to carcinoid tumors, POMC is processed normally, mimicking ACTH production from the pituitary. Glucocorticoid and corticotropin-releasing hormone (CRH) receptors may be present on bronchial carcinoids. Differences in tumor aggressiveness, POMC processing, and the presence of feedback receptors lead to the differences in presentation.

Terzolo M, Reimondo G, Ali A, et al: Ectopic ACTH syndrome: Molecular bases and clinical heterogeneity. Ann Oncol 12:S83–S87, 2001.

13. **How is the diagnosis of ECS made?**

An elevated 24-hour urinary-free cortisol level and serum ACTH level confirm the presence of Cushing's syndrome due either to Cushing's disease (i.e., pituitary hypersecretion of ACTH) or to ECS. If ECS is secondary to small cell carcinoma, the distinction is usually not difficult: the atypical presentation, hypokalemia, and, frequently, the advanced stage of cancer aid in the diagnosis. Cortisol levels are not suppressed, even by high-dose dexamethasone. When the ECS is due to a carcinoid tumor, the distinction is more challenging. The presentations are similar, the tumor is indolent and often difficult to locate radiographically, and endocrine testing can be misleading (see question 12). Magnetic resonance imaging (MRI) of the pituitary gland, inferior petrosal vein sampling, ^{111}In-octreotide scanning, and positron emission tomography have been useful adjunctive tests.

14. **How is ECS treated?**

ECS secondary to carcinoid tumors should be cured by surgical resection of the tumor. Medical management is used to treat the ECS in small cell carcinoma as resection is not an option. Medications that inhibit steroid biosynthesis such as metyrapone and ketoconazole, as well as somatostatin analogues such as octreotide, have been used. Bilateral adrenalectomy can also be considered. Retinoic acid and targeted methylation of POMC promoter regions are being studied as therapeutic options.

Newell-Price J: Proopiomelanocortin gene expression and DNA methylation: Implications for Cushing's syndrome and beyond. J Endocrinology 177:365–372, 2003.

Paez-Pereda M, Kovalovsky D, Hopfner U, et al: Retinoic acid prevents experimental Cushing syndrome. J Clin Invest 108:1123–1131, 2001.

Van den Bruel A, Bex M, Van Dorpe J, et al: Occult ectopic ACTH secretion due to recurrent lung carcinoid: Long-term control of hypercortisolism by continuous subcutaneous infusion of octreotide. Clin Endocrinol 49:541–546, 1998.

Winquist EW, Laskey J, Crump M, et al: Ketoconazole in the management of paraneoplastic Cushing's syndrome secondary to ectopic adrenocorticotropin production. J Clin Oncol 13:157–164, 1995.

KEY POINTS: MOST-COMMON PARANEOPLASTIC NEUROLOGIC SYNDROMES

1. Autonomic dysfunction

2. Cancer-associated retinopathy

3. Lambert–Eaton myasthenic syndrome

4. Paraneoplastic encephalomyelitis

   - Paraneoplastic limbic encephalitis

   - Paraneoplastic cerebellar degeneration

   - Opsoclonus–myoclonus

   - Anti-Hu antibody syndrome

5. Sensory and motor neuropathies

15. **Describe the features of anti-Hu antibody syndrome.**
    Anti-Hu antibody syndrome (also known as the encephalomyelitis/subacute sensory neuropathy syndrome) occurs in patients with small cell carcinoma with high-titer anti-Hu antibodies in their serum and cerebrospinal fluid (CSF). The syndrome often presents before the diagnosis of the cancer, with a sensory neuropathy or manifestation of encephalomyelitis (limbic, cerebellar, or brainstem), progressing to a diffuse encephalomyelopathy with sensory and autonomic deficits. Sensory neuropathy has been found in 74% of patients, motor neuron dysfunction in 20%, limbic encephalopathy in 20%, cerebellar symptoms in 15%, brainstem symptoms in 14%, and autonomic dysfunction in 10%.

    Dalmau J, Graus F, Rosenblum MK, et al: Anti-Hu-associated paraneoplastic encephalomyelitis/sensory neuronopathy. A clinical study of 71 patients. Medicine 71:59–72, 1992.

16. **What are the features of Lambert–Eaton myasthenic syndrome (LEMS)?**
    LEMS presents with proximal muscle weakness, affecting the lower extremities more than the upper. Fatigue, depressed deep tendon reflexes, and autonomic features such as dry mouth and ptosis are common. A transient increase in strength can be seen with exercise. Electromyography shows a low baseline muscle action potential that increases with repeated stimulation. The syndrome often develops prior to the diagnosis of cancer (typically small cell carcinoma). It is the most common neurologic paraneoplastic syndrome (with 3% prevalence in small cell carcinoma).

    Elrington GM, Murray NMF, Spiro SG, et al: Neurological paraneoplastic syndromes in patients with small cell lung cancer. A prospective survey of 150 patients. J Neurol Neurosurg Psychiatry 54:764–767, 1991.
    O'Neill JH, Murray NM, Newsom-Davis J: The Lambert-Eaton myasthenic syndrome. A review of 50 cases. Brain 111:577–596, 1988.

17. **Describe the clinical features of hypertrophic pulmonary osteoarthropathy.**
    Hypertrophic pulmonary osteoarthropathy presents with clubbing of the digits, bilateral symmetrical periosteal new bone formation affecting mainly the long bones of the distal extremities, a noninflammatory arthritis, thickness of the subcutaneous soft tissue in the distal extremities, and evidence of autonomic dysfunction. When present in patients with lung cancer, a non–small cell carcinoma tends to be found.

CHAPTER 60

BENIGN NEOPLASMS OF THE LUNG

Karen Wesenberg, MD, and Melvin Morganroth, MD

1. **What percentage of primary neoplasms are benign?**

   Approximately 2–5% of primary lung tumors are benign. However, most solitary pulmonary nodules (SPNs) are neither benign nor malignant neoplasms. Most benign nodules are granulomas or inflammatory in nature; only 10–20% are benign tumors. When looking specifically at SPNs, older age, positive smoking history, and residence outside the Southwest and Midwest increase the likelihood of malignancy to 30–50%.

   Ginsberg MS, Griff SK, Go BD, et al: Pulmonary nodules resected at video-assisted thoracoscopic surgery: Etiology in 426 patients. Radiology 213:277–282, 1999.

2. **What are the symptoms of benign pulmonary neoplasms?**

   The symptoms depend largely on the anatomical location of the lesion. Intratracheal tumors are frequently asymptomatic but may cause wheezing, cough, or dyspnea, often misdiagnosed as asthma. Endobronchial tumors are more frequently symptomatic secondary to obstruction-causing pneumonias, bronchiectasis from recurrent infections, wheezing, atelectasis, or hyperinflation. Hemoptysis may occur. Parenchymal or peripheral lesions are by far the most common and are usually asymptomatic. Consequently, most benign lung tumors are discovered incidentally on routine chest x-ray or computed tomography (CT) scan.

KEY POINTS: SYMPTOMS OF BENIGN LUNG TUMORS

1. Endobronchial tumors cause wheezing or atelectasis.

2. Parenchymal tumors are usually asymptomatic.

3. **When is an SPN considered benign?**

   An SPN is defined as a well-circumscribed round or oval lesion less than 3 cm in diameter. In general, all SPNs should be considered malignant until proven otherwise. Nodules are considered benign if there is no growth of the lesion over 2 years on chest x-ray or CT scan. Organized patterns of calcification within the nodule such as popcorn, lamellar concentric rings of calcium, or central or homogenous dense calcification are classic radiographic signs that are associated with a low likelihood of malignancy. However, radiographic stability must be demonstrated, either with serial films or by obtaining old radiographs.

   Lillington GA: Solitary pulmonary nodules: new wine in old bottles. Curr Opin Pulmon Med 7:242–246, 2001.

4. **What imaging modalities are available to evaluate SPNs?**

   As imaging techniques continue to improve and detect even smaller nodules, the prevalence of benign lesions will rise, creating a need for a less-invasive means of determining whether a lesion is benign or malignant. CT is very useful as a first approach to the SPN as it can detect patterns of calcification and can determine if other nodules are present. Collimation is best at 5 mm for detecting nodules with adequate sensitivity and specificity.

Positron emission tomography (PET) imaging with 18F2-fluoro-2-deoxyglucose (FDG) exploits the increased glucose metabolism of neoplastic cells and is useful in differentiating between benign and malignant lesions. Prospective studies confirm a sensitivity of 90–98% for lesions at least 1.5 cm in diameter. False-negative PET scans can occur with malignancies with less mitotic activity such as carcinoid or bronchial alveolar cell carcinoma. Smaller nodules also have a significant false-negative rate and lesions (<5 mm) are usually assessed for malignancy by change in size over 6 months on a follow-up CT scan rather than by a PET scan. Any inflammatory process can have increased FDG uptake, so false-positive PET scans are also possible, decreasing their specificity for malignancy.

Gould MK, Maclean CG, Kuschner WG, et al: Accuracy of positron emission tomography for diagnosis of pulmonary nodules and mass lesions: A meta-analysis. JAMA 285:914–924, 2001.

5. **What is the most common benign pulmonary neoplasm?**
The most common benign pulmonary neoplasm is a pulmonary hamartoma. Unfortunately, hamartomas can increase in size over a 2-year period and can be confused with malignant nodules. Hamartomas are mesenchymal tumors that originate from undifferentiated multipotential cells in the connective tissue of bronchial walls. Histologically, hamartomas consist of collagen, smooth muscle, cartilage, and fat. Generally, hamartomas occur as solitary tumors, although, rarely, they can present as multiple pulmonary nodules. Peak incidence is in the sixth to seventh decade of life, with a predilection for men by a ratio of 2:1 to 3:1. Pulmonary hamartomas usually occur as peripheral intraparenchymal nodules and are subsequently asymptomatic. Endobronchial hamartomas are rare, accounting for <8% of all hamartomas.

6. **How is a hamartoma diagnosed?**
Hamartomas have a classic radiographic appearance as well-demarcated peripheral nodules with an average diameter of 1.5 cm. Margins are sharp and may be lobulated. Popcorn calcification occurs in less than 20% of hamartomas. CT findings include fat attenuation, with or without calcification. CT-guided biopsy can establish the diagnosis in approximately 85% of cases, with low overall morbidity and mortality. Malignant transformation has not been reported with hamartoma, and local recurrences are rare.

KEY POINTS: FEATURES OF HAMARTOMA

1. Solitary parenchymal nodule

2. Sharp margins, often lobulated

3. Fat attenuation, with (20%) or without calcification

4. Mesenchymal tumor

5. Average diameter of 1.5 cm

7. **What are bronchial carcinoids?**
Bronchial carcinoids are thought to arise from neuroendocrine Kulchitsky's cells located in the bronchial mucosa; they account for approximately 2% of primary lung tumors. Well-differentiated pulmonary neuroendocrine tumors (i.e., typical carcinoids) behave in an indolent manner, with metastasis reported in less than 15% of cases. Subsequently, the 5-year survival rate is generally greater than 90%.

Typical carcinoids are included in this chapter because of this indolent behavior, but they should not be considered benign. Surgical resection is indicated, if possible, when they are discovered. Pulmonary carcinoids belong to a spectrum of neuroendocrine tumors, of which small cell lung cancer is the most malignant. Atypical carcinoids have an intermediate grade but are clearly malignant and require aggressive therapy.

8. **Who gets bronchial carcinoids?**
   Bronchial carcinoids are generally seen in adults in their mid 40s and occur equally in men and women. Although there is no association with smoking in patients with typical carcinoids, there is a correlation with smoking in patients with atypical carcinoids and small cell carcinoma.

9. **How do bronchial carcinoids present?**
   The majority of pulmonary carcinoids are perihilar in location, with approximately 75% being endobronchial tumors. Patients often present with obstructive symptoms such as recurrent pneumonia, cough, hemoptysis, or chest pain. Occasionally, patients may present with carcinoid syndrome, resulting from vasoactive substances released by the tumor.

10. **How are carcinoids diagnosed?**
    Because of their endobronchial location, carcinoids are generally seen on bronchoscopy. Endobronchial lesions can be seen on CT, especially if three-dimensional (3-D) airway reconstruction (i.e., virtual bronchoscopy) is done, but bronchoscopy is still the procedure of choice. They often appear to be reddish-brown, which gives them a hypervascular appearance. Bronchoscopists were reluctant to biopsy these lesions because they were thought to be at increased risk of hemorrhage during the procedure. However, studies have shown that these lesions can be safely biopsied if care is taken.

11. **What is the carcinoid syndrome?**
    Carcinoid syndrome occurs in 1–4% of patients with carcinoid tumors and always reflects metastasis of the tumor, usually to the liver. The syndrome is caused by the production of high levels of 5-hydroxytryptamine that enter the systemic circulation and cause severe flushing, hypotension, anxiety, nausea, and vomiting. The difference between metastatic abdominal carcinoids and metastatic thoracic carcinoids is that the systemic symptoms are much more profound in thoracic tumors.

    Kulke MH, Mayer RJ: Carcinoid tumors. N Engl J Med 340:858–867, 1999.

12. **List the differences between typical and atypical carcinoids.**
    See Table 60-1.

13. **Does a pulmonary carcinoid produce any paraneoplastic syndromes?**
    Yes. Although carcinoid syndrome is rare (occurring in <1%) in bronchial carcinoid, paraneo-plastic syndromes due to hormonal production are relatively common. Corticotropin (i.e., adrenocorticotropic hormone [ACTH]), antidiuretic hormone, growth-hormone releasing factor, pancreatic polypeptide, gastrin-releasing peptide, vasoactive intestinal peptide, calcitonin, and serotonin have been reported. ACTH production may lead to Cushing's syndrome. Refractory hypertension and hypokalemia? Think carcinoid!

    Limper AH, Carpenter PC, Scheithauer B, et al: The Cushing syndrome induced by bronchial carcinoid tumors. Ann Intern Med 117:209–214, 1992.

14. **Describe tracheobronchial papillary tumors.**
    Tracheobronchial tumors most commonly occur in young children in the larynx and are generally squamous papillomas. Human papillomavirus has been implicated in their develop-ment. Tracheobronchial papillomas tend to cause central symptoms (i.e., cough, wheezing, stri-dor, or hemoptysis). These tumors are generally benign and tend to regress before adolescence without treatment. In adults, these tumors can undergo malignant transformation and generally are removed either endobronchially, with a laser, or through surgery. There is a significant

TABLE 60-1. DIFFERENCES BETWEEN TYPICAL AND ATYPICAL CARCINOIDS		
Feature	**Typical Carcinoid**	**Atypical Carcinoid**
Gender difference	None	None
Age (years)	40s	50s
Smoking	No association	60% occur in smokers
Frequency	75% of carcinoids	25% of carcinoids
Location in the lung	Usually central	Usually peripheral
Radiographic appearance	Well circumscribed; can be associated with obstructive pneumonia and atelectasis	Spiculated or smooth margins; may show evidence of necrosis or hilar adenopathy
Lymph node involvement	Rare (7%)	45%
Metastasis	Almost never	20%
Malignant potential	Low	High
5-year survival rate	>90%	40–60%

From Cooper WA, Thourani VH, Gal AA, et al: The surgical spectrum of pulmonary neuroendocrine neoplasms. Chest 119(1):14–18, 2001; and Kulke MH, Mayer RJ: Carcinoid tumors. N Engl J Med 340:858–867, 1999.

recurrence rate after removal, and multiple resections can result in airway strictures and upper airway obstruction.

Grillo HC, Mathisen DJ: Primary tracheal tumors: Treatment and results. Ann Thorac Surg 49:69–77, 1990.

15. What are teratomas?

Teratomas are included in the differential diagnosis of anterior mediastinal masses, in addition to thymomas, thyroid cancers, and lymphomas. Teratomas are very rarely seen within the pulmonary parenchyma. They contain every embryonic cell line (i.e., endoderm, mesoderm, and ectoderm) and arise from the third pharyngeal pouch. These tumors may have a malignant component. When the diagnosis of teratoma is considered, the possibility of a metastatic lesion from the gonads should be ruled out. Teratomas are more commonly seen in younger patients, between the ages of 20 and 30 years, and occur equally in men and women.

16. What are pulmonary tumorlets?

These represent a benign localized neuroendocrine cell proliferation, <3 mm in diameter, adjacent to small bronchioles. They are usually associated with damaged and ecstatic small airways. Pulmonary tumorlets often manifest as a subcentimeter pulmonary nodule (or nodules) on CT. Pulmonary tumorlets very likely represent hyperplastic cells. They are more common in older women.

Ginsberg MS, Akin O, Berger DM, et al: Pulmonary Tumorlets: CT findings. Am J Roentgenol 183(2):293–296, 2004.

17. Do intrapulmonary lymph nodes exist?

Yes. Intrapulmonary lymph nodes have been described on thin-section CT. The nodules are distributed throughout all lung fields and are located abutting or in close proximity to the visceral pleura. They are well circumscribed, homogenous, round or ovoid, and smaller than 12 mm in size. Benign intrapulmonary lymph nodes have been described in patients with known primary lung cancer. Therefore, these small nodules should not be considered metastases unless this is pathologically proven.

Oshiro Y, Kusumoto M, Moriyama N, et al: Intrapulmonary lymph nodes: Thin-section CT features of 19 nodules. J Comput Assist Tomogr 26(4):553–557, 2002.

Tsunezuka Y, Sato H, Hiranuma C, et al: Intrapulmonary lymph nodes detected by exploratory video-assisted thoracoscopic surgery: Appearance of helical computed tomography. Ann Thorac Cardiovasc Surg 6(6):369–372, 2000.

18. **Provide a framework to help remember all of the benign tumors of the lung.**

There are many rare types of benign lung tumors. Most can be classified by location, as follows:

Tracheobronchial:	Papillomatosis
	Adenoma
	Granular cell myoblastoma
	Endobronchial hamartoma
	Lipoma (almost always endobronchial)
Solitary parenchymal:	Hamartoma
	Sclerosing hemangioma
	Leiomyoma
	Neurofibroma
	Teratoma
	Benign clear cell tumor
	Plasma cell granuloma
	Endometrioma
Multiple parenchymal:	Metastasizing leiomyoma
	Pulmonary tumorlets
	Chondromas

Allan J: Rare solitary benign tumors of the lung. Semin Thorac Cardiovasc Surg 15(3):315–322, 2003.

Allen M: Multiple benign lung tumors. Semin Thorac Cardiovasc Surg 15(3):310–314, 2003.

Murray JF, Nadel JA: Textbook of Respiratory Medicine, 3rd ed. Philadelphia, W.B. Saunders, 2000.

CHAPTER 61

PULMONARY METASTATIC DISEASE

R. Hal Hughes, MD, and Stephanie M. Levine, MD

1. How common are pulmonary metastases?

At autopsy, evidence of lung metastases is seen, either grossly or microscopically, in 30–40% of patients with extrathoracic primary tumors. However, only 10–30% of these are recognized before death. Although many tumor types may metastasize to the lungs, the malignancies that are most consistently associated with pulmonary metastases are malignant melanomas; genitourinary, colorectal, breast, and head and neck carcinomas; soft-tissue and osteogenic sarcomas; and germ cell neoplasms.

Burt M: Pulmonary metastases. In Fishman AP (ed): Pulmonary Diseases and Disorders, 3rd ed. New York, McGraw-Hill, 1998.

Luce JA: Metastatic malignant tumors. In Murray JF, Nadel JA (eds): Textbook of Respiratory Medicine, 3rd ed. Philadelphia, W.B. Saunders, 2000.

KEY POINTS: COMMON TUMORS THAT CAUSE LUNG METASTASES

1. Melanomas

2. Genitourinary cancers

3. Sarcomas

4. Germ cell tumors

5. Colon cancers

6. Breast cancers

2. Describe the usual radiographic patterns of pulmonary metastatic disease.

Solitary and multiple metastatic nodules tend to occur in the periphery of the lungs, presumably because they spread hematogenously. The lower and middle lung fields are involved more commonly because these are the zones of greatest blood flow. Often, the multiple metastatic lesions are bilateral, are well circumscribed, and occur in varying sizes. Chest computed tomography (CT) is understandably superior in detecting small metastases involving the subpleural, apical, and costophrenic angle regions, as well as in assessing mediastinal lymphadenopathy.

Lymphangitic carcinomatosis often simulates interstitial pulmonary edema, insofar as it has irregular, coarse bronchovascular markings and prominent septal or Kerley's B lines. However, the linear pattern may have a nodular component, thus creating a coarse reticulonodular pattern. High-resolution CT in these patients may show an increased number of irregular, thickened septal lines arranged in polyhedral patterns. The lines predominate in the central chest and may be termed *Kerley's A lines*. Often, knot-like thickening or beading occurs along the course of the lines; this is the most specific finding for lymphangitic carcinomatosis.

3. **Which primary extrathoracic tumor can result in *solitary* pulmonary metastases?**

   It is estimated that 25% of all metastases to the lung are solitary. Moreover, 3–5% of all solitary pulmonary nodules (SPNs) are actually solitary metastases. The most common tumor types that result in solitary metastases are colon carcinomas (usually rectosigmoid), head and neck carcinomas, sarcomas (especially osteogenic), renal cell and breast carcinomas, testicular neoplasms, and melanomas. On rare occasions, bladder and hepatocellular carcinomas present as solitary pulmonary metastases.

   Naidich DP, Webb WR, Muller NL, et al: Computed Tomography and Magnetic Resonance of the Thorax, 3rd ed. Philadelphia, Lippincott-Raven, 1999.
   Pugatch RD: Radiologic evaluation in chest malignancies: A review of imaging modalities. Chest 107:294S–297S, 1995.

KEY POINTS: COMMON TUMORS THAT CAUSE SOLITARY PULMONARY METASTASES

1. Colon carcinomas

2. Sarcomas

3. Renal carcinomas

4. Breast carcinomas

5. Germ cell tumors

6. Melanomas

---

4. **What primary extrathoracic tumor types occur as *multiple* pulmonary metastases?**

   Although multiple metastases may present in numerous forms, the following radiographic patterns may suggest certain tumor types:

   - **Cannonball** lesions are associated with colorectal and renal cell carcinomas, sarcomas, melanomas, choriocarcinomas, and testicular tumors.
   - **Miliary** patterns are noted with medullary thyroid carcinomas, melanomas, renal cell carcinomas, and ovarian carcinomas.
   - **Cavitary** masses are most commonly seen with squamous cell carcinomas of any origin (but usually head and neck tumors in males and genitalia-related tumors in females), colon carcinomas, osteogenic sarcomas, and (rarely) pancreas or bladder carcinomas. Osteogenic sarcomas are commonly associated with pneumothoraces, which may be the initial presentation of this disease.
   - **Calcified** metastases are unique to osteogenic sarcomas, chondrosarcomas, and synovial cell sarcomas.

5. **Which primary extrathoracic malignancies are associated with lymphangitic pulmonary metastases?**

   The most common tumor types are breast, pancreatic, gastric, and colon carcinomas. Less commonly, germ cell tumors (especially testicular), prostate carcinomas, and cervical carcinomas metastasize in this fashion. Lung carcinomas and lymphomas are intrathoracic malignancies that can present with a lymphangitic pattern.

6. **What are the common clinical manifestations of lymphangitic spread of carcinoma to the lungs?**
Dyspnea often begins insidiously and, characteristically, progresses rapidly, during which time pulmonary function tests may reveal decreased diffusion capacity, reduced lung volumes and lung compliance, and hypoxemia. Cough is also a frequent complaint and is usually nonproductive.

7. **Name the extrathoracic tumors that metastasize endobronchially.**
Renal cell carcinoma, breast carcinoma, melanoma, and colorectal carcinoma all occur commonly. Occasionally other tumors, such as cervical carcinoma, uterine carcinoma, Kaposi sarcoma, and other sarcomas, are found endobronchially.

KEY POINTS: COMMON TUMORS THAT CAUSE ENDOBRONCHIAL METASTASES

1. Renal cell carcinomas

2. Breast carcinomas

3. Melanomas

4. Colorectal carcinomas

8. **Which extrathoracic tumor types are associated with pleural effusions?**
The most common malignancies presenting with pleural effusions are breast, pancreatic, gastric, ovarian, and renal cell carcinomas. Lymphangitic carcinomatosis is also often associated with pleural effusion.

9. **How is metastatic disease of the lung usually diagnosed?**
Sputum cytology may be positive in up to 35% of patients; the yield is higher with larger masses and endobronchial disease. Fiberoptic bronchoscopy with transbronchial biopsy is especially useful if patients have hemoptysis, localized wheezing, or radiographs suggesting atelectasis or diffuse infiltrates. Bronchoalveolar lavage may be diagnostic of a metastatic tumor, especially when lymphangitic spread has occurred. Transthoracic fine-needle aspiration or biopsy is often diagnostic with peripheral lesions or lymphangitic spread. Aspiration of wedged capillary blood by pulmonary artery catheters has been reported to be diagnostic for lymphangitic carcinomatosis when cytologic examination of the buffy coat is performed. Newer techniques such as radiolabeled monoclonal antibodies directed toward specific primary tumor antigens may ultimately be useful.

Masson RG, Krikorian J, Lukl P, et al: Pulmonary microvascular cytology in the diagnosis of lymphangitic carcinomatosis. N Engl J Med 321:71–76, 1989.

10. **Does a new SPN discovered after a primary extrathoracic tumor has been found always represent metastatic disease?**
The answer often depends on the primary tumor pathology. SPNs after resection of sarcomas or melanomas are 10 times more likely to represent a metastasis than a second primary tumor. However, new SPNs after genitourinary or colorectal primaries have a 50% chance of being a metastasis. Those after head and neck tumors are twice as likely to be new primaries.

11. **What are the criteria for surgical resection of pulmonary metastases?**
    Most authors agree on the following criteria:
    - The primary tumor is controlled.
    - There is no other evidence of extrathoracic metastatic disease.
    - The metastatic lung disease is amenable to complete resection.
    - The patient is physiologically able to tolerate the proposed surgery.
    - There is no other effective systemic therapy.

    More controversial issues regarding the potential success of metastasectomies include a smaller number of lung nodules, a longer disease-free interval (defined as the time from diagnosis of the primary cancer to the appearance of pulmonary metastases), a longer tumor doubling time, smaller-sized nodules, and unilateral (versus bilateral) metastatic disease.

    Belal A, Salah E, Hajjar W, et al: Pulmonary metastasectomy for soft tissue sarcomas: Is it valuable? J Cardiovasc Surg 42:835–840, 2001.

    Rusch VW: Pulmonary metastasectomy: Current indications. Chest 107:322S–330S, 1995.

    Todd TR: Pulmonary metastasectomy: Current indications for removing lung metastases. Chest 103:401S–403S, 1993.

    Todd TR: The surgical treatment of pulmonary metastases. Chest 112:287S–290S, 1997.

12. **What are the usual surgical approaches for metastasectomies?**
    The majority of cases require single or multiple wedge resections or a limited segmentectomy. Lobectomies are required in approximately 25% of cases, and pneumonectomies in only 8%. A combination of lobectomy with wedge resection can also be performed. New techniques such as laser or needle-tipped electrocautery have been used successfully in some instances. Video-assisted thoracoscopic surgery (VATS) has been used more recently, but it relies heavily on CT findings, which limits its use to staging in some cases. For bilateral resections, either a median sternotomy or a "clam shell" thoracotomy (i.e., a bilateral anterior thoracotomy with a transverse sternotomy) is used in selected patients. The reported surgical mortality of pulmonary metastasectomies is 1%.

    Cheng LC, Chiu CSW, Lee JWT: Surgical resection of pulmonary metastases. J Cardiovasc Surg 39:503–507, 1998.

    Downey RJ: Surgical treatment of pulmonary metastases. Surg Oncol Clin North Am 8:341, 1999.

13. **What factors are important in the success of surgical resections of pulmonary metastases?**
    The overall success of these surgeries is directly related to the type of tumor; in many cases, a smaller number (i.e., ≤3) of nodules (particularly solitary metastases), a longer tumor doubling time, smaller-sized lesions (i.e., ≤3 cm), unilateral (versus bilateral) involvement, and a longer disease-free interval (i.e., ≥36 months) portend a better prognosis, but these latter variables have not been consistently shown to affect outcome in all studies. The completeness of the resection is also a key factor in survival. For colon carcinoma, a normal carcinoembryonic antigen (CEA) prior to surgery may also portend a better survival following metastasectomy.

    Marincola FM, Mark J: Selection factors resulting in improved survival after surgical resection of tumors metastatic to the lungs. Arch Surg 125:1387–1393, 1990.

    Matsuzaki Y, Shimizu T, Edagawa M, et al: "The Law of 3": Prognostic parameters for resected metastatic pulmonary tumors. Ann Thorac Cardiovasc Surg 9:290–294, 2003.

    Pastorino U, Buyse M, Friedel G, et al: Long-term results of lung metastasectomy: Prognostic analyses based on 5206 cases. J Thorac Cardiovasc Surg 113:37–49, 1997.

    Rena O, Casadio C, Viano F, et al: Pulmonary resection for metastases from colorectal cancer: Factors influencing prognosis. Twenty-year experience. Eur J Cardiothorac Surg 21:906–912, 2002.

    Robert JH, Ambrogi V, Mermillod B, et al: Factors influencing long-term survival after lung metastasectomy. Ann Thorac Surg 63:777–784, 1997.

14. **How successful are surgical resections of pulmonary metastases?**

In large series of patients undergoing metastasectomy for varying histologic diagnoses, 2-, 5-, and 10-year survival rates are 50–69%, 36–48%, and 26–35%, respectively, but these vary widely by tumor histology. For example, patients with metastasectomy for teratomas and other germ cell tumors have the best prognosis, with a 10-year survival rate approaching 70%. Patients with metastatic disease from soft tissue sarcomas undergoing metastasectomy have an overall 5-year survival rate ranging between 20% and 38%, but most series show improved survival with less than five nodules, a disease-free interval of more than 1 year, and a tumor doubling time of more than 40 days. Patients undergoing metastasectomy for colorectal carcinoma have an overall 5-year survival rate of 20–58%, with a trend toward longer survival in those with a solitary metastasis 3 cm or less in size or with normal preoperative CEA levels.

Melanomas tend to metastasize to extrathoracic locations, but when metastases are limited to the lungs, patients undergoing metastasectomies have a poorer prognosis than those reported for other tumor types; however, they can still have 5-year survival rates of 5–33%. There is a better prognosis with two or fewer nodules and a disease-free interval of more than 1 year. Disease recurrence is common, and further surgical resections may have to be performed.

Rarely, metastatic tumors may regress spontaneously without any specific therapy, as has been reported with renal cell carcinoma, trophoblastic carcinoma, and transitional cell carcinoma of the bladder. Some studies suggest that the addition of adjunctive chemotherapy, particularly in patients with breast or colorectal metastases, may result in improved survival.

Monteiro A, Arce N, Bernardo J, et al: Surgical resection of lung metastases from epithelial tumors. Ann Thorac Surg 77:431–437, 2004.

Mountain CF, McMurtrey MJ, Hermes KE: Surgery for pulmonary metastasis: A 20-year experience. Ann Thorac Surg 38:323–330, 1994.

Okumura S, Kondo H, Tsuboi M, et al: Pulmonary resection for metastatic colorectal cancer: Experiences with 159 patients. J Thorac Cardiovasc Surg 112:867–874, 1996.

Saito Y, Omiya H, Kohno K, et al: Pulmonary metastasectomy for 165 patients with colorectal carcinoma: A prognostic assessment. J Thorac Cardiovasc Surg 124:1007–1013, 2002.

van Halteren HK, van Geel AN, Hart A, et al: Pulmonary resection for metastases of colorectal origin. Chest 107:1526–1531, 1995.

WEBSITES

http://www.ctsnet.org/doc/7455
http://www. emedicine.com/radio/byname/lung-metastases.htm
http://www.thoracicrad. org/STR_Archive/PostGraduatePapers/LibshitzHI.html

BIBLIOGRAPHY

Fraser RG, Muller NL, Colman N, et al: Diagnosis of Diseases of the Chest, 4th ed. Philadelphia, W.B. Saunders, 1999.

ACUTE RESPIRATORY FAILURE

Hyun Joo Kim, MD, and David H. Ingbar, MD

CHAPTER 62

1. Define acute respiratory failure (ARF), and list the common causes.

ARF is characterized by an inability to maintain adequate oxygenation, ventilation (i.e., CO_2 excretion), or both, that develops over a short period of time. For practical purposes, the onset usually occurs over several hours or days. Subacute respiratory failure usually occurs over several weeks to 2 months.

The oxygenation criterion defining ARF is either a PaO_2 of less than 50–55 mmHg or an arterial oxygen saturation by pulse oximetry of less than 85% on room air. Some authorities say patients with less-severe relative hypoxemia (compared with the expected normal PaO_2) have respiratory insufficiency, but this term is not well defined.

The ventilation criterion defining acute respiratory failure is a $PaCO_2$ greater than 50 mmHg or an increase of more than 10 mmHg over the baseline $PaCO_2$.

ARF has many causes including infection (from pneumonia), pulmonary edema, diffuse alveolar hemorrhage, lobar atelectasis, airway obstruction (mechanical or from asthma or chronic obstructive lung disease [COPD]), neuromuscular or chest wall disease, pulmonary embolism, drug overdose, sleep disordered breathing, massive pleural effusion, pneumothorax, and ascites. Sometimes ARF is superimposed on chronic respiratory failure, as often occurs in exacerbations of COPD.

2. How can the causes of ARF be classified for practical clinical use?

ARF can be classified into hypercapnic respiratory failure, defined by a very high $PaCO_2$, or by hypoxemic respiratory failure, with a very low PaO_2. Hypercapnic ventilatory failure commonly occurs due to problems in the function of the respiratory muscles (i.e., "pump failure"), including diaphragm paralysis, or is due to decreased ventilatory drive, as happens in drug overdose or myxedema coma. Oxygenation failure usually occurs because of problems with alveolar disease (i.e., pulmonary edema or acute lung injury), severe ventilation-perfusion (V/Q) mismatching (in COPD and asthma), or loss of functional alveolar–capillary surface area (from pulmonary emboli, vasculitis, emphysema, or interstitial fibrosis).

Many diseases have abnormalities of both oxygenation and ventilation. For example, COPD often has both hypoxemia and hypercapnia. In most COPD patients with hypercapnia, minute ventilation is actually increased above normal, so the inability to excrete CO_2 really is due more to the inability to compensate for very inefficient alveolar ventilation rather than to pump failure *per se*.

The chest radiograph provides another way to classify ARF. The common causes of ARF can be divided into those with a normal versus an abnormal chest radiograph. ARF with normal lung parenchyma on chest radiograph often is due to COPD, asthma, pulmonary embolism, or neuromuscular dysfunction. In contrast, infection, pulmonary edema, atelectasis, very large pleural effusions, and pneumothorax result in abnormalities on the radiograph.

3. What is the prognosis for a patient with ARF?

In a recent multicenter international study, the overall in-hospital mortality rate for patients with ARF was 44%. Another recent European study found that the 90-day mortality for patients with ARF was 41%. Obviously the prognosis in a specific individual is a function of the specific etiology, the severity of pulmonary dysfunction, other acute medical conditions, and concomitant

KEY POINTS: CONTRIBUTORS TO HYPERCAPNIA

1. In patients with hypercapnic acute respiratory failure, remember to think about contributions from disorders of ventilatory drive, diaphragm dysfunction, and neuromuscular weakness.

2. Reversible causes include myxedema, alkalemia, hypophosphatemia, critical illness polyneuropathy, and myasthenic crisis.

underlying lung or systemic disease. Patients with ARF caused by sepsis had average survival rates (46%), whereas those with ARF due to pneumonia or post-shock lung injury had higher survival rates (63% and 67%, respectively). Factors associated with poor survival included greater severity of lung injury, an inspired fraction of oxygen (FiO_2) requirement ≥ 80% on the ventilator, a peak inspiratory pressure on the ventilator > 50 cmH$_2$O, longer periods of mechanical ventilation, and concomitant multiorgan failure.

Afessa B, Morales IJ, Scanlon PD, Peters SG: Prognostic factors, clinical course, and hospital outcome of patients with chronic obstructive pulmonary disease admitted to an intensive care unit for acute respiratory failure. Crit Care Med 30(7):1610–1615, 2002.

Blivet S, Philit F, Sab J, et al: Outcome of patients with idiopathic pulmonary fibrosis admitted to the ICU for respiratory failure. Chest 120(1):209–212, 2001.

Luhr OR, Antonsen K, Karlsson M, et al: Incidence and mortality after acute respiratory failure and acute respiratory distress syndrome in Sweden, Denmark, and Iceland. Am J Respir Crit Care Med 159:1849–1861, 1999.

Nevins ML, Epstein SK: Predictors of outcome for patients with COPD requiring invasive mechanical ventilation. Chest 119(6):1840–1849, 2001.

Vasilyev S, Schaap RN, Mortensen JD: Hospital survival rates of patients with acute respiratory failure in modern respiratory intensive care units. Chest 107:1083–1088, 1995.

Vincent JL, Sakr Y, Ranieri VM: Epidemiology and outcome of acute respiratory failure in intensive care unit patients. Crit Care Med 31(4 Suppl):S296–S299, 2003.

4. **How can the clinician monitor a patient for development of ARF?**
In order to monitor a patient, the clinician should follow vital signs, the lung examination, oxygenation (i.e., arterial blood gas [ABG] or oxygen saturation), the chest radiograph, and the function of vital end-organs (especially central nervous system and kidney function). Clues to the development of ARF include complaints of dyspnea, cough, chest tightness, or chest pain. Physical exam may reveal tachycardia, tachypnea > 25–30 breaths/minute, diffuse crackles in pulmonary edema, or signs of lobar consolidation in pneumonia. Cyanosis is not a very reliable physical exam finding because it is very observer dependent and, in the best circumstances, requires > 5 gm% of desaturated hemoglobin. Because some patients with severe hypoxemia have no shortness of breath, only by measuring blood gas levels can respiratory failure be excluded. Laboratory assessment by ABG analysis is essential because oximetry cannot detect hypercapnia. In addition, with supplemental oxygen therapy, it may be easy to achieve an oxygen saturation above 92%, even when a very large alveolar-to-arterial (A-a) gradient is present, indicating incipient respiratory failure. The chest radiograph also is a critical assessment tool that may demonstrate abnormalities such as tension pneumothorax, diffuse alveolar infiltrates, lobar atelectasis, or large effusions.

5. **How do you calculate the A-a gradient?**
The alveolar-to-arterial oxygen gradient is calculated based on the measured PaO_2 and $PaCO_2$ and the alveolar PO_2 (PAO_2), which is calculated from FiO_2. The A-a gradient is calculated using the alveolar gas equation, as follows:

A-a gradient = $PAO_2 - PaO_2 - 1.25(PaCO_2)$

A-a gradient = $[FiO_2$ (atmospheric pressure − water pressure)$] − PaO_2 − 1.25(PaCO_2)$
At sea level, atmospheric pressure is 760 mmHg, so
$$PAO_2 = FiO_2 (760 − 47)$$
For room air with an FiO_2 of 0.21,
$$PAO_2 = 0.21 \times 713 = 150$$
$$\text{A-a gradient} = 150 − PaO_2 − 1.25(PaCO_2)$$
The A-a oxygen gradient normally is 8–15 mmHg, but it increases with age because the PaO_2 decreases with age as V/Q mismatch gradually increases.

6. **Name the five mechanisms of hypoxemia.**
   1. **Shunt:** This occurs when areas of lung are perfused, but not ventilated, leading to hypoxemia that does not correct with increasing FiO_2. Shunt can be anatomic, as seen with an arterio-venous malformation, or physiologic, as occurs with alveolar flooding or collapse in acute lung injury. Shunt does not correct with 100% FiO_2 because the alveoli do not participate in gas exchange. The lesion opposite of shunt is dead space, or alveoli that are ventilated but not perfused, which occurs in pulmonary emboli. However, dead space does not cause hypoxemia because the blood does not flow to these regions. In clinical situations, some-times the "venous admixture" is calculated. In this estimation, one calculates the fraction of shunt that would account for the size of the A-a gradient *if* all the hypoxemia were due to shunt physiology.
   2. **V/Q mismatch:** The normal lung has alveoli that exist at a range of V/Q ratios. V/Q mismatch refers to hypoxemias resulting from an abnormal extent of V/Q mismatching. Two types of mismatches coexist: (1) alveoli that are normally ventilated but poorly perfused (i.e., high V/Q units), and (2) alveolar areas that are normally perfused but poorly ventilated (i.e., low V/Q units). The extreme of the former units is dead space, whereas the extreme of the latter is shunt. Low V/Q units contribute much more to hypoxemia. This type of hypoxemia usually improves relatively easily with supplemental oxygen because a small change in FiO_2 leads to a big increase in the PAO_2 in the poorly ventilated alveoli, significantly increasing oxygenation of the red blood cells traveling past these alveoli.
   3. **Diffusion block:** This is an uncommon cause of hypoxemia that results from marked thickening of the interstitial tissue between the alveolar space and the capillary. In the past, this mechanism was believed to operate in patients with interstitial lung disease. However, recently, capillary destruction has been recognized as probably being more important as a cause of hypoxemia in these diseases. Diffusion block may cause hypoxemia when patients with interstitial disease exercise, when the time that red blood cells spend in the capillaries decreases to the point at which there is incomplete equilibration with PAO_2. Among pulmonary function tests, the diffusing capacity for carbon monoxide (DLCO) measures the overall functional alveolar–capillary surface area, and the measurement incorporates problems in diffusion, loss of capillaries, and incomplete equilibration.
   4. **Low FiO_2:** At high altitudes at which FiO_2 is less than 21%, low FiO_2 causes hypoxemia, as indicated in the alveolar gas equation.
   5. **Hypoventilation:** In a patient with normal lungs, a decrease in total and alveolar ventilation increases the $PACO_2$ while decreasing PAO_2, as predicted by the alveolar gas equation. This occurs in patients with decreased respiratory drive (as happens with narcotic overdoses), neuromuscular disease, or sleep apnea.

   Henig NR, Pierson DJ: Mechanisms of hypoxemia. Respir Care Clin North Am 6(4):501–521, 2000.

7. **Can the A-a gradient help to determine the mechanism of hypoxemia?**
   The A-a gradient may delineate the mechanism of hypoxemic ARF. For example, a normal A-a gradient indicates hypoventilation or low FiO_2, whereas an increased A-a gradient indicates shunt, V/Q mismatch, or decreased diffusing capacity as the mechanism. Because it helps deter-mine whether the lung parenchyma is functioning normally, this calculation is particularly useful

in patients with a drug overdose who hypoventilate but also may have components of chemical or bacterial aspiration pneumonia or atelectasis.

8. **What are the consequences of hypercapnia?**
   Hypercapnia may lead to the following:
   - Hypoxemia
   - Acidemia
   - Tachycardia
   - Decreased work of breathing as a consequence of hypoventilation
   - Decreased blood pressure (but the secondary release of systemic catecholamines counterbalances this tendency)
   - Changes in cerebral vascular autoregulation

   Hypercapnia causes cerebral vasodilation, which in turn increases cerebral CO_2 washout, thus reducing the effect of hypercapnia on the brain by lowering cerebral PCO_2 and cerebral acidosis. Some of these effects of hypercapnia always are present, whereas others are more variable. Some recent data suggest that there may be some beneficial effects of hypercapnia.

   Laffey JG, Kavanagh BP: Carbon dioxide and the critically ill—Too little of a good thing? Lancet 354(9186):1283–1286, 1999.

9. **What are the indications for endotracheal intubation or mechanical ventilation?**
   The decisions to initiate mechanical ventilation and to intubate a patient may be linked, or they may be independent. Endotracheal intubation is beneficial in patients with inadequate oxygenation or ventilation during conventional therapy, but also is indicated—even without mechanical ventilation—in some patients for upper airway obstruction, airway protection, or secretion management. Conversely, noninvasive ventilation sometimes is sufficient to allow mechanical ventilation without intubation (*see* Question 10).

   Often, the clinical judgment decision in choosing the time when intubation is necessary is difficult. In some patients who are rapidly deteriorating or who are tiring out and do not have prospects for a rapid reversal and improvement, intubation should be done early and under controlled circumstances. Patients who are slowly deteriorating or who are likely to rapidly improve with the initiation of therapy (i.e., those with acute congestive heart failure or untreated asthma) sometimes may be carefully observed and repeatedly assessed before the decision to intubate is made. Most patients who cannot maintain oxygenation (i.e., with PaO_2 < 60 mmHg and FiO_2 ≥50%) or ventilation (i.e., with a rising $PaCO_2$ with worsening acidemia) should be seriously considered for intubation.

   Other clues suggesting the need for intubation include fatigue from increased work of breathing, manifested by increased respiratory rate, heart rate, and paradoxical or dyskinetic motion of the abdominal muscles. Airway protection also may be needed for a patient who is somnolent or lethargic or at high risk of aspiration. Examples include patients with neurologic disorders, hepatic encephalopathy, or drug overdoses, as well as some individuals undergoing upper gastrointestinal (GI) endoscopy or lavage with a large-bore gastric tube. Careful serial assessment of the gag reflex is important. Rarely, patients may need intubation for secretion management because they are unable to clear increased secretions caused by an acute bronchitis or pneumonia superimposed on severe chronic lung disease or neuromuscular disease.

10. **When is noninvasive ventilation reasonable to consider?**
    Noninvasive ventilation (NIV) refers to positive-pressure mechanical ventilation using a face or nasal mask, which sometimes may avoid or delay the need for endotracheal intubation. Several modalities can be utilized noninvasively, including continuous positive airway pressure (CPAP), bilevel positive airway pressure (bilevel-PAP), pressure-support ventilation (PSV), and pressure-control ventilation (PCV). CPAP provides positive pressure throughout the respiratory cycle and thus helps in avoiding atelectasis and maintaining airway and alveolar recruitment.

A tightly fitting face or nasal mask is required to maintain positive end-expiratory pressure (PEEP). Bilevel-PAP allows independent setting of the inspiratory and expiratory pressures, and the inspiratory pressure may be triggered to augment the patient's spontaneous inspiration, or it may work independently. PSV assists the patient's spontaneous inspiratory efforts without necessarily imposing PEEP and is more comfortable for some patients. PCV is similar to PSV in supporting only inspiration but does not require patient triggering or effort.

The advantages of NIV include avoidance of endotracheal intubation and its complications, patient comfort, and preservation of speech and swallowing when nasal ventilation is used. The principal disadvantages of NIV include the difficulty some patients have in keeping on a tight-fitting device and, with a face mask, the inability to talk, eat, or swallow, as well as the risk of aspiration due to vomiting with increased air in the stomach.

Contraindications to the use of NIV include an inability to swallow, large amounts of secretions, claustrophobia, vomiting, and the inability to remove the mask if necessary. In general, nasal mask NIV is better tolerated than a full face mask, but nasal NIV is difficult to use at high inspiratory pressures.

11. Can noninvasive ventilation prevent endotracheal intubation?

Noninvasive ventilation can be used continuously in the tenuous patient or, intermittently, for short- or long-term therapy. Recent studies have demonstrated that NIV reduces the need for intubation in patients with ARF of various etiologies. It also may shorten the length of hospital stays and the in-hospital mortality in patients with COPD and severe cardiogenic pulmonary edema. Much of this benefit probably results from a decreased incidence of nosocomial pneumonia. Intermittent chronic use of these modes also provides respiratory muscle rest, which may avoid gradual deterioration and worsening chronic respiratory failure in patients with neuromuscular diseases.

Brochard L: Noninvasive ventilation for acute respiratory failure. JAMA 288(8):932–935, 2002.

Keenan SP, Sinuff T, Cook DJ, Hill NS: Does noninvasive positive pressure ventilation improve outcome in acute hypoxemic respiratory failure? A systematic review. [Review] Critical Care Medicine. 32(12):2516–2523, 2004.

Liesching T, Kwok H, Hill NS: Acute applications of noninvasive positive pressure ventilation. Chest 124(2):699–713, 2003.

Lightowler JV, Wedzicha JA, Elliott MW, Ram FS: Noninvasive positive pressure ventilation to treat respiratory failure resulting from exacerbations of chronic obstructive pulmonary disease: Cochrane systematic review and meta-analysis. BMJ 326(7382):185, 2003.

Schortgen F, Lefort Y, Antonelli M, et al: Treatment of acute hypoxemic nonhypercapnic respiratory insufficiency with continuous positive airway pressure delivered by a face mask: A randomized controlled trial. JAMA 284(18):2352–2360, 2000.

Sinuff T, Cook DJ, Randall J, Allen CJ: Evaluation of a practice guideline for noninvasive positive-pressure ventilation for acute respiratory failure. Chest 123(6):2062–2073, 2003.

12. What other therapies exist for ARF?

Treatment of ARF is a combination of supportive care and treating the specific cause of the ARF. Thus, the clinician should use antibiotics for pneumonia, diuretics and vasodilators for pulmonary edema, or bronchodilators and glucocorticoids for obstructive lung disease.

In addition, supplemental oxygen therapy, support of blood pressure, correction of electrolyte abnormalities, adequate nutrition, and prophylaxis for deep venous thrombosis are strongly encouraged. Other intensive care unit (ICU) measures include maintaining elevation of the head of the bed unless specifically contraindicated since this reduces the risk of aspiration and nosocomial pneumonia.

Practically speaking, it is very important to have detailed information about a patient's prior pulmonary status. In particular, baseline ABG measurements are helpful in determining the best possible $PaCO_2$ to expect when the patient's pulmonary function has completely improved. A common mistake in ventilated patients is overventilation so that their $PaCO_2$

is "normal" but is at a level that is significantly lower than their baseline chronic hypercapnia. Their kidneys then excrete bicarbonate, and, when weaning starts and the PaCO$_2$ rises because of limited optimal lung function, respiratory acidosis occurs. Similarly, in patients with chronic lung disease, prior pulmonary function testing data is helpful as it can suggest whether a specific patient is likely to meet the standard weaning criteria or whether a trial of extubation may be appropriate even if the patient does not meet the standard criteria.

Glucocorticoids benefit some specific, rare causes of ARF such as acute eosinophilic pneumonia. There has been recent interest in the use of steroids for persistent inflammation in the fibroproliferative phase of acute respiratory distress syndrome (ARDS). Although there is no benefit in early ARDS, the use of steroids given in the late fibroproliferative phase has been controversial. In one small study, patients given steroids during this time period had a better survival when compared to those given placebo (87% overall mortality vs. 37%), but this finding has not been confirmed in a large multicenter trial.

Helium–oxygen gas mixtures can improve ventilation in some patients with turbulent airflow due to airway obstruction. The density of helium is significantly less than that of nitrogen, and, consequently, the flow is greater in situations in which there is nonlinear flow. Initially, this therapy was used for upper airway obstruction, and then its use spread to patients with severe asthma exacerbations. More recently, it is being studied for use in patients with COPD and early status asthmaticus.

Nebulized prostacyclin or inhaled nitric oxide serve as local lung vasodilators that augment pulmonary blood flow to the ventilated alveoli receiving the gas. This can increase oxygenation by improving matching of lung perfusion with ventilation. Inhaled nitric oxide can significantly improve gas exchange in some patients, but it has not led to group survival advantage in ARDS or other adult lung diseases. Nitric oxide is relatively expensive, and there can be rebound worsening upon its withdrawal. Careful, controlled studies have not yet been done with prostacyclin.

Arnal JM, Jean P: Use of heliox in patients with severe exacerbation of chronic obstructive pulmonary disease. Crit Care Med 29(12):2322–2324, 2001.

Jantz MA, Sahn SA: Corticosteroids in acute respiratory failure. Am J Respir Crit Care Med 160:1079–1100, 1999.

Peigang Y, Marini JJ: Ventilation of patients with asthma and chronic obstructive pulmonary disease. Curr Opin Crit Care 8(1):70–76, 2002.

13. **Why are perioperative patients at risk for respiratory failure?**
    Patients in the perioperative period are susceptible to atelectasis, infection, and blood clotting, each of which can lead to ARF. Factors predisposing to the development of postoperative atelectasis include obesity, supine positioning, upper abdominal incision, ascites/peritonitis, airway secretions, fluid overload, and anesthesia. The chest radiograph is helpful in deciding how

KEY POINTS: MONITORING OF GAS EXCHANGE

1. A normal A-a gradient in a hypoxemic patient usually indicates that the lungs themselves are working normally and that the patient has a problem with ventilatory drive or neuromuscular respiratory muscle pump function.

2. Venous blood gas values are impossible to interpret if they are not drawn from a central mixed venous site.

3. A rising mixed venous oxygen saturation is not necessarily a sign of improvement; often, it is caused by worsening sepsis with shunting of peripheral blood flow past tissue beds.

aggressively to treat atelectases (i.e., in determining whether a bronchoscopy is necessary). If air bronchograms are present on the radiograph, then bronchoscopy usually is not beneficial because the proximal airways are patent and the patient normally can be managed with bronchodilators, aggressive chest physiotherapy, mobilization, and frequent suctioning. In contrast, if air bronchograms are absent, then bronchoscopy may be helpful in diagnosing and treating an obstructing plug or copious secretions in the airways if respiratory care maneuvers are not sufficient.

Marini JJ, Pierson DJ, Hudson LD: Acute lobar atelectasis: A prospective comparison of fiberoptic bronchoscopy and respiratory therapy. Am Rev Respir Dis 119:971–978, 1979.

Overend TJ, Anderson CM, Lucy S, et al: The effect of incentive spirometry on postoperative pulmonary complications: A systematic review. Chest 120(3):971–978, 2001.

14. **What systemic complications often develop in patients with acute respiratory failure?**
See Table 62-1. In addition to systemic complications, there are many potential complications related to the presence of an endotracheal tube and positive pressure ventilation, such as barotrauma, endotracheal tube problems, tracheal stenosis or dilatation, nosocomial sinusitis or otitis, self-extubation, and laryngeal trauma.

15. **What should be done routinely to prevent these complications of ARF?**
It is important to carefully monitor the patient with ARF. Symptoms and physical exam should be assessed at least every day. In patients who are sedated and paralyzed, sedatives and paralytics should be stopped daily if possible to assess the patient's neurologic status, pain in different regions, and level of sedation. This reduces oversedation and shortens ICU stay and cost. Blood pressure must be optimized to maintain adequate perfusion of end-organs, and vasopressors should be used if blood pressure cannot be maintained with intravenous fluid administration alone. Renal function should be kept optimal with fluids or diuretics. Since patients with ARF are at risk for cardiac complications, the cardiac rhythm should be monitored continuously. In addition, routine laboratory tests should be obtained daily until the patient's condition is stabilized. These tests include electrolyte, blood urea nitrogen and creatinine, liver function, hemoglobin, white blood cell count, and platelets (as heparin-associated thrombocytopenia is often seen even with the use of heparin flushes alone). Cultures of blood, sputum, and urine, along with any cultures of other drainage sites, should be obtained if the patient develops a fever. For intubated or critically ill patients, a daily chest radiograph is useful in looking for worsening pulmonary status.

Ventilated patients should have daily assessment of their secretions and measurement of the airway peak and static pressures, the presence of auto-PEEP, the minute ventilation, and the actual respiratory rate and achieved tidal volume. In some institutions, more complete respiratory parameters, including peak negative inspiratory pressure and spontaneous respiratory rate, tidal volume, and vital capacity, are assessed daily in patients who are not paralyzed. The endotracheal tube cuff pressure should also be checked at least daily to help avoid high pressures that can cause tracheomalacia or late tracheal stenosis.

Some specific preventive measures include routine use of prophylaxis for deep venous thrombosis and stress GI bleeding; daily measurement of endotracheal cuff pressure; daily assessment of endotracheal tube positioning; provision of adequate nutrition, beginning early in the ICU stay; adequate sedation or restraint, if necessary; ensuring adequate sleep in a day–night cycle; and physical therapy.

16. **List the advanced modes of ventilation.**
Recent advances in ventilator therapy have provided additional options in the management of critically ill patients with ARF who are difficult to ventilate or oxygenate. These include the following:
- PCV
- Inverse ratio ventilation (IRV)

TABLE 62-1. SYSTEMIC COMPLICATIONS OF ACUTE RESPIRATORY FAILURE

Cardiopulmonary

Deep venous thrombosis

Pulmonary emboli

Myocardial ischemia

Cardiac arrhythmias

Nosocomial pneumonia

Atelectasis

Neuromuscular

Delirium

Stupor and coma

"Intensive care unit psychosis"

Critical illness polyneuropathy

Contractures

Muscle weakness

Infectious

Line sepsis

Abscesses

Nosocomial pneumonia

Decubitus ulceration

Other infections (e.g., urinary tract infection)

Gastrointestinal

Acute gastric ulceration or inflammation with hemorrhage

Malnutrition

Complications of enteral and parenteral nutrition

Acalculous cholecystitis

Drug-associated hepatic dysfunction

Renal

Acute renal failure (due to hypoperfusion, acute tubular necrosis, or nephrotoxic drugs)

Hypomagnesemia

Hypophosphatemia

Electrolyte disorders

- Proportional-assist ventilation (PAV)
- Airway pressure release ventilation (APRV)
- High-frequency ventilation (HFV)
- Split lung ventilation

- Permissive hypercapnia
- Lung-protective strategy

17. **What is the most commonly used new advanced mode of ventilation?**

PCV. In this mode, the clinician sets an inspiratory pressure and the inspiratory time or fraction (i.e., the percent of the cycle length), and the set pressure is maintained without guaranteeing a delivered tidal volume. The actual tidal volume delivered is primarily a function of the lung compliance and, consequently, may change with altered lung compliance (caused by a mucus plug, pneumothorax, or pulmonary edema). PCV may be set to have a higher mean intrathoracic pressure than conventional volume ventilatory modes, increasing the functional residual capacity and keeping more alveoli open. It also provides greater inspiratory flow during early inspiration, which may aid in popping open more alveoli and allowing better distribution of the inspired gas over the time of inspiration. Consequently, PCV may help patients with inhomogeneous lung disease or acute lung injury.

The major disadvantage of PCV is the lack of a guaranteed tidal volume. Newer ventilators offer this backup option and also have sensitive triggering of PCV breaths by patient inspiration. It is very important that the personnel managing the patient understand that with tension pneumothorax, the airway pressure does not increase in PCV—instead, there is a drop in tidal volume—and that decreases in tidal volume should prompt rapid assessment by chest radiograph.

18. **What is IRV?**

IRV refers to mechanical ventilation in which the inspiratory-to-expiratory (I:E) ratio is reversed to > 1. This allows a longer time at higher intrathoracic pressure for alveoli to fill with oxygen and less time during expiration for alveoli to collapse. IRV may be beneficial in patients with acute lung injury who are difficult to oxygenate with conventional mechanical ventilation. It also may help patients with heterogeneous lung disease. Possible consequences of IRV include hypotension from the increased mean intrathoracic pressure and increased auto-PEEP and hypercapnia from the decreased expiratory time. IRV is not a comfortable mode of ventilation and usually requires that the patient be paralyzed or heavily sedated.

19. **Explain PAV.**

PAV is a recent experimental mode that is used only in spontaneously breathing patients. PAV is designed to optimize the relationship between patient effort and ventilator response by adjusting inspiratory pressure to patient effort. This allows the patient to better control his or her breathing pattern and minute ventilation. PAV provides greater patient comfort, lower peak airway pressures, and improved control over respiratory pattern.

20. **How does APRV work?**

APRV is being used primarily for patients with ARDS. Patients breathe spontaneously while being maintained at a relatively high intrathoracic pressure, allowing oxygenation, followed by the intrathoracic pressure being released to allow CO_2 excretion. Although this mode of ventilation is feasible in ARDS patients, in series of patients studied to date, it does not clearly augment survival. There may be major benefits in selected individuals, but the method of selecting these specific patients is not known.

21. **What is HFV?**

HFV uses very small tidal volumes with high respiratory rates and is available in multiple variants with different respiratory frequencies and delivery mechanisms. Minute ventilation is maintained by using very high rates. Some patients may benefit from improved healing of bronchopleural fistulas or more uniform distribution of ventilation, leading to improved gas exchange. However, in large randomized series of patients with ARF, HFV has not demonstrated any benefit over other modes of ventilation, and barotrauma still occurs. The theoretical benefit of a lower risk of barotrauma with smaller tidal volumes has not been clinically substantiated, possibly because the alveolar pressure may be much higher than the measured proximal airway pressure.

22. **How is split lung ventilation accomplished?**
Split lung ventilation refers to differential ventilation of the lungs accomplished by blocking one main bronchus while ventilating the other lung, Alternately, with a double lumen endotracheal tube, split lung ventilation allows each lung to be ventilated and inspected separately. This approach may be useful in the setting of unilateral massive hemoptysis, a large bronchopleural fistula, or radically unequal degrees of lung injury.

23. **What other modes of advanced ventilation might sometimes be warranted?**
In some patients with very high airway resistance (e.g., asthma) or a high risk of ventilator-induced lung injury, the clinician accepts the trade-off of a higher $PaCO_2$ than normal in return for decreasing the risk of barotraumas incurred by trying to normalize the $PaCO_2$. This "strategy" is termed permissive hypercapnia. It has been applied in patients with asthma and, more recently, in those with ARDS. Patients generally tolerate hypercapnia and the potential respiratory acidosis fairly well, although clinicians typically become nervous when the arterial pH is below 7.25. It remains unclear whether there are subtle positive or negative effects of hypercapnia or respiratory acidosis in these conditions. In patients with neurosurgical trauma, hypercapnia should be avoided due to the cerebral vasodilatation that results.

In mechanical ventilation of patients with ARDS, there have been conflicting studies about the benefit of using a "lung protective strategy." Typically, this strategy has included relatively high PEEP levels, relatively small tidal volumes, and avoidance of airway pressures above 35 cmH$_2$O. In the multicenter NIH-sponsored ARDS Network study, which utilized a 6 mL/kg ideal body weight in the low tidal volume group, the relative mortality was reduced by 25% in spite of worse oxygenation over the first several days. There remains some debate about what constitutes the optimal "low tidal volume" and the relative importance of the tidal volumes and the airway pressure limitation. It also is unclear whether most ventilator-induced lung damage is incurred from overdistention of relatively compliant alveoli or is from the sheer stress of frequent opening and closing of surfactant-depleted alveoli during the respiratory cycle.

Artigas A, Bernard GR, Carlet J, et al: The American-European Consensus Conference on ARDS. Part 2: Ventilatory, pharmacologic, supportive therapy, study design strategies, and issues related to recovery and remodeling. Acute respiratory distress syndrome. Am J Respir Crit Care Med 157(4 Pt 1):1332–1347, 1998.

Brower RG, Rubenfeld GD: Lung-protective ventilation strategies in acute lung injury. Crit Care Med 31(4 Suppl):S312–S316, 2003.

Delclaux C, L'Her E, Alberti C, et al: High-frequency oscillatory ventilation for acute respiratory distress syndrome in adult patients. Crit Care Med 31(4 Suppl):S317–323, 2003.

Hickling KG: Permissive hypercapnia. Respir Care Clin North Am 8(2):155–169, 2002.

Marcy TW, Marini JJ: Inverse ratio ventilation in ARDS: Rationale and implementation. Chest 100:494–504, 1991.

Messerole E, Peine P, Wittkopp S, et al: The pragmatics of prone positioning. Am J Respir Crit Care Med 165(10):1359–1363, 2002.

Navalesi P, Costa R: New modes of mechanical ventilation: proportional assist ventilation, neurally adjusted ventilatory assist, and fractal ventilation. Curr Opin Crit Care 9(1):51–58, 2003.

CHAPTER 63

ACUTE RESPIRATORY DISTRESS SYNDROME

Ellen L. Burnham, MD, and Marc Moss, MD

1. **What is acute respiratory distress syndrome (ARDS)?**
   ARDS is a unique form of acute lung injury that occurs with a variety of diagnoses, including sepsis, trauma, and the aspiration of gastric contents. Pathologically, ARDS is characterized by a nonspecific pattern of diffuse alveolar damage in association with a proteinaceous alveolar edema. Because the left ventricular filling pressure is not elevated in ARDS, this syndrome is sometimes identified as noncardiogenic pulmonary edema.

   Ware LB, Matthay MA: The acute respiratory distress syndrome. New Eng J Med 342:1334–1349, 2000.

2. **Describe the postulated pathogenesis of ARDS.**
   Investigators have artificially divided the pathogenesis of ARDS into three phases: initiation, amplification, and injury. During initiation, the precipitating event, such as sepsis, triggers a general inflammatory response involving endotoxin, tumor necrosis factor, interleukin-1, and other cytokines. Subsequently, during amplification, effector cells such as neutrophils are recruited, activated, and retained in the endothelial cell bed of the lung, from which they migrate into the pulmonary parenchyma. Finally, during injury, these effector cells release harmful substances, such as superoxide anion and hydrogen peroxide, that damage the surrounding lung tissue.

KEY POINTS: AMERICAN–EUROPEAN CONSENSUS CONFERENCE DEFINITION OF ARDS

1. Acute onset of illness

2. PaO_2-to-FiO_2 ratio of 200 (regardless of positive end-expiratory pressure)

3. Bilateral infiltrates seen on frontal chest radiograph

4. Pulmonary artery wedge pressure of 18 mmHg or less when measured, or no clinical evidence of left atrial hypertension

3. **What is the difference between ARDS and acute lung injury (ALI)?**
   In 1994, the American–European Consensus Conference on ARDS established uniform definitions for ARDS and ALI. ALI is a mild form of lung injury with the same pathogenesis as ARDS. The criteria for ALI are the same as those for ARDS except that the PaO_2-to-FiO_2 ratio is 300 or less (i.e., ALI has less-severe hypoxemia).

   Bernard GR, Artigas A, Brigham KL, et al: Report of the American-European Consensus Conference on Acute Respiratory Distress Syndrome: Definitions, mechanisms, relevant outcomes, and clinical trial coordination. Am J Respir Crit Care Med 151:818–824, 1994.

4. **How common is ARDS?**
   Several authors have reported on the incidence of ALI and ARDS. These studies estimate the incidence of ALI to be 20–50 cases per 100,000 person-years, with 18–25% of these cases

meeting criteria for ALI but not for ARDS. The variation in results probably reflects differences in the methodologies used to calculate the incidence. Utilizing data from the screening logs of the Acute Respiratory Distress Syndrome Network (ARDSnet) and data from the American Hospital Association, the annual incidence of ALI in the United States is between 17.3 and 64.2 per 100,000 inhabitants per year.

Frutos-Vivar F, Nicolas N, Estaban A: Epidemiology of acute lung injury and acute respiratory distress syndrome. Curr Op Crit Care 10:1–6, 2004.

Goss CH, Brower RG, Hudson LD, et al: Incidence of acute lung injury in the United States. Crit Care Med 31:1607–1611, 2003.

5. **Give examples of direct and indirect lung injuries that can predispose a patient to develop ARDS.**
   Direct lung injury resulting in ARDS is caused by factors insulting the lungs through the airway; indirect lung injury causing ARDS affects the lungs through the release of mediators into the bloodstream from an extrapulmonary focus of inflammation (Table 63-1).

TABLE 63-1.　DIRECT VERSUS INDIRECT LUNG INJURY	
Direct Lung Injury	**Indirect Lung Injury**
Pneumonia	Sepsis
Aspiration	Severe trauma with multiple fractures
Pulmonary contusion	Drug overdose
Reperfusion injury	Cardiopulmonary bypass
Near-drowning	Burns
Fat emboli	Pancreatitis

6. **Describe the computed tomography (CT) scan appearance of the lungs in a patient with ARDS.**
   Despite diffuse infiltrates on plain chest radiographs, CT scanning reveals patchy areas of dense infiltrates and areas of normal-appearing lung tissue. Posterior and gravitationally dependent areas of the lung are more infiltrated than nondependent areas (Fig. 63-1). With the addition of positive end-expiratory pressure (PEEP), a portion of the consolidated lung parenchyma can be recruited for gas exchange. In ARDS secondary to indirect lung injury, infiltrates are typically more diffuse and uniform, whereas in indirect lung injury, the CT infiltrate pattern may be more asymmetric.

7. **Which diagnoses are more likely to be associated with ARDS development?**
   The incidence of ARDS has been consistently highest in patients with sepsis (40%), trauma (10–34%), and aspiration (10–36%). In addition, it has been reported that chronic alcohol abuse increases the risk of ARDS in patients with an at-risk diagnosis.

Moss M, Bucher B, Moore FA, et al: The role of chronic alcohol abuse in the development of acute respiratory distress syndrome in adults. JAMA 275:50–54, 1996.

8. **How quickly do patients develop ARDS?**
   Most patients develop ARDS within 5 days of their acute event. For patients with sepsis, the onset of ARDS is rapid: more than 50% develop ARDS within a 24-hour period. For trauma patients, ARDS develops slightly more slowly: less than 33% develop ARDS within 24 hours. This may be due in part to the ability to pinpoint the exact time of a traumatic incident relative to

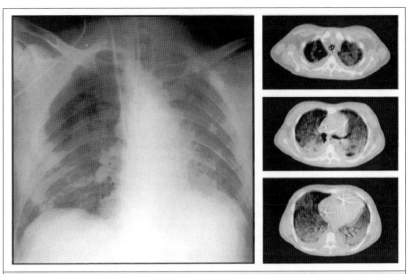

Figure 63-1. Anteroposterior chest x-ray and CT scans (at the apex, hilum, and base) in ARDS from sepsis. Images were taken at 5 cmH$_2$O end-expiratory pressure. The chest x-ray shows diffuse ground-glass opacification, sparing the right upper lung. The CT scans show inhomogeneous disease and both the craniocaudal and sternovertebral gradients. (Adapted from Gattinoni L, Caironi P, Pelosi P, Goodman LR: What has computed tomography taught us about the acute respiratory distress syndrome? Am J Respir Crit Care Med 164:1701–1711, 2001.)

the development of ARDS. In contrast, patients may have been septic for several days before seeking medical attention.

9. **What is the optimal mode of mechanical ventilation for patients with ARDS?**
   The primary goal of mechanical ventilation in patients with ARDS is to achieve ventilation and oxygenation that will adequately support all organ systems. Based on evidence that large tidal volumes and high airway pressures produce barotrauma to the lung both macroscopically (e.g., pneumothorax) and microscopically (e.g., alveolar edema), strategies in mechanical ventilation have been redirected. Protective ventilation strategies have been examined with the goal of decreased barotrauma and reduced alveolar collapse. A landmark study by the ARDSnet investigators reported

KEY POINTS: STANDARD VENTILATOR SETTINGS FOR PATIENTS WITH ARDS

1. Set tidal volume at 6 cc/kg of ideal body weight.

2. Limit plateau pressures to 30 cmH$_2$O.

3. Set respiratory rate to maintain an acceptable pH (with a goal of 7.25 and greater), but a higher partial pressure of carbon dioxide (pCO$_2$) may be tolerated (i.e., permissive hypercapnia).

4. Give additional PEEP as necessary to wean FiO$_2$ (with a goal of 60%), but there is no optimal value.

a significant decrease in hospital mortality (i.e., a 9% absolute decrease) when patients with ARDS were ventilated with lower tidal volumes, compared to traditional ventilation.

Brower RG, Matthay MA, Morris A, et al: Ventilation with lower tidal volumes as compared with traditional tidal volumes for acute lung injury and the acute respiratory distress syndrome. N Engl J Med 342:1301–1308, 2000.

10. **What is the optimal level of PEEP for patients with ARDS?**
In a recent multicenter trial, the effect of higher PEEP (mean = 13.2 ± 3.5 cmH$_2$O) versus lower PEEP (mean = 8.3 ± 3.2 cmH$_2$O), combined with the lower tidal volume ventilation strategy, did not appear to impact mortality or the number of ventilator-free days. Although it did not appear to affect mortality, the use of PEEP is still warranted in those situations in which it is difficult to oxygenate a patient despite the administration of high levels of supplemental oxygen.

Brower RG, Lanken PN, MacIntyre N, et al: Higher versus lower positive end-expiratory pressures in patients with the acute respiratory distress syndrome. N Eng J Med 351:327–336, 2004.

11. **Is there any proven therapy for ARDS?**
Although a variety of therapeutic modalities have been tested in patients at risk for ARDS and in those with documented ARDS, there is presently no standard medical treatment for ARDS. Ketoconazole and lisofylline have been the therapies most recently examined in well-designed prospective randomized clinical trials. Both trials were stopped early due to lack of efficacy. A recent multicenter randomized placebo-controlled trial revealed that inhaled nitric oxide in patients with ALI resulted in short-term oxygenation improvements but had no substantial impact on the duration of ventilatory support or mortality. To promote better outcomes, it is important in ARDS patients to provide care that has been proven to prevent complications, such as deep venous thrombosis and ulcer prophylaxis, as well as ensuring appropriate antimicrobial coverage.

Taylor RW, Zimmerman JL, Dellinger RP, et al: Low dose inhaled nitric oxide in patients with acute lung injury: A randomized controlled trail. JAMA 291:1603–1609, 2004.

12. **What is the mortality rate of patients with ARDS?**
The mortality rate for patients with ARDS varies between 30% and 50%. Recently, the ARDS network study of ventilatory strategies reported a further decline in ARDS mortality to 31% by utilizing a low tidal volume ventilation strategy. Additionally, the mortality of patients with ARDS appears to be increased in the elderly and in those with cirrhosis.

Ely EW, Wheeler AW, Thompson BT, et al: Recovery rate and prognosis in older persons who develop acute lung injury and the acute respiratory distress syndrome. Ann Int Med 136(1):25–36, 2002.

Milberg JA, Davis DR, Steinberg KP, Hudson LD: Improved survival of patients with acute respiratory distress syndrome (ARDS): 1983–1993. JAMA 273:306–309, 1995.

13. **What are the causes of death in patients with ARDS?**
Classically, the causes of mortality in patients with ARDS have been divided into early causes (within 72 hours) and late causes (after 72 hours). The original presenting illness or injury causes the majority of early deaths. Late deaths were most commonly caused by sepsis syndrome (36%) and cardiac dysfunction (23%). Irreversible respiratory failure was responsible for only 16% of late deaths. However, more recent studies have reported that irreversible respiratory failure is becoming a more common cause of late mortality in patients with ARDS and can account for up to 40% of all deaths.

Luhr LR, Antonsen K, Karlsson M, et al: Incidence and mortality after acute respiratory failure and acute respiratory distress syndrome in Sweden, Denmark, and Iceland. Am J Respir Crit Care Med 159:1849–1861, 1999.

14. **Do ARDS survivors have long-term sequelae from their illness?**
In a prospective cohort study, there was no difference in long-term mortality between ARDS survivors and matched controls. However, ARDS survivors have a significantly reduced quality

of life when compared to critically ill patients who had an equivalent severity of illness. The largest impairment is in physical function and pulmonary symptoms and limitations. Survivors of ARDS have a persistent functional disability as much as 1 year after discharge that is largely related to extrapulmonary conditions such as muscle wasting and weakness.

Davidson TA, Caldwell ES, Curtis JR, et al: Reduced quality of life in survivors of acute respiratory distress syndrome compared with critically ill control patients. JAMA 281:354–360, 1999.

Herridge MS, Cheung AM, Tansey CM, et al: One-year outcomes in survivors of the acute respiratory distress syndrome. N Eng J Med 348:683–693, 2003.

15. **How long does it take for pulmonary function to normalize in ARDS survivors?**
Decreased diffusing capacity and restrictive defects are the most commonly observed pulmonary function testing (PFT) abnormalities. The majority of improvements in PFTs occur in the first 3 months after extubation. However, PFTs have been reported to be abnormal in 50% of patients at 6 months after extubation and in 25% of patients at 1 year. The best predictors of persistently abnormal PFT results are increased FiO_2, higher levels of PEEP, and decreased static pulmonary compliance during the acute clinical course of ARDS.

16. **Does the inflammatory cascade postulated to cause ARDS produce injury to other organs?**
ARDS must be viewed as the pulmonary expression of a systemic disease. The inflammatory cascade and effector cells that are postulated to be involved in the pathogenesis of ARDS also affect other organ systems. Clinically, in acutely ill patients, a pattern of progressive organ dysfunction called the multiple-organ dysfunction syndrome (MODS) has been described. The other organ systems commonly affected in MODS include the renal, hepatic, cardiovascular, hematologic, and central nervous systems.

17. **What prognostic markers are available in ARDS?**
Many markers in plasma and bronchoalveolar lavage (BAL) have been examined for their efficacy in predicting outcomes in ARDS, typically in small cohorts of patients. Variables independently associated with mortality are qualitative or are not specific for pulmonary pathophysiology. Some examples of these include sepsis as a risk factor, multiorgan failure, age, and cirrhosis. Most recently, elevation of the ratio of dead space to total space (V_D/V_T) measured in the early phase of ARDS has been shown to correlate with mortality in a prospective clinical trial. Although this is cumbersome to measure, it is the most pulmonary-specific marker of outcomes to date.

Nuckton TJ, Alonso JA, Kallet RH, et al: Pulmonary dead-space fraction as a risk factor for death in the acute respiratory distress syndrome. N Eng J Med 346:1281–1286, 2002.

18. **When should steroids be used in the treatment of ARDS?**
Well-designed randomized prospective multicenter trials have shown no benefit from high-dose glucocorticoid administration in *early* ARDS. Later in the course of ARDS, collagen deposition occurs in the lung, which can rapidly progress to fibrosis, termed the *fibroproliferative phase* of ARDS (Fig. 63-2). One small randomized prospective study reported an improvement in mortality when glucocorticoids were given after 7 days of unresolving ARDS. A multicenter randomized controlled trial (the Late Steroid Rescue Study [LaSRS]) reported no clear mortality benefit in patients who received late corticosteroids. However, it may be beneficial to replace physiologic doses of steroids in critically ill individuals with ARDS who have relative adrenal insufficiency.

Meduri GU, Headley AS, Golden E, et al: Effect of prolonged methylprednisolone therapy in unresolving acute respiratory distress syndrome. JAMA 280:159–165, 1998.

19. **What is the proper fluid management in patients with ARDS?**
Endothelial cell damage in patients with ARDS results in an increase in the lung's microvascular permeability, with fluid flux across the capillary membrane related primarily to the hydrostatic

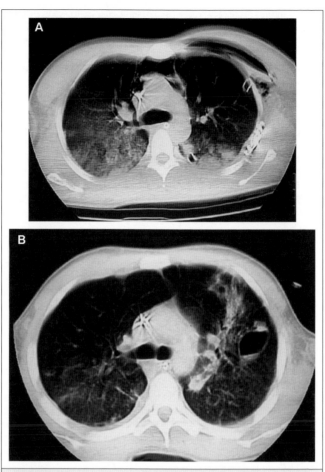

Figure 63-2. CT scans of a patient with ARDS due to multiple trauma. *A,* a CT scan through the carina 5 days after severe trauma, showing diffuse ground-glass opacification, greater on the right than the left. There is a nondependent-to-dependent gradient. Incidentally noted is pneumomediastinum and a chest tube draining a pneumothorax. *B,* 5 days later, ground-glass opacification has a more reticular pattern. There is now a pneumatocele in the left mid-lung and increasing atelectasis adjacent to it. (Adapted from Gattinoni L, Caironi P, Pelosi P, Goodman LR: What has computed tomography taught us about the acute respiratory distress syndrome? Am J Respir Crit Care Med 164:1701–1711, 2001.)

pressure. Elevations in the microvascular hydrostatic pressure lead to increases in extravascular lung water content, further pulmonary damage, and, potentially, a need for higher FiO_2. A reasonable strategy for patients with ARDS would be to reduce pulmonary microvascular hydrostatic pressure to minimize the accumulation of extravascular lung water, but this must be balanced with the need for adequate volume resuscitation to maintain oxygen delivery to other vital organs.

20. **Should pulmonary artery catheters be routinely placed in patients with ARDS?**
    Placement of a pulmonary artery catheter (PAC) to measure pulmonary capillary wedge pressure (PCWP) can be useful in patients with ARDS to assess volume status. However, two different studies demonstrate no survival benefit from the use of PACs in critically ill patients, including those with ARDS. An ongoing trial will help provide more information to answer this question. In general, one should utilize all information derived from a PAC (not just the PCWP) in a systematic fashion and perhaps should have a definite question in mind that the PAC could help answer prior to placement of this device in a patient with ARDS.

    Connors AF, Speroff T, Dawson NV, et al: The effectiveness of right heart catheterization in the initial care of critically ill patients. JAMA 276:889–897, 1996.

    Richard C, Warszawski J, Anguel N, et al: Early use of the pulmonary artery catheter and outcomes in patients with shock and acute respiratory distress syndrome: A randomized controlled trial. JAMA 290:2713–2720, 2003.

21. **Does prone positioning improve outcomes in patients with ARDS?**
    An improvement in oxygenation has been reported when patients with ARDS are turned from a supine to a prone position due to a more uniform gravitational distribution of pleural pressures and an improvement in ventilation/perfusion (V/Q) mismatching. Several recent clinical trials have demonstrated that patients with ARDS have a significant improvement in oxygenation in the prone position that may persist after returning to a supine position. None of the studies has proven a survival benefit, and the optimal duration of prone positioning remains unclear. Nevertheless, prone positioning may be useful in patients who are difficult to oxygenate with routine mechanical ventilatory techniques.

    Guerin C, Gaillard S, Lemasson S, et al: Effects of systematic prone positioning in hypoxemic acute respiratory failure: A randomized controlled trial. JAMA 292(19):2379–2387, 2004.

CHAPTER 64

AIRWAY MANAGEMENT

Mark P. Hamlin, MD, MS, and Mitchell H. Tsai, MD, MS

1. **What equipment should you have ready before you intubate a patient?**
   Remember the acronym **SOAP:**

   S = Suction: A suction source, placed by your right hand to allow immediate suctioning in case of gastric reflux into pharynx

   O = Oxygen: Oxygen source, with appropriate adaptors, bag, and mask attached

   A = Airway: A prestocked intubation box, containing, at a minimum,
   - Oral/nasal airways
   - Endotracheal tubes
   - A laryngoscope and blades (e.g., Miller and Macintosh blades)
   - Spare batteries (and, for older laryngoscopes, spare bulbs)
   - Stylets, lubricants, and topical anesthetics
   - An end-tidal carbon dioxide detector

   P = Pharmaceuticals and paralytics: IV access, induction agents, and neuromuscular blocking agents

2. **How should you evaluate the patient's airway?**
   Many classifications have been devised to predict the feasibility of intubation based upon a patient's physical characteristics. The Mallampati classification (Fig. 64-1) grades the visibility of posterior structures in the oropharynx during the opening of the mouth, with lower grades correlated with greater ease of placing an endotracheal tube. However, even patients with a Mallampati Class I or II airway can still be difficult to intubate.

   Mallampati SR, Gatt SP, Gugino LD, et al: A clinical sign to predict difficult tracheal intubation: A prospective study. Can J Anaesth 32:429–434, 1985.

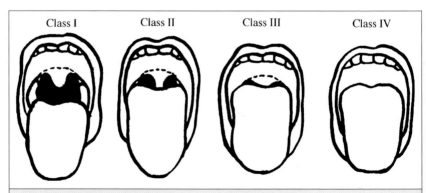

Figure 64-1. The Mallampati classification.

3. **What warning signs of a difficult airway may be found with a brief physical examination before intubation?**
    - **Short mandible:** A short mandible limits laryngoscope displacement of the tongue into the submandibular space. An inability to place three fingers laterally between the tip of the chin and the thyroid cartilage is concerning.
    - **Small mouth opening:** Ask the patient to open his or her mouth wide. The distance between the upper and lower teeth should be greater than three fingerbreadths. A small mouth opening may limit access and make it difficult to place airway equipment.
    - **Prominent incisors or overbite:** Ask the patient to bite his or her upper lip using his or her lower teeth. An inability to displace the lower jaw an adequate distance can interfere with laryngoscopy. Moreover, large incisors can physically obstruct the blade of the laryngoscope and the visualization of the vocal cords.
    - **Cervical spine immobility or instability:** A trauma patient in a cervical collar is the clearest example. Arthritis, osteoporosis, and ankylosing spondylitis are other well-known causes of limited mobility. Prior surgical history of cervical fusion may be unknown, but a linear paratracheal scar on the neck is suggestive. Beware of situations associated with cervical instability, including trisomy 21 syndrome (i.e., Down syndrome) and rheumatoid arthritis.
    - **History of a difficult intubation:** Examine the patient's chart carefully. If the patient has a past surgical history, the anesthesia record should provide concise, clear information about previous airway manipulation. Most anesthesiologists will document the laryngoscope blade type and size, the endotracheal tube size, and the degree of vocal cord visualization. If the patient has a known difficult airway and requires equipment outside the realm of your skills and practice, consult an anesthesiologist.

    Cormack RS, Lehane J: Difficult tracheal intubation in obstetrics. Anaesthesia 39:1105–1111, 1984.

KEY POINTS: WARNING SIGNS OF A POSSIBLY DIFFICULT INTUBATION

1. Short mandible

2. Small mouth opening

3. Prominent incisors or overbite

4. Cervical spine immobility or instability

5. History of a difficult intubation

4. **Describe bag mask ventilation.**
    The ability to ventilate a patient is the first step in the management of that patient's airway. Using your left hand, your third, fourth, and fifth fingers should be placed along the patient's left mandible. (Your fifth finger should be on the angle of the mandible, and your third finger should be at the mentum.) Your thumb and index fingers should be placed along the superior and inferior aspects of the face mask. *Lift* the mandible into the mask with your third, fourth, and fifth fingers, and ensure that the mask forms a seal with the patient's face using your thumb and index finger. The force applied by your thumb and index finger should directly oppose the force generated by your remaining three fingers. Simply pushing the mask down onto the face of the patient will displace the tongue posteriorly and will occlude the airway.

5. **You have difficulty ventilating the patient. What maneuvers can you perform to alleviate the upper airway obstruction?**

   Both the chin lift and jaw thrust displace the anterior musculature of the oropharynx and hypopharynx forward and allow for easier mask ventilation. Two-hand, two-person mask ventilation can be used when it is difficult to obtain a seal with the mask around the patient's face. This technique is similar to one-hand mask ventilation: the right hand merely mirrors the positions of the left hand. The second person is responsible for ventilating the patient with the bag. Also, an oral or nasal airway can be inserted. These devices displace the tongue anteriorly and create a conduit for the passage of air.

6. **When should you *not* use oral and nasal airways?**

   Both oral and nasal airways should be used judiciously. Avoid nasal airways in head trauma patients (because of the possibility of a cribiform fracture) and parturients (because the airway mucosa is friable and prone to bleeding). In conscious patients, oral airways may elicit a strong gag reflex, causing vomiting.

7. **The patient has a beard. Are there any tricks to prevent leakage around the mask during ventilation?**

   Sterile surgical lubricant or lidocaine ointment applied judiciously around the perimeter of the mask prior to its placement on the face will form a seal and facilitate a more airtight fit.

8. **How do you size oral and nasal airways?**

   Size can be estimated by placing an oral airway between the corner of the patient's mouth and the tragus of the ipsilateral ear; the tips of the oral airway should approximate this distance. Similarly, a nasal airway should be measured between the nares and ipsilateral tragus. Remember, judicious application of lidocaine ointment or Surgilube can facilitate placement of a nasal airway.

9. **What is the sniffing position?**

   In the sniffing position, the patient's neck is flexed and the head is extended. This position aligns the nasopharyngeal, oropharyngeal, and laryngeal axes (Fig. 64-2) of the patient. It may be difficult to determine whether the patient is placed in the optimal position when viewed from the head of the bed. Oftentimes, standing at the side of the bed provides a better perspective (when there is time). Remember, the patient should look like he or she is sniffing a flower held in an outstretched hand.

   Benumof JL: Clinical Procedures in Anesthesia and Intensive Care. Philadelphia, JB Lippincott, 1991, pp. 115–148.

10. **What can you do to facilitate intubation in a morbidly obese patient?**

    Many obese patients can have adipose distribution on the upper back. In this case, if the obese patient were to lie supine on a flat surface, his or her head would drop back (with extension at the lower cervical spine), causing misalignment of the oral, pharyngeal, and tracheal axes. Building a ramp of folded blankets, towels, or pillows on the bed to raise both the upper back and the head can help to realign the axes and to improve laryngoscopic grade.

11. **How do you manipulate the laryngoscope?**

    Laryngoscopes are gently held with the left hand. The right hand should be free to position the patient's head, to open the patient's mouth using the scissor maneuver (with the thumb on the lower teeth and the third finger on the upper teeth), to perform the BURP maneuver (see question 13) if necessary, and to insert the endotracheal tube. Remember that the force on the laryngoscope should be directed in line with the handle rather than levering back. This common error in inexperienced operators worsens the laryngoscopic view and risks dental injury.

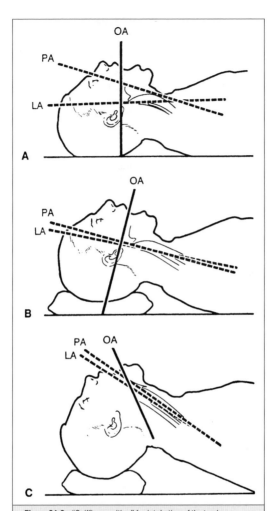

Figure 64-2. "Sniffing position" for intubation of the trachea. **A,** Successful exposure of the glottic opening using direct laryngoscopy requires alignment of the oropharyngeal axis (OA), nasopharyngeal axis (PA), and laryngeal axis (LA). **B,** Elevation of the head with pads under the occiput, with the shoulders remaining on the table, aligns the PA and LA. **C,** Subsequent head extension of the atlantooccipital joint serves to create the shortest distance and straightest line from the incisor teeth to the glottic opening. (From Stoelting RK, Miller RD: Airway management and tracheal intubation. In: Basics of Anesthesia, 4th ed. New York, Churchill Livingstone, 2000, p 150.)

12. **How are Macintosh and Miller blades manipulated?**
    The Macintosh blade is inserted on the right side of the mouth and advanced while gently sweeping across to the midline. The tip of the Macintosh blade is designed to be inserted anterior to the epiglottis into the vallecula; anterior and caudal displacement of the blade brings the vocal cords into view (similar to theater curtains being raised to reveal the stage behind).

The Miller blade is advanced in the midline past the tip of the epiglottis, and the tip of the blade is used to lift the epiglottis anteriorly to visualize the vocal cords.

13. **What is the BURP maneuver?**
The BURP maneuver was first described by Dr. Richard Knill in 1971. The acronym stands for **b**ackward, **u**pward, **r**ightward **p**ressure and refers to the displacement of the larynx during laryngoscopy. Specifically, the thyroid cartilage should be directed with your right hand (or by the hand of an experienced assistant) "posteriorly against the cervical vertebrae, superiorly as far as possible, and slightly laterally to the right." The maneuver can be employed to improve the view of the glottis, and multiple studies have demonstrated that grade III (with no view of the vocal cords) laryngoscopy can be changed to grade I or II by its application.

Knill RL: Difficult laryngoscopy made easy with a "BURP." Can J Anesth 40(3):279–282, 1992.

14. **When would you use the Sellick maneuver (or "cricoid pressure")?**
The Sellick maneuver describes pressure placed on the patient's cricoid cartilage in an effort to occlude the esophagus, which lies posterior to the trachea. Cricoid pressure should be instituted in patients who have full stomachs (e.g., from recent food ingestion, pregnancy, or bowel obstruction) and who have a history of gastroesophageal reflux.

15. **What size endotracheal tube should you select ?**
Select an endotracheal tube with an internal diameter of 7.0–7.5 mm for females and a tube with an internal diameter of 7.5–8.0 mm for males. These are guidelines; always have endotracheal tubes a half-size larger and smaller readily available. Remember to check the cuff on the endotracheal tube prior to intubation. The cuff should be insufflated with approximately 10 mL of air and should be pinched. The presence of a leak will result in gradual cuff deflation. Placing an endotracheal tube with a cuff leak, although not life-threatening, may expose the patient to additional airway trauma and the possibility of a lost airway.

16. **How do you confirm proper endotracheal tube placement?**
Confirmation of proper endotracheal tube placement is a multistep process:
- **End-tidal carbon dioxide ($ETCO_2$) detector:** This remains the current gold standard. After the endotracheal tube is inserted and the cuff is inflated, an $ETCO_2$ detector should be inserted between the end of the tube and the bag. A color change in the detector over a series of 5–6 breaths indicates tracheal placement. Remember that esophageal intubation can result in

---

KEY POINTS: TECHNIQUES FOR CONFIRMATION OF PROPER ENDOTRACHEAL TUBE PLACEMENT

1. End-tidal carbon dioxide ($ETCO_2$) detector (the current gold standard)

2. Auscultation of breath sounds over the left and right lung fields (lateral to the midclavicular line) and the stomach

3. Fiberoptic bronchoscopy

4. A bulb aspiration detection device

5. Repeat laryngoscopy, with direct visualization of the endotracheal tube as it passes through the vocal cords

6. Standard anterior–posterior chest radiographs (does not rule out esophageal placement)

early positive color changes on $ETCO_2$ detectors, followed by their gradual disappearance after several breaths.

- **Physical exam:** Additional confirmation includes auscultation of breath sounds, which should be performed over the left and right lung fields (lateral to the midclavicular line) and the stomach.
- **Other techniques:** other ways to confirm proper placement include fiberoptic bronchoscopy, a bulb aspiration detection device, repeat laryngoscopy with direct visualization of the endotracheal tube as it passes through the vocal cords, and standard anterior–posterior chest radiographs.

Always be vigilant.

17. **True or false: Tracheal intubation in a patient in cardiac arrest may result in no color changes in an $ETCO_2$ detector.**
    True. Cardiac arrest results in cessation of blood flow not only from the heart to the periphery but also in blood return from the periphery to the lungs. The lack of blood flow to the lungs will severely limit the body's ability to ventilate (or remove) carbon dioxide. The lack of carbon dioxide in the lungs results in little or no color change in an $ETCO_2$ detector.

18. **How far should you insert the endotracheal tube?**
    All endotracheal tubes are marked with centimeter markings on the side indicating distance to the tip. General guidelines for the securing of endotracheal tubes (measured at the lips) are 21 cm for adult females and 23 cm for adult males. Endobronchial intubation (i.e., the tube being advanced too far) usually occurs in the right mainstem bronchus, resulting in breath sounds transmitted in the right lung fields and the absence of sounds in the left. It can also present as wheezing or high inflation pressures. When the endotracheal tube is not advanced far enough and the cuff is inflated at the level of the vocal cords, vocal cord injury and tube dislodgement are possible. Remember, when intubating a patient, the endotracheal tube should be continually visualized until the cuff is advanced past the vocal cords.

19. **What is cuff palpation, and when should you use this technique?**
    A quick bedside technique to determine proper placement of the endotracheal tube is cuff ballottement. This technique involves applying intermittent pressure in the suprasternal notch while holding the pilot balloon partially compressed in the other hand. The endotracheal tube should be advanced and withdrawn until maximum counterpressure is felt in the pilot balloon. This method should only be used to verify endotracheal tube position and to decrease the risk of endobronchial intubation. It should not be used to confirm proper intubation of the trachea (see question 16).

    Pollard RJ, Lobato EB: Endotracheal tube location verified reliably by cuff palpation. Anesth Analg 81:135–139, 1995.

20. **How does neck movement alter endotracheal tube position?**
    The characteristics that may affect the position of the tube include sex, height, and neck position. Neck flexion may result in right mainstem bronchial intubation, and neck extension may result in accidental extubation. An easy way to remember which way the tip of the endotracheal tube travels with the neck movement is the saying, "The hose follows the nose." A flexed neck brings the nose closer to the thorax; an extended neck moves the nose away from the thorax.

21. **What are the two most common injuries that occur during intubation?**
    Dental injury is common when the laryngoscope is mishandled, when the patient has large incisors or a severe overbite, and during a difficult intubation (i.e., repeated attempts). With proper technique (pulling force in line with the handle of the laryngoscope), dental injuries are rare even in difficult intubations. Corneal abrasions occur when the patient's eyes are not protected or when the eyelids are displaced during intubation. Name tags hanging from pockets are a common culprit.

22. **When should you consider using an induction agent?**
The placement of an airway in a patient in cardiac arrest supersedes any pharmacotherapy. However, during an elective intubation, an amnestic and analgesic should be considered to provide patient comfort and to blunt the extreme elevations in heart rate and blood pressure that can occur during laryngoscopy. Agents include benzodiazepines, opioids, barbiturates, and nonbarbiturate anesthetics (i.e., propofol, ketamine, and etomidate). The recommended dosing regimens are beyond the scope of this chapter, but familiarity with these medications will facilitate a clinician's ability to provide a smooth, comfortable, and gentle intubation.

23. **When would you consider using a paralytic agent?**
Paralytic agents act at the neuromuscular junction, specifically, the nicotinic cholinergic receptors. They can be subdivided into depolarizing and nondepolarizing agents. Depolarizing neuromuscular blocking agents act by binding to the active sites on the nicotinic receptors, whereas nondepolarizing agents prevent the binding of acetylcholine to the nicotinic receptors. These drugs are often used to facilitate tracheal intubation by relaxing neck and laryngeal musculature. Remember the drawbacks: neuromuscular blocking agents have no analgesic or amnestic properties, and once they are administered, the patient will be unable to assist with ventilation in the event of a failed intubation. It is easy to turn an elective or urgent situation into a true emergency by removing a patient's respiratory effort.

24. **What are the advantages of succinylcholine, a depolarizing agent?**
Succinylcholine (1–1.5 mg/kg IV) remains the paralytic agent with the fastest onset (usually 30 seconds) and the shortest duration (about 3–5 minutes).

25. **What are some side effects and contraindications to succinylcholine?**
Succinylcholine binds to the active site and causes immediate depolarization of the muscle cells. This is caused by a rapid efflux of potassium ions from the intracellular to the extracellular space. In normal patients, there is a transient rise in serum potassium without clinical significance. However, in patients with preexisting hyperkalemia, a small rise in potassium could have catastrophic effects. Some patients have the risk of developing extremely large elevations of serum potassium after succinylcholine administration, including spinal cord injury or stroke with residual paralysis, muscular dystrophy, recent crush injury, and burns. Other side effects of succinylcholine include bradycardia, elevated intraocular pressure, masseter spasm, and triggering of malignant hyperthermia.

26. **You are unable to intubate the patient after multiple attempts. What should you do next?**
Remember, repeated attempts with direct laryngoscopy without any procedural changes will only lead to airway trauma.
- Change something (e.g., blade, operator, or head position).
- Bag-mask the patient while you are contemplating how to proceed. Improving a patient's oxygen saturation from 85% to 97% will give you a considerable time advantage while you are manipulating the airway.
- Consider an advanced technique.
- The inability to ventilate and intubate a patient is a true emergency. You should immediately summon assistance from an anesthesiologist and a surgeon.

27. **List several advanced techniques for obtaining an airway.**
- Laryngeal mask airway (LMA)
- Intubating LMA
- Flexible fiberoptic scope (through a nare, the mouth, or an LMA)
- Rigid fiberoptic scope (Bullard or Wu)
- Lighted stylet

- Blind nasal intubation
- Transtracheal jet ventilation
- Retrograde wire intubation
- Emergency cricothyrotomy

These techniques should be attempted only by persons experienced in their use. Do what you know!

28. **How would you intubate a patient with an unstable cervical fracture?**
   Flexion or extension of the neck in this patient may result in further or permanent neurologic damage. If the decision is made to use direct laryngoscopy, an assistant should be designated to maintain the neck with in-line stabilization. Traction should be avoided because of the possibility of atlantooccipital dissociation. Laryngoscopy should be performed gently, with minimal movement of the neck. Other alternatives include awake nasal intubation, flexible or rigid fiberoptic scopes, light wands, or intubating LMAs.

29. **Are there any published guidelines regarding the management of a patient with a difficult intubation?**
   In 1992 (with an update in 2002), the American Society of Anesthesiologists (ASA) established the Practice Guidelines for Management of the Difficult Airway. These provide an excellent overview of the issues and the systematic approach to management. They are available for review through the ASA Web site (http://www.asahq.org).

BIBLIOGRAPHY

1. Morgan GE, Mikhail MS, Murray MJ: Clinical Anesthesiology, 3rd ed. New York, McGraw-Hill, 2002.
2. Rosenblatt WH: Airway management. In Barash PG, Cullen BF, Stoelting RK (eds): Clinical Anesthesia, 4th ed. Philadelphia, Lippincott Williams & Wilkins, 2001, pp. 595–638.
3. Stoelting RK, Hiller SC: Pharmacology & Physiology in Anesthetic Practice, 4th ed. Philadelphia, Lippincott Williams & Wilkins, 2006.

CHAPTER 65

TRACHEOSTOMY

John E. Heffner, MD

1. **When is tracheostomy performed for critically ill patients?**
   Tracheostomy provides direct access to the airway just below the first or second tracheal rings. The four indications for tracheostomy are as follows:
   1. Maintenance of an airway for patients with functional or mechanical upper airway obstruction
   2. Provision of airway access for suctioning retained secretions
   3. Management of aspiration in patients with glottic dysfunction
   4. Management of patients who require long-term airway access for ventilatory support
   Advances in tube design and the advent of percutaneous tracheostomy performed at the bedside have expanded the application of tracheostomy, which now represents the most commonly performed surgical procedure for critically ill patients. From 10–24% of mechanically ventilated patients undergo this procedure.

   Esteban A, Anzueto A, Alia I, et al: How is mechanical ventilation employed in the intensive care unit? An international utilization review. Am J Respir Crit Care Med 161(5):1450–1458, 2000.
   Heffner JE: Tracheotomy application and timing. Clin Chest Med 24:389–398, 2003.

2. **How is tracheostomy performed?**
   A tracheostomy can be performed as an *open surgical tracheostomy* or as a *percutaneous tracheostomy*. An open surgical tracheostomy provides tracheal access through an incisional tracheostoma that enters the trachea between cartilaginous rings. The stoma tract is temporary and closes spontaneously after the tracheostomy tube is removed. This procedure is well tolerated, with a mortality rate below 1% for even the most critically ill patients. Percutaneous tracheostomy is a general term that refers to several different techniques that insert a standard or modified tracheostomy tube between the second and third tracheal rings using a Seldinger technique and either a device to cut and spread the trachea or forceps or dilator instruments to cannulate and dilate tracheal tissue between cartilaginous rings. Currently, the percutaneous dilational tracheostomy (PDT) technique of Ciaglia is most commonly performed in the intensive care unit (ICU). With this technique, one inserts a needle and guidewire below the first tracheal ring, followed by a single dilator that increases in caliber from its tip to its base, where it matches the diameter of a tracheostomy tube. This shape, which simulates a rhinoceros horn, and the dilator's blue color impart the procedure's name, the "Ciaglia Blue Rhino technique." A tracheostomy tube loaded over a tapered introducer is then inserted through the dilated stoma tract into the tracheal airway.

   Bliznikas D, Baredes S: Percutaneous tracheostomy. Available at http://www.emedicine.com/ent/topic682.htm.
   de Boisblanc BP: Percutaneous dilational tracheostomy techniques. Clin Chest Med 24(3):399–407, 2003.
   Walts PA, Murthy SC, DeCamp MM: Techniques of surgical tracheostomy. Clin Chest Med 24:413–422, 2003.

3. **Which is the preferred tracheostomy technique for critically ill patients?**
   Multiple studies have compared the safety, speed, and relative benefits of open surgical tracheostomy and PDT in critically ill patients. Results to date confirm that both procedures can be performed safely with acceptable complications when performed by appropriately skilled and experienced clinicians. The PDT technique is completed faster, but time differences are not clinically important. Also, less bleeding may occur with PDT because the

dilational procedure allows stoma tissue to compress venous vessels against the tracheostomy tube to tamponade any "bleeders." Again, clinical significance of this benefit is minor. Because PDT can be performed at the bedside, considerable cost savings derive from omitting an operating room charge. Some centers, however, perform open surgical tracheostomy by the bedside, which obviates this relative advantage of PDT. On the basis of existing studies, both procedures remain acceptable options for critically ill patients who require elective placement of a tracheostomy.

Massick DD, Yao S, Powell DM, et al: Bedside tracheostomy in the intensive care unit: A prospective randomized trial comparing open surgical tracheostomy with endoscopically guided percutaneous dilational tracheotomy. Laryngoscope 111(3):494–500, 2001.

Wu JJ, Huang MS, Tang GJ, et al: Percutaneous dilatational tracheostomy versus open tracheostomy—A prospective, randomized, controlled trial. J Chin Med Assoc 66(8):467–473, 2003.

4. **What other techniques exist to place a tube into the trachea?**
    Although elective tracheostomies can be performed safely in critically ill patients, their use in emergency settings is associated with high rates of complications, including cardiopulmonary arrest due to misplaced tubes. In this setting, cricothyroidotomy is the preferred procedure. Cricothyroidotomy places a tracheostomy tube through the cricothyroid space, which lies between the laryngeal cartilage and the cricoid cartilage. Because this space is relatively superficial to the anterior surface of the neck, cricothyroidotomy can be completed quickly, with a high rate of successful placement into the airway despite unstable circumstances during respiratory emergencies. A high rate of subglottic stenosis, however, requires the cricothyroidotomy to be converted to a tracheostomy by standard techniques once the patient stabilizes.

    A minitracheostomy represents an additional technique for cannulating the trachea for patients who require periodic airway suctioning but can breathe through their native airway. This technique entails placement of a small-caliber (i.e., 4-mm inner diameter) tube into the trachea by a Seldinger technique, which allows insertion of a suction catheter. The tube can be capped when not in use. Short-term placement of minitracheostomies can assist patients who have retained secretions and poor ability to cough after thoracic surgery.

    Wright CD: Minitracheostomy. Clin Chest Med 24(3):431–435, 2003.

    Wright MJ, Greenberg DE, Hunt JP, et al: Surgical cricothyroidotomy in trauma patients. South Med J 96(5):465–467, 2003.

5. **What are the most serious immediate complications of PDT? How can they be prevented?**
    In its original description, PDT was a "blind" technique that required an operator to insert a guidewire, dilator, and tracheostomy tube into the airway using only palpation and knowledge of anatomic landmarks as guides. This technique resulted occasionally in airways misplaced adjacent to the trachea or into the retrotracheal space when tubes transited the trachea and perforated its posterior wall. Modifications to the procedure employed fiberoptic bronchoscopy to visualize insertion of the needle and guidewire into the airway. The addition of bronchoscopy has markedly decreased the incidence of tube misplacement. Some centers now use ultrasound or capnography to monitor needle and tracheostomy tube placement, with results similar to bronchoscopy.

    Hinerman R, Alvarez F, Keller CA: Outcome of bedside percutaneous tracheostomy with bronchoscopic guidance. Intens Care Med 26(12):1850–1856, 2000.

    Winkler WB, Karnik R, Seelmann O, et al: Bedside percutaneous dilational tracheostomy with endoscopic guidance: Experience with 71 ICU patients. Intens Care Med 20(7):476–479, 1994.

6. **Should PDT be avoided in any patients?**
    PDT was first applied electively to critically ill patients in a conservative manner as experience with this relatively new procedure was being gained. Initial contraindications included age less than 16 years, bleeding diatheses, heavily calcified tracheal rings, previous tracheostomy, acute

cervical trauma, high positive end-expiratory pressure (PEEP) requirements, and abnormalities of cervical anatomic landmarks such as obesity or thyromegaly. Reports now exist, however, of safe and successful performance of PDT in many of these settings. At present, no absolute contraindications exist to the procedure, with patient selection being guided by the knowledge and experience of the operator. Ultrasound, used to guide needle insertion, can assist the procedure for patients with abnormal cervical anatomy.

Beiderlinden M, Groeben H, Peters J: Safety of percutaneous dilational tracheostomy in patients ventilated with high positive end-expiratory pressure (PEEP). Intens Care Med 29(6):944–948, 2003.

Mansharamani NG, Koziel H, Garland R, et al: Safety of bedside percutaneous dilatational tracheostomy in obese patients in the ICU. Chest 117(5):1426–1429, 2000.

Meyer M, Critchlow J, Mansharamani N, et al: Repeat bedside percutaneous dilational tracheostomy is a safe procedure. Crit Care Med 30(5):986–988, 2002.

7. **How are the complications of tracheostomy categorized?**
Both open surgical tracheostomy and PDT can cause serious complications, which are categorized as intraoperative, early postoperative, and late. Every clinician managing patients with tracheostomy requires clear knowledge of these complications and measures to monitor for their occurrence.

8. **Summarize the major complications of tracheostomy.**
See Table 65-1.

TABLE 65-1. COMPLICATIONS OF TRACHEOSTOMY		
Intraoperative	**Early Postoperative**	**Late**
Cardiorespiratory arrest	Hemorrhage	Tracheal stenosis
Hemorrhage	Subcutaneous emphysema	Tracheoesophageal fistula
Pneumothorax and pneumomediastinum	Inadvertent decannulation	Tracheoinnominate fistula
	Wound infection	Tracheocutaneous fistula
Recurrent laryngeal nerve injury	Pneumonia	Tracheal ring fracture and herniation
Tracheoesophageal fistula	Tube obstruction	

9. **When should tracheostomy be performed for intubated, ventilator-dependent patients?**
Frequent complications of open surgical tracheostomy in the 1960s encouraged physicians to delay its use for ventilator-dependent patients until they had remained intubated for 2–3 weeks. Many clinicians would reluctantly perform tracheostomy at this time because of concerns that translaryngeal intubation longer than 2–3 weeks would cause subglottic stenosis unless the patient was converted to a tracheostomy. Refinements in tracheostomy techniques and improvements in procedural quality control have diminished complications and allowed earlier performance of the procedure. Also, no data have clearly confirmed a correlation between duration of translaryngeal intubation and risks for subglottic stenosis.

Consequently, the modern approach eschews calendar watching with conversion to tracheostomy after a specific duration of intubation, and instead promotes an anticipatory approach. This approach recommends tracheostomy when a specific patient appears likely to require long-term ventilation and can experience the benefits of the procedure, which requires clinicians to predict the likely duration of mechanical ventilation and to have a clear understanding of the benefits that tracheostomy can provide.

Multiple clinical trials have attempted to identify an ideal time to perform tracheostomy in specific categories of mechanically ventilated patients, such as those with trauma. Many of these studies demonstrate improved outcomes in terms of ICU length of stay and risk for pneumonia in those patients who undergo a routine early tracheostomy, within the first several days of intubation, as compared with those patients who are converted to tracheostomy after 7 days. Most of these studies, however, had significant design flaws that introduced extensive bias. Most observers have accepted the conclusion that physicians no longer need to delay tracheostomy because of inherent risks, but rather can apply it when the benefits appear to justify the risks.

Heffner JE: Timing of tracheotomy in mechanically ventilated patients. Am Rev Respir Dis 147:768–771, 1993.

Heffner JE, Hess D: Tracheostomy management in the chronically ventilated patient. Clin Chest Med 22(1):55–69, 2001.

10. **What are the potential benefits of tracheostomy?**
Little data exist to confirm and quantify the benefits of tracheostomy, but experienced clinicians propose that carefully selected patients can have improved outcomes when converted to a tracheostomy. Many of these benefits derive from improved patient comfort after placement of tracheostomy, which allows weaning of analgesics and sedatives, all of which have inherent risks for critically ill patients. These risks include altered mental status, prolonged ventilation, and ventilator-associated pneumonia. A tracheostomy also presents to the patient a lower resistance to airflow, as compared to translaryngeal intubation, which may facilitate spontaneous breathing during weaning trials. No data demonstrate that patients have a higher likelihood of weaning successfully after performance of a tracheostomy, but patients with borderline ventilatory status probably do benefit in this regard because of decreased work of breathing and better removal of airway secretions by suctioning. Other benefits of tracheostomy may be obtained in selected patients.

Banner MJ, Blanch PB, Kirby RR: Imposed work of breathing and methods of triggering demand-flow, continuous positive airway pressure system. Crit Care Med 21:183–190, 1993.

KEY POINTS: POTENTIAL BENEFITS OF TRACHEOSTOMY

1. Lower airway resistance, which may promote weaning from mechanical ventilation

2. Lower risk of nosocomial pneumonia in patient subgroups

3. Earlier transfer of ventilator-dependent patients to a non–intensive care unit setting

4. Improved oral nutrition

5. The ability to communicate verbally

6. Improved airway suctioning

7. Increased comfort

8. Greater patient mobility

9. Removal of endotracheal tube and its associated risks for direct endolaryngeal injury

10. A more secure airway, which decreases the risk of inadvertent decannulation

Heffner JE: The role of tracheotomy in weaning. Chest 120(6 Suppl):477S–481S, 2001.

Jaeger JM, Littlewood KA, Durbin CG Jr: The role of tracheostomy in weaning from mechanical ventilation. Respir Care 47(4):469–480, 2002.

Moscovici da Cruz V, Demarzo SE, Sobrinho JB, et al: Effects of tracheotomy on respiratory mechanics in spontaneously breathing patients. Eur Respir J 20(1):112–117, 2002.

11. **How common and serious are the long-term complications of tracheostomy?**
It is difficult to study the long-term effects of tracheostomy performed in critically ill patients because many patients with critical illnesses or serious underlying chronic conditions do not survive in the long term, and those who do survive are often lost for follow-up. Nevertheless, existing studies indicate that tracheostomy done by either PDT or the open surgical technique has low risks for serious long-term complications. However, maintenance of this low risk requires meticulous attention to management details such as avoiding overinflation of the tube cuff, anchoring of the ventilator hose to avoid traction of the tube on tracheal mucosa, and appropriate surgical technique. The most common complication is tracheal stenosis at the stoma site. Most instances, however, are not sufficiently severe to cause respiratory compromise. Patients who experience persistent dyspnea or difficulty clearing secretions after decannulation of a tracheostomy should be evaluated for tracheal stenosis even if their symptoms can be explained by underlying lung disease such as chronic obstructive pulmonary disease. Tracheal stenosis at the cuff site has been rare since the advent of high-volume, low-pressure tube cuffs.

12. **What is a tracheoesophageal fistula?**
A tracheoesophageal fistula is a rare complication of tracheostomy that usually results from overinflation of a tracheostomy cuff or pressure of the curved region of the tube against the posterior tracheal wall. This pressure on tracheal mucosa causes formation of a fistula from the trachea to the esophagus. The fistula may be difficult to diagnose because clinical manifestations may simulate more-common conditions. Among patients still receiving mechanical ventilation, fistulae may cause increased airway secretions and aspiration of tube feedings. Also, ventilator breaths may insufflate the esophagus, causing excessive bowel gas. After weaning from mechanical ventilation, patients with fistulae may experience increased cough, sputum production, and dyspnea. The diagnosis requires a high index of suspicion and careful visualization of the airway and esophagus with bronchoscopy and esophagoscopy to adequately exclude the diagnosis. Chest computed tomography (CT) may assist in some settings.

Reed MF, Mathisen DJ: Tracheoesophageal fistula. Chest Surg Clin North Am 13(2):271–289, 2003.

13. **What is a tracheoinnominate fistula?**
A tracheoinnominate fistula occurs rarely in patients who undergo a tracheostomy. Most often, the tracheostomy is placed overly low so that the tip of the tube overlies the region of the trachea crossed by the innominate artery. Anterior abutment of the tracheostomy tube tip causes tracheal erosion and submucosal infection, which erodes into the innominate artery. Such patients present with herald hemorrhages that can suddenly progress to massive airway hemorrhage and acute asphyxia. Patients suspected of a tracheoinnominate fistula should undergo cautious airway visualization in a setting in which an immediate thoracotomy can be performed if manipulation of the tracheostomy tube releases a tamponading effect of the cuff resulting in massive hemorrhage.

Allan JS, Wright CD: Tracheoinnominate fistula: Diagnosis and management. Chest Surg Clin North Am 13(2):331–341, 2003.

14. **Can patients converted to a tracheostomy eat?**
After weaning from mechanical ventilation, patients with a tracheostomy in place develop problems with swallowing that may promote aspiration and interfere with eating. The tracheostomy tube interferes with normal swallowing by anchoring the hyoid bone and the larynx, thereby preventing their normal elevation during swallowing, which is the physiologic mechanism for closing

the airway and preventing aspiration. Also, an inflated tracheostomy tube cuff may interfere with esophageal motility and cause retrograde flow of ingested material into the pharynx. Before initiating an oral diet, patients with a tracheostomy should undergo a systematic assessment to identify any swallowing disorders and the presence of aspiration.

Dikeman KJ, Kazandjjan MS: Communication and swallowing management of tracheostomized and ventilator-dependent adults. Clifton Park, NY, Thomson Delmar Learning, 2003.

15. **How can patients with a tracheostomy talk?**
In contrast to a translaryngeal endotracheal tube, a tracheostomy tube provides opportunities for patients to communicate verbally. Transient deflation of a tracheostomy cuff with the application of PEEP allows an airway leak that exits through the native airway, allowing patients to whisper words. Specialized "talking tubes" have a cannula through which a flow of gas can enter the airway above the cuff, allowing airflow across the vocal cords and articulated speech. Because a tracheostomy tube frees the pharynx of appliances, an electrolarynx applied to the submandibular space can allow patients to turn the vibratory tone into understandable speech by mouthing words. For spontaneously breathing patients, a one-way valve (i.e., a Passy–Muir valve) can be placed on the tracheostomy tube, which allows inspiration through the tube and exhalation through the native airway. Patients can then speak normally during exhalation.

16. **When can a tracheostomy tube be removed?**
Most patients recovering from respiratory failure require a step-wise approach to remove a tracheostomy tube to avoid failure of decannulation. Assessment for decannulation begins when patients have demonstrated the ability to breathe spontaneously for 48 hours. The patient's ability to avoid aspiration is assessed by deflating the tracheostomy tube cuff and observing for frank aspiration. Upper airway narrowing is excluded by deflating the tube cuff and occluding the tube lumen to evaluate the patient's ability to breathe through the native airway. The ability to breathe around a tube or through a fenestrated tube has a high positive predictive value for the exclusion of upper airway narrowing.

Patients who pass the above tests can be observed for the ability to breathe for 30 minutes with a plugged tracheostomy tube and a deflated cuff. Most patients who pass this breathing trial can be successfully decannulated. Failure of the trial indicates the need for daily reevaluations. Borderline patients may benefit from serial downsizing of their tracheostomy tube or periodic closure of the tracheal stoma with a stoma plug, which allows spontaneous weaning trials and clearance of the trachea of the obstructive effects of the tracheostomy tube. An interdisciplinary tracheostomy decannulation team can accelerate successful weaning.

Ceriana P, Carlucci A, Navalesi P, et al: Weaning from tracheotomy in long-term mechanically ventilated patients: Feasibility of a decisional flowchart and clinical outcome. Intensive Care Med (5):845–848, 2003.

Heffner JE: The technique of weaning from tracheostomy. Criteria for weaning: Practical measures to prevent failure. J Crit Illn 10:729–731, 1995.

Rumbak MJ, Graves AE, Scott MP, et al: Tracheostomy tube occlusion protocol predicts significant tracheal obstruction to air flow in patients requiring prolonged mechanical ventilation. Crit Care Med 25(3):413–417, 1997.

CHAPTER 66

NONINVASIVE VENTILATION

Nicholas S. Hill, MD

1. **What is noninvasive ventilation?**

   Noninvasive ventilation (NIV) refers to the provision of mechanical ventilatory assistance without the need for an invasive (i.e., endotracheal) airway. Over the past 15 years, it has assumed an important role in the management of both acute and chronic forms of respiratory failure.

   Mehta S, Hill NS: Noninvasive ventilation. State of the art. Am J Respir Crit Care Med 163:540–557, 1998.

2. **What types of noninvasive ventilation are there?**

   In the past, noninvasive ventilation was delivered mainly using so-called "body" ventilators, such as negative pressure ventilators, that would assist ventilation by intermittently applying a negative pressure external to the thorax and abdomen, helping the lungs to expand. Such devices have largely been abandoned; now, the main means of assisting ventilation is through positive pressure techniques applied to the upper airway by a mask (or interface). Currently, we deliver positive pressure to the upper airway using continuous positive airway pressure (CPAP), which applies a steady pressure but does not actively assist inhalation, and noninvasive positive-pressure ventilation (NPPV), which consists of a higher pressure during inhalation to actively provide ventilatory assistance, usually combined with positive end-expiratory pressure (PEEP).

3. **What is BiPAP?**

   BiPAP is a proprietary name for certain respiratory assistance devices manufactured by Respironics, Inc. (Murrysville, PA) that have become popular for provision of NIV, but the name is often used generically to refer to any portable positive pressure device designed to deliver NPPV. Some clinicians prefer the term "bilevel devices" to refer to this class of portable pressure-limited devices. These are blower-based units that fluctuate between higher inspiratory pressures and lower expiratory pressures (hence the name "bilevel") and that have single limb ventilator circuits. Because they have sensitive flow triggers and cycle into expiration in response to decreases in inspiratory flow, they function essentially as pressure support ventilators. However, it is important to keep in mind that bilevel ventilation delivered through portable pressure devices and pressure support ventilation delivered through critical care ventilators use different terminologies. With bilevel ventilation, the inspiratory positive airway pressure (IPAP) and expiratory positive airway pressure (EPAP) are absolute pressures, and the difference between them is the level of pressure support. With critical care ventilators, the level of pressure support is added to PEEP. Thus, a pressure support of 10 cmH_2O and a PEEP of 5 cmH_2O are equivalent to an IPAP of 15 cmH_2O and an EPAP of 5 cmH_2O.

4. **Why has NPPV assumed an important role in the management of acute respiratory failure?**

   NIV has theoretical advantages over invasive mechanical ventilation. Intubation traumatizes the upper airway, possibly causing bleeding, vomiting, or laceration of the trachea or esophagus. Once an endotracheal tube is in place, it is a source of continual irritation and requires suctioning to maintain a clear airway, compounding the trauma. In addition, the risk of nosocomial infection, including health care–acquired pneumonia, rises in proportion to the duration of intubation (an estimated 1–3% per day). Furthermore, intubation is uncomfortable for patients, requiring sedation and analgesia, which add to potential complications and may slow weaning and extubation. By avoiding these potential complications, NIV may improve outcomes by shortening duration of intubation and stays in the intensive care unit (ICU) and hospital as well as reducing mortality rates. The evidence that NIV lowers rates of hospital-acquired infections compared to invasive mechanical ventilation is quite strong. However, NIV must be used selectively if these outcomes are to be realized, as discussed below.

5. Can CPAP alone help patients with acute respiratory failure?

CPAP alone offers important benefits for patients with chronic obstructive pulmonary disease (COPD) or congestive heart failure (CHF). Patients presenting with exacerbations of COPD usually have dynamic hyperinflation, failing to empty their lungs prior to the next inspiration because of expiratory flow limitation. They have positive end-expiratory alveolar pressure, a condition referred to as intrinsic PEEP or auto-PEEP. In order to initiate their next breath or to trigger a ventilator, they must overcome this "inspiratory threshold load" and lower alveolar pressure to subatmospheric levels. The application of extrinsic CPAP (or PEEP), as long as it is below the level of auto-PEEP, counterbalances the inspiratory threshold load and alleviates dyspnea by reducing the work necessary to initiate the next breath.

In patients with CHF, CPAP increases functional residual capacity (FRC), helping to reopen flooded alveoli, thereby reducing shunt and ventilation-perfusion (V/Q) mismatching and improving oxygenation, an effect that can be quite dramatic. This can also improve lung compliance, the work of breathing, and the sensation of dyspnea. When the cardiac ventricles are enlarged and hypocontractile, increased intrathoracic pressure can have salutary hemodynamic effects by diminishing venous return (and reducing preload) and lowering afterload by reducing transmyocardial pressure.

6. What does NPPV add to the effects of CPAP?

NPPV refers to the provision of ventilatory support during inspiration using either pressure- or volume-limited breaths, usually superimposed on positive expiratory pressure. If the ventilator is adequately synchronized, the patient will usually reduce his or her breathing effort, allowing the ventilator to assume at least part of the work of breathing and reducing the sensation of dyspnea, usually more than with CPAP alone. Inspiratory ventilatory support may also augment tidal volume, allowing for more effective elimination of CO_2 and reversal of respiratory failure.

7. What masks (interfaces) are used to deliver NPPV?

NPPV is delivered using a wide array of nasal full-face masks (which seal over the nose and mouth) and oral devices. In addition, a mask that resembles a hockey goalie's mask, which seals on the perimeter of the face, is available, and, in some European countries, a clear plastic cylindrical helmet is used that fits over the head and seals on the shoulder girdle. In the acute setting, studies indicate that the full-face mask is best tolerated initially because air leaks through the mouth are less of a problem. Masks used in the acute setting must be inexpensive and disposable or reusable. Nasal masks are better for speaking, coughing, and even eating, and, in the long-term setting, they are rated as more comfortable by patients. When patients begun with full-face masks in the acute setting are to remain on NPPV as outpatients, some clinicians transition them to nasal masks. Oral devices are commercially available and are most often used in the long-term setting, but less often than nasal or full-face masks. They are sometimes used to facilitate initiation of NPPV in the acute setting.

Kwok H, McCormack J, Cece R, et al: Controlled trial of oronasal versus nasal mask ventilation in the treatment of acute respiratory failure. Crit Care Med 31(2):468–473, 2003.

8. What ventilators are used for NPPV?

Recent surveys show that portable pressure-limited "bilevel" ventilators are used for the vast majority of outpatient applications of NPPV, both in the United States and in Europe. Portable volume-limited ventilators may be used as well, but these compensate less well for leaks, are heavier, and have more alarms, which become a nuisance unless the patient is dependent on mechanical ventilation nearly all the time. However, they offer the advantage of "stacking" multiple breaths to achieve higher inflation volumes and greater cough flows in patients with neuromuscular diseases.

Bilevel ventilators have also become popular to deliver NPPV in the acute care setting, although critical care ventilators—those designed mainly for invasive mechanical ventilation—are commonly used as well. With the exception of models designed specifically for acute applications of NPPV that have oxygen blenders, oxygen supplementation with most bilevel ventilators requires connecting oxygen tubing directly to the mask or ventilator circuit, and even at the maximum oxygen flow rate recommended by the manufacturer (15 L/min), FiO_2 does not exceed 50%. Thus, although bilevel devices function as well as or even better than critical care ventilators with regard to triggering, cycling, and flow delivery, they should not be used for patients with hypoxemic respiratory failure unless equipped with oxygen blenders.

9. What about rebreathing?

Bilevel ventilators, by virtue of their single ventilator circuit, are subject to rebreathing unless CO_2 is eliminated through their fixed exhalation ports during exhalation. Using sufficient expiratory pressure (≥ 4 cmH_2O), special nonrebreathing valves, or masks with the exhalation port situated in the mask over the bridge of the nose will minimize rebreathing.

Schettino GPP, Chatmongkolchart S, Hess D, Kacmarek RM: Position of exhalation port and mask design affect CO2 rebreathing during noninvasive positive pressure ventilation. Crit Care Med 31:2178–2182, 2003.

10. What are the indications for NPPV in the acute care setting?

Evidence has accumulated to support the use of NPPV for patients with a number of different forms of respiratory failure (Table 66-1). Multiple randomized controlled trials and meta-analyses (level A evidence) have demonstrated that NPPV more rapidly improves vital signs and gas exchange and avoids intubation compared to conventional therapy in patients with respiratory failure due to COPD exacerbations or acute cardiogenic pulmonary edema or in association with immunocompromised states. In these patients, NPPV should be considered the ventilatory modality of first choice unless there are contraindications. Level B evidence supports the use of NPPV in a variety of other forms of respiratory failure, including asthma and severe community-acquired pneumonia occurring in COPD patients or in the postoperative setting after lung resection. NPPV can be used for these latter conditions, but firm guidelines cannot be proffered in the absence of more data. For entities supported by level C evidence (case series or conflicting evidence), NPPV can be tried, but cautious monitoring is advised.

A partial list of conditions in which NPPV is unlikely to be of benefit or may even be harmful is also found in Table 66-1. Unless dealing with single-organ-system failure, controllable secretions, and a highly cooperative patient, NPPV should probably not be used for acute respiratory distress syndrome (ARDS) or for severe pneumonia in non-COPD patients.

Lightowler JV, Wedzicha JA, Elliott MW, Ram FS: Non-invasive positive pressure ventilation to treat respiratory failure resulting from exacerbations of chronic obstructive pulmonary disease: Cochrane systematic review and meta-analysis. BMJ 326(7382):185–189, 2003.

Mehta S, Jay GD, Woolard RH, et al: Randomized prospective trial of bilevel versus continuous positive airway pressure in acute pulmonary edema. Crit Care Med 25:620–628, 1997.

11. How are candidates for NPPV selected?

Once potential recipients for NPPV are identified, patients should be selected using guidelines that are pragmatic but have not been validated in prospective studies. Selection involves a simple two-step process, the first step of which is to identify patients at risk of needing intubation based on simple clinical observations of respiratory compromise and gas exchange disturbance (Table 66-2). The second step is to exclude patients who would be at high risk of failure or who simply cannot be managed noninvasively. These include patients having a frank respiratory arrest, uncooperative patients, and those who cannot cope with their secretions. The idea is to take advantage of a window of opportunity, intervening with NPPV when ventilatory assistance is needed but before the patient becomes too acutely ill to succeed.

TABLE 66-1. NONINVASIVE POSITIVE-PRESSURE VENTILATION INDICATIONS ACCORDING TO LEVEL OF EVIDENCE, AS DETERMINED BY DIAGNOSIS, CATEGORY OF ACUTE RESPIRATORY FAILURE, OR BOTH

Level A evidence (multiple randomized controlled trials, meta-analyses, or both)
- Acute hypercapnic respiratory failure in COPD
- Cardiogenic pulmonary edema
- Acute respiratory failure in immunocompromised patients
- Facilitation of weaning (COPD)

Level B evidence (a single randomized controlled trial or multiple uncontrolled or historically controlled series)
- Asthma
- Community-acquired pneumonia (with COPD)
- Extubation failure (COPD)
- Hypoxemic respiratory failure
- Do-not-intubate patients (COPD and CHF)
- Postoperative respiratory failure

Level C evidence (case series or conflicting evidence)
- Acute respiratory distress syndrome (ARDS)
- Community-acquired pneumonia (non-COPD)
- Cystic fibrosis
- Facilitation of weaning or extubation failure (non-COPD)
- Obstructive sleep apnea or obesity hypoventilation
- Trauma
- Upper airway obstruction

NPPV not advised
- Acute deterioration in the end stage
- Interstitial fibrosis
- Severe ARDS with multiple-organ dysfunction syndrome (MODS)
- Postoperative upper airway or esophageal surgery
- Upper airway obstruction with a high risk for occlusion

12. **Are there predictors of NPPV failure?**
    Yes. Predictors of NPPV failure include a high Acute Physiology and Chronic Health Evaluation (APACHE) II score (i.e., ≥29), a low pH (i.e., <7.25), a low Glasgow Coma Score (i.e., <11), excessive tachypnea (i.e., >35 breaths/min), severe hypercarbia (i.e., >92 mmHg), an inability to cooperate or to coordinate breathing with the ventilator, excessive air leaking, and lack of teeth, which makes it harder to get a good seal (Table 66-3). The more of these predictors that

TABLE 66-2.   SELECTION GUIDELINES: NONINVASIVE VENTILATION FOR PATIENTS WITH ACUTE RESPIRATORY FAILURE

Step 1. Identify patients who may need intubation.

1. Symptoms and signs of acute respiratory distress:
   - Moderate to severe dyspnea, *and*
   - Respiratory rate > 24 breaths/min,[*] accessory muscle use, and paradoxical breathing
2. Gas exchange abnormalities
   - $PaCO_2$ > 45 mmHg; pH < 7.35, *or*
   - PaO_2-to-FiO_2 ratio < 200

Step 2. Exclude those in whom noninvasive ventilation would be risky.

1. Respiratory arrest
2. Medical instability (i.e., hypotensive shock, uncontrolled cardiac ischemia, arrhythmias, or upper gastrointestinal bleeding)
3. Inability to protect airway (impaired cough or swallowing mechanism)
4. Excessive secretions
5. Agitation or uncooperativeness
6. Recent upper airway or esophageal surgery
7. Facial trauma or burns or anatomic abnormalities interfering with mask fit

[*]Respiratory rate >30 breaths/min in patients with hypoxemic respiratory failure

TABLE 66-3.   PREDICTORS OF NONINVASIVE POSITIVE-PRESSURE VENTILATION FAILURE IN ACUTE RESPIRATORY FAILURE

- Advanced age
- Greater acuity of illness (a new simplified acute physiology score [SAPS II] ≥ 29)
- Inability to cooperate (Glasgow Coma Score < 11)
- Inability to coordinate breathing with ventilator
- Air leaking from lack of dentition
- Severe hypercarbia ($PaCO_2$ > 92 mmHg)
- Acidemia (pH < 7.25)
- Failure to improve gas exchange, pH, and heart and respiratory rates within the first 2 hours[*]

[*]Most powerful predictor

are present at initiation, the more likely NPPV will fail. Even better at predicting failure, however, is the persistence of these predictors after 2 hours of NPPV. Lack of improvement in at least some of these predictors at that point would indicate the need for intubation. A recent study that associated increased mortality with delayed intubation has underlined the importance of not persisting too long with a failed attempt at NPPV.

13. **How do I initiate NPPV in acute respiratory failure?**

Select a mask that fits properly and is comfortable for the patient. Allow cooperative patients to hold the mask in place to impart control. Connect the mask to the ventilator, initially at low pressures (8–12 cmH_2O inspiratory and 4–5 cmH_2O expiratory) to facilitate adaptation. With volume-limited modes, a tidal volume of 10–15 mL/kg is used, higher than with invasive venti-lation because of the need to compensate for leaks and dead space of the mask exceeding that of an endotracheal tube. Reassure the patient, offering explanations at each step and pointing out that success will mean no need for an endotracheal tube. If using a mode with a backup rate, select one that will allow spontaneous breathing, usually 12–16 breaths/min. Oxygen sup-plementation, through either an oxygen blender or a tube attached to the mask or ventilator circuit, should be adjusted to maintain a target oxygen saturation, usually >90–92%.

It is important to adjust pressures promptly once patients have become comfortable with the initial settings. Because the difference between the inspiratory and expiratory pressures is the pressure support, and because this pressure is responsible for decreasing respiratory distress and facilitating the elimination of CO_2, the inspiratory pressure should be increased as tolerated, usually to pressures between 12 cmH_2O and 20 cmH_2O. The expiratory pressure can be increased (usually to a maximum of 8 cmH_2O) to facilitate triggering in patients with auto-PEEP or to treat hypoxemia. Remember that increases in expiratory pressure must be accompanied by increases in inspiratory pressure if the level of pressure support is to be maintained. For uncooperative patients, sedation may be helpful, administered judiciously using small doses of benzodiazepines and narcotics. Initiation of NPPV is usually more labor intensive than invasive mechanical ventilation, but only until adaptation is successful, and improved outcomes in appropriate patients make it worthwhile.

14. **How do I monitor patients receiving NPPV in the acute setting?**

Patients started on NPPV in the acute setting require close monitoring, as dictated by the acuity of their illness. Just because they avoided intubation does not mean that they require a lower level of attention, so unless they have stabilized and can tolerate lengthy periods (>30 min) without mask ventilation, they should be placed in an ICU or step-down unit. Subjective responses are important initially, particularly comfort and respiratory distress (see Table 66-3). Respiratory rate and stern-ocleidomastoid muscle activity should be diminishing, and abdominal paradox (if present) should be abolished. Synchrony with the ventilator is important, and air leaks should be minimized. (Remember that bilevel ventilators have fixed leaks through the exhalation port to eliminate CO_2.) Oximetry should be monitored continuously at first, and blood gases should be obtained periodically (usually within the first hour or two, and then as clinically indicated, to ascertain changes in $PaCO_2$).

15. **How about gastric tubes?**

Although gastric tubes were recommended routinely in the past for patients receiving full-face mask ventilation, the risk of vomiting into the mask and aspirating appears to be quite small, and this is no longer recommended. Feeding tubes are usually unnecessary because most patients receiving NPPV are able to tolerate periods of time off the device to permit eating by mouth. For patients too ill to eat, a feeding tube can be inserted nasally, but it should be a small-bore tube to minimize leaking under the mask seal and the potential for facial trauma.

16. **How should NPPV for acute respiratory failure be discontinued?**

No controlled trials have yet examined this question. Most clinicians await patient stabilization as indicated by adequate oxygenation (O_2 saturation > 90% on $FiO_2 \leq 40\%$ or equivalent; expiratory pressure ≤ 5 cmH$_2$O) and amelioration of respiratory distress (respiratory rate ≤ 24) during ventilator use. The patient is then removed from assisted ventilation and is observed while breathing supplemental O$_2$ as needed. Patients who develop increasing respiratory distress or deterioration of gas exchange are placed back on NPPV at the previous settings and are allowed to rest for a few hours, with weaning tried again periodically. Alternatively, some investigators lower the inspiratory pressure, as with pressure support weaning. Some patients, particularly those with cardiogenic pulmonary edema, who may improve rapidly, remove the mask themselves when they feel ready to breathe unassisted.

17. **What are the indications for NPPV in chronic respiratory failure?**
NPPV is indicated when symptomatic nocturnal hypoventilation develops in a wide variety of slowly progressive neuromuscular disorders such as limb girdle muscular dystrophy, postpolio syndrome, and multiple sclerosis. Ideally, assisted ventilation is started before the

---

TABLE 66-4.   SELECTION GUIDELINES FOR NONINVASIVE POSITIVE-PRESSURE VENTILATION USE IN CHRONIC RESPIRATORY FAILURE

1. Symptoms of hypoventilation or poor sleep
   - Morning headache or fatigue
   - Daytime hypersomnolence
   - Pulmonary function testing abnormalities
   - FVC ≤ 50% of predicted, maximal inspiratory pressure ≤ 60 cmH$_2$O, or gas exchange abnormalities
2. Evidence of nocturnal hypoventilation (O$_2$ saturation ≤ 88% for ≥ 5 min) or daytime hypercapnia (PaCO$_2$ ≥ 45 mmHg)*
3. Appropriate condition
   - Slowly progressive neuromuscular disorder
   - Chest wall deformities
   - Obstructive sleep apnea unresponsive to CPAP
   - Obesity-related hypoventilation
   - Idiopathic hypoventilation
   - Cystic fibrosis
   - Chronic obstructive pulmonary disease
4. Relative contraindications:
   - A compromised ability to protect the airway
   - An inability to clear secretions
   - An uncooperative or unmotivated patient
   - Inadequate resources for long-term support
   - A need for continuous ventilatory support (NPPV may be used for appropriate candidates)

*Based on Medicare guidelines.

development of daytime hypercapnia to better control symptoms and to minimize the likelihood of a respiratory crisis before the patient can adequately adapt to NPPV. Medicare guidelines also permit initiation when the forced vital capacity (FVC) is ≤50% of predicted or when maximal inspiratory pressure is below 60 cmH$_2$O, even in the absence of symptoms. Patients with severe kyphoscoliosis or central hypoventilation are also good candidates. Obstructive sleep apnea with hypoventilation or obesity-hypoventilation syndrome with persistent hypercapnia despite nasal CPAP therapy are also appropriate indications, although the very obese may require high inspiratory pressures. Obesity hypoventilators constituted the largest and most rapidly growing subgroup of patients receiving home NPPV, according to a recent survey from Switzerland (Table 66-4).

Use of long-term NPPV in patients with COPD is controversial (*see* Question 21), but it has been used successfully in cystic fibrosis patients with hypercapnic respiratory failure as a bridge to potential lung transplantation. Relative contraindications for long-term NPPV include the inability to protect the airway, the inability to cooperate with the technique, or inadequate financial or caregiver resources. Patients needing continuous ventilatory support are usually managed with invasive mechanical ventilation, although some can be managed successfully for many years using noninvasive techniques.

18. How do you initiate and help patients adapt to long-term NPPV?

There is no universally accepted way to initiate NPPV for chronic respiratory failure. Some clinicians prefer initiation during a brief hospital admission to permit close patient monitoring and adjustment of the ventilator. Others favor titration of pressures in the sleep laboratory to eliminate apneas and hypopneas. As long as the patient has fairly stable respiratory insufficiency, others may prefer to initiate the patient at home, gradually increasing pressures as tolerated (starting with low initial pressures, i.e., 8–10 cmH$_2$O inspiratory and 3–4 cmH$_2$O expiratory), sometimes waiting weeks or even months while the patient adapts. Initially, patients may tolerate the mask only for an hour at a time. Many complain of discomfort related to the mask or air pressure and have difficulty becoming accustomed to the sensation of a foreign object on their face. However, over time, they gradually become tolerant of the higher pressures (i.e., inspiratory pressure ranging up to 20 cmH$_2$O or more) associated with improvements in nocturnal and daytime gas exchange and resolution of symptoms. Daytime PaCO$_2$ need not be normalized, and some patients tolerate daytime PaCO$_2$s in the 50- or even 60-mmHg range with good control of symptoms as long as they use NPPV during sleep to avoid worsening of hypoventilation.

19. What are the potential complications of NPPV?

If candidates for NPPV are carefully selected, the modality is safe and most complications are minor. The most frequently encountered complications are mask related. Discomfort, nasal dryness, and congestion are common, sometimes occurring in the same patient. Remedies for nasal dryness include use of nasal saline or humidification; for congestion, topical decongestants, steroids, and oral antihistamine–decongestant combinations can be used.

Other frequently encountered complications with standard nasal masks include eye irritation, caused by air leaking under the mask seal, and nasal bridge redness or ulceration, caused by excessive mask pressure, often during attempts to reduce air leaking. Although some earlier reports have observed nasal ulceration in up to 40% of patients treated with NPPV in the acute setting, minimizing strap tension, switching to newer masks with softer silicone seals, and the routine use of artificial skin over the bridge of the nose have rendered it an unusual occurrence. Acneiform rashes that develop at areas of mask and skin contact may respond to topical steroids or antibiotics. Gastric insufflation and flatulence are also common but are rarely severe enough to warrant discontinuation, probably because insufflation pressures are usually low. Aspiration is a rare complication as long as NPPV is reserved for patients who can adequately protect their airway.

Some patients (15–30%, in most studies) cannot tolerate NPPV, usually because of discomfort from mask or air pressure, and less often because of claustrophobia. The clinician should be willing to make frequent adjustments, to try different interfaces, and to not give up too easily. Coaching, encouragement, and judicious use of sedation may be helpful in achieving patient tolerance. For patients with chronic respiratory failure who are unable to tolerate the mask or who fail to improve after an adequate trial of NPPV, alternative noninvasive ventilators (e.g., body ventilators) may be successful. For patients with acute respiratory failure, intubation is usually necessary if NPPV fails.

20. **When should humidification be used with NPPV?**
Although there are few published reports examining this question, humidification probably enhances tolerance and is recommended for NPPV applications of more than 6–12 hours. Humidification may also reduce the increase in nasal resistance induced by the high flow rates associated with air leaks. Humidification should certainly be tried in patients complaining of nasal or mouth dryness who fail to respond to local measures such as the use of nasal saline. Complaints of dryness are more common during the winter months or in arid climates and are associated with air leaking, particularly through the mouth. When patients are using bilevel ventilators, heat and moisture exchangers (i.e., artificial noses) should be avoided because of interference with triggering and cycling of the ventilator.

21. **How common is air leakage during NPPV? How much does it compromise efficacy, and what should be done about it?**
NPPV circuits are leaky by design. Some leaks are intentional, as is the case with exhalation valves to reduce rebreathing on portable pressure-limited ventilators. However, unintentional leaks are also common, depending on the type of mask or interface used. With nasal ventilation, some leaking occurs around the mask, but most occurs through the mouth. Full-face masks and mouthpieces also are associated with leaking (through the nose with the latter). These leaks may interfere with ventilator triggering and cycling and may be enough to impair ventilator efficacy. Most of the time, however, patients do well with NPPV despite air leaking and may have nearly normal sleep quality.

The consequences of air leaking may depend partly on the ventilator mode used. Some pressure-limited ventilators sustain inspiratory airflow to compensate for leaks and to maintain mask pressure. Volume-limited ventilators are unable to alter inspiratory airflow in response to leaks, but air leaks may still be compensated for by an increase in tidal volume. Chin straps may reduce leaking through the mouth but do not eliminate it. Full-face masks may be used if air leaks through the mouth with nasal masks are excessive, but oronasal masks may seal poorly on the chin. If so, a mouthpiece or total-face mask can be considered.

22. **When should NPPV be used for hypoxemic respiratory failure?**
Although a number of controlled studies have demonstrated improved outcomes when patients with hypoxemic (type 1) respiratory failure have been managed noninvasively, there is wide agreement that NPPV is less successful for these patients than for those with hypercapnic (type 2) respiratory failure. In addition, some have objected to the breadth of the hypoxemic respiratory failure category, comprising ARDS, pneumonia, and cardiogenic pulmonary edema. Overall, favorable findings could reflect benefit in one subgroup and obscure harm to another. Thus, clinicians are cautioned to select patients with hypoxemic respiratory failure very carefully when using NPPV and to monitor them closely. Also, more faith should be placed in studies that examine the individual subgroups.

Ferrer M, Esquinas A, Leon M, et al: Noninvasive ventilation in severe hypoxemic respiratory failure. A randomized clinical trial. Am J Respir Crit Care Med 168:1438–1444, 2003.

23. **Compare CPAP versus NPPV for acute cardiogenic pulmonary edema.**
Both CPAP and NPPV (the combination of positive expiratory pressure and an inspiratory pressure boost) are effective in alleviating respiratory distress, improving vital signs and gas

exchange, and avoiding intubation in patients with acute cardiogenic pulmonary edema, especially those with hypercapnia. A few studies have compared the two directly, a notable early one observing an increase in the myocardial infarction rate in the NPPV patients. Subsequent studies have not confirmed this observation (although they were careful to exclude patients with active ischemia or acute infarctions). CPAP has some potential advantages, in that it can be administered using less-sophisticated, cheaper equipment, and patient–ventilator synchrony is not an issue. By incorporating inspiratory assistance, however, NPPV may more rapidly alleviate dyspnea, lower $PaCO_2$ (in retainers), and improve oxygenation. However, the studies have not shown that NPPV reduces intubation, mortality rates, or lengths of hospital stays better than CPAP. Since these global outcomes appear to be similar between the two modes, current recommendations are to begin with CPAP (although NPPV will work as well) and to add inspiratory pressure support if the patient remains dyspneic or is found to be hypercarbic.

Nava S, Carbone G, DiBattista N, et al: Noninvasive ventilation in cardiogenic pulmonary edema: A multicenter randomized trial. Am J Respir Crit Care Med 168(12):1432–1437, 2003.

24. **What is the role of NPPV in weaning from invasive mechanical ventilation?**
Several studies have shown that patients who are extubated early and are placed on NPPV before they meet standard extubation criteria have higher eventual weaning rates and fewer pneumonias, spend less time on the ventilator and in the ICU, and have lower mortality rates than controls who remain intubated and are weaned in the routine fashion. The evidence supporting this approach is now considered level A. However, caution is advised when planning an early extubation. This approach is mainly for COPD patients, who constituted most of the patients in the studies. Candidates should be excellent candidates for NPPV otherwise, medically stable with intact cough and minimal secretions and able to breathe comfortably using pressure support settings that will be used during NPPV, and should not have been a difficult intubation.

Even more controversial is the use of NPPV to treat extubation failure, the occurrence of respiratory failure after an extubation according to standard criteria. Extubation failure is known to impart a poor prognosis; mortality rates exceed 40% in some studies. Thus, it has been proposed that use of NPPV to avoid reintubation might lower these. However, a few randomized, controlled trials have failed to show benefit using this approach, and one large multinational trial showed an excess ICU mortality attributable to NPPV thought to be related to a delay in needed intubation. It is notable that these trials had few COPD patients (approximately 10%) and that there was a tendency for reduced reintubations in the COPD subgroup of the multinational trial, which had too few patients to show statistical significance. Currently, the best recommendation is not to use NPPV routinely to prevent extubation failure, but when patients with extubation failure, mainly those with COPD, appear otherwise to be good NPPV candidates, a trial is reasonable with the proviso that needed intubation is not unduly delayed if there is no improvement within the first 2 hours.

Esteban A, Frutos-Vivar F, Ferguson ND, et al: Noninvasive positive-pressure ventilation for respiratory failure after extubation. N Eng J Med 350(24):2452–2460, 2004.
Ferrer M, Esquinas A, Arancibia F, et al: Noninvasive ventilation during persistent weaning failure. A randomized controlled trial. Am J Respir Crit Care Med 168:70–76, 2003.

25. **Should NPPV be used for patients with severe, stable COPD?**
As discussed above, NPPV has proven effective in avoiding intubation and in improving global outcomes in patients with acute respiratory failure due to COPD exacerbations. However, despite studies extending back more than 2 decades (with the earlier ones using negative pressure ventilation), it remains unclear how beneficial NIV is in patients with severe, stable COPD (meaning those who are in their stable state with severe airway obstruction and marked functional limitations). The current evidence (based on a few randomized controlled trials, the most recent from Italy) suggests that symptomatic patients (with fatigue, morning headaches,

and hypersomnolence) with substantial chronic CO_2 retention (i.e., daytime $PaCO_2 \geq 50$ mmHg), sleep-disordered breathing or frequent nocturnal desaturations despite O_2 supplementation, poor tolerance of O_2 supplementation with greater CO_2 retention, or frequent hospitalizations (e.g., "revolving door" or "frequent flyer" patients) are most likely to benefit.

Anticipated benefits include amelioration of symptoms, a lower increase in CO_2 retention over time, a better quality of life, and, possibly, fewer hospitalizations. Even when patients appear to be good candidates, successful adaptation is a challenge, with as few as 50% of patients continuing to use the therapy after 6 months, even when initiated under ideal circumstances in a chronic ventilator unit.

CHAPTER 67

TRADITIONAL INVASIVE VENTILATION

Gregory Diette, MD, and Roy Brower, MD

1. **How do hypercapnic and hypoxic respiratory failure differ? When is mechanical ventilation needed in each?**

   Hypercapnic respiratory failure means there is inadequate ventilation (i.e., movement of air in and out of the lungs), and it is marked by an increase in $PaCO_2$. It may be caused by disorders of the central nervous system (CNS), peripheral nerves, muscles, airways, lung parenchyma, and chest wall. When hypercapnic respiratory failure is acute, $PaCO_2$ increases over a relatively short time (i.e., minutes to hours) and arterial pH decreases. Clinical signs may include agitation, tachypnea, accessory muscle use, cyanosis, and decline of consciousness. In such cases, mechanical ventilation may be necessary to prevent death.

   Hypoxic respiratory failure is marked by inadequate arterial oxygenation (i.e., PaO_2 or oxyhemoglobin saturation). This frequently occurs despite adequate spontaneous ventilation (i.e., normal or even low $PaCO_2$). Mechanical ventilation is sometimes helpful in managing hypoxemia, even though ventilation may be adequate. For example, in acute respiratory distress syndrome (ARDS), positive end-expiratory pressure (PEEP) may be useful for improving arterial oxygenation. In addition, by assuming some or all of the work of breathing, the ventilator may reduce the oxygen cost of breathing, allowing utilization of blood oxygen by other critical organs such as the brain and the heart.

2. **What are some causes of hypercapnic respiratory failure?**

   Disorders of the CNS with diminished respiratory drive
   - General anesthesia
   - Narcotic or barbiturate overdose
   - Brainstem stroke or trauma

   Disorders of the spinal cord
   - High cervical spinal cord trauma
   - Cervical myelitis
   - Amyotrophic lateral sclerosis

   Disorders of peripheral nerves and muscles
   - Myasthenia gravis
   - Guillain–Barré syndrome
   - Neuromuscular blockade
   - Poliomyelitis
   - Muscular dystrophy

   Disorders of the thoracic cage with increased chest wall stiffness
   - Kyphoscoliosis
   - Morbid obesity

   Disorders of the lung parenchyma (increased lung stiffness)
   - Pulmonary fibrosis
   - Sarcoidosis

   Disorders of airways
   - Asthma
   - Chronic obstructive pulmonary disease (COPD)
   - Cystic fibrosis
   - Bronchiolitis obliterans

3. **In addition to recognizing respiratory failure, what else should be considered before initiating mechanical ventilation?**

First, how rapid is the decline in respiratory status? Chronic hypercapnic respiratory failure is generally not an indication for mechanical ventilation. For example, a COPD patient with a $PaCO_2$ of 80 mmHg, an arterial pH of 7.37, and a PaO_2 of 65 mmHg on FiO_2 of 0.30 has adequate metabolic compensation for the hypercapnia and probably does not require mechanical ventilation. In contrast, a patient with acute asthma whose $PaCO_2$ has risen from 35 mmHg to 53 mmHg while in the emergency department may need mechanical ventilation to prevent further deterioration, which could lead to death.

Second, can more conservative measures reverse respiratory failure without resorting to intubation and mechanical ventilation? For example, hypoventilation from opiate overdose may be reversed rapidly with an intravenous injection of naloxone.

Third, is mechanical ventilation consistent with the patient's overall care goals? For example, some patients with terminal illness may request that mechanical ventilation not be used.

4. **What are the usual modes of mechanical ventilation?**
   - Assist-control (A-C)
   - Synchronized intermittent mandatory ventilation (SIMV)
   - Pressure support (PS)
   - Pressure control (PC)

   Tobin MJ: Principles and Practice of Mechanical Ventilation. New York, McGraw-Hill, 1994, pp. 191–318.
   http://www.ccmtutorials.com/rs/mv

5. **What is A-C ventilation?**

In this mode of ventilation, clinicians select a minimum respiratory rate, tidal volume, and inspiratory flow rate. If the patient makes no or very weak inspiratory efforts, then the ventilator provides "controlled" breaths by blowing air into the patient's lungs at the prescribed flow rate until the prescribed tidal volume is achieved.

The time interval between controlled breaths is determined by the respiratory rate selected by the clinician. If the patient makes an adequate inspiratory effort during this interval, the machine responds by blowing air at the prescribed inspiratory flow rate until the prescribed tidal volume is achieved (Fig. 67-1). This is an "assisted" breath. If a patient's intrinsic respiratory rate exceeds the minimum rate for controlled breaths, all breathing will be assisted. With assisted breaths, the work of breathing is shared between the patient and the ventilator. With either assisted or controlled breaths, the tidal volume is the same regardless of patient effort.

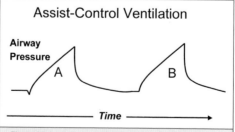

Figure 67-1. Assist-control ventilation. Breath A is an assisted breath. The initial downward airway pressure deflection represents the patient's inspiratory effort, before the ventilator begins its positive pressure assist. Breath B is delivered by the ventilator when no inspiratory effort is detected.

A-C ventilation is often the mode chosen immediately after initiation of mechanical ventilation. It is useful when the intent is to have the ventilator assume most or all of the work of breathing, as in neuromuscular blockade, respiratory muscle fatigue, or profound neuromuscular weakness.

6. **How does the ventilator "know" that a patient is trying to initiate a breath?**
   The ventilator monitors pressure at or near the endotracheal tube. A patient's efforts to inspire cause the pressures in the airways to fall below the level at end-expiration, before the beginning of the inspiratory effort. If the airway pressure falls below a trigger threshold, the ventilator responds by raising airway pressure to assist the inspiratory effort. Typically, the trigger threshold is set to 1–2 cmH$_2$O below the airway pressure at end-expiration.

7. **What is SIMV?**
   As in the A-C mode, with SIMV, clinicians select a minimum respiratory rate, tidal volume, and inspiratory flow rate. If there are no or very weak inspiratory efforts, the ventilator provides controlled breaths in the same manner as in the A-C mode. Unlike A-C, however, SIMV does not assist any patient inspiratory efforts above the minimum. For any additional attempts to inspire, the patient must breathe on his or her own (Fig. 67-2). For example, if the clinician-selected minimum respiratory rate is 6 breaths per minute (bpm) and the patient makes inspiratory efforts 20 times per minute, only 6 bpm will be assisted by the ventilator; the remaining 14 breaths will be unassisted. The size of the unassisted breaths will be whatever the patient can achieve on his or her own.

   The term *synchronized* means that the machine-assisted breaths occur during patient efforts, if any. As with the A-C mode, the SIMV ventilator monitors airway pressure at or near the endotracheal tube to detect the onset of the patient's inspiratory efforts. Synchronization prevents ventilator-delivered breaths from occurring in the middle of a patient-initiated breath.

   SIMV was initially developed for weaning, to allow the frequency of assisted breaths to be gradually reduced while the patient resumes an increasing proportion of the work of breathing. SIMV may also be useful in patients requiring substantial ventilatory assistance but whose respiratory rates are too high.

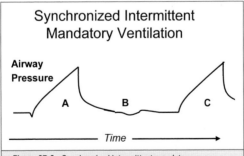

Figure 67-2. Synchronized intermittent mandatory ventilation. Breath A is an assisted breath, triggered by the patient's effort. Breath B is a spontaneous, unassisted breath. Breath C is delivered by the ventilator when no inspiratory effort is detected.

8. **What is PS ventilation?**
   In the PS mode, the ventilator responds to a patient's inspiratory effort by raising pressure at or near the endotracheal tube to a clinician-selected level, such as 15 cmH$_2$O above the airway pressure level at end-expiration (Fig. 67-3). The ventilator maintains this pressure until the

end of the patient's inspiratory effort, at which point airway pressure returns to the appropriate level for expiration (either 0 or the PEEP level, if any). The respiratory rate is determined entirely by the patient.

PS ventilation is often used as an alternative to A-C or SIMV. In the PS mode, the patient has more control over inspiratory flow rate, tidal volume, and duration of inspiration. If the patient feels more dyspneic, he or she may take larger tidal volumes at more rapid inspiratory flow rates. If dyspnea or requirements for ventilation decrease, he or she may take smaller breaths at lower flow rates. This is in contrast to the stereotyped breaths provided in A-C or SIMV. Hence, breathing may be more comfortable on PS.

Many clinicians also use PS for weaning. When used for this purpose, the level of PS is gradually reduced in steps (usually over several hours), allowing the patient to gradually resume the work of breathing with each breath.

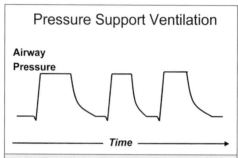

Figure 67-3. Pressure support ventilation. Each breath is supported by the ventilator after an inspiratory effort by the patient (signified by the brief downward deflections in airway pressure). The ventilator responds to the patient's efforts by raising airway pressure to the clinician-selected level. Airway pressure is maintained at this level until the end of the patient's inspiratory effort. The intervals between breaths and the duration of inspiration are variable.

9. **Are there contraindications to PS ventilation?**
In the PS mode, the ventilator delivers positive pressure only in response to a patient's inspiratory efforts. Therefore, important contraindications to PS ventilation are inadequate respiratory drive and very weak inspiratory effort. These may occur in patients with disorders of the brainstem or of the nerves and muscles.

10. **What is the right amount of PS?**
When the intent is to assume most of the work of breathing, the right level of PS is one at which the patient is comfortable and is receiving adequate ventilation. Comfort can be assessed from the respiratory rate (<25–30 bpm is usually acceptable) and the level of effort the patient makes with each breath. Use of accessory muscles, diaphoresis, and intercostal retractions are signs of excessive (and uncomfortable) effort. Higher levels of PS are usually necessary when the compliance of the respiratory system is low (as in ARDS), the airway resistance is high (as in asthma or COPD), or the patient is able to make only weak inspiratory efforts (as in neuromuscular diseases). A useful starting level of pressure support is approximately 10–15 cmH$_2$O. Adjustments in this level should be made quickly (within minutes) after assessing the patient's comfort and adequacy of ventilation.

KEY POINTS: VENTILATOR SETTINGS THAT CLINICIANS MUST CHOOSE

1. Ventilator mode

2. Tidal volume (if using assist-control, pressure-regulated volume control, auto-flow, or adaptive pressure ventilation) or inspiratory airway pressure (if using pressure control or pressure support)

3. FiO_2

4. Positive end-expiratory pressure

5. Minimum respiratory rate (if using assist-control, pressure-regulated volume control, auto-flow, adaptive pressure, or pressure control ventilation)

11. **What is PC mode?**

PC is similar to PS in that the ventilator raises the pressure at or near the endotracheal tube to a physician-selected level, such as 15 cmH_2O above the level at end-expiration. In PC mode, the physician also prescribes a minimum respiratory rate and the duration of inspiration. If a patient on PC has no inspiratory effort, the ventilator will cycle at the rate prescribed by the physician. The tidal volume will depend primarily on the inspiratory increment in airway pressure and the compliance of the patient's lungs and chest wall. If a patient makes inspiratory efforts, the ventilator will respond to the efforts in a manner similar to pressure support mode (Fig. 67-4). In this situation, tidal volume depends on the intensity of the patient's inspiratory efforts in addition to the increment in airway pressure and the lung and chest wall compliance.

PC is sometimes used in patients with acute lung injury or ARDS because physicians are concerned that the ventilator may actually worsen lung injury by causing overdistention or excessive stretch of some lung tissues. The terms *barotrauma* and *volutrauma* are frequently used to describe this problem. Limiting the pressure that the ventilator generates with each breath in PC may reduce risks of barotrauma or volutrauma. Similar beneficial effects can be achieved in the

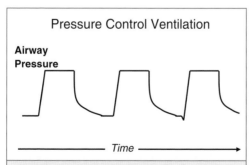

Figure 67-4. Pressure control ventilation. Each breath is supported by the ventilator, which raises airway pressure above the end-expiratory airway pressure by an amount prescribed by the physician. The duration of each inspiration is also prescribed by the physician. In the first two breaths, the ventilator has cycled according to the minimum rate prescribed by the physician. The third breath was triggered by patient effort.

A-C mode by lowering the tidal volume until the airway pressure during inspiration decreases below the limit considered safe.

12. **What is pressure-regulated volume control (PRVC)?**

This is a hybrid mode in which a clinician prescribes a tidal volume (and also a minimum respiratory rate, PEEP, and FiO_2). The ventilator then determines empirically the level of airway pressure that must be applied to generate the prescribed tidal volume. Once this airway pressure is identified, the ventilator continues to apply this pressure during inspiration and monitors the resulting tidal volumes. If tidal volumes subsequently fall below or rise above the prescribed tidal volume, the ventilator increases or decreases, respectively, the inspiratory pressure to restore the tidal volume back to the prescribed level. Similar hybrid modes go by different names including "auto-flow" and "adaptive pressure ventilation."

With these hybrid modes, the ventilator functions as if it is in a PC mode with each breath. However, unlike the PC mode, with these hybrid modes, the ventilator monitors tidal volumes and automatically adjusts inspiratory airway pressure to maintain tidal volumes at the prescribed level.

For the same tidal volume, peak inspiratory airway pressures tend to be lower with PC (and hybrid modes) than with the volume A-C mode. The reason for this difference is that with PC (and hybrid) modes, inspiratory flow is rapid in early inspiration but then decreases to low levels at end-inspiration. The lower peak inspiratory pressures with PC and PRVC may help to avoid frequent high-pressure alarms (see questions 27 and 28). However, this should not be interpreted to mean the risks of barotrauma or volutrauma are lessened with these modes. These risks are related to mechanical forces that result from volumes delivered to alveoli and small bronchioles.

13. **In a paralyzed patient, what minute ventilation can be expected with each of the following ventilator settings:**
    A. A-C, tidal volume = 750 mL, minimum respiratory rate = 10 bpm?
    B. SIMV, tidal volume = 750 mL, minimum respiratory rate = 10 bpm?
    C. PS, 20 cmH_2O?

    A. 7.5 liters/min. The patient will receive 10 bpm of 750 mL. All breaths will be controlled.

    B. 7.5 liters/min. The patient will receive 10 bpm of 750 mL. There will be no additional unsupported breaths. In paralyzed patients, A-C and SIMV are identical.

    C. None! PS only supports breaths initiated by the patient. A patient who is unable to make an inspiratory effort will receive no ventilation in the PS mode. (Most, but not all, ventilators have volume-cycled backup modes that automatically turn on when apnea occurs.)

14. **In a patient making 20 inspiratory efforts per minute, what ventilation can be expected with each of the following settings:**
    A. A-C, tidal volume = 750 mL, minimum respiratory rate = 10 bpm?
    B. SIMV, tidal volume = 750 mL, minimum respiratory rate = 10 bpm?
    C. PS, 10 cmH_2O?

    A. 15 liters/min. Each inspiratory effort will be assisted, and each tidal volume will equal 750 mL. The minute ventilation will be 20 bpm × 0.75 liters/breath = 15 liters/min.

    B. >7.5 liters/min. It is not possible to know the exact amount. Ten breaths of 750 mL will be assisted by the ventilator. The volume of the other 10 spontaneous breaths will be determined by patient effort and the mechanics of the lungs and chest wall. Each spontaneous breath may be a different tidal volume and can be less than, equal to, or greater than 750 mL.

    C. Impossible to calculate. We know the respiratory rate will be 20 bpm, but we do not know the size of the tidal volumes. The three factors that determine tidal volume in patients on PS are (1) the level of pressure support, (2) the amount of patient effort (i.e., muscle force), and (3) the lung mechanics (i.e., the resistance of the airways and the compliance of the lungs and chest wall). Minute ventilation can be assessed in patients on PS by observing the tidal volumes and multiplying by the rate. Most ventilators report the size of each tidal volume at the end of each breath. Many ventilators also report a value for minute ventilation.

15. **What are static compliance and plateau pressure?**
Static compliance of any structure represents its distensibility (i.e., how easy is it to increase its volume). In mathematic terms, compliance equals the change in volume divided by the change in transmural pressure. Static compliance of the respiratory system represents the combined distensibility of the lungs and chest wall.
It is easy to measure this compliance in a patient on a ventilator by dividing the tidal volume by the change in alveolar pressure that occurs from end-expiration to end-inspiration. The alveolar pressure at end-expiration is usually the same as the pressure at the endotracheal tube (0 or the level of PEEP). The pressure in the alveoli at end-inspiration is measured by occluding the expiratory conduit from the ventilator at the end of the tidal volume inspiration and waiting approximately 0.5–1.0 sec. The pressure that the ventilator reports after this brief interval is called the **plateau pressure** and represents the average pressure in the alveoli at end-inspiration.
Static compliance of the respiratory system is then calculated as follows:

$$\text{Static compliance} = (\text{tidal volume})/(\text{plateau pressure} - \text{PEEP})$$

For example, if the tidal volume = 600 mL, PEEP = 5 cmH_2O, and plateau pressure = 25 cmH_2O, then the respiratory system compliance is

$$600 \text{ mL}/(25 \text{ } cmH_2O - 5 \text{ } cmH_2O) = 30 \text{ mL}/cmH_2O$$

Normal respiratory system compliance for an average-sized adult is approximately 80–100 mL/cmH_2O. Conditions associated with low respiratory system compliance are pulmonary edema (cardiogenic and noncardiogenic), severe pneumonia, pulmonary fibrosis, kyphoscoliosis, and marked obesity.

Kreit JW, Eschenbacher WL: The physiology of spontaneous and mechanical ventilation. Clin Chest Med 9:11–21, 1988.

16. **What is PEEP used for?**
When no PEEP is applied, the ventilator allows airway pressure to fall to atmospheric pressure during expiration. When PEEP is applied, the ventilator maintains airway pressure at the physician-selected level of PEEP during expiration. PEEP is helpful for maintaining arterial oxygenation in many patients in whom intrapulmonary shunt causes hypoxemia, as in ARDS. PEEP improves oxygenation in these patients by stabilizing alveoli that tend to collapse. This may allow adequate arterial oxygenation without using potentially toxic concentrations of inspired oxygen (FiO_2). In some patients, PEEP may be necessary to maintain oxygenation even with high levels of FiO_2.

17. **How much PEEP should be used in patients with hypoxemic respiratory failure?**
PEEP can have deleterious effects. For example, risks of pneumothorax and other forms of barotrauma may increase when PEEP is applied because the airway pressures and distending forces in the lungs increase. Cardiac output also decreases when PEEP is applied because pressures in the chest rise, impeding venous return. When cardiac output decreases, delivery of oxygen to peripheral tissues decreases. Because of these and other deleterious effects of PEEP, most clinicians use only enough PEEP to achieve adequate oxygenation (i.e., oxyhemoglobin saturation of approximately 90%) at levels of FiO_2 that are believed to be safe (approximately ≤ 50–70%). Recently, some investigators have recommended using additional amounts of PEEP in patients with ARDS to prevent injurious mechanical forces associated with opening and reclosing of the unstable alveoli.

Shapiro BA, Cane RD, Harrison RA: Positive end-expiratory pressure therapy in adults with special reference to acute lung injury: A review of the literature and suggested clinical correlations. Crit Care Med 12:127–141, 1984.

18. **What is continuous positive airway pressure (CPAP)?**

With CPAP, a constant level of positive pressure throughout inspiration and expiration. Like PEEP, CPAP stabilizes alveoli that tend to collapse. It is useful when intrapulmonary shunt causes hypoxemia.

Some clinicians use CPAP during weaning when hypoxemia is still a problem but ventilatory assistance is not required. Also, setting the ventilator to CPAP = 0 cmH_2O will allow a patient to breathe on his or her own but still be connected to the ventilator circuit and its alarms.

http://www.ccmtutorials.com/rs/mv/page14.htm

19. **What is auto-PEEP?**

Auto-PEEP (synonymous with intrinsic PEEP) is when the pressure in the alveoli at the end of expiration exceeds pressure at the airway opening (i.e., the endotracheal tube in a patient receiving positive pressure ventilation). Normally, the pressure in the alveoli at the end of expiration equals the pressure at the airway opening (i.e., the mouth or endotracheal tube). However, in some patients there is insufficient time for the respiratory system to empty down to the normal relaxation volume (i.e., normal functional residual capacity). This is common in patients with airflow obstruction, as occurs in asthma. Rapid respiratory rates and large tidal volume also contribute to the development of auto-PEEP.

Rossi A, Polese G, Brandi G, Conti G: Intrinsic positive end-expiratory pressure (PEEPi). Intens Care Med 21:522–536, 1995.

20. **What are the effects of auto-PEEP?**

Auto-PEEP can have deleterious effects on the respiratory and circulatory systems. Venous return and cardiac output decrease because, as with external PEEP, the pressures in the chest surrounding the heart rise. Auto-PEEP also increases pulmonary vascular resistance because the high alveolar pressures tend to compress alveolar capillaries. This increases the work of the right ventricle to pump blood through the pulmonary circulation.

The work required to trigger the ventilator increases when there is auto-PEEP because the inspiratory muscles must first contract with enough force to lower alveolar pressure to 0 (or the external level of PEEP) before the ventilator can detect the inspiratory effort. Consider a patient with auto-PEEP of 7 cmH_2O (i.e., alveolar pressure at end-expiration 7 cmH_2O greater than the pressure in the endotracheal tube) and a ventilator trigger threshold of 1 cmH_2O below atmospheric pressure. This patient must generate 8 cmH_2O of negative pressure with his or her inspiratory muscles before the pressure in the endotracheal tube decreases to the trigger threshold. In contrast, if this patient had no auto-PEEP, the ventilator could be triggered with only 1 cmH_2O of negative pressure.

21. **How do you detect auto-PEEP in a ventilated patient?**

Auto-PEEP is not typically measured or reported by the ventilator. To measure auto-PEEP in a patient on a ventilator, briefly occlude the exhalation port of the ventilator a moment before the next inspiration would occur. When the exhalation port is occluded, any expiratory airflow ceases and the pressure the ventilator measures and displays on its manometer equals the pressure everywhere throughout the ventilator tubes, bronchi, and alveoli. Hence, this pressure equals auto-PEEP. This is, unfortunately, difficult to perform, especially in patients with rapid respiratory rates.

22. **How can auto-PEEP be minimized or eliminated?**

There are three general approaches to managing auto-PEEP:
1. Treat any reversible airway constriction and inflammation. By so doing, airway resistance may decrease, leading to increased expiratory flow rates.

2. Decrease tidal volume. This maneuver may cause hypercapnia, which may have deleterious effects that must be considered relative to those of auto-PEEP.
3. Increase the time available for exhalation. This can be accomplished in two ways: (1) shorten the duration of inspiration by increasing the inspiratory flow rate or (2) decrease the respiratory rate. To lower the respiratory rate, it may be necessary to sedate the patient. As with decreased tidal volume, the decreased respiratory rate may lead to hypercapnia.

KEY POINTS: WAYS TO REDUCE AUTO–POSITIVE END-EXPIRATORY PRESSURE

1. Treating reversible causes of airway constriction or inflammation

2. Decreasing tidal volume

3. Decreasing respiratory rate

4. Increasing exhalation time by shortening the duration of inspiration

23. **What do all those ventilator alarms do?**
The alarms on the ventilator are designed to alert people caring for the patient that there may be a harmful situation. The alarms are grouped according to three main functions, as shown in Table 67-1.

TABLE 67-1. VENTILATOR ALARMS	
Type of Alarm	**Implication of Alarm**
Inadequate ventilation	
Low exhaled volume	Air leak or disconnected tubes
Low minute ventilation	Air leak or low respiratory rate or tidal volumes
Low airway pressure	Air leak
Apnea	Loss of patient respiratory drive or disconnection from ventilator
Harmful physiology	
High airway pressure	Increased risk of barotrauma or mucus plug
High respiratory rate	Patient is agitated, or there is risk of overventilation or auto-PEEP
High inspiration-to-expiration time ratio (>1)	Consider adjusting the inspiratory flow rate or respiratory rate
Failure of the ventilator	
Power disconnect	Check the power supply
Low back-up battery	Check the back-up battery
Low pressure at the oxygen inlet	Check the oxygen supply

24. **Why are the ventilator alarms always going off?**

Each ventilator alarm has a threshold value that is set by the therapist or clinician depending on specific characteristics of individual patients. Serious consequences may result if problems are not quickly recognized and corrected, so alarms' thresholds are usually set at levels that make them very sensitive to potential problems. Unfortunately, in practical terms, high sensitivity usually comes at the expense of decreased specificity. Thus, the tradeoff for detecting all or nearly all dangerous situations is having to respond to many false alarms.

25. **What is peak inspiratory pressure?**

Peak inspiratory pressure is the highest pressure that occurs during the inspiratory portion of the cycle, usually at or near the end of inspiration. High peak inspiratory airway pressures usually reflect either narrowed airway (i.e., high airway resistance) or decreased respiratory compliance (i.e., stiff lungs or chest wall). Common causes of airway narrowing are bronchospasm (as in asthma and bronchitis), bronchial obstruction from secretions, or kinking of the endotracheal tube. Causes of decreased respiratory system compliance include ARDS, pulmonary edema, kyphoscoliosis, marked obesity, and tension pneumothorax. Peak inspiratory pressures also tend to rise, sometimes to alarming levels, when high inspiratory flow rates are used.

26. **Why do we have a high peak inspiratory pressure alarm?**

When a high peak pressure alarm is first heard, each of the potential causes should be considered quickly. Sometimes, a problem such as excessive secretions, a kinked endotracheal tube, or pneumothorax can be identified and rectified quickly. At other times, it is impossible to intervene to quickly decrease the peak inspiratory pressure without causing other, perhaps worse, problems. For example, in severe asthma, the high airway pressures are likely attributable to the high airway resistance and high inspiratory flow rates (selected to allow sufficient time for exhalation). If the peak flow rate is reduced, auto-PEEP will be worse. Under such circumstances, the best solution may be to increase the alarm threshold to decrease the number of subsequent false alarms.

27. **What causes a low exhaled volume alarm?**

The exhaled volume alarm is designed to sound when the volume of air that comes out during exhalation is less than a lower-limit threshold. If a patient is receiving a volume-cycled breath, this alarm should suggest that there is a leak in the system, allowing part of the intended tidal volume to escape without entering the patient's lungs. This may be caused by malposition of the endotracheal tube, a ruptured or inadequately inflated endotracheal cuff, or a disconnection of the endotracheal tube from the ventilator tubing. If a patient is on a pressure-cycled mode (i.e., PC or PS), this alarm may sound if the tidal volumes are lower than some minimal acceptable volume. This may signify that the patient is too weak to ventilate sufficiently at the current pressure setting.

CHAPTER 68

ALTERNATIVE INVASIVE VENTILATORY STRATEGIES

Septimiu D. Murgu, MD, and Catherine S. H. Sassoon, MD

1. **Why are alternative invasive ventilatory strategies needed? Name some of these strategies.**

   The use of conventional modes of mechanical ventilation in very ill patients may (1) fail to provide adequate gas exchange; (2) prevent direct control of patient effort, causing patient–ventilator asynchrony; (3) fail to prevent lung injury due to overdistention and under-recruitment of lung units; or (4) fail to maintain cardiac output due to high intrathoracic pressure. Alternative ventilatory strategies include pressure-controlled inverted ratio ventilation (PC-IRV), permissive hypercapnia (PH), airway pressure release ventilation (APRV), closed-loop ventilation, high-frequency ventilation (HFV), and partial liquid ventilation (PLV). Before discussing alternative ventilatory strategies, we will discuss the basic characteristics of a mechanical breath.

KEY POINTS: ALTERNATIVE LUNG-PROTECTIVE VENTILATION STRATEGIES

1. Alternative lung-protective ventilation strategies (LPVSs) include pressure-controlled inverted ratio ventilation (PC-IRV), APRV, high-frequency ventilation (HFV), and partial liquid ventilation (PLV).

2. PC-IRV and APRV are considered lung protective because the pressure limit is set, preventing alveolar overdistention, and its maintenance optimizes alveolar recruitment.

3. HFV is an extreme form of LPVS that uses subdead space tidal volumes and high levels of positive end-expiratory pressure (PEEP).

4. PLV uses perfluorocarbons, which, through their properties, act as a "liquid PEEP" to reopen collapsed alveoli.

5. There are insufficient data to support the use of these strategies over conventional mechanical ventilation with low tidal volumes.

---

2. **What are the basic characteristics of a ventilator breath?**

   A ventilator breath can be divided into three variables: the trigger, the target (i.e., the limit), and the cycle. The trigger variable initiates a breath. It is either controlled (by machine timer, called time-triggering) or assisted (by patient effort). The latter may be a pressure trigger (i.e., the patient's effort produces a pressure drop in the ventilator circuit) or a flow trigger (i.e., the patient's effort draws gas out of a continuous flow through the ventilator circuit). The gas delivery target, or limit, governs the gas flow; it is either a set flow or a set inspiratory pressure. The cycle terminates the breath. The breath is turned off when a certain set volume, time, flow, or pressure is reached (Fig. 68-1). Advances in ventilator technology have introduced new triggering and cycling methods to improve patient–ventilator synchrony and, potentially, patient comfort.

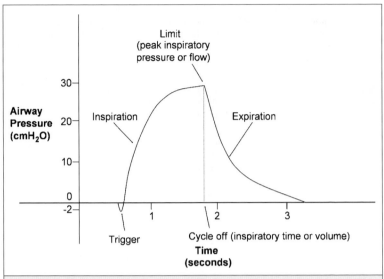

Figure 68-1. Airway pressure waveform of a mechanical breath during assist-control volume-cycled ventilation. The patient's inspiratory effort creates a pressure drop (the trigger variable) in the airway that the ventilator senses. The machine then delivers a breath of a predetermined flow (the limit variable) and volume (the cycle-off variable). The "limit" stops the breath from increasing, and the "cycle-off" switches the breath from inspiration to expiration.

3. **Explain PC-IRV and its indications.**

    PC-IRV is positive-pressure ventilation, in which the ventilator delivers a breath until a set target pressure and inspiratory time (I) greater than expiratory time (E) are reached, at which point the ventilator cycles off. During normal respiration, I is about one-half to one-third of E, so that I:E = 1:2 to 1:3.

    PC-IRV reverses the normal respiratory timing pattern, and the tidal volume (V_T) varies with each breath, depending on lung compliance and airway resistance. To maintain a constant V_T, volume-cycled ventilation with a low peak flow rate can be used, with or without an inspiratory pause, to achieve a goal similar to that of PC-IRV. However, most clinicians use PC-IRV to confine the peak pressure and to avoid lung overdistention.

    PC-IRV may benefit patients with acute respiratory distress syndrome (ARDS) and acute lung injury (ALI) who have poor oxygenation. These patients may manifest high peak airway pressures due to severely decreased lung compliance. Peak airway pressures of greater than 30 cmH$_2$O have been associated with parenchymal lung injury. Because PC-IRV sets a target pressure, it decreases elevated airway pressures. It also increases mean airway pressure, places all alveoli under the same sustained pressure, and improves oxygenation while preventing hyperinflation of the more compliant alveoli.

4. **Name some disadvantages of PC-IRV.**

    The higher mean airway pressure achieved during PC-IRV can decrease venous return and lower cardiac output if left ventricular preload is inadequate. In this mode, tidal volume varies depending on lung compliance, resistance, and patient effort. Therefore, if the volume alarms are not set properly, hypoventilation and acidosis may occur and go undetected. The higher the I:E ratio, the higher the potential for air trapping, resulting in intrinsic positive end-expiratory pressure (PEEPi). PEEPi is the end-expiratory elastic recoil pressure at the end of exhalation, which may cause barotrauma, decrease cardiac output, and increase work of breathing. Because of the mode's unnatural I:E ratio, patients may not tolerate PC-IRV without heavy sedation and, possibly, paralysis.

Vines DL, Peters JI: Pressure control ventilation in acute lung injury. Clin Pulm Med 8:231–237, 2001.

5. **What is permissive hypercapnia (PH)?**
   In patients with ARDS, mechanical breaths may cause lung injury and worsen outcome through repetitive overstretching and cyclic recruitment–derecruitment of collapsed lung areas. To reduce mechanotrauma and its resulting inflammatory effects, ventilator-associated lung injury may be limited by permitting hypoventilation. This invariably involves reduced V_T, and generally leads to elevated $PaCO_2$, an approach that has been termed "permissive hypercapnia." This lung-protective ventilation strategy (LPVS) has been shown to improve survival in ARDS patients.

6. **Does hypercapnia, *per se,* contribute to the beneficial effects seen in LPVSs?**
   Current thought attributes the protective effect of LPVSs solely to reductions in lung stretch and permits hypercapnia to achieve this goal. There are no human data on the direct effects of hypercapnic acidosis independent of ventilator strategy. An analysis of patients enrolled in the ARDSnet study demonstrated that permissive hypercapnia reduced mortality in patients randomized to the higher V_T (12 mL/kg); however, no additional effect was seen in patients randomized to receive the lower V_T (6 mL/kg). To date, there are insufficient clinical data to suggest that hypercapnia should be independently induced outside the context of a protective ventilatory strategy.

7. **Is hypercapnia safe? Name some of the concerns associated with it.**
   In many studies of patients undergoing permissive hypercapnia, a pH below 7.2 appeared to be well tolerated. There are case reports of survival after exposure to extreme levels of CO_2, but hypercapnia, acidosis, or both may exert deleterious effects that require consideration when applying this strategy in a clinical context. Some well-recognized deleterious effects of hypercapnic acidosis are illustrated in Table 68-1.

TABLE 68-1.   ADVERSE EFFECTS AND RELATIVE CONTRAINDICATIONS OF PERMISSIVE HYPERCAPNIA
1. Attenuated neutrophil respiratory burst and superoxide production and increased tissue nitration (suggested to be a key mechanism of tissue damage in inflammatory conditions)
2. Neurologic injury, cerebral vasodilation, and increased intracranial pressure, contraindicating it in patients with cerebral edema or high intracranial pressure
3. An increased adrenergic response, which results in sweating, anxiety, and tachycardia, with a risk of precipitating arrhythmias
4. Reduced systemic vascular resistance and cardiac contractility, making low cardiac output states a relative contraindication to permissive hypercapnia
5. Constriction in the pulmonary vasculature, enhanced hypoxic vasoconstriction, and increased pulmonary vascular resistance, making it relatively contraindicated in pulmonary hypertension
6. Intense renal vasoconstriction and avid tubular sodium reabsorption, causing depressed glomerular filtration and increased fluid retention

KEY POINTS: PERMISSIVE HYPERCAPNIA

1. PH is an inherent component of LPVS.

2. PH should not be independently induced outside of LPVS.

3. Contraindications to PH include elevated intracranial pressure, pulmonary hypertension, and low cardiac output.

4. No long-term outcome data support the practice of buffering hypercapnic acidosis.

8. **How does one manage a patient with ARDS and a contraindication to permissive hypercapnia?**
Clinical scenarios in which ARDS coexists with increased intracranial pressure, pulmonary hypertension, or low cardiac output are not unusual. These conditions suggest the use of LPVS without allowing CO_2 to rise significantly. This can be accomplished by reducing dead space ventilation through techniques like tracheal gas insufflation (TGI). A lower tracheal cannula that provides a constant or intermittent fresh gas flow can flush out gas containing CO_2. By reducing dead space, TGI has been shown to decrease the need for V_T without excessive hypercapnia or acidemia. However, routine TGI use in intensive care warrants further investigation.

9. **Should one buffer hypercapnic-induced acidosis in ARDS patients?**
The clinical practice of buffering hypercapnic acidosis in ARDS remains controversial. Bicarbonate may further raise systemic CO_2 levels under conditions of hypoventilation and may worsen intracellular acidosis because the CO_2 produced when bicarbonate reacts with the hydrogen ion diffuses readily across cell membranes, whereas bicarbonate does not. An alternative to bicarbonate, tris-hydroxymethyl aminomethane (THAM), may be used for buffering in acidemia. THAM penetrates cells easily and can buffer pH changes and simultaneously can reduce PCO_2. THAM rapidly decreases hemodynamic alterations and restores myocardial contractility in ARDS patients with hypercapnic acidosis. However, no long-term clinical outcome data support this practice.

Acute Respiratory Distress Syndrome Network: Ventilation with lower tidal volumes as compared with traditional tidal volumes for acute lung injury and the acute respiratory distress syndrome. N Engl J Med 342:1301–1308, 2000.

Laffey JG, O'Croinin D, McLoughlin P, et al: Permissive hypercapnia—role in protective lung ventilatory strategies. Intens Care Med 30:347–356, 2004.

Martinez-Perez M, Bernabe F, Pena R, et al: Effects of expiratory tracheal gas insufflation in patients with severe head trauma and acute lung injury. Intens Care Med 30:2021–2027, 2004.

Nahum A: Tracheal gas insufflation as an adjunct to mechanical ventilation. Respir Care Clin North Am 8:171–185, 2002.

Sevransky JE, Levy MM, Marini JJ: Mechanical ventilation in sepsis-induced acute lung injury/acute respiratory distress syndrome: An evidence-based review. Crit Care Med 32:S548–S553, 2004.

10. **Name another mode of mechanical ventilation that limits peak airway pressure.**
Airway pressure release ventilation is a bilevel continuous positive airway pressure (CPAP) ventilation with brief, regular, intermittent releases from high to low pressures, which allows spontaneous breaths between and during the airway pressure releases (Fig. 68-2). The clinician sets the upper and lower CPAP levels, pressure-release frequency, and either the inspiratory or the pressure-release time. Depending on the set pressure-release frequency, alveolar ventilation is augmented by intermittently releasing the upper to lower positive pressure levels, simulating expiration and clearing the CO_2. The elevated baseline pressure facilitates oxygenation. Like other pressure-limited ventilation modes, APRV is affected by lung compliance and resistance, making it necessary to monitor tidal volume.

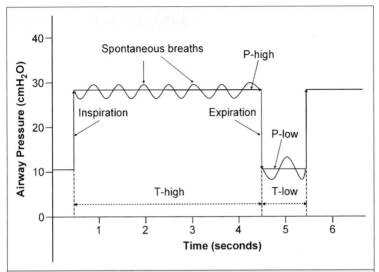

Figure 68-2. Airway pressure release ventilation. T-high and T-low represent the lengths of time that high airway pressure (P-high) and low airway pressure (P-low) are maintained, respectively. The T-high can be set greater or less than T-low (the release time). The set variables are the P-high and P-low, the T-high and T-low, and the pressure release frequency. Unsupported spontaneous breaths are permitted throughout the entire ventilatory cycle.

11. **Is APRV better than conventional mechanical ventilation for patients with ARDS?**
    Initially, APRV has been shown to (1) improve alveolar ventilation with lower airway pressure; (2) require lower minute ventilation, suggesting that it results in less dead space ventilation; (3) improve ventilation-perfusion (V/Q) matching; (4) lead to fewer adverse hemodynamic effects and organ perfusion; (5) allow spontaneous breathing throughout the entire ventilatory cycle; and (6) require less sedation and lead to less paralysis. APRV can be considered an LPVS because the set high-pressure limit prevents alveolar overdistention, and its maintenance optimizes alveolar recruitment and may prevent low-volume lung injury. However, except for its lower inspiratory pressure, APRV has similar effects to conventional mechanical ventilation in its application in patients with ARDS.

    Frawley PM, Habashi NM: Airway pressure release ventilation: Theory and practice. AACN Clin Issues 12:234–246, 2001.
    Putensen C, Zech S, Wrigge H, et al: Long-term effects of spontaneous breathing during ventilatory support in patients with acute lung injury. Am J Respir Crit Care Med 164:43–49, 2001.
    Varpula T, Valta P, Niemi R, et al: Airway pressure release ventilation as a primary ventilatory mode in acute respiratory distress syndrome. Acta Anaesthesiol Scand 48:722–731, 2004.

12. **What is closed-loop mechanical ventilation? Name some of these systems.**
    In closed-loop ventilation, all ventilator operations are automatically controlled by the ventilator's response to changes in patient respiratory mechanics or gas exchange. Totally independent closed-loop systems currently do not exist. Examples of closed-loop systems are listed in Table 68-2, and we will discuss the first five modes of ventilation listed.

    Branson RD, Johannigman JA, Campbell RS, Davis K Jr: Closed-loop mechanical ventilation. Respir Care 47:427–451, 2002.

TABLE 68-2. CLOSED-LOOP MECHANICAL VENTILATION SYSTEMS

Proportional assist ventilation (PAV)

Neurally adjusted ventilatory assist (NAVA)

Adaptive support ventilation (ASV)

Automatic tube compensation (ATC)

Dual control breath-to-breath (pressure-regulated volume control or autoflow)

Dual control within breath (volume assured pressure support [VAPS] and pressure augmentation [PA])*

Volume support (VS) and variable pressure support (VPS)*

Pressure support controlled by airway occlusion pressure*

Automode (volume support with pressure regulated volume control) and variable pressure support with variable pressure control*

*Not discussed in this chapter; *see* Branson RD, Johannigman JA, Campbell RS, Davis K Jr: Closed-loop mechanical ventilation. Respir Care 47:427–451, 2002.

13. **Describe the concept of proportional-assist ventilation (PAV).**

PAV is a form of synchronized partial ventilatory assistance in which the ventilator generates pressure in proportion to the patient's instantaneous effort. The more the patient pulls, the more pressure the machine generates. PAV's operational principle follows the equation of motion; that is, the pressure applied by the respiratory muscles (P_{mus}) to the system is used to overcome the elastic (E) and resistive (R) forces. E is proportional to the volume (V) displacement, whereas R is proportional to the flow rate ($\dot{V}$); thus, $P_{mus} = (ExV) + (Rx\dot{V})$. During PAV, the equation becomes $P_{mus} = (ExV) + (Rx\dot{V}) + PEEPi - P_{aw}$ [1], where PEEPi is the end-expiratory elastic recoil pressure that the respiratory muscles must overcome at the onset of inspiration to trigger the ventilator and P_{aw} is the pressure applied by the ventilator. Rearranging this equation, the ventilator-applied pressure is $P_{aw} = (ExV) + (Rx\dot{V}) + PEEPi - P_{mus}$.

During PAV, the ventilator instantaneously delivers positive pressure throughout inspiration in proportion to patient-generated volume (i.e., volume assist [VA], cmH_2O/L) and flow (flow assist [FA], $cmH_2O/L/sec$). The VA and FA levels are adjustable settings. To select the appropriate settings, PAV requires knowledge of patient respiratory mechanics that is not easily obtained. Fortunately, noninvasive measuring techniques have been developed to continuously

KEY POINTS: CLOSED-LOOP MECHANICAL VENTILATION

1. Represents the control of ventilator output variables based on input variables

2. Includes the following modes: proportional assist ventilation, adaptive support ventilation, automatic tube compensation, and pressure-regulated volume control or volume control plus, among others

3. Mimics more closely the ventilatory control and response of human physiology, thus improving patient–ventilator interaction and comfort

4. Shows little evidence of clinical benefit in terms of mechanical ventilation duration, mortality, and resource use

assess elastance and resistance, allowing VA and FA gains to be adjusted accordingly. PAV entails no target flow, volume, or pressure and, consequently, improves patient–ventilator interaction.

Vitacca M: New things are not always better: Proportional assist ventilation vs. pressure support ventilation. Intens Care Med 29:1038–1040, 2003.

14. **What is the clinical difference between PAV and pressure-support ventilation (PSV) or assist-control (AC) ventilation?**
   During PAV, flow and volume vary breath by breath, indicating a more physiologic breathing pattern. This is in contrast to PSV or AC ventilation, in which the ventilator delivers a set inspiratory pressure or flow, respectively. In PSV or AC, when patient ventilatory demand increases in response to the fixed settings, the ventilator is unable to meet the patient's flow demand. PAV's improved synchrony between patient effort and the ventilator results in better subjective comfort at a significantly lower mean airway pressure than PSV. However, in terms of gas exchange and unloading the work of breathing, PAV and PSV are comparable.

Vitacca M: New things are not always better: Proportional assist ventilation vs. pressure support ventilation. Intens Care Med 29:1038–1040, 2003.

15. **What is neurally adjusted ventilatory assist (NAVA)?**
   NAVA is a form of partial ventilatory support in which diaphragm electrical activity triggers the ventilator and provides a means of continuous ventilatory assistance in proportion to the neural drive both within and between breaths. Thus, the ventilator triggering is independent of respiratory mechanics. Because the ventilator is triggered directly by the diaphragm's electrical activity, the synchrony between neural and mechanical (i.e., ventilator) inspiratory time is guaranteed both at the onset and at the end of inspiration, regardless of PEEPi, air leaks, and alterations in respiratory mechanics. However, NAVA requires an intact neural pathway from the respiratory center to the diaphragm. Currently, NAVA is not available for clinical use and remains an investigational tool.

Navalesi P, Costa R: New modes of mechanical ventilation: proportional assist ventilation, neurally adjusted ventilatory assist, and fractal ventilation. Curr Opin Crit Care 9:51–58, 2003.

16. **What is adaptive support ventilation (ASV), and how does it work?**
   ASV is a minute ventilation (MV)-controlled mode governed by a closed-loop algorithm that maintains the clinician-preset MV in accordance with the patient's respiratory activity. In the absence of spontaneous respiratory activity, ASV delivers pressure-controlled ventilation, but it switches to pressure support when spontaneous breathing resumes. Changes in the patient's ventilatory condition induce increases or decreases in the pressure support level without human intervention.

   The ASV algorithm determines the optimal breathing pattern by applying the "minimum work of breathing" concept. This concept suggests that the patient breathes at a V_T and respiratory rate (f) that maintain acid–base balance and oxygenation while minimizing the elastic and resistive loads on the respiratory system according to the equation $f = \sqrt{[1 + 4\pi^2 RC_e (V_A/V_D) - 1]/2\pi^2 RC_e}$, in which RC_e is the expiratory time constant and V_A and V_D are alveolar and dead space volume, respectively. The clinician sets the patient's ideal body weight (to determine the dead space), the high-pressure alarm, PEEP, FiO_2, and inspiratory pressure-rise-time and flow-cycle-off variables for the pressure-support breaths.

17. **What are the benefits and limitations of ASV?**
   ASV is capable of titrating the degree of ventilatory support from initiation to maintenance to discontinuation of mechanical ventilation. On initial ventilator settings, for achieving similar arterial blood gas values to conventional mechanical ventilation, ASV was associated with a lower V_T, peak inspiratory pressure, and V_D/V_T ratio and a higher respiratory rate. ASV adapts to patient changes in lung mechanics and inspiratory effort, and thus improves patient–ventilator

interaction and potentially facilitates weaning. ASV's limitations include its inability to detect and to respond to changes in serial or alveolar dead space, requiring close monitoring of arterial blood gases. ASV selects a breathing pattern with a low V_T and a high respiratory rate. In patients with chronic obstructive pulmonary disease, it may result in inadequate lung emptying, with consequent air trapping. Furthermore, ASV responds to increased patient effort by reducing inspiratory pressure, which may be inappropriate when patient effort and work of breathing are excessive. However, ASV's potential advantages in patient outcome, number of ventilator days, and resource use deserve further investigation.

Branson RD, Johannigman JA, Campbell RS, et al: Closed-loop mechanical ventilation. Respir Care 47:427–451, 2002.

Campbell RS, Branson RD, Johannigman JA: Adaptive support ventilation. Respir Care Clin North Am 7:425–440, 2001.

Petter AH, Chiolero RL, Cassina T: Automatic "respirator/weaning" with adaptive support ventilation: The effect on duration of endotracheal intubation and patient management. Anesth Analg 97:1743–1750, 2003.

Sulzer CF, Chiolero R, Chassot PG, et al: Adaptive support ventilation for fast tracheal extubation after cardiac surgery: A randomized controlled study. Anesthesiology 95:1339–1345, 2001.

18. What is automatic tube compensation (ATC)? How does it work?

During mechanical ventilation, the resistance of the endotracheal tube (ETT) imposes additional work of breathing for the spontaneously breathing patient. ATC is a ventilatory mode that applies the necessary pressure support during spontaneous breathing to overcome the ETT's resistance at each instantaneous flow rate throughout the breathing cycle. In the ATC mode, the ventilator continuously calculates the pressure drop across the ETT due to frictional energy loss using a mathematical prediction model for turbulent flow based on the clinician's input of the internal tube diameter and the instantaneous flow measurement.

19. Explain the differences between ATC and PSV.

In the spontaneously breathing patient, flow is highly variable within each breath and between breaths, either because of physiologic variations in the breathing pattern or because of the altered breathing control. The same applies to the flow-dependent pressure drop across the ETT. PSV applies a constant positive pressure, making it impossible to precisely correct intra-breath or breath-to-breath compensation for tube resistance. Furthermore, PSV is restricted to compensating during the inspiratory phase. During expiration, the ETT can limit flow and produce dynamic overinflation. ATC can overcome this problem by lowering pressure support during expiration, improving breathing comfort. ATC also produces better extubation outcomes than does PSV or T-piece ventilation. Similarly, the predictive power of the ratio of respiratory rate to V_T (f/V_T) for successful extubation, measured at the end of the spontaneous breathing trial, is better with ATC than without.

20. What are ATC's clinical implications?

ATC should be viewed as a new ventilatory support component that can either stand alone or be combined with conventional modes. Adding ATC to another mode poses a potential risk of overassistance; thus, the primary support level should be reduced. Reduction in the ETT cross-sectional area, caused by secretions, kinking, or external compression, can result in underestimation of the pressure drop along the tube. In that case, ATC undercompensates for tube resistance, and hypoventilation may occur. A bedside procedure has been proposed to determine current specific coefficients of the ETT *in situ* and includes inserting a pressure-measuring catheter into the ETT to spot-check the tracheal pressure (P_{trach}) measurement, followed by an online least-squares fit procedure with subsequent correction for removing the pressure-measuring catheter. If this maneuver is periodically performed at the bedside, accurate P_{trach} calculation should be guaranteed. This method's utility in clinical practice remains to be determined.

Cohen JD, Shapiro M, Grozovski E, et al: Automatic tube compensation-assisted respiratory rate to tidal volume ratio improves the prediction of weaning outcome. Chest 122:980–984, 2002.

Elsasser S, Guttmann J, Stocker R, et al: Accuracy of automatic tube compensation in new-generation mechanical ventilators. Crit Care Med 31:2619–2626, 2003.

Guttmann J, Haberthur C, Mols G: Automatic tube compensation. Respir Care Clin North Am 7:475–501, 2001.

Haberthur C, Lichtwarck-Aschoff M, Guttmann J: Continuous monitoring of tracheal pressure including spot-check of endotracheal tube resistance. Technol Health Care 11:413–424, 2003.

21. **What is dual-control breath-to-breath pressure-limited time-cycled ventilation?**

This mode is commercially available on different ventilators as pressure-regulated volume control (PRVC), volume control plus (VC+), adaptive pressure ventilation, auto-flow, or variable pressure control. It uses V_T exiting from the ventilator as a feedback control to continuously adjust the pressure limit. All breaths are time- or patient-triggered, pressure-limited, and time-cycled.

This mode's advantages are the positive attributes of pressure-limited ventilation with constant V_T and the automatic pressure limit reduction as lung mechanics improve. However, any errors in V_T measurements will result in decision errors. Furthermore, if the patient's demand increases, the pressure level may diminish when support is most necessary, and oxygenation may decrease. Studies show that peak inspiratory pressure is significantly lower during PRVC than during volume-cycled ventilation. PRVC has not been shown to improve mechanical ventilation duration or mortality.

Branson RD, Johannigman JA, Campbell RS, Davis K Jr: Closed-loop mechanical ventilation. Respir Care 47:427–451, 2002.

22. **What is HFV? Name some clinical uses of HFV.**

The term HFV refers to positive pressure mechanical ventilation that delivers a high frequency of small (usually subanatomic dead space) V_Ts. There are three types of HFV: high-frequency positive pressure ventilation (HFPPV), high-frequency jet ventilation (HFJV), and high-frequency oscillatory ventilation (HFOV). Each mode's characteristics and some clinical applications are summarized in Table 68-3.

HFOV is the only HFV mode approved by the Food and Drug Administration (FDA) for treating ARDS. HFOV ventilation is not dependent on bulk gas transport, so V_T and f become less meaningful. In fact, the normal relationship between alveolar ventilation ($\dot{V}_A$) and f, V_T, and V_D [$\dot{V}_A = f \times (V_T - V_D)$], no longer applies when V_T is less than V_D. Gas transport differs from conventional mechanical ventilation, and oxygenation is achieved by increasing mean airway pressure to effect alveolar recruitment similar to PEEP.

23. **What is the rationale behind the use of HFOV in ARDS?**

The current best practice for ventilation in ARDS is the LPVS using low V_T (6 mL/kg) with a plateau pressure less than 30 cmH$_2$O to avoid lung overdistention and PEEP to prevent alveolar collapse at the end of expiration. HFOV can be considered an extreme form of LPVS that uses subdead space V_T and high PEEP levels. Several HFOV trials in adults with ARDS showed consistent improvement in the PaO$_2$:FiO$_2$ ratio. However, a recent meta-analysis showed that there is not enough evidence to conclude whether HFV reduces mortality or long-term morbidity in children and adults with ALI or ARDS. Future studies should compare HFOV to conventional mechanical ventilation with low V_T, the standard practice for ARDS. Until then, HFOV should be used as a rescue therapy in patients with severe ARDS with high distending lung pressure exceeding 35 cmH$_2$O who are not responding to conventional therapy.

Bartz RR: What is the role of high-frequency ventilation in adult respiratory distress syndrome? Respir Care Clin North Am 10:329–339, 2004.

Bouchut JC, Godard J, Claris O: High-frequency oscillatory ventilation. Anesthesiology 100:1007–1012, 2004.

McLuckie A: High-frequency oscillation in acute respiratory distress syndrome (ARDS). Br J Anaesth 93:322–324, 2004.

Wunsch H, Mapstone J: High-frequency ventilation versus conventional ventilation for treatment of acute lung injury and acute respiratory distress syndrome. Cochrane Database Syst Rev CD004085, 2004.

TABLE 68-3. CHARACTERISTICS AND CLINICAL APPLICATIONS OF HIGH-FREQUENCY VENTILATION

Type of HFV	Mechanism	VT (mL/kg)	Frequency (Hz)	Comments and Clinical Use
HFPPV	Positive pressure ventilation using high inspiratory flow through a circuit with low internal compliance	3–4	1–2	Airway surgery
HFJV	Delivers small tidal volumes under high pressure to the airway; uses a small catheter to produce high-velocity jets at a set frequency and inspiratory time	2–5	2–16	Upper airway surgery, large bronchopleural fistula, and extracorporeal lithotripsy
HFOV	The gas flow is oscillated by a piston-like device close to the airway opening; the air column in the proximal airways is compressed and decompressed, and distally no net transfer of gas takes place	1–3	3–5	Infant respiratory distress syndrome and ARDS, and intraoperative use for various pediatric thoracic and abdominal procedures

ARDS = acute respiratory distress syndrome, HFV = high-frequency ventilation, HFJV = high-frequency jet ventilation, HFPPV = high-frequency positive pressure ventilation, HFOV = high-frequency oscillatory ventilation.

24. **Describe the concept of liquid ventilation.**

In ALI, the surface tension at the lung's air–liquid interface is increased because the pulmonary surfactant system is damaged, causing alveolar collapse, atelectasis, increased right-to-left shunt, and hypoxemia. Liquid ventilation has been developed with the goal of eliminating the air-to-liquid interface by filling the lung with a fluid in which oxygen and carbon dioxide are highly soluble. Perfluorocarbons (PFCs) are biologically and chemically inert substances that have these physical properties and have been used to improve gas exchange and lung mechanics in respiratory failure. PFCs are dense and gravitate to the dependent parts of the lungs to reopen collapsed alveoli, acting as liquid PEEP. They improve the matching of ventilation to perfusion by compressing the pulmonary vessels in the dependent lung regions, thus diverting blood flow toward the nondependent aerated lung; they also have been shown to have anti-inflammatory properties in the alveolar space. There are two types of liquid ventilation: (1) total liquid ventilation, in which a device is used to liquid-ventilate PFC-filled lungs; and (2) PLV, which uses conventional gas ventilation together with PFC instillation of the functional residual capacity. Recent clinical activities have focused on PLV.

Davies MW, Sargent PH: Partial liquid ventilation for the prevention of mortality and morbidity in pediatric acute lung injury and acute respiratory distress syndrome. Cochrane Database Syst Rev CD003845, 2004.

Kaisers U, Kelly KP, Busch T: Liquid ventilation. Br J Anaesth 91:143–151, 2003.

25. **What clinical conditions warrant PLV use?**

In young patients, PLV resulted in a significantly rapid discontinuation of mechanical ventilation and a trend toward more ventilator-free days. However, in a large multicenter trial of adult patients with ALI, PLV did not improve the number of ventilator-free days or the 28-day all-cause mortality rate. Furthermore, a recent meta-analysis found no evidence to support or refute PLV use in children with ALI or ARDS. Animal studies suggest that lung disease could be treated by PFCs in aerosol or vapor form. Future research may clarify whether this approach has any advantages over true liquid ventilation.

CHAPTER 69

WEANING

Anthony M. Cosentino, MD, FACP, FACCP

1. **The procedure by which mechanical ventilation is discontinued is often referred to as "weaning." Is this term appropriate?**

   If weaning refers to a process during which mechanical ventilation is gradually withdrawn, the term is probably inappropriate. Mechanical ventilation for an episode of acute respiratory failure unrelated to neuromuscular diseases can usually be discontinued without a period of weaning. The term *discontinuation* is preferred.

   ACCP/AARC/SCCM Task Force: Evidence-based guidelines for weaning and discontinuing mechanical ventilatory support. Chest 120(Suppl 16):375S–484S, 2001. (See recommendation 3.)

2. **When can efforts to discontinue ventilation be initiated?**

   Patients should exhibit some clinical and radiologic evidence of reversal of the underlying cause for the respiratory failure, adequate oxygenation with an FiO_2 of 0.4, hemodynamic stability, and an intact respiratory center and muscular apparatus.

   ACCP/AARC/SCCM Task Force: Evidence-based guidelines for weaning and discontinuing mechanical ventilatory support. Chest 120(Suppl 16):375S–484S, 2001. (See recommendation 3.)

3. **Which indices are generally regarded as having the best negative and positive predictive values to assess the likelihood of successful discontinuation of mechanical ventilation?**

   Yang and Tobin demonstrated that simple is best. The ratio of tidal volume (V_T) to respiratory rate (f) was the best predictor of successful discontinuation, and the maximum inspiratory pressure at residual volume (PI_{max}) and f:V_T ratios were the best predictors of failure. Furthermore, a value of 100 is easy to remember, which is fortunate because that is the magic ratio that separates success from failure. The PI_{max} was only marginally superior in sensitivity to the f:V_T ratio, but the former lacked specificity.

   Alvisi et al, in a study of subjects with chronic obstructive pulmonary disease (COPD), found that the ratio of the change in inspiratory pressure (ΔPI) to the maximum inspiratory pressure (MIP), combined with compliance, rate, oxygenation, and PI_{max} (CROP), is superior.

   Alvisi R, Volta CA, Beghini ER, Melic-Emili J: Predictors of weaning outcomes in chronic obstructive pulmonary disease patients. Eur Resp J 15:656–662, 2000.
   Yang KL, Tobin MJ: A prospective study of indexes predicting the outcome of trials of weaning from mechanical ventilation. N Engl J Med 324:1445–1450, 1991.

4. **The positive predictive value of the f:V_T ratio was 80%; in other words, 20% required reintubation. Why?**

   Epstein and colleagues demonstrated that most of the subjects who required reintubation were in congestive heart failure, a process for which f:V_T is physiologically or temporally unlikely to predict success or failure. Listen for the telltale third heart sound.

   The results of Epstein and of Alvisi et al. demonstrate that "one size may not fit all." (*Cf.* Procrustes, "he who stretches," a bandit from Attica killed by Theseus in Greek mythology.)

   Epstein SD: Etiology of extubation failure and the predictive nature of the rapid shallow breathing index. Am J Respir Crit Care Med 152:545–549, 1995.

5. **What assessment and ventilator strategies best identify the patient who is ready to discontinue mechanical ventilation?**

Weaning strategies have included intermittent mandatory ventilation (IMV) without pressure support, IMV with declining levels of pressure support, and assist-control with daily unassisted spontaneous breathing trials. IMV without pressure support now is outmoded. Declining pressure support continues to have many advocates but, in the author's opinion, lacks physiologic foundation and is, in fact, a throwback to the concept that weaning should be gradual. The Lung Failure Collaborative Group concluded that assist-control ventilation with a once-daily spontaneous breathing trial (SBT) was superior. A tube trial with or without 7 cmH$_2$O pressure support was equivalent. It is recommended that a spontaneous breathing trial of 30–120 minutes be performed once daily. Sedation may need to be discontinued.

Esteban A, Alia I, Cordo F, et al: Extubation outcome after spontaneous breathing trials with T-tube or pressure support ventilation. Am J Respir Crit Care Med 156:459–465, 1997.

Esteban A, Frutos F, Tobin MJ, et al, for the Spanish Lung Failure Collaborative Group: A comparison of four methods of weaning patients from mechanical ventilation. N Eng J Med 332:345–350, 1995.

Kress JP, Pholman AS, O'Connor MF, Hall JB: Daily interruption of sedative infusions in critically ill patients undergoing mechanical ventilation. N Engl J Med 342:1471–1477, 2000.

Vallverdu I, Calaf N, Subirana M, et al: Clinical characteristics, respiratory functional parameters, and outcome of a two hour T-piece trial in patients weaning from mechanical ventilation. Am J Resp Crit Care Med 158:1855–1862, 1998.

6. **Your patient has just failed an SBT. What next?**

Resume mechanical ventilation with a mode that ensures comfort (e.g., assist-control) without excess sedation. Rest the respiratory muscles. Reverse what can be reversed (e.g., fluid overload), and try again in 24 hours.

ACCP/AARC/SCCM Task Force: Evidence-based guidelines for weaning and discontinuing mechanical ventilatory support. Chest 120(Suppl 16):375S–484S, 2001. (See recommendation 6.)

Vassilakopolous T, Zakinthynos S, Roussos C: The tension time index and the frequency/tidal volume ratio are the major pathophysiologic determinants of weaning failure and success. Am J Respir Crit Care Med 158:378–385, 1998.

KEY POINTS: ACUTE PHASE OF LIBERATION

1. Need not be a gradual process

2. Should include a daily spontaneous breathing trial

3. F:V$_T$ ratio is the best predictive value for success and failure

4. Should include a daily T-tube trial, not to exceed 2 hours

5. Beware of resistances in ventilator circuitry

6. Spontaneous breathing may aggravate chronic heart failure

7. **Subjects with left ventricular dysfunction often prove difficult to remove from mechanical ventilation. How does mechanical ventilation improve left ventricular function?**

An increase in intrapleural pressure may result in a decrease in venous return in the normal heart and, thus, a decrease in cardiac output. Patients with a dilated heart are maximally preloaded (i.e., are at the flat part of their Starling–Sarnoff curves) and do not experience this effect. However, an increase in intrapleural pressure also decreases left ventricle (LV) afterload and thus facilitates LV performance. Afterload is wall tension during systole. Wall tension is represented as the transmural pressure across the LV (i.e., the aortic root pressure minus pleural pressure) $\times$ radius $\times 2h^{-1}$, where h = thickness. Thus, an increase in pleural pressure results in a decrease in transmural pressure and a decrease in afterload.

Lemaire F, Teboul JL, Cinotti L, et al: Acute left ventricular dysfunction during unsuccessful weaning from mechanical ventilation. Anesthesiology 69:171–179, 1988.

Permutt S: Circulatory effects of weaning from mechanical ventilation: The importance of transdiaphragmatic pressure. Anesthesiology 691:157–160, 1988.

8. **What is the role of noninvasive positive pressure ventilation for respiratory failure after extubation?**
This strategy has its advocates. However, a multicenter randomized trial of 221 patients showed no difference in the need for reintubation or mortality in unselected patients with respiratory failure after extubation.

Esteban A, Frutos-Vivar F, Ferguson ND, et al: Noninvasive positive-pressure ventilation for respiratory failure after extubation. N Engl J Med 350:2452–2460, 2004.

9. **What sources of resistance in the ventilator circuitry may contribute to a failed SBT?**
It is customary to perform SBTs through the ventilator circuitry. Resistances to airflow may be encountered in the humidifier, in the inspiratory valve, and in the expiratory valves. Effort expended in opening a valve is not counted as work (i.e., pressure $\times$ flow) but will be reflected in the pressure-time product. Expiratory resistance may contribute to intrinsic positive end-expiratory pressure (PEEP) and hyperinflation. A properly constructed PEEP valve should not impose a flow resistance.

Sassoon CS, DelRosario N, Fei R: Influence of pressure and flow triggered synchronous intermittent mandatory ventilation on inspiratory muscle work. Crit Care Med 22:1933–1941, 1994.

Sassoon CS, Light RW, Lodia R, et al: Pressure-time product during CPAP, PSV, and T-piece during weaning from mechanical ventilation. Am Rev Resp Dis 143:469–475, 1991.

10. **What clinical finding may suggest intrinsic PEEP and hyperinflation?**
A paradoxical pulse. Lung hyperinflation competes with the heart for the pericardial space and thus effectively produces cardiac tamponade.

McGregor M: Pulsus paradoxus. N Eng J Med 301:480–482, 1979.

Pepe PE, Marin JJ: Occult positive end expiratory pressure in mechanically ventilated patients with flow obstruction: The auto PEEP effect. Am Rev Respir Dis 126:166–170, 1982.

11. **What is the median duration of mechanical ventilation required by patients in medical intensive care and coronary care units? What is the rate of reintubation after a successful SBT and termination of ventilator support?**
The study of Ely et al is probably representative of the problem. In their study, mechanical ventilation was required for 2–11 days. Reintubation was required in fewer than 11% of patients, and prolonged mechanical ventilation was required in 6% of subjects in whom early extubation was attempted by protocol, versus 13% in a control group.

Ely EW, Baker AM, Dunagan DP, et al: Effect on the duration of mechanical ventilation of identifying patients capable of breathing spontaneously. N Engl J Med 335:1864–1869, 1996.

12. **What is the definition of prolonged mechanical ventilation, according to the U.S. Health Care Financing Administration?**
Ventilation for an excess of 21 days.

Cohen IL, Booth FV: Cost containment and mechanical ventilation in the United States. New Horiz 2:283–290, 1994.

13. **List three probable causes for failure to successfully discontinue mechanical ventilation.**
   - **Severe congestive heart failure:** There are encouraging reports that noninvasive continuous positive airway pressure (CPAP) may improve LV performance.
   - **Oropharyngeal dysfunction:** Earlier tracheotomy may mitigate this problem, but data are lacking.
   - **Intensive care unit (ICU) neuromuscular syndrome:** Sometimes called critical illness polyneuropathy. Lesions have been identified at the neuromuscular junction, the muscle, and the peripheral nerve.

      Deem S, Lee CM, Curtis JR: Acquired neuromuscular disorders in the intensive care unit. Am J Respir Crit Care Med 168:735–739, 2003.
      Heffner JE, Casey K, Hoffman C: Care of the mechanically ventilated patient with a tracheotomy. In Tobin MJ (ed): Principles and Practice of Mechanical Ventilation. New York, McGraw-Hill, 1994.
      Yan AT, Bradley D, Liu PP: The role of continuous positive airway pressure in the treatment of congestive heart failure. Chest 120:1675–1685, 2001.

KEY POINTS: PROLONGED FAILURE TO DISCONTINUE MECHANICAL VENTILATION

1. Heart failure, often with normal ejection fraction

2. Suspect glossopharyngeal dysfunction and aspiration

3. ICU neuromuscular syndrome related to sepsis, glycemic control, corticosteroids, and neuromuscular blocking agents

14. **What factors have been implicated in the development of the syndrome of critical illness polyneuropathy?**
   - Neuromuscular blocking agents
   - Corticosteroids
   - Prolonged time in the ICU and on mechanical ventilation
   - Hyperglycemia
   - Sepsis
   - Insulin, which may be neuroprotective

      Hund E: Myopathy in critically ill patients. Crit Care Med 27:2544–2547, 1999.
      Segredo V, Caldwell JE, Matthay MA, et al: Persistent paralysis after long term administration of vecuronium. N Engl J Med 327:524–528, 1992.
      Witt NJ, Zochodue DW, Bolton CF, et al: Peripheral nerve function in sepsis and multiple organ failure. Chest 99:176–184, 1991.
      Van den Berghe C, Wouters PJ, Bouillon R, et al: Outcome benefit of intensive insulin therapy in the critically ill: Insulin dose versus glycemic control. Crit Care Med 31:359–366, 2003.

15. **Where is the best place to care for such patients?**
   It is recommended that patients who require prolonged mechanical ventilation be cared for in special facilities designed for long-term efforts to discontinue mechanical ventilation.

      ACCP/AARC/SCCM Task Force Evidence-based guidelines for weaning and discontinuing mechanical ventilatory support. Chest 120(Suppl 16):375S–484S, 2001. (*See* recommendation 11.)

16. **What strategy is recommended to achieve discontinuation from mechanical ventilation in these long-term ventilator-dependent patients?**
   A weaning strategy is in fact recommended for these patients. No specific regimen has proven to be superior.

Scheinhorn DJ, Chao DC, Stearn-Hassenpflug M, et al: Post-ICU mechanical ventilation : Treatment of 1123 patients at a regional weaning center. Chest 111:1654–1659, 1997.

17. **How long a period of gradual withdrawal from mechanical ventilation is considered to be compatible with ultimate success?**
A period of 3–6 months. More than half are weaned. Overall survival at 1 year after discharge is 38%.

Scheinhorn DJ, Chao DC, Stearn-Hassenpflug M, et al: Post-ICU mechanical ventilation: Treatment of 1123 patients at a regional weaning center. Chest 111:1654–1659, 1997.

CHAPTER 70

CHRONIC VENTILATORY SUPPORT

Mary Gilmartin, BSN, RRT, AE-C, and Enrique Fernandez, MD

1. **Define chronic ventilatory support.**

   A long-term ventilator-assisted individual (VAI) requires mechanical ventilatory assistance for more than 6 hours a day for more than 3 weeks after all acute illnesses have been maximally treated and after multiple weaning attempts by an experienced respiratory care team have been unsuccessful. This definition takes into account the following issues:

   1. The chronic medical condition and the component or components of the respiratory system that has been affected (e.g., bony thorax, peripheral or central nervous system, respiratory muscles, and/or lungs)
   2. The reason ventilator assistance was initiated
   3. Length of time that ventilatory assistance is used on a daily basis, and the total duration of the assistance
   4. Whether there is a possibility of weaning the patient after a program of rehabilitation

   Make BJ: Epidemiology of long-term ventilatory assistance. In Hill N (ed): Long-Term Mechanical Ventilation. New York, Marcel Dekker, 2001, pp 1–17.

2. **What are the goals of chronic ventilatory support?**

   According to the guidelines for long-term mechanical ventilation published by a task force of the American College of Chest Physicians, the goals of chronic ventilatory support, either in the home or elsewhere, are as follows:

   - Extending life
   - Enhancing the quality of life
   - Providing an environment that will enhance individual potential
   - Reducing morbidity
   - Improving physical and physiologic function
   - Cost-effectiveness

   Make BJ, Hill NS, Goldberg AI, et al: Mechanical ventilation beyond the intensive care unit: Report of a consensus conference of the American College of Chest Physicians. Chest 113(suppl):289S–344S, 1998.

3. **Are there economic benefits to placing chronically ventilated patients in a homecare setting?**

   The costs of home ventilator care will vary depending on factors such as the mode of ventilation (i.e., tracheostomy versus noninvasive ventilation), the hours of ventilation per day, the complexity and severity of the patient's condition, the necessary medication and supplies, the need for skilled nursing care, self-care ability, the family's ability to provide care, the cost of utilities, funding sources, and lost wages by homecare providers. There is a lack of good data to determine actual costs of home care; past reports have used different methodologies to determine the costs. When sending patients home, we must not only look at the costs of care but also at what is best for the patient and the family.

   Downes JJ, Parra MM: Costs and reimbursement issues in long term mechanical ventilation of patients at home. In Hill N (eds): Long-term mechanical ventilation. New York, Marcel Dekker, 2001, pp 353–374.

4. **What are the characteristics of patients who require long-term ventilation?**

   - Absence of or significantly impaired spontaneous breathing efforts, as seen in central disorders such as a stroke, in central alveolar hypoventilation, or in high spinal cord injuries.

- Consequences of a major insult to the respiratory system, as seen with acute respiratory distress syndrome (ARDS) or with postoperative complications.
- A chronic respiratory disorder that precipitates recurrent episodes of acute respiratory failure. Such disorders include chronic obstructive pulmonary disease (COPD), postpolio sequelae, or kyphoscoliosis.
- Progressive neuromuscular disorders such as muscular dystrophy or amyotrophic lateral sclerosis.

5. **List the key factors that can potentially influence survival.**
   - Patient selection, based on underlying disease, disease severity, comorbid illness, patient wishes, family support, age, and respiratory function
   - The clinical setting in which the patient was ventilated (i.e., emergently vs. semi-elective)
   - Methods of ventilation, such as invasive ventilation by tracheostomy, noninvasive positive-pressure ventilation (NPPV), negative pressure, or other modes such as a pneumobelt or rocking bed
   - The site of care (i.e., an intensive care unit [ICU], a hospital, a skilled nursing facility, or home)

   Langmack EL, Make BJ: Survival of individuals receiving long-term mechanical ventilation. Respir Care Clin 8:355–377, 2002.

6. **Which patients are the best candidates for long-term mechanical ventilation used as life support?**
   In general, a good candidate is young and otherwise healthy except for an isolated disorder of the respiratory system that limits ventilation. Patients with slowly progressive or stable disorders such as kyphoscoliosis, diaphragmatic paralysis, sequelae of poliomyelitis, or traumatic high cervical spinal cord injury are good candidates. Because not all neuromuscular disorders progress slowly, the decision to ventilate must be individualized and discussed at length with each patient in a timely manner.

   There is still controversy regarding the use of long-term ventilation for patients with primary pulmonary diseases. Management of patients with COPD, for example, is complicated by advanced age, cor pulmonale, severe dyspnea, and fluctuations in airflow obstruction with resultant hypercapnia and hypoxemia. Recent studies have shown that in selected patients with stable COPD, the use of noninvasive ventilation controls hypoventilation and improves daytime arterial blood gases, sleep quality, and health status. Patients who have the greatest reduction in overnight CO_2 are most likely to benefit from long-term support. Patients with cystic fibrosis and bronchiectasis are also considered poor candidates for chronic ventilatory support because of their copious secretions and frequent infections. NPPV, however, has been used in patients with cystic fibrosis who are awaiting lung transplantation. In some small studies of long-term ventilation in cystic fibrosis patients, there was an improvement in body mass index, arterial blood gases, and quality of sleep. Patients with pulmonary fibrosis are not good candidates for long-term mechanical ventilation because of dyspnea, the increased work of breathing, and the need for higher oxygen concentrations and high inflating pressures.

   Brooks D, De Rosie J, Mousseau M, et al: Long term follow-up of ventilated patients with thoracic restrictive or neuromuscular disease. Can Respir J 9:99–106, 2002.
   Buyse B, Meersseman W, Demedts M: Treatment of chronic respiratory failure in kyphoscoliosis: Oxygen or ventilation? Eur Respir J 22:525–528, 2003.
   Efrati O, Moday-Moses D, Barak A, et al: Long-term non-invasive positive pressure ventilation among cystic fibrosis patients awaiting lung transplantation. Isr Med Assoc J 6:527–530, 2004.
   Fauroux B, Hart N, Lofaso F: Non invasive mechanical ventilation in cystic fibrosis: Physiological effects and monitoring. Monaldi Arch Chest Dis 57:268–272, 2002.
   Finder JD, Birnkrant D, Carl J, et al: Respiratory care of the patient with Duchenne muscular dystrophy: ATS consensus statement. Am J Respir Crit Care Med 170:456–465, 2004.

Gonzalez C, Ferris G, Diaz J, et al: Kyphoscoliotic ventilatory insufficiency: Effects of long-term intermittent positive pressure ventilation. Chest 124:857–862, 2003.

Wedzicha JA, Muir JF: Noninvasive ventilation in chronic obstructive pulmonary disease, bronchiectasis and cystic fibrosis. Eur Respir J 20:777–784, 2002.

7. **List the important criteria for successful chronic ventilator support at home.**
For optimal long-term ventilation at home, the patient should be clinically and physiologically stable for several weeks before hospital discharge, and he or she should also be emotionally stable. In addition, the following conditions should be met:
- Major organ systems are stable
- No acute infections
- FiO_2 of ≤ 0.40, positive end-expiratory pressure (PEEP) ≤ 5 cmH$_2$O
- Dyspnea controlled or absent
- Acid–base and metabolic stability
- Acceptable arterial blood gas levels
- Stable ventilatory settings with tracheostomy or noninvasive ventilation
- Minimal fluctuations in airway resistance and compliance
- Peak pressure varies ±5 cmH$_2$O or less
- Patient will be able to take in adequate nutrition at home
- Ability to clear secretions and protect the airways
- Management at home expected to be stable, without the need for readmission within at least 1 month
- Patient willing and able to participate in care or has capable caregivers
- Patient and family have a good understanding of the ventilator and its accessory equipment

Donat WE, Hill NS: Sites of care for long-term mechanical ventilation. In Hill N (ed): Long-Term Mechanical Ventilation. New York, Marcel Dekker, 2001, pp 19–37.

8. **What factors determine outcomes for patients undergoing chronic ventilatory support?**
The outcomes depend on many factors including the underlying disease, comorbid diseases, effects on survival, and the health status and quality of life of the patient. Reported series indicate that patients with neuromuscular diseases and skeletal conditions experience a better outcome from long-term mechanical ventilation than patients with chronic primary pulmonary diseases.

In one study of 259 patients with COPD ventilated through a tracheostomy at home, the survival rate for the overall study population was 70% at 2 years, 44% at 5 years, and 20% at

KEY POINTS: IMPORTANT EDUCATIONAL NEEDS OF VENTILATOR-ASSISTED INDIVIDUALS

1. Understanding the ventilator function and troubleshooting the ventilator for problems

2. Tracheostomy care and suctioning

3. Use of the manual resuscitator bag

4. Procedures for emergency situations such as a dislodged tracheostomy tube, an obstructed airway, cuff leaks, ventilator failure, and power failure

5. Maintaining the equipment, including cleaning, changing the ventilator circuits, and checking for leaks in the system

10 years. For those aged less than 65 years, use of an uncuffed cannula and a PaO_2 of more than 55 mmHg on room air during the first 3 months after tracheostomy were the variables that most closely correlated with survival for more than 5 years.

Muir JF, Girault C, Cardinaud JP, et al: Survival and long-term follow-up of tracheostomized patients with COPD treated by home mechanical ventilation. A multicenter French study in 259 patients. Chest 106:201–209, 1994.

Simonds AK: Outcomes of long-term mechanical ventilation. In Hill N (ed): Long-Term Mechanical Ventilation. New York, Marcel Dekker, 2001, pp 471–500.

9. **How does ventilatory muscle fatigue contribute to chronic respiratory failure?**
   Muscle fatigue is a condition in which there is a loss in the capacity for developing the force, the velocity of muscle contraction, or both, resulting from muscle activity under a load, which is reversible by rest. Progressive muscle fatigue is an important contributor to the development of respiratory failure. The load imposed on respiratory muscles by any chronic respiratory disease frequently worsens with time and increases the work of breathing. Consequently, a higher proportion of the maximal force that the respiratory muscles can develop is required for each breath. When the ventilatory load can no longer be supported, chronic respiratory muscle fatigue develops, followed by hypercapnic respiratory failure.

   Celli BR: Pathogenesis of chronic respiratory failure and effects of long-term mechanical ventilation on respiratory muscle function. In Hill NS (ed): Long-Term Mechanical Ventilation. New York. Marcel Dekker, 2001, pp 39–57.

10. **How are patients with ventilatory muscle fatigue best managed?**
    Regardless of the mechanism of fatigue, rest is the best treatment. It allows the ventilatory muscles to recover from the fatigue, which improves their contractile force and endurance. Rest interrupts the vicious circle of progressive and continuous blood gas deterioration, which further worsens respiratory muscle performance.

    Clinical signs of ventilatory muscle fatigue can be reduced or eliminated after a period of controlled ventilation, which rests ventilatory muscles. Prolonged daily intermittent use of positive-pressure ventilation reverses fatigue, contributes to the stabilization of the clinical course, restores sleep, prevents recurrent episodes of hypercapnic respiratory failure, and increases functional capacity.

    Goldstein RS, DeRosie JA, Avendana MA, et al: Influence of non-invasive positive pressure ventilation in respiratory muscles. Chest 99:408–415, 1991.

    Celli BR: Pathogenesis of chronic respiratory failure and effects of long-term mechanical ventilation on respiratory muscle function. In Hill NS (ed) Long-Term Mechanical Ventilation. New York, Marcel Dekker, 2001, pp 39–57.

11. **List the criteria for elective intermittent ventilation in chronic respiratory failure.**
    Clinical criteria
    - Slowly progressive, irreversible respiratory failure caused by neuromuscular diseases, thoracic wall deformities, or COPD (in amyotrophic lateral sclerosis, bulbar function should be intact for noninvasive ventilation)
    - Frequent readmission to hospital for respiratory failure
    - Deterioration after successful weaning
    - Obesity hypoventilation or idiopathic hypoventilation
    - Dyspnea, increasing tachypnea, or paradoxical or dyssynchronous breathing
    - Cor pulmonale despite conventional treatment
    - A motivated and cooperative patient with intact upper airway function and minimal secretions
    Pulmonary function criteria
    - Vital capacity (VC) < 50% predicted (mainly in progressive neuromuscular disease)
    - Forced expiratory volume in 1 second (FEV_1) < 25% predicted

- PaCO$_2$ > 45 mmHg, or nocturnal hypoventilation (i.e., O$_2$ saturation < 88% for > 5 consecutive minutes)

    Leger P, Hill NS: Long-term mechanical ventilation for restrictive thoracic disorders. In Hill NS (ed): Long-Term Mechanical Ventilation. New York, Marcel Dekker, 2001, pp 105–150.

12. **What are some of the potential complications associated with long-term ventilation by tracheostomy?**
    - Tracheal stenosis
    - Accidental decannulation
    - Airway and stomal granulation tissue formation
    - Mucus plugging
    - Aspiration
    - Tracheoesophageal fistula (rare)
    - Equipment malfunction
    - Tracheomalacia
    - Infection
    - Esophageal compression at the cuff site
    - Malnutrition
    - Caregiver fatigue

    Wright SE, VanDahm K: Long-term care of the tracheotomy patient. Clin Chest Med 24:473–487, 2003.

13. **What are the goals for intermittent elective mechanical ventilation?**
    - To preserve or increase the functional capacity for daily living activities
    - To alleviate symptoms and signs
    - To decrease the rate of clinical deterioration
    - To avoid acute respiratory failure

KEY POINTS: SITE OR TYPE OF DEFECT CAUSING RESPIRATORY FAILURE

1. Ventilatory drive abnormalities

2. Neural transmission to the ventilatory muscles

3. Genetic or congenital myopathies

4. Bony thorax abnormalities

5. Lung and airway disorders

14. **How is elective long-term mechanical ventilation delivered?**
    Initially, elective long-term mechanical ventilation may be delivered noninvasively. Patients with progressive disorders eventually may require a tracheostomy, which is usually performed when respiratory failure has progressed to the point at which ventilatory assistance is needed for more than 16 hours daily. Other patients with swallowing disorders, chronic aspiration, intolerance to noninvasive ventilation, or an inability to adequately ventilate with noninvasive ventilation will require a tracheostomy.

15. **Can I send my patient home on the critical care ventilator we use?**
    No! A patient that requires a critical care ventilator is not a candidate for home care. The most common ventilator type used for invasive ventilation in the home is a portable volume-limited

ventilator. The earlier versions of these ventilators did not incorporate PEEP, and the oxygen needed to be "bled" into the system. This is not a problem because a candidate for home care should not require a precise or high FiO_2. All of the portable ventilators have adequate alarms and an internal battery, and can be attached to an external battery. More recently, portable ventilators have become more sophisticated and can provide volume- or pressure-targeted modes, PEEP, and a more precise FiO_2.

Kacmarek RM: New ventilator options for long-term mechanical ventilation in the home. In Hill NS (ed): Long-Term Mechanical Ventilation. New York, Marcel Dekker, 2001, pp 375–409.

16. **When I see a ventilated patient on television, I do not see the airway secured to the patient's neck or face. Is that okay?**
No, the tracheostomy tube needs to be secured. It is best to use Velcro ties that can be easily adjusted to the patient's neck. The ties should only be loose enough to allow one to two fingers between the tie and the neck.

17. **What factors are predictors of success with home ventilation?**
There are several predictors of a successful outcome of home ventilator care. The following predictors should be carefully evaluated before home mechanical ventilation is initiated:
- The coping styles of the patient (ideally, the patient should be optimistic, motivated, flexible, and adaptable)
- The patient's ability to learn
- The patient's ability to direct others
- The primary diagnosis
- Clinical and physiologic stability
- Comorbidity
- The mode of ventilation and the ventilator settings
- Homecare support
- Age
- Nutritional status
- Aspiration potential
- The team caring for the patient (i.e., the physicians and primary caregivers)
- Ease of equipment maintenance and supply

Gilmartin M; Transitions from the intensive care clinic to home: Patient selection and discharge planning. Respir Care 39:456–480, 1994.

18. **What is the importance of discharge planning?**
Well-coordinated discharge planning is the key to the successful placement of a ventilator-dependent patient in the home; this requires a team of individuals that should include the patient and family in addition to a physician, nurse, respiratory therapist, social worker, physical therapist, occupational therapist, speech therapist, and nutritionist, as well as psychiatric services.
    The homecare company and equipment should be selected and completed before discharge. Regardless of who is on the team, communication among team members is essential; they should meet on a regular basis and should discuss short-term goals, the progress of the patient, and the family's concerns. With the patient and family present, the physician should discuss specific issues regarding treatment and discharge, using language that ensures understanding.

19. **How should patients undergoing home ventilation be monitored?**
A stable patient should only require intermittent monitoring in the homecare setting. The level of monitoring required for each patient should be determined prior to discharge. Good communication among the family, the homecare company, and the physician is the key to successful home ventilator care (Table 70-1).

TABLE 70-1.   MONITORING NEEDS OF PATIENTS UNDERGOING HOME VENTILATION

Patient monitoring

- Saturation obtained by pulse oximetry (SpO_2), intermittently
- Arterial blood gases, intermittently
- Clinical status (i.e., vital signs, lung sounds, and sputum production), intermittently
- Compliance, intermittently
- Airway resistance, before and after bronchodilation, intermittently
- Presence of intrinsic PEEP, intermittently
- End-tidal pressure of carbon dioxide (PET_{CO_2}), intermittently by a therapist
- Spontaneous ventilatory parameters (for selected patients), including tidal volume, vital capacity, and maximum inspiratory pressure
- Tracheostomy site, daily
- Tracheostomy cuff pressure and volume, intermittently

Equipment monitoring

- Ventilator function, at routine therapist visits
- Alarm setting, daily
- Alarm function, daily
- Peak inspiratory pressure, daily and at routine therapist visits
- Ventilator settings, daily, including machine-delivered tidal volume (V_T), rate, sensitivity, FiO_2 (monthly and at routine therapist visits), flow rate, and inspiratory time
- System leaks, daily
- System integrity, daily
- Hours of use, at routine therapist visits
- Inlet filters, per manufacturer's recommendations
- Bacteria filters, monthly
- Accessory equipment function

From Gilmartin M: Monitoring in the home and the outpatient setting. In Kacmarek RM, Hess D, Stoller JK (eds): Monitoring in Respiratory Care, St. Louis, Mosby, 1993, pp 767–787.

OXYGEN THERAPY

Rebecca L. Meredith, BS, RRT, and James K. Stoller, MD, MS

CHAPTER 71

1. When should supplemental oxygen be prescribed?

Long-standing hypoxemia can cause many adverse effects, including pulmonary hypertension, cor pulmonale, erythrocytosis, reduced exercise tolerance, neuropsychiatric impairment, and, most importantly, decreased survival. The clinical impact of long-standing hypoxemia and the benefits of supplemental oxygen have been most extensively studied in patients with chronic obstructive pulmonary disease (COPD).

For example, the combined results from the British Medical Research Council and the American Nocturnal Oxygen Therapy Trial (NOTT) studies demonstrated that the use of supplemental oxygen was associated with enhanced survival and improved neuropsychiatric well-being in hypoxic patients with COPD. Use of oxygen for 15 hours per day was associated with better survival rates, as compared with not using oxygen at all, but a longer duration of daily use (i.e., approximately 19 hours per day) was associated with still better survival than that seen with use for 12 hours daily.

On the basis of these findings, oxygen is recommended to be used as close to 24 hours per day as possible for appropriate candidates. For patients with hypoxemia caused by COPD, aggressive treatment with bronchodilators and antibiotics (if needed for airway infections) has been shown to improve oxygenation and can obviate the need for supplemental oxygen in up to 40% of individuals. The need for supplemental oxygen should be reestablished, and the dose of oxygen required should be assessed periodically, perhaps every 6 months.

Cottrell JJ, Openbrier D, Lave JR, et al: Home oxygen therapy: A comparison of 2- vs. 6-month patient re-evaluation. Chest 107:358–361, 1995.

Oakes D: Therapeutic modalities. In Clinical Practitioners' Guide to Respiratory Care. Rockville, MD, Health Educator Publishers, 1988, pp 143–159.

O'Donohue WJ: Indications for long-term oxygen therapy and appropriate use. In O'Donohue WJ (ed): Long-Term Oxygen Therapy: Scientific Basis and Application. New York, Marcel Dekker, 1995, pp 53–68.

Petty TL: Historical highlights of long-term oxygen therapy. Respir Care 45:29–36, 2000.

Tarpy SP, Celli BR: Long-term oxygen therapy. N Engl J Med 333:710–714, 1995.

Tiep BL: Long-term home oxygen therapy. Clin Chest Med 11:505–521, 1990.

2. List the indications for prescribing long-term oxygen therapy.

Continuous oxygen

- Resting room air $PaO_2 < 55$ mmHg or $SaO_2 < 88\%$
- Resting $PaO_2 = 56–59$ mmHg or $SaO_2 < 89\%$ in the presence of any of the following:
    - Edema suggesting congestive heart failure or P pulmonale on ECG
    - Erythrocytosis (i.e., hematocrit 56% or more)
- Resting $PaO_2 > 59$ mmHg or $SaO_2 > 89\%$ (reimbursable only with additional documentation justifying the oxygen prescription and a summary stating that more conservative therapy has failed)

Noncontinuous oxygen*

- Oxygen flow rate and number of hours per day must be specified
- During exercise: $PaO_2 < 55$ mmHg or $SaO_2 < 88\%$ with a low level of exertion
- During sleep: $PaO_2 < 55$ mmHg or $SaO_2 < 88\%$ with associated complications (i.e., pulmonary hypertension, daytime somnolence, or cardiac arrhythmias)

- More than a 5% fall in saturation during sleep
* Supportive evidence less definite than that for continuous oxygen. These are criteria for Medicare reimbursement for noncontinuous oxygen.

MEDICARE REQUIREMENTS FOR LONG-TERM OXYGEN THERAPY

- The laboratory, *not* the oxygen supplier, must measure PaO_2 or SaO_2 (or both).
- The patient must have optimal medical management and must be clinically stable before certification.
- The physician must complete a medical necessity form.
- There must be recertification and retesting in 61–90 days if the patient has an initial PaO_2 of 56–59 mmHg and a saturation of 89%. All other patients need recertification after 12 months but require no retesting.
- Certification should be revised when the prescription is changed.

http://www.goldcopd.org

Kacmarek RM: Supplemental oxygen and other medical gas therapy. In Pierson DJ, Kacmarek RM (eds): Foundations of Respiratory Care. New York, Churchill Livingstone, 1992, pp 859–889.

O'Donohue WJ: Indications for long-term oxygen therapy and appropriate use. In O'Donohue WJ (ed): Long-Term Oxygen Therapy: Scientific Basis and Application. New York, Marcel Dekker, 1995, pp 53–68.

Plummer AL: The role of the home oxygen provider in education, assessment, and quality improvement. In O'Donohue WJ (ed): Long-Term Oxygen Therapy: Scientific Basis and Application. New York, Marcel Dekker, 1995, pp 197–217.

Stoller JK, Hoisington E, Auger G: A comparative analysis of arranging in-flight oxygen aboard commercial air carriers. Chest 115:991–995, 1999.

Tarpy SP, Celli BR: Long-term oxygen therapy. N Engl J Med 333:710–714, 1995.

Tiep BL: Long-term home oxygen therapy. Clin Chest Med 11:505–521, 1990.

KEY POINT: INDICATIONS FOR CONTINUOUS SUPPLEMENTAL OXYGEN

1. Resting room air $PaO_2 < 55$ mmHg or $SaO_2 < 88\%$

2. Resting $PaO_2 < 55$ mmHg or $SaO_2 < 88\%$

3. Resting $PaO_2 = 56–59$ mmHg or $SaO_2 < 89\%$ in the presence of any of the following:

   - Edema suggesting congestive heart failure or P pulmonale on electrocardiogram.

   - Erythrocytosis (i.e., hematocrit 56% or more).

4. Resting $PaO_2 > 59$ mmHg or $SaO_2 > 89\%$, reimbursable only with additional documentation justifying the oxygen prescription and a summary that more conservative therapy has failed

3. **Should supplemental oxygen be prescribed during sleep?**
   For individuals with resting daytime hypoxemia, supplemental oxygen should be provided during sleep as part of the goal of providing oxygen for as close to 24 hours a day as possible. For COPD patients with nocturnal hypoxemia (i.e., $SaO_2 < 88\%$ or $PaO_2 \leq 55$ mmHg) but adequate oxygenation during wakefulness (i.e., $PaO_2 > 60$ mmHg), the benefits of supplemental oxygen are less clear, but many clinicians prescribe oxygen when symptoms ascribable to hypoxemia are present (e.g., pulmonary hypertension, cardiac arrhythmias, or disrupted sleep with daytime hypersomnolence).

4. **Should supplemental oxygen be prescribed during exercise?**
   Although hypoxemia is less frequently the cause of exercise limitation than is reaching ventilatory or cardiovascular limits, patients with hypoxemia during exercise (i.e., $PaO_2 \leq 55$ mmHg or

$SaO_2 \leq 88\%$) may benefit from using supplemental oxygen during exercise. In this circumstance, supplemental oxygen may reduce minute ventilation, improve ventilatory muscle function, lessen dyspnea, and improve endurance. As such, many clinicians will prescribe oxygen to eligible individuals during exercise. The liter flow rates are best determined by exercise studies with intermittent blood gas sampling through an indwelling arterial line. Although less invasive, pulse oximetry measurements of oxygen saturation during exercise can be misleading, causing oxygen to be prescribed when not needed and also leading to undertreatment of hypoxemia.

Oakes D: Therapeutic modalities. In Clinical Practitioners' Guide to Respiratory Care. Rockville, MD, Health Educator Publishers, 1988, pp 143–159.

Tarpy SP, Celli BR: Long-term oxygen therapy. N Engl J Med 333:710–714, 1995.

5. **Should supplemental oxygen be prescribed for individuals with hypoxemia due to causes other than COPD?**
   Yes. Although the indications and benefits of supplemental oxygen have been studied best for individuals with COPD, other hypoxemic individuals should also be considered as candidates for supplemental oxygen. Examples of such patients include those with idiopathic pulmonary fibrosis, kyphoscoliosis, or cystic fibrosis.

Petty TL: Historical highlights of long-term oxygen therapy. Respir Care 45:29–36, 2000.

Zielinski J: Long-term oxygen therapy in conditions other than chronic obstructive pulmonary disease. Respir Care 45:172–176, 2000.

6. **How should an oxygen prescription be written?**
   Once the need for supplemental oxygen is established, a prescription can be written. It should include:
   - The qualifying arterial blood gas
   - The type of delivery system to be used (e.g., a stationary system, portable or ambulatory equipment, or an oxygen-conserving device)
   - The delivery device (i.e., a nasal cannula, a transtracheal catheter, or a mask)
   - The liter flow under specific conditions (i.e., sleep, rest, and exercise)
   - The patient's diagnosis

   The physician is responsible for all forms and documentation. A Health Care Financing Administration (HCFA) form 494 (Certificate of Medical Necessity: Oxygen) must be filled out for all Medicare patients and for some third-party payers. Oxygen prescriptions are unique in that the patient generally receives oxygen therapy before the home medical equipment (HME) company has a properly written prescription. Therefore, it is often the HME company's responsibility to ensure that the patient has a proper oxygen prescription on file for reimbursement to take place.

Plummer AL: The role of the home oxygen provider in education, assessment, and quality improvement. In O'Donohue WJ (ed): Long-Term Oxygen Therapy: Scientific Basis and Application. New York, Marcel Dekker, 1995, pp 197–217.

7. **Is supplemental oxygen recommended during commercial air travel?**
   As evidence of Dalton's law of gases, conditions inside the cabin of a commercial airplane in flight expose travelers to conditions of hypobaric hypoxia; in other words, because the ambient pressure is decreased, the inspired oxygen tension is decreased. The specific ambient pressure within the plane depends on the altitude and the properties of the plane itself, but U.S. Federal Aviation Administration rules require that the pressure inside the cabin remain below the equivalent of 8000 feet (except for brief ascents to a 10,000-foot equivalent to avoid bad weather). Under conditions of hypobaric hypoxia, arterial oxygen tension falls in travelers. Because of the theoretic risks of hypoxemia, especially when SaO_2 falls below 90%, supplemental oxygen has been recommended for air travelers when their resting PaO_2 is predicted to be 50 mmHg during flight, so clinicians should attempt to predict whether an individual traveler's PaO_2 is likely to fall below 50 mmHg during air flight. For patients with normocapnic, stable COPD,

several regression equations are available that help to predict the traveler's in-flight PaO_2, the most recent of which is as follows:

$$\text{Predicted } PaO_2 \text{ at } 8000 \text{ ft} = 0.294 \, (PaO_2 \text{ on room air at sea level})$$
$$+ 0.086 \, (FEV_1\% \text{ predicted}) + 23.211$$

Where FEV_1 is the forced expiratory volume in 1 second.

This calculation requires measurement of the traveler's room air resting PaO_2 and FEV_1 (without a bronchodilator). Alternative methods for predicting the traveler's in-flight PaO_2 include measuring the PaO_2 while the traveler breathes a hypoxic gas mixture (i.e., 15.1% oxygen) meant to simulate the hypoxia during air travel or measuring of the PaO_2 under actual hypobaric conditions (e.g., a hypobaric chamber or an actual ascent to altitude). Practical constraints make these approaches unattractive, thereby favoring use of the regression equation. However, for patients with pulmonary diseases other than normocapnic, stable COPD (e.g., restrictive diseases or hypercapnic COPD), no predictive equations are available, and clinicians must either prescribe supplemental in-flight oxygen empirically or must determine the traveler's actual PaO_2 under hypoxic conditions (i.e., by breathing a hypoxic gas or by measuring PaO_2 under actual hypobaric conditions).

Dillard TA, Moores LK, Bilello KL, et al: The preflight evaluation: A comparison of the hypoxia inhalation test with hypobaric exposure. Chest 107:352–357, 1995.

Stoller JK: Oxygen and air travel. Respir Care 45:214–221, 2000.

8. **How is oxygen arranged for air travelers?**
Once the decision has been made to prescribe supplemental oxygen during air flight, the traveler must arrange for in-flight oxygen to be supplied by the airline. Current regulations by the U.S. Federal Aviation Administration prohibit travelers from bringing their own oxygen supplies for use in the airline cabin. Furthermore, individual airlines vary regarding the type of oxygen system they supply (generally they supply cylinders, and occasionally they offer concentrators [i.e., the Air Sep Lifestyle Portable Oxygen Concentrator]), the liter flow and delivery device (e.g., cannula or mask), the cost of providing oxygen (which is not covered by Medicare, even if the traveler qualifies for supplemental oxygen under Medicare guidelines), and the advance time needed to arrange for oxygen. As a result, it is important for the traveler to know the specific policy of the airline on which travel is planned. Notwithstanding individual variation among airlines, several general rules apply, as follows:

- Arrangements for oxygen must be made well in advance of the actual trip, usually allowing at least 3 days prior to domestic trips.
- Although the specific airline may wish its medical department to speak with the traveler's physician, a written prescription for oxygen by the traveler's physician is advised. The prescription should specify the liter flow and the duration of oxygen needed.
- Travelers should bring along their own nasal tubing in extra length.
- A seat near the bathroom is advised to minimize motion and time off from supplemental oxygen.
- Traveling on a nonstop direct flight is advised to minimize travel time and the expense of receiving oxygen (because some air carriers charge for each leg of a connecting flight, at least with cylinders).
- Traveling during business hours is advised, especially if the traveler requires supplemental oxygen on arrival at the airport and at the travel destination. Oxygen supplied by the airline stops when the traveler leaves the plane, so for travelers requiring supplemental oxygen at sea level (or if the travel destination is at high altitude), interaction with an oxygen vendor on arrival must be arranged separately.
- Most airlines have medical departments that can provide specific information about the carrier's oxygen policy.

Stoller JK: Oxygen and air travel. Respir Care 45:214–221, 2000.

Stoller JK, Hoisington E, Auger G: A comparative analysis of arranging in-flight oxygen aboard commercial air carriers. Chest 115:991–995, 1999.

9. **What systems exist to provide supplemental oxygen for use at home?**

Oxygen in the home is often delivered by nasal cannula at low flow rates of 2–4 L/min. Patients often require several different systems for use at home, for example, for use around the house (where an oxygen concentrator and a long connecting delivery tube may work well), during excursions outside the home (when a liquid oxygen portable carrier or a smaller tank such as an E-type cylinder is especially suitable), and during exercise in the home. There are three delivery systems currently available for use in the home: compressed-oxygen cylinders, liquid oxygen systems, and oxygen concentrators. Hybrid systems allow an oxygen canister to be transfilled from a reservoir or an oxygen concentrator. Liquid oxygen systems and compressed oxygen cylinders are available for travel.

Compressed oxygen is provided in high-pressure cylinders. They are large and heavy and can cause injury because of their high pressure if the valve end of the tank is damaged. Generally, size H or G tanks are used, with a duration of use of 57.5 and 39.2 hours, respectively, at 2 L/min. Several links of oxygen tubing can be attached to the tank in order to provide (limited) patient mobility. Smaller tanks, sizes D and E, are available for use during travel; their durations of use at 2 L/min are 2.9 and 5.1 hours, respectively. Combining the smaller units with an oxygen-conserving device may extend the duration of available oxygen to as long as 8 hours. Compressed gas systems generally require frequent visits from the homecare company. If the patient is unable to change the regulator, visits may be required every other day.

Liquid oxygen systems offer several advantages over compressed oxygen cylinders, particularly for patients who are active. Stationary systems of liquid oxygen weigh 240 pounds and provide 7 days of continuous oxygen at 2 L/min. Portable liquid systems can be refilled easily from the larger stationary systems; they weigh less and will last four times longer than compressed oxygen cylinders at a given flow rate. The major disadvantage of liquid oxygen systems is their high cost. Oxygen itself is relatively inexpensive, but the cost of specialized home stationary units and delivery trucks dramatically increases the cost. As a result, liquid oxygen is often available only in large metropolitan areas. Liquid oxygen is stored at −183°C; as the tanks warm up, the oxygen expands, requiring pressure-relief valves, which waste unused oxygen. Coupling devices for the stationary and portable systems made by different manufacturers may not be compatible, which further increases the cost. An advantage of liquid systems is that patients may fill their own tanks from the stationary system, but this poses the risk of thermal burns if the liquid oxygen is accidentally poured on the skin. Therefore, as a precaution, gloves should always be worn when transfilling cylinders.

Oxygen concentrators are electric devices that use either a molecular sieve or a semiperme-able membrane. The molecular sieve separates oxygen from the air for delivery to the patient and returns nitrogen to the atmosphere. This device can deliver more than 90% oxygen at flows of up to 4 L/min. The membrane-type concentrator is primarily permeable to oxygen and water vapor. These units function at a low level of efficiency, delivering oxygen concentrations of only 40%. Both types weigh approximately 35 pounds and operate on wall current. Therefore, they are used as stationary sources of oxygen in the home. Periodic refilling of the device is not necessary, although periodic preventive maintenance is required. Compressed oxygen cylinders and an electric generator should be available as a backup in areas prone to frequent power failures. Delivered oxygen concentrations should be analyzed on a monthly basis.

As a recent innovation, some concentrators are now available with a unit on top that can transfill a compressed oxygen tank for use outside the home. These units weigh approximately 10 pounds and, at 2 L/min with an oxygen-conserving device, will provide oxygen for 8 hours. Without a conserving device, the supply may last for only 2.5 hours. Advantages of the device include versa-tility and the possibility of limiting the need for home visits to service liquid systems, although these systems are currently expensive (~$5000) and are not currently reimbursed by Medicare.

Development of a portable oxygen concentrator remains an attractive goal. To date, one such device exists, which uses membrane technology to provide 1 L/min of 40% oxygen for 1 hour. The device weighs 10 pounds, but flow rate and limited supply duration make it clinically impractical for most uses at this time.

Another new development is a device that produces liquid oxygen by diversion of 1 L/min flow from a cryocooler device. Further assessment and experience with this system are needed before it can be endorsed.

Kacmarek RM: Delivery systems for long-term oxygen therapy. Respir Care 45:84–92, 2000.

Kacmarek RM: Oxygen delivery systems for long-term oxygen therapy. In O'Donohue WJ (ed): Long-Term Oxygen Therapy: Scientific Basis and Application. New York, Marcel Dekker, 1995, pp 219–234.

Tiep BL: Long-term home oxygen therapy. Clin Chest Med 11:505–521, 1990.

10. **What is the cost of supplemental oxygen?**
Medicare provides a set monthly fee (now approximately $193/month) for reimbursement to vendors of supplemental oxygen, regardless of the oxygen system used. As a result, the least expensive oxygen system is generally provided by the oxygen vendor unless otherwise specified by the physician's oxygen prescription. Most patients require a stationary source, usually a concentrator, for use in the home. Concentrators are relatively inexpensive (at approximately $2200 per unit) and require regular maintenance. Patients not confined to bed should have a system to supply oxygen when they are outside their home.
Compressed gas or liquid oxygen systems are available as portable devices. Liquid oxygen has a higher cost (at approximately $3500/unit) for a stationary system that can be the primary oxygen source and also can fill smaller cylinders for use outside the home. Compressed oxygen tanks cost approximately $350 each and require frequent refilling by the homecare company.

Dunne PJ: The demographics and economics of long-term oxygen therapy. Respir Care 45:223–238, 2000.

11. **What is an oxygen delivery device?**
Oxygen delivery devices are the conduits through which oxygen flows from the oxygen source (e.g., the tank or concentrator) to the patient. Such delivery devices can be divided into two major categories: low-flow and high-flow systems. Low-flow systems are not intended to meet the patient's total inspiratory requirements. Oxygen concentrations delivered by these devices vary with ventilatory rate and tidal volume. For example, if the tidal volume is large, the inspired FiO_2 is lower; if the tidal volume is small, the inspired FiO_2 increases. A high-flow system has a reservoir and a total gas flow that supplies the patient's inspiratory requirements. The ventilatory rate and tidal volume have no effect on inspired oxygen concentrations.

Adamo J, Mehta AC, Stelmach KA, et al: The Cleveland Clinic's initial experience with transtracheal oxygen therapy. Respir Care 35:153–160, 1990.

Huber GL, Carter R, Mahajan VK: Transtracheal oxygen therapy. In O'Donohue WJ (ed): Long-Term Oxygen Therapy: Scientific Basis and Application. New York, Marcel Dekker, 1995, pp 257–309.

Kacmarek RM: Oxygen delivery systems for long-term oxygen therapy. In O'Donohue WJ (ed): Long-Term Oxygen Therapy: Scientific Basis and Application. New York, Marcel Dekker, 1995, pp 219–234.

KEY POINTS: AVAILABLE OXYGEN SYSTEMS

1. Compressed oxygen

2. Liquid oxygen

3. Oxygen concentrator devices

12. **What oxygen delivery devices are available?**
See Table 71-1.

13. **Is humidification of supplemental oxygen necessary?**
Medical gases are essentially anhydrous (i.e., without water) and therefore require artificial humidification. Over the years, whether supplemental oxygen should be humidified has been

TABLE 71-1. OXYGEN DELIVERY DEVICES AND FiO₂ CAPABILITIES

Delivery System	Description	L/min Flow Rate Delivers FiO₂	Complications
Nasal cannula	Flow rate of 1–6 L/min (except for two new systems that provide higher flow [up to 40 L/min] with humidification; see question 15) Delivers approximately 4%/L Prongs insert 1 cm into each nostril Comfortable and inexpensive Patient can eat and talk	1 L/min = 24% 2 L/min = 28% 3 L/min = 32% 4 L/min = 36% 5 L/min = 40% 6 L/min = 44%	Delivered FiO_2 depends on tidal volume and ventilatory rate Nasal passages must be patent Easily dislodged May irritate nasal passages and eyes at higher flow rates
Simple mask*	Flow rate of 5–8 L/min Clear plastic Must fit tightly on patient's face	5–8 L/min = 50–60%	Need a minimum of 5 L/min to adequately flush carbon dioxide and avoid rebreathing Must fit securely to patient's face to avoid entrainment of room air and dilution of inspired FiO_2; increased risk of aspiration Less comfortable than nasal cannula Easily removed
Partial rebreathing mask*	Flow rate of 6–10 L/min Clear plastic mask that incorporates reservoir bag into system to deliver oxygen concentrations >60%	6–10 L/min = 55–70%	Flow should be sufficient to keep reservoir bag inflated on inspiration Other complications same as those for simple mask
Nonrebreathing mask*	Flow rate of 10–12 L/min Clear plastic mask with reservoir bag and two one-way valves (one on the mask and one between the reservoir bag and the mask)	10–12 L/min = 80–100%	Flow should be sufficient to keep reservoir bag inflated on inspiration Other complications same as for simple mask

Continued

TABLE 71-1. OXYGEN DELIVERY DEVICES AND FiO₂ CAPABILITIES—CONT'D

Delivery System	Description	L/min Flow Rate Delivers FiO_2	Complications
Venturi mask**	Flow rates are variable	2 L/min = 24%	Same as for simple mask
	Clear plastic mask with different adapters that determine FiO_2	3 L/min = 28%	
	Provides exact oxygen concentrations	4 L/min = 31%	
	Inspired concentrations do not vary with ventilatory rate and tidal volume	6 L/min = 35%	
		8 L/min = 40%	
	Delivery device of choice for patients with chronic obstructive pulmonary disease, depending on hypoxic drive	10 L/min = 45%	
		12 L/min = 50%	
		14 L/min = 55%	

*Low-flow system (i.e., does not meet total patient demand)
**High-flow system (i.e., meets total patient demand)
Adapted from Oakes D: Therapeutic modalities. In Clinical Practitioners' Guide to Respiratory Care. Rockville, MD, Health Educator Publications, 1988, pp 143–159; Ryerson CG, Block AJ: Oxygen as a drug: Chemical properties, benefits and hazards of administration. In Burton GG, Hodgkin JE (eds): Respiratory Care. 2nd ed. Philadelphia, J.B. Lippincott, 1984, pp 395–415; Tarpy SP, Celli BR: Long-term oxygen therapy. N Engl J Med 333:710–714, 1995; and Waugh JP, Granger WM: An evaluation of two new devices for nasal high-flow oxygen therapy. Respir Care 49: 902–906, 2004.

debated. Current standards indicate that humidification of inhaled gas should be provided when flows are ≥ 4 L/min or when the patient requests humidification.

When gas reaches body temperature, ambient pressure, and saturation with water vapor (BTPS), it has an absolute humidity of 43.9 mgH$_2$O/L of gas. An unheated bubble humidifier producing a water vapor content of 13.5 mgH$_2$O/L would cause a deficit of 30.4 mgH$_2$O/L that must be met by the body, thereby predisposing the patient to drying and dehydration. Thus, at higher flow rates, the risk that loss of airway moisture could cause problems and side effects increases. Such side effects of inadequate humidification include decreased ciliary activity, squamous epithelial changes, dehydration and thickening of secretions, atelectasis, tracheitis, and heat loss.

American Association for Respiratory Care: AARC Clinical Practice Guideline: Oxygen therapy for adults in the acute care facility: 2002 revision and update. Respir Care 47: 717–720, 2002.

Branson, RD: The nuts and bolts of increasing arterial oxygenation: Devices and techniques. Respir Care 38: 672–686, 1993.

Waugh JP, Granger WM: An evaluation of two new devices for nasal high-flow oxygen therapy. Respir Care 49: 902–906, 2004.

14. **Can high-flow oxygen be administered through nasal cannula?**
Until recently, gas flows through nasal cannula have been limited to 6 L/min because of the challenges of humidifying nasal oxygen at higher rates. As such, to date, nasal cannula have been considered a low-flow delivery device. However, two new devices are available that can deliver high-flow humidified gas through nasal cannula. Specifically, one product (Salter Labs, Inc.) is a nonheated nasal cannula and bubble humidifier capable of flows up to 15 L/min. The second device, called Vapotherm 2000i (Vapotherm, Inc., Stevensville, MD), is a high-flow gas delivery device that heats and humidifies gas for delivery through a nasal cannula, face mask, tracheostomy mask, or other traditional device. The Vapotherm has a high-flow cartridge providing 5–40 L/min at > 95% relative humidity; the low-flow cartridge has a range of 1–8 L/min at >95% relative humidity.

The American Society for Testing and Materials (ASTM) specifies that humidification systems must provide an output of at least 10 mgH$_2$O/L (equivalent to 60% relative humidity) and, if the upper airway is bypassed, the output must be at least 33 mgH$_2$O/L. In a recent study, both of the aforementioned devices exceeded the minimum humidification standards at higher-than-traditional flow, thereby meeting ASTM standards. The Salter device achieved 72.5–78.7% relative humidity at 5–15 L/min with 17.3–14.2 mgH$_2$O/L. The Vapotherm device achieved 99.9% relative humidity at 5–40 L/min with 42.6–44.0 mgH$_2$O/L.

The ability of these nasal cannula systems to exceed the average adult peak inspiratory flow (30 L/min) allows them to be classified as high-flow systems, thereby challenging the traditional classification of the nasal cannula as a low-flow device. Further research is needed to determine the optimal clinical role of these high-flow nasal cannula.

Waugh JP, Granger WM: An evaluation of two new devices for nasal high-flow oxygen therapy. Respir Care 49:902–906, 2004.

15. **What are oxygen-conserving devices?**
Delivery of oxygen to the alveoli occurs during the first sixth of the inspiratory cycle. Oxygen delivered throughout the remainder of the respiratory cycle is wasted. Oxygen-conserving devices have been developed with the intent of eliminating "wasted" oxygen flow and maximizing the efficiency of oxygen supply devices. These oxygen-conserving devices generally provide adequate oxygenation at rest, with exercise, and during sleep; conserve oxygen; are more comfortable for the patient; and generally are more economical.

Three types of oxygen-conserving devices are currently available: reservoir systems, demand delivery systems, and transtracheal catheters. One type of reservoir system uses the nasal cannula as the reservoir. Such reservoir nasal cannulas have a pouch that stores 20 mL of oxygen during the expiratory phase, to be delivered at the beginning of the following inspiration as a bolus. In contrast, demand delivery systems sense inspiration and deliver an inspiratory bolus of oxygen. Finally, transtracheal catheters are inserted directly into the trachea, thereby bypassing the cephalad anatomic dead space and using the upper airways as a reservoir for oxygen during end-expiration. Placement of transtracheal catheters requires an office procedure that is usually performed by a pulmonologist or an otolaryngologist. Oxygen-conserving devices have gained great popularity because they reduce the amount of oxygen used, decrease the cost of oxygen, and provide the patient with increased mobility and independence.

Adamo J, Mehta AC, Stelmach KA, et al: The Cleveland Clinic's initial experience with transtracheal oxygen therapy. Respir Care 35:153–160, 1990.

Tiep BL, Lewis MI: Oxygen conservation and oxygen conserving devices in chronic lung disease. Chest 92:263–272, 1987.

Weill D, Make B: Oxygen-conserving devices. In O'Donohue WJ (ed): Long-Term Oxygen Therapy: Scientific Basis and Application. New York, Marcel Dekker, 1995, pp 235–256.

16. **List the advantages and disadvantages of different oxygen-conserving devices.**
See Table 71-2.

17. **How are oxygen-conserving devices paid for or reimbursed?**
Medicare reimbursement rates for home oxygen therapy are based on local costs, independent of the device used. The rate of reimbursement is set for users with liter-flow rates of 1–4 L/min, although Medicare reimbursement is adjusted for very low or very high flow rates. For example, if the liter flow is less than 1 L/min, the rate of reimbursement is reduced to 50% of the base cost, whereas liter flow rates of more than 4 L/min raise the reimbursement rate to 150% of the base rate. Unfortunately, the new reimbursement regulations have discouraged the use of oxygen-conserving devices, particularly transtracheal oxygen, which often operates at less than 1 L/min. The decision to provide an oxygen-conserving service is often influenced greatly by whether or not funding can be secured; a conserving device may be deferred unless reimbursement is available.

Dunne PJ: The demographics and economics of long-term oxygen therapy. Respir Care 45:223–238, 2000.

18. **How is oxygen therapy monitored and adjusted?**
Oxygen therapy should be monitored and adjusted periodically based on careful patient assessment. Oxygen therapy is best monitored by arterial blood gas or pulse oximetry measurements with target values of $PaO_2 \geq 60$ mmHg and a pulse oximetry measurement $(SpO_2) \geq 90\%$. Readings of SaO_2 and SpO_2 generally correlate within ±2% at rest. As a way of verifying the reliability of pulse oximeter measurements, the palpated pulse or heart rate derived from the electrocardiogram (ECG) and the heart rate displayed on the pulse oximeter should agree within ±5 beats. If pulse oximetry does provide accurate readings of saturation, it is preferred for titrating oxygen at rest. In this way, use of pulse oximetry can decrease the number of samples needed for arterial blood gas measurement.

McCarthy K, Decker M, Strohl KP, et al: Pulse oximetry. In Kacmarek RM, Hess D, Stoller JK (eds): Monitoring in Respiratory Care. St. Louis, Mosby Yearbook, 1993, pp 309–347.

19. **Are there risks associated with providing supplemental oxygen?**
Yes. The risks associated with oxygen use relate to the possible effects of oxygen on ventilatory control, the morbidity associated with various oxygen delivery devices, and the risks related to using a combustible substance like oxygen. With regard to effects of supplemental oxygen on ventilation, some patients with hypoxemia experience hypoventilation when supplemental oxygen is used. Two mechanisms have been proposed as the cause of hypoventilation: (1) suppression of the hypoxic drive to breathe in individuals dependent on hypoxic drive as the major ventilatory drive and (2) increased dead space ventilation caused by increased pulmonary perfusion after relief of alveolar hypoxia. Individuals likely to experience hypercapnia when using supplemental oxygen are those with fixed, severe airflow obstruction and preexisting hypercapnia.

Other risks associated with using oxygen relate to the devices through which oxygen is delivered. A nasal cannula can cause irritation of the nasal mucosa or the skin over the ears, epistaxis

TABLE 71-2. OXYGEN-CONSERVING DEVICES

Type	Cost	Advantages	Disadvantages
Reservoir nasal cannula	Low (approximately $25 per unit)	Reliable, easy to initiate and use, 33–50% oxygen conservation	Not aesthetically pleasing for the patient Frequent replacement needed
Demand delivery system	High (approximately $800–950 per unit)	Greatest degree of conserving oxygen of available systems (87%)	Mechanical failure possible Complicated technology (although it is easy to use)
Transtracheal catheter	High (approximately $700 for initial placement and $98 per replacement catheter, generally required every 3 months)	Aesthetically pleasing for patient Requires special care (i.e., hidden from sight) Decreases work of breathing Patients are more compliant with oxygen use Does not easily become dislodged during sleep	Requires dexterity and tolerance of minor annoyances and complications

Adapted from Tarpy SP, Celli BR: Long-term oxygen therapy. N Engl J Med 333:710–714, 1995; and Weill D, Make B: Oxygen-conserving devices. In O'Donohue WJ (ed): Long-Term Oxygen Therapy: Scientific Basis and Application. New York, Marcel Dekker, 1995, pp 235–256.

resulting from drying of the nasal mucosa, and psychologic unease about public exposure of one's oxygen dependence. Complications accompanying transtracheal oxygen are frequent but usually minor. These include infection at the insertion site, catheter displacement requiring reinsertion, cough, cephalad misplacement of the catheter between the vocal cords, and bleeding and tracheal obstruction related to collection of inspissated mucus on the catheter. Finally, individuals using supplemental oxygen must avoid close exposure to open flames (e.g., stove burners or cigarettes) because oxygen supports combustion and can promote fire.

Specific delivery systems may pose certain risks. For example, the pressure within compressed gas cylinders can exceed safe levels when ambient temperatures surpass 70°F. As the temperature rises, a safety valve opens, releasing oxygen into the air, creating a fire hazard. Also, liquid delivery systems store oxygen at very low temperatures (i.e., −297°F). Hazards are related to the transfer of liquid oxygen from a large tank to a smaller portable one. The process can expose the patient or caregiver to liquid oxygen, incurring a risk of frostbite or burn.

Benditt JO: Adverse effects of low-flow oxygen therapy. Respir Care 45:54–61, 2000.

Kacmarek RM: Supplemental oxygen and other medical gas therapy. In Pierson DJ, Kacmarek RM (eds): Foundations of Respiratory Care. New York, Churchill Livingstone, 1992, pp 859–889.

Ryerson GG, Block AJ: Oxygen as a drug: Chemical properties, benefits and hazards of administration. In Burton GG, Hodgkin JE (eds): Respiratory Care, 2nd ed. Philadelphia, J.B. Lippincott, 1984, pp 395–415.

20. **How should patients receiving supplemental oxygen be transported within the hospital?**

Transport of a patient receiving oxygen therapy within the hospital demands specific attention to patient assessment and FiO_2 requirements. Once the need for oxygen has been established by arterial blood gas analysis or pulse oximetry, transport should be planned carefully so that all necessary equipment and personnel are available. Patients receiving low-flow oxygen at 1–6 L/min can be transported using a portable liquid vessel of oxygen, often available from the patient transportation department at larger institutions. Higher flows (i.e., more than 6 L/min) require the use of a compressed gas cylinder, usually size E. The cylinder should be checked to ensure that it is full before the transport is begun; full cylinders contain 2200 pounds per square inch (psi) and will provide oxygen for 1.7 hours at a flow rate of 6 L/min. Clinically unstable patients ideally should have a portable pulse oximeter in place while undergoing diagnostic tests or transport to other areas of the institution. Because transporting a sick patient incurs some risk, the benefits of the diagnostic test or treatment for which transport is needed must always justify the trip.

CHAPTER 72

LUNG TRANSPLANTATION

Marie M. Budev, DO, MPH, and Janet R. Maurer, MD, MBA

1. **Summarize the history of lung transplantation.**

   The first human lung transplant was performed in 1963 by Dr. James Hardy at the University of Mississippi in a recipient with lung cancer. This recipient died within 18 days of the transplant, not of graft failure, but rather from kidney failure. Over the next 20 years, more than 40 lung transplants were performed worldwide, but only two patients survived more than 1 month. Factors that contributed to the lack of success in the early history of lung transplantation included defective healing of the bronchial anastomoses, lack of medical and surgical knowledge of the complications associated with organ transplantation, and inadequate immunosuppressive agents.

   The introduction of cyclosporine was a pivotal point in the history of lung transplantation. In 1983, Dr. Joel Cooper performed the first successful single lung transplant using a technique to prevent bronchial ischemia, a "vascularized" omental wrap. In the past 15 years, lung transplantation has been an accepted therapy for end-stage lung and pulmonary vascular diseases. Success came with improved surgical techniques and improved knowledge of posttransplantation complications and management.

   More than 16,000 lung transplants were performed through 2002; overall, the number of double lung transplants has increased 83% since 1983 and now exceeds the number of single lung transplants.

   http://www.ishlt.org

2. **How does the bilateral sequential lung transplant procedure differ from an *en bloc* lung transplant?**

   The first double lung transplant was performed as an *en bloc* procedure, in which two lungs were transplanted as a group (or *en bloc*) with a single tracheal anastomosis and a single vascular anastomosis. However, *en bloc* double lung transplantation seemed to have a higher rate of death with anastomotic necrosis because of the large amount of donor airway that lacked an adequate amount of vascular supply. Bilateral sequential lung transplantation is essentially two separate unilateral transplants, done one after the other, each with separate bronchial and vascular anastomoses.

DONOR ISSUES

3. **What is a non–heart-beating donor?**

   The concept of utilizing lungs from a donor whose circulation has ceased is defined as a non–heart-beating donation. Typically, a potential donor with irreversible severe central nervous system (CNS) dysfunction is removed from life support to allow cessation of vital functions before organ retrieval begins. A number of centers have now had limited experiences with this donor pool with good outcomes. Non–heart-beating donors provide an opportunity to increase the overall donor supply.

   de Perrot M, Weder W, Patterson GA, et al: Strategies to increase limited donor resources. Eur Resp J 23:477–482, 2004.

4. **Which patients are candidates for a living lobar transplantation?**
   Most living lobar transplants have been performed in cystic fibrosis patients. But patients
   with other diseases, including pulmonary hypertension, pulmonary fibrosis, and obliterative
   bronchiolitis, have also undergone living lobar transplantation.

   In living lobar transplantation, one donor provides a right lower lobe and a second donor provides a left lower lobe to the recipient. Perioperative mortality, morbidity, and long-term survival
   are comparable to outcomes reported in cadaveric donor transplants.

   Starnes VA, Barr ML, Woo M: A decade of living lobar transplantation. Recipient outcomes. J Thorac
   Cardiovasc Surg 4:1283–1288, 2004.

5. **What types of donor complications can occur with living lobar transplant?**
   Complications in donors include phrenic nerve paralysis, loss of right middle lobe function, and
   bronchial strictures. No increase in mortality in the living lobar donor group has been noted,
   despite an increase in morbidity.

   de Perrot M, Weder W, Patterson GA, et al: Strategies to increase limited donor resources. Eur Resp J
   23:477–482, 2004.

KEY POINTS: LUNG TRANSPLANTATION

1. Lung transplantation is indicated for patients with end-stage lung disease and pulmonary
   vascular diseases who demonstrate declining function despite optimal medical therapy.

2. Critically ill patients in extreme clinical situations are rarely appropriate candidates for lung
   transplantation.

3. A large disparity exists between the number of potential recipients and the number of donor
   organs available, and many patients die on waiting lists. Early referral is key. A new organ
   allocation system will use parameters reflecting medical urgency, deemphasizing waitlist time.

4. Extension of donor criteria has increased the donor organ pool without significant impact on
   postoperative morbidity and mortality.

6. **What are the criteria that define a standard donor?**
   - Aged ≤ 55 years
   - Smoking history < 20 pack-years
   - Clear chest x-ray
   - $PaO_2 \geq 300$ mmHg at $FiO_2 = 1.0$, positive end-expiratory pressure (PEEP) = 5 cmH$_2$O
   - No aspiration or evidence of sepsis
   - No significant chest trauma or contusions
   - Absence of purulent secretions on bronchoscopy
   - Absence of organisms on Gram–Weigert stain and cultures
   - Length of intubation ≤ 48 hours
   - No previous cardiac surgery

   de Perrot M, Weder W, Patterson GA, et al: Strategies to increase limited donor resources. Eur Resp J
   23:477–482, 2004.

7. **What is an extended, or marginal, donor?**
   To increase the donor pool, the standard donor criteria have been liberalized, without a significant impact on postoperative morbidity or mortality. The criteria for an extended, or marginal, donor
   include age >55 years, a smoking history >20 pack-years, prolonged mechanical ventilation, a posi-

tive Gram–Weigert stain on sputum or bronchoalveolar lavage (BAL) samples, and limited infiltrates on chest x-ray.

de Perrot M, Weder W, Patterson GA, et al: Strategies to increase limited donor resources. Eur Resp J 23:477–482, 2004.

RECIPIENT SELECTION ISSUES AND THE PRETRANSPLANTATION PERIOD

8. **When should patients be referred for lung transplantation?**
   Candidates should have significant limitations in functional capacity, such that their current activity levels significantly impact on their quality of life. Traditionally, transplant pulmonologists have looked at the median 2-year posttransplant survival and have compared this to the projected survival of the patient's underlying primary condition.

   A newly devised allocation system for donor organs will involve more parameters that reflect medical urgency and a greater need for transplantation, while deemphasizing time waited on the list. This revised listing and allocation may eventually reduce the practice of placing candidates on the waiting list too early during their disease stage in an effort to accrue time.

   http://www.ustransplant.org

9. **Which patients are candidates for lung transplantation?**
   Candidates for lung transplantation should not have conditions that limit rehabilitation potential or comorbid medical conditions with organ damage. Relative contraindications to lung transplantation include symptomatic osteoporosis, nonambulatory status, severe cachexia or obesity, or unresponsive psychosocial or compliance issues. Presence of panresistant bacteria, including *Pseudomonas aeruginosa,* previously was felt to be a relative contraindication to transplantation of the cystic fibrosis patient, but recent data have demonstrated that this does not impact outcomes. Absolute contraindications include significant nonpulmonary end-organ damage, infection with hepatitis C with evidence of cirrhosis, presence of hepatitis B antigens, infection with human immunodeficiency virus (HIV), substance abuse within 6 months of listing, and malignancy within 2 years (with the exception of some skin cancers).

   Age criteria for lung transplantation are 65 years for single lung transplantation, 60 years for double lung transplantation, and 55 years for heart-lung transplantation. The specific disease considerations and eligibility criteria are listed in Table 72-1.

10. **Which type of transplant is appropriate for which type of disease?**
    Three types of transplants are now possible for lung transplant candidates: heart-lung; bilateral lung, or double lung; and unilateral, or single, lung. The most common indication for a single lung transplant (approximately 60%) is chronic obstructive pulmonary disease. Other indications include pulmonary fibrosis and primary or secondary pulmonary hypertension. Uncommon disease indications include lymphangioleiomyomatosis, histiocytosis X, and sarcoidosis.

    Bilateral transplants are most commonly performed for bronchiectasis, cystic fibrosis, and pulmonary hypertension.

    Heart-lung transplants, rare due to organ shortage, are reserved for patients with combined parenchymal and cardiac disease and for patients with Eisenmenger's syndrome.

11. **Why can patients with bronchiectasis receive only bilateral lung transplants?**
    In candidates with chronic infections, the native lungs serve as reservoirs for infection; therefore, both organs must be removed, or infection would rapidly disseminate when the patient is immunosuppressed. In rare cases, candidates with bronchiectasis may receive a single lung transplant, with pneumonectomy of the other lung.

TABLE 72-1. ELIGIBILITY CRITERIA FOR SPECIFIC DISEASES

Chronic obstructive lung disease or pulmonary fibrosis

- $FEV_1 < 25\%$ predicted, *and/or*
- Symptomatic progressive disease on $PCO_2 \geq 55$ mmHg, *and/or*
- Medical therapy (i.e., vital capacity [VC] < 60–70%,* elevated pulmonary artery pressure [PAP]-predicated and DLCO < 50–60%)

Cystic fibrosis and/or bronchiectasis and/or pulmonary hypertension

- $FEV_1 < 30\%$ predicted
- Symptomatic progressive disease
- $PCO_2 > 50$ mmHg despite prostacyclin therapy
- Rapid change in clinical status: New York Heart Association (NYHA) III or IV
- Other useful data: cardiac index < 2L, RAP > 15 mmHg, or mean PAP > 55 mmHg*

---

* These criteria are currently undergoing review and revision, and updated criteria should be available in the near future.
Modified from Maurer JR, Frost AE, Estenne M, Higenbottam T, Glanville AR: International Guidelines for the Selection of Lung Transplant Candidates. The International Society for Heart and Lung Transplantation, the American Thoracic Society, the American Society of Transplant Physicians, the European Respiratory Society. J Heart Lung Transplant 17:703–709, 1998.

---

12. **How is it determined which lung is selected to be transplanted in a unilateral transplant?**

    Perfusion scans determine the relative perfusion. The less-perfused side is transplanted in most cases. If a candidate has excessive surgical risk due to previous major thoracic surgery or other abnormalities, the side involved may be avoided. Alternatively, large cystic areas or other parenchymal changes may mark a native lung for transplant because of the risk of posttransplant infections, hyperinflation, and so forth.

13. **What is included in the preoperative management of lung transplant candidates?**

    Before transplant, many programs require enrollment in pulmonary rehabilitation. If patients become nonambulatory, they may be considered too ill to survive transplant and may be removed from the waiting list.

14. **Is the use of noninvasive positive pressure ventilation a contraindication to transplantation?**

    The use of noninvasive positive pressure ventilation is not a contraindication to transplantation. In general, patients on mechanical ventilatory support who are nonambulatory are not candidates for lung transplantation.

15. **What work-up is needed to determine if an individual is a candidate for lung transplantation?**

    Potential candidates undergo pulmonary function testing, a chest x-ray, a computed tomography (CT) scan of the chest, an echocardiogram, a 6-minute walk test or another exercise study, a stress cardiac study, and, possibly, left- and right-heart catheterization. In addition, routine blood work, antiviral serologies, tissue typing, and creatinine clearance are obtained. Bone mineral density should also be measured. Other preventive health screenings should be completed as part of the work for transplantation (e.g., sigmoidoscopy or colonoscopy, mammography, Pap smear, and dental clearance).

16. **What is the most common indication for retransplantation?**
Retransplantation is most commonly performed for chronic graft rejection or bronchiolitis obliterations. Retransplantation remains controversial. Early survival after retransplantation is reduced compared with that after the first transplant. Recurrent chronic rejection has been observed at a frequency similar to that seen after first transplant. Ventilator independence, ambulatory status, retransplantation after 1991, and prior experience of the transplant center are predictors of a good outcome after retransplantation.

Novick RJ, Stitt LW, Al-Kattan K, et al: Pulmonary retransplantation: Prediction of graft function and survival in 230 patients: Pulmonary retransplant registry. Ann Thorac Surg 65:227–234, 1998.

NONINFECTIOUS COMPLICATIONS AFTER TRANSPLANTATION

17. **What is the pulmonary reimplantation response?**
New grafts often develop noncardiogenic pulmonary edema within minutes to hours after the blood supply is reestablished. This process has been called the pulmonary reimplantation response or reperfusion injury. It is believed to be secondary to the effects of free oxygen radicals and various inflammatory cytokines produced after rewarming of the ischemic donor lung. Other factors include surgical trauma, denervation, and lymphatic disruption. This syndrome nearly always manifests in the first 48–72 hours after the transplant; pulmonary processes beginning after this interval should be investigated for other causes, including infection.

Radiographs show perihilar to diffuse infiltrates, and marked hypoxemia is seen. The differential diagnosis includes fluid overload, cardiogenic pulmonary edema, rejection, infection, and, occasionally, atelectasis.

18. **When does acute rejection occur? How is it diagnosed?**
Acute rejection occurs in approximately half of patients in the first year. This high rate of acute rejection is attributed to (1) lack of human leukocyte antigen (HLA) matching; (2) graft exposure to the external environment and to various inhaled agents including fumes, toxins, and infectious agents, which may trigger acute rejection; and (3) lung grafts containing many donor antigen-presenting cells. Acute rejection can be asymptomatic or present with nonspecific symptoms or findings including shortness of breath, fatigue, fever, cough, dyspnea, crackles, a fall in the forced expiratory volume in 1 second [FEV_1], and, occasionally, infiltrates or pleural effusions. The gold standard for diagnosing acute rejection is by histology using transbronchial biopsies, although noninvasive measurements of daily home spirometric measurements of FEV_1 may be helpful in the early detection of rejection. Overall, lung function is neither very sensitive nor specific for the diagnosis of acute rejection. There are no sensitive and specific surrogate markers of acute rejection.

Knoop C, Haverich A, Fischer S: Immunosuppressive therapy after human lung transplantation. Eur Respir J 23:159–171, 2004.

19. **What is the relationship between acute and chronic rejection?**
Acute rejection is rarely lethal. However, the numbers of episodes and the severity of acute rejection are risk factors for the subsequent development of chronic rejection. Acute rejection is treated intravenously with steroid pulses, specifically with up to three doses with 1 gram or 500 mg of methylprednisolone per day, usually followed by an increase in the oral prednisone dose, with a subsequent taper over 2–3 weeks. If acute rejection is recurrent or resistant to steroids on

repeat biopsies, changes in the patient's immunosuppressive regimen should be considered. In particularly refractory cases, antithymocyte or antilymphocyte preparations may be used. In rare cases of hyperacute cellular rejection, high-dose intravenous immunoglobulin (IVIG) therapy has been reported to be effective.

Knoop C, Haverich A, Fischer S: Immunosuppressive therapy after human lung transplantation. Eur Respir J 23:159–171, 2004.

INFECTIOUS COMPLICATIONS AFTER LUNG TRANSPLANTATION

20. **What is the reason that infection rates are higher in lung transplant recipients, as compared with other solid-organ transplant populations?**
It is likely that infection rates among lung transplant recipients are higher compared to other solid organ transplant populations because of exposure of the graft to the external environment, more intense immunosuppression, and impaired posttransplant pulmonary clearance mechanisms.

Maurer JR, Tullis E, Grossman RF, et al: Infectious complications following isolated lung transplantation. Chest 101:1056–1059, 1992.

21. **Which factors predispose lung transplant recipients to early bacterial infections?**
Bacterial pneumonia is most frequent in the first posttransplant month, with a reported incidence of 16%. Risk factors include high levels of immunosuppression, the need for prolonged mechanical ventilatory support, a blunted cough reflex due to pain, a disruption of lymphatic flow, ischemic injury to the bronchial mucosa, and impairment of mucociliary clearance. The most-common organisms include gram-negative rods of the Enterobacteriaceae family and *Pseudomonas* spp., as well as *Staphylococcus aureus* and *Haemophilus influenzae.*

Weill D, Dey GC, Hicks RA, et al: A positive donor gram stain does not predict outcome following lung transplantation. J Heart Lung Transplant 21:555–558, 2002.

22. **Does the presence of *Burkholderia cepacia* in cystic fibrosis patients affect survival outcomes after transplant?**
The presence of *Burkholderia cepacia* has been associated with a high risk of severe and often deadly postoperative infections, leading to 1-year survival rates of 50%, compared to 83% in patients without *B. cepacia*. Strain-specific virulence factors, in particular genomovar III, have been associated with an excessive risk of deadly infections.

Aris RM, Routh JC, LiPuma JJ, et al: Lung transplantation for cystic fibrosis patients with *Burkholderia cepacia* complex. Survival linked to genomovar type. Am J Respir Crit Care Med 164:2102–2106, 2001.

23. **What is the role of antimicrobial prophylaxis?**
   - **Bacterial:** Broad-spectrum antibiotics are used for a few days postoperatively in most patients and for as long as 2 weeks in patients with bronchiectasis. The length of treatment is usually determined by sensitivities found on preoperative sputum cultures.
   - **Viral:** Anti-cytomegalovirus (CMV) prophylaxis with ganciclovir or hyperimmune globulin (or both) or valacyclovir is used by most programs. However, the emergence of resistant strains has led some programs to use preemptive therapy instead of prophylaxis, depending on viral DNA levels.
   - **Fungal:** The emergence of fungal infections, especially *Aspergillus* infections, has led to near-universal prophylaxis against these infections with either aerosolized amphotericin or oral azoles. Length of prophylaxis varies.
   Trimethoprim–sulfamethoxazole prophylaxis is used in virtually all programs and is very effective in preventing *Pneumocystis carinii* and other bacterial infections.

24. **What is the most common viral pathogen in the posttransplant period?**
    The CMV is the most common viral pathogen encountered in the posttransplant period. CMV infection has been associated with an increased risk for bacterial and fungal suprainfections and has been implicated as a possible risk factor in the development of chronic rejection or bronchiolitis obliterans syndrome (BOS). Recipients seronegative for CMV who acquire infection from seropositive donors are at greatest risk for developing severe invasive disease and pneumonia. A diagnosis of CMV pneumonia is established by the presence of viral inclusion bodies on lung biopsy or on cytologic specimens obtained by bronchoalveolar lavage, but the sensitivity of these findings is low.

    Ettinger NA, Bailey TC, Trulock EP, et al: Cytomegalovirus infection and pneumonitis: Impact after isolated lung transplantation. Am Rev Respir Dis 147:1017–1023, 1993.

25. **What is the agent of choice for ganciclovir-resistant strains of CMV?**
    Ganciclovir-resistant strains occur at an incidence of approximately 5% but have not been associated with decreased survival. Risk factors include an increased number of CMV infections, an increased cumulative exposure to ganciclovir, and the use of antilymphocyte antibodies and daclizumab. Foscarnet is the agent of choice for ganciclovir-resistant disease but is limited in its use due to its nephrotoxicity.

    Bhorade SM, Lurain NS, Jordan A, et al: Emergence of ganciclovir resistant cytomegalovirus in lung transplant recipients. J Heart Lung Transplant 21:1274–1282, 2002.

26. **Are the other herpes viruses a threat to lung transplant?**
    Primary Epstein–Barr virus (EBV) infections occur in seronegative recipients who receive a seropositive graft. These recipients are at greatest risk for developing posttransplantation lymphoproliferative disorder (PTLD). A mononucleosis-like syndrome with fever, chills, myalgias, pharyngitis, and adenopathy is a sign of primary infection. This may be followed in weeks to months by manifestations of PTLD.

    Aris RM, Maia DM, Neuringer IP, et al: Post transplantation lymphoproliferative disorder in the Epstein-Barr virus-naïve lung transplant recipient. Am J Respir Crit Care Med 154:1712–1717, 1996.

27. **Is there a role for influenza vaccine in lung transplant recipients?**
    Influenza vaccine is recommended for lung transplant recipients, although the humoral immune response and the cell-mediated immune response to influenza vaccine may be poor. Nevertheless, there is little risk from vaccination, and the potential benefits are obvious. In addition, the community-acquired respiratory viral infections, including respiratory syncytial virus, parainfluenza, influenza, and adenovirus, may play a role in the development of bronchiolitis obliterans syndrome. These infections have important clinical implications, and strategies—for example, avoidance of children with upper respiratory infections (URIs), early treatment with antivirals, and so forth—to prevent or to modify viral infection should be followed.

    Khalifah AP, Hachem RR, Chakinala MM, et al: Respiratory viral infections are a distinct risk for bronchiolitis obliterans syndrome and death. Am J Respir Crit Care Med 170:181–187, 2004.
    Mazzone PJ, Mossad SB, Mawhorter SD, et al: Cell mediated immune response to influenza vaccination in lung transplant recipients. J Heart Lung Transpl 23:1175–1181, 2004.
    Mazzone PJ, Mossad SB, Mawhorter, SD, et al: The humoral immune response to influenza vaccination and lung transplantations. Eur Respir J 18:971–976, 2001.

28. **What is the most serious fungal infection in the posttransplant period?**
    Invasive aspergillosis is the most serious and life-threatening infection in the lung transplant recipient. Aspergillosis occurs in approximately 5% of patients, usually within the first year post transplant. Symptoms are nonspecific and include fever, cough, pleuritic pain, and hemoptysis. Radiographically, pulmonary aspergillosis may appear as a single or multiple cavitary lesions or nodules or as a consolidation with a pathopneumonic "halo sign" (i.e., a rim of ground-glass attenuation surrounding the nodular opacity on chest CT). Amphotericin B is the treatment of

choice for invasive aspergillosis, but a new triazole, voriconazole, was shown to have superior efficacy and less toxicity than amphotericin B in a large randomized trial.

Gordon SM, Avery RK: Aspergillosis in lung transplantation: incidence, risk factors, and prophylactic strategies. Transpl Infect Dis 3:161–167, 2001.

Herbrecht R, Denning DW, Patterson TF, et al: Voriconazole versus amphotericin B for primary therapy of invasive aspergillosis. N Engl J Med 347:408–415, 2002.

IMMUNOSUPPRESSION IN LUNG TRANSPLANTATION

29. **What is the role of induction immunosuppression after lung transplantation?**
The rationale for using induction therapy after lung transplantation includes the following:
- Lung transplant recipients are considered to be at high risk for rejection.
- Induction therapy levels allow a comfortable time frame to achieve target levels of calcineurin inhibitors without exposing the patient to significant risks of early rejection.
- Induction therapy allows renal function to recover from postoperative stress.

However, the use of induction therapy after lung transplant remains controversial as its benefits have not clearly been established. Arguments against its use include increased infection rate, a possible increased PTLD rate, and the high cost of these drugs.

Meyers BF, Lynch J, Trulock EP, et al: Lung transplantation: A decade of experience. Ann Surg 230:362–371, 1999.

30. **What is the standard immunosuppressive regimen after lung transplantation?**
The majority of lung transplant recipients receive a triple-drug maintenance regimen including a calcineurin inhibitor (either cyclosporine or tacrolimus), a cell-cycle inhibitor (either mycophenolate mofetil or azathioprine), and steroids. Steroid withdrawal is uncommon, even 5 years after transplantation. The superiority of one calcineurin agent over another has not been established to date.

Knoop C, Haverich A, Fischer S: Immunosuppressive therapy after human lung transplantation. Eur Respir J 23:159–171, 2004.

KEY POINTS: MEDICAL ISSUES AND IMMUNOSUPPRESSION ✔ IN LUNG TRANSPLANTATION

1. The rate of acute rejection in lung transplantation is as high as 54% early in the transplant period.

2. The most common posttransplant issues include nephrotoxicity, hypertension, osteoporosis, gastrointestinal complications including peptic ulcer disease, and malignancies including nonmelanoma skin cancers, followed by posttransplant lymphoproliferative disease.

3. Infection and BOS are the leading causes of early and late mortality in lung transplant recipients.

4. Current maintenance immunosuppressive strategies are three-pronged and include calcineurin inhibitors, cell-cycle inhibitors, and steroids. The role of sirolimus, a unique new immunosuppressant, is not yet clearly defined.

5. Insidious infection, which can often be treated, can mimic BOS and must be ruled out before the diagnosis of chronic rejection is made.

31. **What is the role of inhaled aerosolized cyclosporine?**
The concept of delivering maintenance immunosuppressant medication directly to the lower respiratory tract, thereby achieving higher levels of drug and avoiding toxicity, has led to the development of techniques to aerosolize cyclosporine A. One small study has reported stabilization of pulmonary function in patients with chronic rejection after treatment with inhaled cyclosporine A.

Iacono AT, Corcoran TE, Griffith BP, et al: Aerosol cyclosporine therapy in lung transplant recipients with bronchiolitis obliterans. Eur Resp J 23:384–390, 2004.

32. **How is sirolimus used in the immunosuppressive regimen?**
Sirolimus (rapamycin) is produced by the actinomycete species *Streptomyces hygroscopicus*, which has a structure remarkably similar to that of tacrolimus. However, sirolimus's immunosuppressive mechanism is entirely different in that it blocks growth-factor-driven cell proliferation of both hematopoietic and nonhematopoietic cells. Sirolimus frequently interacts with cyclosporine pharmacokinetically and may increase cyclosporine A levels and promote toxicity if administered simultaneously.

Knoop C, Haverich A, Fischer S: Immunosuppressive therapy after human lung transplantation. Eur Respir J 23:159–171, 2004.

CHRONIC REJECTION

33. **What is obliterative bronchiolitis?**
Obliterative bronchiolitis (OB) is considered to be chronic rejection in lung allografts. It begins as an airway injury—either an immune injury or an infection—that produces airway inflammation, resulting in a fibroproliferative response, which leads to obstruction and destruction of the pulmonary bronchioles. This process can occur either rapidly or over a number of years and usually involves distortion of the bronchioles and narrowing, plugging, and eventual obliteration of the airway, with resulting severe obstructive airway disease. In some cases of OB, bronchiectasis or bronchial malacia may complicate the clinical situation and predispose the patient to infection. It is rare for patients to regain lost function after developing OB.

34. **What is the BOS?**
Acute rejection is usually diagnosed by transbronchial biopsy, but the opposite is true for obliterative bronchiolitis lesions. Sensitivity for BOS by transbronchial biopsy has been reported to be less than 50%. Therefore, a relatively specific clinical syndrome with distinct pulmonary function findings has been developed to categorize lung function related to presumed OB (Table 72-2). This system recognizes, but does not require, a histologic diagnosis of OB.

A potential stage of BOS (0-p) has also been added to the original staging classification to detect early deterioration in allograft function that might prestage BOS stage 1; it is defined as a 10–19% decrease in FEV_1 or a 25% or more decrease in the forced expiratory flow at 25–75% of forced vital capacity (FEF_{25-75}) from baseline.

Clinical features of BOS usually occur after 6 months and may be subtle. The onset is often insidious and is heralded by a vague feeling of unwellness, fatigue, and mild shortness of breath. A flulike illness may proceed the deterioration in lung function. Sometimes the only sign of BOS is an asymptomatic fall in the FEV_1. Once again, airflow obstruction rarely improves spontaneously or even with enhanced immunosuppression; however, the course of disease can be quite variable, and many patients with BOS enjoy many years of slowly declining or stable lung function. Because of other complications and insidious infection that can mimic BOS, it is a diagnosis of exclusion. Therefore, bronchoscopy is often necessary to rule out other causes.

Hachem RR, Murali MM, Yusen RD, et al: The predictive value of bronchiolitis obliterans syndrome stage 0-p. Am J Respir Crit Care Med 169:468–472, 2004.

TABLE 72-2.	CATEGORIES OF BRONCHIOLITIS OBLITERANS SYNDROME	
Stage	Verbal Description	FEV_1 (% Predicted)
0	No significant abnormality	80% or more
1	Mild BOS	66–80%
2	Moderate BOS	51–65%
3	Severe BOS	50% or less

35. How is BOS treated?

The treatment of established chronic rejection is difficult. Current strategies include the following:

- Changing medications within the therapeutic class (e.g., changing from cyclosporine A to tacrolimus or substituting mycophenolate mofetil for azathioprine, or both)
- Adding inhaled immunosuppressants
- Temporarily augmenting the net immunosuppression by using high-dose methylpred-nisolone, by adding antilymphocytic therapy such as antithymocyte globulin or OKT3 (the brand name for muromonab-CD3), or by adding methotrexate or cyclophosphamide
- Applying immunomodulating therapies, including total lymphoid irradiation or photopheresis (rarely used)
- Using azithromycin (a recent and promising, but as yet unproven, approach)

Knoop C, Haverich A, Fischer S: Immunosuppressive therapy after human lung transplantation. Eur Respir J 23:159–171, 2004.

Verleden GM, Dupont LJ: Azithromycin therapy for patients with bronchiolitis obliterans syndrome after lung transplantation. Transplantation 77:1465–1467, 2004.

LIFE AFTER TRANSPLANTATION

36. What happens to lung function after transplantation?

Patients with bilateral lung transplants achieve near-normal lung function, and those with unilateral transplants can achieve up to 60% of normal lung function. PaO_2 increases to near-normal values in many patients. Patients have significant increases in their lung function values, usually during the 3 months postoperatively, but improvements may continue over the first year.

37. How does the patient's quality of life change after transplant?

The lung transplant patient's quality of life improves markedly after transplant, even in the face of many drugs with multiple toxicities that the patient will have to take throughout his or her life. In one survey, satisfaction with physical and emotional health was rated good or excellent by more than 80%, and satisfaction with life exceeded more than 70%.

Studer SM, Levy RD, McNeil K, et al: Lung transplant outcomes: A review of survival, graft function, physiology, health related quality of life and cost effectiveness. Eur Resp J 24:674–685, 2004.

38. What are the outcomes of lung transplant?

The best survival rates are in patients with chronic obstructive pulmonary disease (COPD), who have 80% 1-year survival and 50% 5-year survival. Other diagnoses have survivals of 70–75% at 1 year and 45–50% at 5 years. Up to 3 years posttransplantation, unilateral and bilateral transplant recipients have similar survivals, but emerging evidence suggests that bilateral transplant recipients may have significantly better survival as they get further and further from transplant.

http://www.unos.org

39. **What common medical complications occur after lung transplantation?**

Renal toxicity occurs in virtually all patients, and 5–10% will develop end-stage disease. Hypertension is also almost universal and requires aggressive antihypertensive management. In rare cases, hemolytic uremic syndrome has been reported. Hyperlipidemia is common, particularly in patient sirolimus and cyclosporine-taking patients. The risk of neoplasm is high after lung transplant. Most common is nonmelanoma skin cancer, followed by PTLD.

Treatments for PTLD have included reduction in immunosuppression, use of rituximab, and, occasionally, chemotherapeutic agents. There is no proven role for antiviral therapy in established PTLD, although recent evidence suggests that prophylactic use of antiviral agents initiated in at-risk patients may reduce the rate of developing PTLD.

Lung cancer has been reported in patients with COPD or idiopathic pulmonary fibrosis (IPF) who have undergone lung transplantation, usually in the native lung, with a reported incidence of 3% in COPD patients and 4% in IPF patients. Post-transplant cancers are often aggressive.

Osteoporosis is common, both pretransplant and post-transplant. It can lead to debilitating fractures or loss of lung function in extreme cases. Gastrointestinal complications include peptic ulcer disease, gastritis, pseudomembranous colitis, cyclosporin-induced gastroparesis, and gastric reflux. Neurologic complications occur in up to one-quarter of transplant patients and are wide-ranging. Some manifestations include tremor, headache, paresthesias seizures, and, rarely, leukoencephalopathy. Other complications include anemia, thrombocytopenia, hypomagnesemia, hypokalemia, pancreatitis, diabetes mellitus (a complication of tacrolimus therapy), gingival hypertrophy (from cyclosporine therapy), and hair loss or growth.

Maurer JR, Tewari S: Nonpulmonary medical complications in the intermediate and long term survivor. Clin Chest Med 18:367–382, 1999.

Niedermeyer J, Hoffmeyer F, Hertenstein B, et al: Treatment of lymphoproliferative disease with rituximab. Lancet 355:499, 2000.

40. **What are the two main causes of death after lung transplantation?**

The main cause of death after lung transplantation is BO, and the second most common is infection. Often, *Aspergillus* spp. infection or pseudomonal infection is the ultimate cause of death in patients who have BO.

PLEURAL EFFUSIONS

Steven A. Sahn, MD

1. **What are the mechanisms responsible for the clinical accumulation of pleural fluid?**

   Pleural effusions accumulate when production of fluid exceeds absorption of fluid from the pleural space. The mechanisms responsible are as follows:
   - An increase in hydrostatic pressure in the microvascular circulation (from congestive heart failure)
   - A decrease in oncotic pressure in the microvascular circulation (from hypoalbuminemia)
   - A decrease in pressure in the pleural space (from atelectasis)
   - Increased permeability of the microvascular circulation (from pneumonia)
   - Impaired lymphatic drainage from the pleural space (from malignancy)
   - Movement of fluid from the abdomen into the pleural space (from cirrhosis)
   - Movement of fluid from an extravascular source (from duropleural fistula)

   Sahn SA: The pleura. Am Rev Respir Dis 138:184–234, 1988.

2. **What is the indication for diagnostic thoracentesis?**

   Diagnostic thoracentesis is performed when a pleural effusion of unknown cause is present. Unless the diagnosis is clinically secure, such as in a patient with classic congestive heart failure with no atypical features, a thoracentesis should be done to definitively or presumptively establish the cause of the effusion.

   Sahn SA: The pleura. Am Rev Respir Dis 138:184–234, 1988.

   Sahn SA: Thoracentesis and pleural biopsy. In Shelhamer J, Pizzo PA, Parrillo JE, et al (eds): Respiratory Disease in the Immunosuppressed Host. Philadelphia, J.B. Lippincott, 1991, pp 118–129.

   Sahn SA: The diagnostic value of pleural fluid analysis. Semin Respir Crit Care Med 16:269–278, 1995.

3. **Are there are absolute contraindications to thoracentesis?**

   No. If clinical judgment dictates that the information gained from pleural fluid analysis may help in diagnosis and therapy, thoracentesis should be done.

   Sahn SA: The pleura. Am Rev Respir Dis 138:184–234, 1988.

   Sahn SA: Thoracentesis and pleural biopsy. In Shelhamer J, Pizzo PA, Parrillo JE, et al (eds): Respiratory Disease in the Immunosuppressed Host. Philadelphia, J.B. Lippincott, 1991, pp 118–129.

4. **What are the relative contraindications to thoracentesis?**

   A bleeding diathesis, anticoagulation therapy, a small amount of pleural fluid, and mechanical ventilation are relative contraindications.

   Sahn SA: The pleura. Am Rev Respir Dis 138:184–234, 1988.

   Sahn SA: Thoracentesis and pleural biopsy. In Shelhamer J, Pizzo PA, Parrillo JE, et al (eds): Respiratory Disease in the Immunosuppressed Host. Philadelphia, J.B. Lippincott, 1991, pp 118–129.

5. **Is the patient on mechanical ventilation at increased risk for pneumothorax with thoracentesis?**

   The patient is probably not at increased risk of a pneumothorax but is at greater risk for developing a tension pneumothorax if the lung is punctured.

   Sahn SA: Thoracentesis and pleural biopsy. In Shelhamer J, Pizzo PA, Parrillo JE, et al (eds): Respiratory Disease in the Immunosuppressed Host. Philadelphia, J.B. Lippincott, 1991, pp 118–129.

6. **What are the complications of diagnostic thoracentesis?**

Pneumothorax is the most common clinically important complication. Other complications include pain at the needle insertion site, bleeding (local, intrapleural, or intra-abdominal), empyema, and spleen or liver puncture.

Sahn SA: Thoracentesis and pleural biopsy. In Shelhamer J, Pizzo PA, Parrillo JE, et al (eds): Respiratory Disease in the Immunosuppressed Host. Philadelphia, J.B. Lippincott, 1991, pp 118–129.

7. **What are the complications of therapeutic thoracentesis?**

Complications of therapeutic thoracentesis include those of diagnostic thoracentesis; however, three other complications are unique to therapeutic thoracentesis: hypoxemia, unilateral pulmonary edema, and hypovolemia. Hypoxemia, which may occur despite relief of dyspnea, results from worsening of ventilation–perfusion relationships in the ipsilateral lung or from clinically occult unilateral pulmonary edema. Patients with an endobronchial obstruction or lung entrapment may develop a precipitous drop in pleural pressure when fluid is removed, thus increasing the likelihood of unilateral pulmonary edema.

Sahn SA: Thoracentesis and pleural biopsy. In Shelhamer J, Pizzo PA, Parrillo JE, et al (eds): Respiratory Disease in the Immunosuppressed Host. Philadelphia, J.B. Lippincott, 1991, pp 118–129.

8. **Which patients are most likely to develop unilateral pulmonary edema after thoracentesis?**

Patients with a mainstem endobronchial lesion causing atelectasis and patients with lung entrapment from malignancy or previous pleural space infection are at risk. When fluid is removed from the pleural space, pleural pressure drops precipitously, increasing the pressure gradient across alveolar capillary vessels and promoting pulmonary edema. The chest radiograph in these patients typically shows a large pleural effusion without contralateral mediastinal shift and suggests an increased risk of developing pulmonary edema.

Sahn SA: Thoracentesis and pleural biopsy. In Shelhamer J, Pizzo PA, Parrillo JE, et al (eds): Respiratory Disease in the Immunosuppressed Host. Philadelphia, J.B. Lippincott, 1991, pp 118–129.

9. **What criteria are used to classify transudates and exudates?**

If any of the following criteria are present, the fluid has a high likelihood of being an exudate, and, conversely, if none of the criteria is present, it has a high likelihood of being a transudate:

- A ratio of pleural fluid total protein to serum total protein greater than 0.5
- Pleural fluid lactate dehydrogenase (LDH) greater than or equal to 0.82 of the upper limit of normal of the serum LDH
- Pleural fluid cholesterol greater than 45 mg/dL

Heffner JE, Brown LK, Barbieri CA: Diagnostic value of tests that discriminate between exudative and transudative pleural effusions: Primary Study Investigators. Chest 111:970–980, 1997.

Light RW, MacGregor MI, Luchsinger PC, et al: Pleural effusion: The diagnostic separation of transudates and exudates. Ann Intern Med 77:507–513, 1972.

Sahn SA: Clinical evaluation of the patient with a pleural effusion. In Bouros (ed): Pleural Disease. New York, Marcel Dekker, 2004, pp 267–286.

Sahn SA: The pleura. Am Rev Respir Dis 138:184–234, 1988.

10. **Why is it important to distinguish transudates from exudates?**

Establishing the presence of a transudate limits the diagnostic possibilities, which are usually discernible from the clinical presentation. Transudates are caused by imbalances in hydrostatic and oncotic pressures and include congestive heart failure, hepatic hydrothorax, nephrotic syndrome, peritoneal dialysis, hypoalbuminemia, constrictive pericarditis, trapped lung, urinothorax, duropleural fistula, and extravascular migration of a central venous catheter with saline infusion. The differential diagnosis of an exudate is more extensive and at times is problematic for the clinician.

Heffner JE, Brown LK, Barbieri CA: Diagnostic value of tests that discriminate between exudative and transudative pleural effusions: Primary Study Investigators. Chest 111:970–980, 1997.

Light RW, MacGregor MI, Luchsinger PC, et al: Pleural effusion: The diagnostic separation of transudates and exudates. Ann Intern Med 77:507–513, 1972.

Sahn SA: Clinical evaluation of the patient with a pleural effusion. In Bouros (ed): Pleural Disease. New York, Marcel Dekker, 2004, pp 267–286.

Sahn SA: The pleura. Am Rev Respir Dis 138:184–234, 1988.

Sahn SA: The diagnostic value of pleural fluid analysis. Semin Respir Crit Care Med 16:269–278, 1995.

11. **Which causes of a pleural effusion should be considered when the pleural fluid total protein is <1.0 gm/dL?**
Consideration should be given to instances when the fluid originates from an extravascular space. Examples include peritoneal dialysis, urinothorax, duropleural fistula, and extravascular migration of a central venous catheter with saline infusion.

Sahn SA: Clinical evaluation of the patient with a pleural effusion. In Bouros (ed): Pleural Disease. New York, Marcel Dekker, 2004, pp 267–286.

KEY POINTS: EFFUSIONS THAT CONSISTENTLY HAVE PLEURAL FLUID TOTAL PROTEIN <1.0 gm/dL

1. Peritoneal dialysis

2. Duropleural fistula

3. Extravascular migration of a central venous catheter with saline infusion

4. Urinothorax

12. **Describe the typical chest radiograph of a patient with pleural effusions from congestive heart failure.**
The chest radiograph shows cardiomegaly, bilateral pleural effusions (more copious on the right than on the left), evidence of interstitial or alveolar edema, and, sometimes, the presence of Kerley's B lines.

Sahn SA: The pleura. Am Rev Respir Dis 138:184–234, 1988.

13. **Do all patients with hepatic hydrothorax have clinical ascites?**
No. Almost all patients with hepatic hydrothorax have clinical ascites, but a number of patients have been reported with large hepatic hydrothoraxes in the absence of clinical ascites. In this situation, virtually all the ascitic fluid that is produced is immediately mobilized into the chest through diaphragmatic defects.

Sahn SA: The pleura. Am Rev Respir Dis 138:184–234, 1988.

14. **What is the best therapeutic option for the patient with a symptomatic hepatic hydrothorax refractory to maximal medical therapy?**
Transjugular intrahepatic portosystemic shunt (TIPS).

Sahn SA: Clinical evaluation of the patient with a pleural effusion. In Bouros (ed): Pleural Disease. New York, Marcel Dekker, 2004, pp 267–286.

15. **What diagnosis is suggested by the presence of a unilateral hemorrhagic exudative pleural effusion in a patient with nephrotic syndrome?**
Pulmonary embolism. Patients with nephrotic syndrome are hypercoagulable and have a 30% incidence of pulmonary embolism resulting from loss of clotting inhibitors in the urine, abnormal platelet aggregation, and volume depletion.

Sahn SA: Clinical evaluation of the patient with a pleural effusion. In Bouros (ed): Pleural Disease. New York, Marcel Dekker, 2004, pp 267–286.

Sahn SA: The pleura. Am Rev Respir Dis 138:184–234, 1988.

Sahn SA: The diagnostic value of pleural fluid analysis. Semin Respir Crit Care Med 16:269–278, 1995.

16. How is the diagnosis of urinothorax established?

Urinothorax, a pleural effusion ipsilateral to an obstructed kidney, is diagnosed by the finding of a pleural fluid or by a serum creatinine ratio greater than 1.0.

Sahn SA: Clinical evaluation of the patient with a pleural effusion. In Bouros (ed): Pleural Disease. New York, Marcel Dekker, 2004, pp 267–286.

Sahn SA: The diagnostic value of pleural fluid analysis. Semin Respir Crit Care Med 16:269–278, 1995.

17. What is a trapped lung? How is it diagnosed?

A trapped lung occurs as a result of a remote inflammatory or infectious process when a fibrous peel does not allow any or allows only a portion of the lung to expand to the chest wall. The most common causes of trapped lung include empyema, rheumatoid pleurisy, uremic pleurisy, and coronary artery bypass grafting (CABG) surgery. Pleural fluid forms because of decreased pleural pressure promoting movement of interstitial fluid into the pleural space until a steady-state pressure is established. This transudate is diagnosed if the lung does not expand following complete removal of fluid at thoracentesis, if the initial pleural liquid pressure is negative, and if the pleural space elastance is greater than or equal to 25 cmH_2O per liter of pleural fluid removed.

Sahn SA: Clinical evaluation of the patient with a pleural effusion. In Bouros (ed): Pleural Disease. New York, Marcel Dekker, 2004, pp 267–286.

18. What pleural fluid criteria suggest that a parapneumonic effusion can be treated successfully with observation and appropriate antibiotic therapy directed at the pneumonia?

A small to moderate nonpurulent, free-flowing pleural fluid with a pH of more than 7.30, a glucose level of more than 60 mg/dL, and an LDH value of less than 700 IU per liter suggests a good outcome without drainage of the pleural space.

Heffner JE: Indications for draining a parapneumonic effusion: An evidence-based approach. Semin Respir Infect 14:48–58, 1999.

Heffner JE, Brown LK, Barbieri C, DeLeo JM: Pleural fluid chemical analysis in parapneumonic effusions: A meta-analysis. Am J Respir Crit Care Med 151:1700–1708, 1995.

Sahn SA: Management of complicated parapneumonic effusions. Am Rev Respir Dis 148:813–817, 1993.

19. Can patients with empyema be treated with antibiotics alone?

No. Empyema (i.e., pus in the pleural space) needs to be treated similarly to pus anywhere in the body (i.e., with appropriate drainage). A contrast-enhanced computed tomography (CT) scan should be done to assess the extent of empyema and the number of loculations before a decision is made about specific therapy. A patient who has a single loculus with minimal pleural enhancement may be drained with a CT-guided chest tube or catheter. Multiloculated empyema usually requires empyemectomy and decortication.

Heffner JE: Indications for draining a parapneumonic effusion: An evidence-based approach. Semin Respir Infect 14:48–58, 1999.

Heffner JE, Brown LK, Barbieri C, DeLeo JM: Pleural fluid chemical analysis in parapneumonic effusions: A meta-analysis. Am J Respir Crit Care Med 151:1700–1708, 1995.

Sahn SA: Management of complicated parapneumonic effusions. Am Rev Respir Dis 148:813–817, 1993.

20. Are there clinical features that suggest that a parapneumonic effusion is complicated?

Yes. All of the following increase the likelihood that a parapneumonic effusion is complicated and requires drainage: prolonged symptoms of pneumonia, alcoholism or other risk factors for aspiration (i.e., anaerobic infection), delayed response to antibiotics, and persistent leukocytosis and fever after several days of antibiotic therapy.

Heffner JE: Indications for draining a parapneumonic effusion: An evidence-based approach. Semin Respir Infect 14:48–58, 1999.

Sahn SA: Management of complicated parapneumonic effusions. Am Rev Respir Dis 148:813–817, 1993.

21. **Does a negative tuberculin skin test exclude the diagnosis of tuberculous pleurisy?**
No. Up to 30% of patients in the acute phase of tuberculous pleurisy have a negative tuberculin skin test with purified protein derivative (PPD). In most, the skin test becomes positive in 6–8 weeks. The negative skin test is the result of transient circulating mononuclear cells that suppress the sensitized T-lymphocyte in the peripheral blood and skin but not in the pleural space.

Sahn SA: Clinical evaluation of the patient with a pleural effusion. In Bouros (ed): Pleural Disease. New York, Marcel Dekker, 2004, pp 267–286.

Sahn SA: The pleura. Am Rev Respir Dis 138:184–234, 1988.

22. **What is the usual pleural fluid lymphocyte percentage in patients with tuberculous pleurisy that has been present for 1–2 weeks?**
Patients with tuberculous pleurisy usually have 90–95% lymphocytes. Other diagnoses with high percentages of pleural fluid lymphocytes (usually > 80%) include chylothorax, lymphoma, yellow nail syndrome, chronic rheumatoid pleurisy, uremic pleurisy, sarcoidosis chronic effusions after CABG surgery, and acute lung rejection.

Sahn SA: Clinical evaluation of the patient with a pleural effusion. In Bouros (ed): Pleural Disease. New York, Marcel Dekker, 2004, pp 267–286.

Sahn SA: The pleura. Am Rev Respir Dis 138:184–234, 1988.

Sahn SA: The diagnostic value of pleural fluid analysis. Semin Respir Crit Care Med 16:269–278, 1995.

23. **What diseases are associated with a low (i.e., less than 7.30) pleural fluid pH?**
The finding of a pleural pH of less than 7.30 narrows the differential diagnosis of the exudative pleural effusion. Empyema, complicated parapneumonic effusion, chronic rheumatoid pleurisy, malignancy, tuberculous pleurisy, acute lupus pleuritis, and esophageal rupture have all been reported with pleural fluid acidosis.

Good JT Jr, Taryle DA, Maulitz RM, et al: The diagnostic value of pleural fluid pH. Chest 78:55–59, 1980.

Sahn SA: Clinical evaluation of the patient with a pleural effusion. In Bouros (ed): Pleural Disease. New York, Marcel Dekker, 2004, pp 267–286.

Sahn SA: The pleura. Am Rev Respir Dis 138:184–234, 1988.

KEY POINTS: EXUDATES ASSOCIATED WITH A PLEURAL FLUID pH < 7.30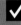

1. Empyema

2. Complicated parapneumonic effusion

3. Chronic rheumatoid pleurisy

4. Esophageal rupture

5. Malignant pleural effusion

6. Tuberculous pleural effusion

7. Acute lupus pleuritis

24. **What is the significance of pleural fluid eosinophilia?**
    Pleural fluid eosinophilia (i.e., a ratio of pleural fluid eosinophils to total nucleated cells greater than 10%) suggests a disease commonly associated with air or blood in the pleural space. The differential diagnosis includes pneumothorax, hemothorax, pulmonary infarction, benign asbestos pleural effusion, parasitic disease, fungal infection, drug reaction, and malignancy.

    Rubins JB, Rubins HB: Etiology and prognostic significance of eosinophilic pleural effusions: A prospective study. Chest 110:1271–1274, 1996.
    Sahn SA: Clinical evaluation of the patient with a pleural effusion. In Bouros (ed): Pleural Disease. New York, Marcel Dekker, 2004, pp 267–286.
    Sahn SA: The pleura. Am Rev Respir Dis 138:184–234, 1988.

25. **Is measurement of pleural fluid glucose a helpful diagnostic test?**
    Yes. Pleural fluid glucose levels less than 60 mg/dL or a pleural fluid-to-serum ratio less than 0.5 narrows the differential diagnosis of exudative effusions to the same diagnoses associated with a low pleural fluid pH, namely, empyema, esophageal rupture, rheumatoid pleurisy, malignancy, tuberculous pleurisy, and lupus pleuritis. Empyema and rheumatoid pleurisy commonly have a pleural fluid glucose concentration less than 30 mg/dL; often concentration is at 0 mg/dL.

    Good JT Jr, Taryle DA, Maulitz RM, et al: The diagnostic value of pleural fluid pH. Chest 78:55–59, 1980.
    Sahn SA: Clinical evaluation of the patient with a pleural effusion. In Bouros (ed): Pleural Disease. New York, Marcel Dekker, 2004, pp 267–286.
    Sahn SA: The pleura. Am Rev Respir Dis 138:184–234, 1988.
    Sahn SA: The diagnostic value of pleural fluid analysis. Semin Respir Crit Care Med 16:269–278, 1995.

KEY POINTS: PLEURAL FLUID GLUCOSE

1. Pleural fluid glucose of 0 mg/dL

   - Empyema.

   - Chronic rheumatoid pleural effusion.

2. Pleural-fluid-to-serum-glucose ratio significantly >1.0

   - Extravascular migration of the central venous catheter with glucose infusion.

   - Esophageal rupture in a patient with oral glucose intake.

   - Peritoneal dialysis.

26. **In the absence of esophageal rupture, what is the most likely diagnosis for a patient with an amylase-rich fluid that is predominantly salivary isoamylase?**
    Malignancy, most likely adenocarcinoma of the lung or ovary. These tumors secrete a salivary isoamylase responsible for this finding.

    Kramer MR, Cepero RJ, Pitchenik AE: High amylase in neoplasm-related pleural effusion. Ann Intern Med 110:567–569, 1989.
    Sahn SA: Clinical evaluation of the patient with a pleural effusion. In Bouros (ed): Pleural Disease. New York, Marcel Dekker, 2004, pp 267–286.

27. **What is the clinical significance of mesothelial cells in pleural fluid?**
    Mesothelial cells are found in small numbers in normal pleural fluid, are prominent in transudative effusions, and vary in exudative effusions. Pleural fluid that contains more than 5% mesothelial cells is unlikely to be caused by tuberculous pleurisy.

Sahn SA: Clinical evaluation of the patient with a pleural effusion. In Bouros (ed): Pleural Disease. New York, Marcel Dekker, 2004, pp 267–286.

28. **Does finding a nonmilky pleural fluid at thoracentesis exclude the diagnosis of chylothorax?**

No. Chylothoraces may be milky, bloody, turbid, or serous. Trauma that produces a hemorrhagic effusion can mask the milky appearance. Malnourished patients or patients who have not eaten a meal recently may present with a turbid or serous effusion. A triglyceride concentration in the pleural fluid greater than 110 mg/dL makes the diagnosis of chylothorax highly likely, whereas a pleural-fluid triglyceride less than 50 mg/dL makes the diagnosis highly unlikely. Finding chylomicrons on lipoprotein electrophoresis of the pleural fluid establishes the diagnosis.

Staats BA, Ellefson RD, Badahn L, et al: The lipoprotein profile of chylous and non-chylous pleural effusions. Mayo Clin Proc 55:700–704, 1980.

29. **What are the characteristic pleural fluid findings in spontaneous esophageal rupture?**

When the esophagus ruptures and the mediastinal pleura is violated, the characteristic findings are a high salivary amylase concentration and a low pleural fluid pH (frequently 6.00); the latter is caused by an anaerobic empyema. Cytology may demonstrate squamous epithelial cells and food particles.

Sahn SA: Clinical evaluation of the patient with a pleural effusion. In Bouros (ed): Pleural Disease. New York, Marcel Dekker, 2004, pp 267–286.

Sahn SA: The pleura. Am Rev Respir Dis 138:184–234, 1988.

Sahn SA: The diagnostic value of pleural fluid analysis. Semin Respir Crit Care Med 16:269–278, 1995.

CHAPTER 74

PNEUMOTHORAX

Milene T. Saavedra, MD, and Michael E. Hanley, MD

1. **How are pneumothoraces classified?**
   Pneumothoraces are classified as either spontaneous or traumatic. Traumatic pneumothoraces result from direct or indirect injury to the chest and are further classified as iatrogenic or noniatrogenic. Spontaneous pneumothoraces occur without obvious cause. They are termed primary if they occur in previously healthy individuals. Secondary spontaneous pneumothoraces occur as complications of underlying lung disease.

   Sahn S, Heffner J: Spontaneous pneumothorax. N Engl J Med 342:868–874, 2000.

2. **What is the differential diagnosis of spontaneous pneumothorax?**
   Patients with pneumothoraces present with acute onset of respiratory symptoms including focal pleuritic chest pain, dyspnea, and dry cough. The differential diagnosis includes musculoskeletal chest pain (i.e., chest trauma, costochondritis, or rib fracture), myocardial ischemia or infarction, pulmonary embolism or infarction, infectious pneumonia, empyema, and viral pleuritis.

3. **List the risk factors for primary spontaneous pneumothorax.**
   - History of smoking (smoking increases the risk of pneumothorax by a factor of 20 in a dose-dependent fashion)
   - Family history of primary spontaneous pneumothorax
   - A tall, thin body habitus, especially in men between the ages of 10 and 30 years

4. **Name some uncommon causes of spontaneous pneumothoraces.**
   - Catamenial pneumothoraces occur in association with menstruation. The two mechanisms that have been proposed for their development are (1) the movement of air from the peritoneal cavity to the pleural cavity through diaphragmatic defects and (2) the development of air in the pleural cavity from pleural endometriosis.
   - Neonatal pneumothoraces occur spontaneously in 1–2% of newborns and may be asymptomatic in 50% of cases.
   - Spontaneous pneumothoraces are a frequent complication in patients with lymphangio-leiomyomatosis (80%) and pulmonary Langerhans cell histiocytosis (30%).

   Glassberg MK: Lymphangioleiomyomatosis. Clin Chest Med 25:573–582, 2004.
   Korom S, Canyurt H, Missbach A, et al: Catamenial pneumothorax revisited: Clinical approach and systematic review of the literature. J Thorac Cardiovasc Surg 128:502–508, 2004.

5. **What are the most common causes of secondary spontaneous pneumothoraces?**
   Chronic obstructive pulmonary disease (COPD) and human immunodeficiency virus (HIV)-related *Pneumocystis jirovecii* pneumonia are the most common etiologies of secondary spontaneous pneumothorax. COPD patients with a forced expiratory volume in 1 second (FEV_1) < 1 L are at the highest risk of pneumothorax. Two to six percent of HIV-seropositive patients develop pneumothorax; 80% of these pneumothoraces occur in patients infected with *Pneumocystis jirovecii* pneumonia.

6. **What procedures are commonly associated with iatrogenic pneumothorax?**
See Table 74-1.

TABLE 74-1. PROCEDURES ASSOCIATED WITH IATROGENIC PNEUMOTHORAX
■ Percutaneous transthoracic needle aspiration, biopsy, or both
■ Subclavian and supraclavicular central venous catheterization
■ Thoracentesis
■ Positive-pressure mechanical ventilation
■ Transbronchial biopsy
■ Closed pleural biopsy
■ Tracheostomy
■ Cardiopulmonary resuscitation

7. **What are the typical clinical manifestations of pneumothorax?**
Chest pain or dyspnea (or both) occur in virtually all patients with pneumothorax. Although symptoms occur acutely in most patients, up to 20% of patients delay seeking medical consultation for more than 7 days. Physical signs include tachycardia and hyperexpansion of the ipsilateral chest with decreased tactile fremitus, hyperresonance, and decrease in or absence of breath sounds.

The clinical diagnosis of a secondary spontaneous pneumothorax can be especially difficult. Although the combined physiologic effects of pneumothorax and underlying lung disease make symptoms more severe, the physical signs of the pneumothorax are frequently masked by those of the underlying lung disease. This is especially true with pneumothoraces complicating COPD.

8. **What are the radiographic appearances of pneumothorax?**
Pneumothorax appears on an upright chest x-ray as a thin pleural edge or stripe with an absence of lung markings between the pleural stripe and the chest wall. These findings may not be present in supine mechanically ventilated patients. Pneumothorax in this setting usually results from barotrauma in nondependent anterior and medial lung segments. Air therefore tends to collect in the anterior part of the chest, producing a "deep sulcus" sign. The deep sulcus sign is inferior displacement of the ipsilateral costophrenic angle due to the presence of air in the costophrenic sulcus.

There are also a number of radiographic abnormalities that may be confused with a pneumothorax. These include radiographic shadows from skin folds and extracorporeal catheters.

KEY POINTS: DIAGNOSIS OF PNEUMOTHORAX

1. Chest pain and dyspnea are the most common symptoms.

2. Physical findings include decreased or absent breath sounds associated with hyperresonant percussion.

3. Definitive diagnosis requires radiographic confirmation.

These abnormalities can usually be differentiated from a pneumothorax by extension of the shadow beyond the chest wall or the presence of lung markings between the shadow and the chest wall. Emphysematous bullae, intrathoracic loops of bowel (due to diaphragmatic hernia-tion or rupture), and dilated loops of bowel that become interposed between the hemidiaphragm and the liver in the setting of bowel obstruction may also mimic the radiographic appearance of pneumothoraces.

Rankine J, Thomas A, Fluechter D: Diagnosis of pneumothorax in critically ill adults. Postgrad Med J 76:399–404, 2000.

9. **What is the role of supplemental oxygen in the management of pneumothorax?**
Reabsorption of pleural air is determined in part by the pressure gradient between the pleural space and pleural capillaries for each gas. If the patient is breathing room air, the sum of the pressure gradients for each gas (assuming the pneumothorax is not under tension) is only 54 mmHg, which results in reabsorption of about 1.25% of the volume of the hemithorax per day. Administration of 100% oxygen decreases the capillary partial pressure of nitrogen (PN_2) and increases the partial pressure of oxygen. However, the decrease in PN_2 is much greater than the increase in the partial pressure of oxygen (PO_2), resulting in a large increase in the net pressure gradient for all gases. Pneumothoraces are reabsorbed four times faster if patients are treated with high concentrations of supplemental oxygen.

10. **Do all pneumothoraces require tube thoracostomy?**
No. Asymptomatic patients with small (i.e., size <15% of the hemithorax) primary spontaneous pneumothoraces or iatrogenic pneumothoraces in patients not being mechanically ventilated may be managed conservatively with oxygen and radiologic observation. Larger primary spontaneous pneumothoraces (i.e., size >15% of the hemithorax), spontaneous secondary pneumothoraces, traumatic pneumothoraces, progressively enlarging pneumothoraces, and pneumothoraces in the setting of mechanical ventilation all require tube thoracostomy.

Baumann MH, Strange C, Heffner JE, et al: Management of spontaneous pneumothorax: An American College of Chest Physicians Delphi consensus statement. Chest 119:590–602, 2001.

Devanand A, Koh MS, Ong TH, et al: Simple aspiration versus chest-tube insertion in the management of primary spontaneous pneumothorax: A systematic review. Respir Med 98:579–590, 2004.

Noppen M: Management of primary spontaneous pneumothorax. Curr Opin Pulm Med 9:272–275, 2003.

11. **What factors determine the size of the chest tube chosen for thoracostomy?**
The size of the chest tube is influenced by the clinical stability of the patient, the size of the pneu-mothorax, and whether the pneumothorax is primary, secondary, or associated with mechanical ventilation.

Baumann MH: What size chest tube? What drainage system is ideal? And other chest tube management questions. Curr Opin Pulm Med 9:276–281, 2003.

KEY POINTS: TREATMENT OPTIONS FOR PNEUMOTHORAX

1. Supplemental oxygen with radiologic observation

2. Simple aspiration

3. Small-bore-tube thoracostomy

4. Large-bore-tube thoracostomy

5. Chemical or mechanical pleurodesis

12. **List the complications of chest tube placement.**
    Pain, pleural infection, hemorrhage, incorrect tube placement (including placement into the lung and bowel), hypotension, and reexpansion pulmonary edema may all occur.

13. **What is the differential diagnosis when a lung does not expand after chest tube placement?**
    The chest tube may be extrathoracic, placed within a major fissure, obstructed with debris, or kinked. Other considerations include a large airway obstruction in the ipsilateral lung, an absence of suction, or the presence of a "trapped lung" due to pleural fibrosis.

14. **What is a tension pneumothorax?**
    A tension pneumothorax occurs when significant positive pressure exists in the pleural space, resulting in severe compression of the ipsilateral lung, contralateral shift of the mediastinum, and caudal depression of the ipsilateral hemidiaphragm. It generally results from a ball or a one-way valve bronchopleural fistula, especially during positive-pressure ventilation. Many patients who have tension pneumothoraces are clinically unstable, with refractory hypoxemia and hypotension.
    Tension pneumothoraces are medical emergencies that require immediate treatment. If a tube thoracostomy tray is not readily available and the patient is hemodynamically unstable, an 18- or 20-gauge angiocatheter should be inserted into the ipsilateral second intercostal space in the midclavicular line to relieve tension and to stabilize the patient pending more definitive therapy.

    Leigh-Smith S, Harris T: Tension pneumothorax—Time for a re-think? Emerg Med J 22:8–16, 2005.

15. **Should a confirmatory chest roentgenogram be obtained before definitive therapy?**
    Generally, a confirmatory chest roentgenogram should be obtained before placement of a tube thoracostomy. However, a chest tube should be placed immediately (without delay for a roentgenogram) if a tension pneumothorax is suspected and the patient is clinically unstable.

16. **Which patients should be considered for pleurodesis?**
    The recurrence rate for primary spontaneous pneumothoraces ranges from 28–52% and increases with each subsequent pneumothorax. Spontaneous secondary pneumothoraces recur at rates of 39–47%. Pleurodesis prevents recurrence by obliterating the pleural space and can be performed either by mechanical scarification during surgery (i.e., thoracoscopy or thoracotomy) or through instillation of chemical sclerosing agents during surgery or through a tube thoracostomy. Pleurodesis of primary spontaneous pneumothoraces is usually reserved until after the first recurrence. Because the physiologic consequences of secondary pneumothoraces are greater, early sclerosis (i.e., after the first occurrence) should be considered.
    Chemical sclerotherapy through a tube thoracostomy does not have high efficacy in patients with persistent air leaks. In the absence of air leaks, chemical sclerotherapy is successful in 75–92% of patients. In contrast, surgical interventions have success rates of 95–100%. For this reason, surgical approaches to prevent recurrence are preferred for most patients. Chemical sclerotherapy is usually reserved for patients who are poor surgical candidates or who are unwilling to undergo surgery.

    Gossot D, Galetta D, Stern JB, et al: Results of thoracoscopic pleural abrasion for primary spontaneous pneumothorax. Surg Endosc 18:466–471, 2004.
    Sedrakyan A, van der Meulen J, Lewsey J, et al: Video assisted thoracic surgery for treatment of pneumothorax and lung resections: Systematic review of randomised clinical trials. BMJ 329:1008, 2004.
    Yim AP, Ng CS: Thoracoscopy in the management of pneumothorax. Curr Opin Pulm Med 7:210–214, 2001.

17. **How is a persistent bronchopleural fistula evaluated?**
    A persistent bronchopleural fistula manifests as a nonresolving "air leak" that is evident after a tube thoracostomy has been performed. Patients with large volume air leaks who have experienced

chest trauma should be emergently evaluated for tracheobronchial lacerations. This is done by direct visualization of the tracheobronchial tree with fiberoptic bronchoscopy. Disruption of the endobronchial mucosa is confirmed either by observation of localized effervescence after application of hydrogen peroxide to suspicious lesions or by appearance in the tracheobronchial tree of methylene blue that has been instilled in the pleural space.

The presence of an external air leak should be excluded in all patients with a persistent bronchopleural fistula. The insertion site of the tube thoracostomy, as well as all external catheter connections, should be inspected visually for leaks. In addition, extrathoracic tube placement (including extrathoracic location of any of the tube's ports) should be excluded by evaluating the tube's position with posteroanterior and lateral chest roentgenograms.

18. How is a persistent bronchopleural fistula managed?

Initial conservative treatment of a persistent bronchopleural fistula is generally indicated because most close spontaneously. Three options are available: (1) continuing current management, (2) increasing the suction applied to the pleural space to -35 cmH$_2$O, or (3) repositioning the chest tube. Successful closure of bronchopleural fistulas after instillation of 50–60 mL of the patient's fresh blood into the pleural space has also been reported. However, the efficacy and safety of this technique (termed a blood patch) have not been studied in a rigorous fashion.

More definitive therapy should be considered if a bronchopleural fistula persists beyond 4–7 days. Patients who are good surgical candidates should undergo surgical closure of the fistula by either thoracoscopy or limited thoracotomy; pleurodesis should also be performed at this time to prevent pneumothorax recurrence. Prolonged chest tube drainage with conversion to an outpatient one-way Heimlich valve, intrabronchial bronchoscopic instillation of materials designed to occlude the fistula (such as a solubilized absorbable gelatin sponge or fibrin and cyanoacrylate-based glues), or instillation of sclerosing agents through the tube thoracostomy should be reserved for patients deemed poor surgical risks or for patients not desiring surgery.

Lang-Lazdunski L, Coonar AS: A prospective study of autologous 'blood patch' pleurodesis for persistent air leak after pulmonary resection. Eur J Cardiothorac Surg 26:897–900, 2004.

Vricella LA, Trachiotis GD: Heimlich valve in the management of pneumothorax in patients with advanced AIDS. Chest 120:15–18, 2001.

19. How do you determine if the tube thoracostomy can be removed?

Removal of the tube thoracostomy should not be considered if a persistent air leak exists. Absence of a visible air leak during inspection of the tube thoracostomy does not guarantee that the leak has resolved because air may bubble out intermittently. Therefore, the tube should be placed under water seal for 4–24 hours when there is no longer a visible leak. The chest tube can generally be safely removed if a subsequent chest roentgenogram demonstrates complete reexpansion of the involved lung. In rare instances, a persistent air leak may not be apparent under water seal because positive-pressure maneuvers such as coughing or talking may vent accumulated air out of the tube thoracostomy. If the physiologic consequences of a recurrent pneumothorax are severe (as in the setting of significant underlying lung disease), it may be prudent not to remove the chest tube until complete reexpansion of the lung has been radiographically demonstrated 4 hours after the tube has been clamped.

CHAPTER 75

MESOTHELIOMA

Y. C. Gary Lee, MBChB, PhD, FCCP, FRACP

1. **What is the incidence of malignant mesothelioma?**

   The global incidence of mesothelioma has risen significantly over the last 50 years. In countries in which restrictions on asbestos use were initiated early in the 1970s (e.g., the United States and Sweden), the incidences of mesothelioma have reached a plateau. In the United States, mesothelioma kills about 3000 patients each year. In most other countries, the incidence of mesothelioma will continue to rise until 2020. Over 250,000 deaths from mesothelioma are expected over the next 35 years from six Western European countries alone.

   Peto J, Decarli A, La Vecchia C, et al: The European mesothelioma epidemic. Br J Cancer 79:666–672, 1999.

2. **From where do mesotheliomas commonly arise?**

   Mesothelioma arises from the mesothelium that lines the serosal cavities of the body. The pleura is the primary site in over 90% of mesotheliomas. Tumor can also arise from the peritoneum (7%) and occasionally from the pericardium (<1%) or the tunica vaginalis testis (rare). Patients with primary peritoneal mesothelioma often had higher asbestos exposure and poorer prognosis than patients with pleural mesothelioma. (The median survivals are 6 and 9 months, respectively.)

3. **What causes mesothelioma?**

   Asbestos is the most-recognized cause of malignant mesothelioma, although up to one-fifth of patients may not have a definite history of asbestos exposure. No threshold of exposure is considered safe. Often, a latency of over 30 years exists between exposure and tumor development. Exposure to Thorotrast, a radiographic contrast material, or to erionite, a natural fibrous zeolite found in Turkey, can also result in mesothelioma. Smoking and thoracic radiotherapy have not been shown to increase the risk of pleural mesothelioma.

   Roushdy-Hammady I, Siegel J, Emri S, et al: Genetic-susceptibility factor and malignant mesothelioma in the Cappadocian region of Turkey. Lancet 357:444–445, 2001.

4. **Who is at risk of developing mesothelioma?**

   Workers with direct occupational exposure to asbestos (e.g., asbestos miners), those who process asbestos into commercial products, and the end-users (e.g., shipbuilders and construction and insulation workers) are all at high risk. Family members of asbestos workers have sometimes developed mesothelioma, presumably because of asbestos fibers brought home on work clothes. Individuals who lived in proximity to factories or mines in which asbestos was prominent have also been reported to have the disease.

   The incidence of mesothelioma increases with age, and most patients present between 50 and 70 years of age. There is a strong male predominance in the incidence of mesothelioma. However, there are no differences in the incidence between males and females after adjusting for occupational exposure.

5. **What dictates the development of mesothelioma after asbestos exposure?**

   The risk of mesothelioma is related to the type of asbestos fibers, the duration and intensity of exposure, and the time from first exposure. Asbestos fibers are categorized into the *amphiboles* (including crocidolite, amosite, and tremolite) and the *serpentine* fibers (i.e., chrysotile). Crocidolite (i.e., blue asbestos) has the highest potency for mesothelioma induction, followed by amosite (i.e., brown asbestos) and then chrysotile (i.e., white asbestos). Asbestos exposure alone cannot adequately predict the risk of eventual mesothelioma development in any individual. The role of other potential contributing factors (e.g., genetic susceptibility) has been postulated but has not yet been convincingly proven.

Testa JR, Jhanwar SC: Genetics of malignant mesothelioma. In Light RW, Lee YCG (eds): Textbook of Pleural Diseases. London, Arnold Press, 2003, pp 120–130.

6. **Is previous polio vaccination a risk factor for the development of mesothelioma?**
   Some of the polio vaccines used in the 1950s were contaminated with simian virus 40 (SV40), a DNA virus that potently induces mesothelioma in laboratory animals, raising concerns that vaccinated individuals are susceptible to development of mesothelioma. Although some researchers have found SV40 in human mesothelioma tissues, a recent study suggested that such results may be false positives from contamination by common laboratory plasmids. The role of SV40 as a possible cofactor for asbestos in the pathogenesis of mesothelioma is controversial. To date, there is a lack of clinical or epidemiologic evidence to support that SV40 or previous polio vaccination causes mesothelioma in humans.

Lopez-Rios F, Illei PB, Rusch V, Ladanyi M: Evidence against a role for SV40 infection in human mesotheliomas and high risk of false-positive PCR results owing to presence of SV40 sequences in common laboratory plasmids. Lancet 364:1157–1166, 2004.

Strickler HD, Goedert JJ, Devesa SS, et al: Trends in U.S. pleural mesothelioma incidence rates following simian virus 40 contamination of early poliovirus vaccines. J Natl Cancer Inst 95:38–45, 2003.

7. **Do patients have to have asbestos-induced pulmonary or pleural diseases for mesothelioma to occur?**
   No. Asbestos-induced pulmonary fibrosis or pleural plaques are not necessary for the development of mesothelioma. It is noteworthy that radiographic evidence of asbestos exposure (e.g., pleural plaques or interstitial fibrosis) are observed in about one-fifth of patients. Hence, the absence of other asbestos-related pleuropulmonary abnormalities does not exclude the diagnosis of mesothelioma.

8. **Is mesothelioma always a malignant disorder?**
   Nowadays, the term "mesothelioma" is only used to describe malignant mesothelioma. In the older literature, the confusing term "benign mesothelioma" was used to describe what is now called solitary fibrous tumor of the pleura, a rare form of tumor that is entirely different from malignant mesothelioma. The development of a solitary fibrous tumor of the pleura has no relation to asbestos exposure; the tumor is usually benign and amenable to surgery, with good long-term prognosis. Symptoms and effusions are uncommon with solitary fibrous tumor of the pleura, which occasionally is associated with hypertrophic osteoarthropathy and intermittent hypoglycemia.

9. **How do patients with malignant mesothelioma commonly present?**
   Symptoms of mesothelioma are nonspecific and are often of gradual onset, resulting in an average delay of 2–3 months between symptom onset and diagnosis. The majority (i.e., >90%) of patients present with a unilateral pleural effusion and associated breathlessness. Weight loss and fatigue are relatively uncommon at the initial presentation but are prominent features in the late stage of the disease.

10. **What is the typical clinical course of malignant mesothelioma?**
    The disease is progressive and relentless. The tumor grows and encases the lung, producing volume loss and functional restriction. Mesothelioma has a high propensity to invade neighboring structures (e.g., the chest wall, mediastinum, and pericardium). Invasion of local structures can result in chest pain, dysphagia, dyspnea, cardiac tamponade, and spinal cord or brachial plexus invasion. Transdiaphragmatic invasion can result in ascites, abdominal pain, or intestinal obstruction. Distant spread of mesothelioma is common at necropsy but is often subclinical.

11. **Can radiologic tests confirm the diagnosis of mesothelioma?**
    No radiologic tests can accurately establish the diagnosis of mesothelioma. A unilateral pleural effusion is often the earliest radiographic feature of malignant pleural mesothelioma. Occasionally, an area of progressive irregular pleural thickening is seen on serial films. As the disease progresses, the affected side contracts and opacifies.
    Computed tomography, magnetic resonance imaging, and positron emission tomography can provide additional information to support a malignant pleural etiology but cannot differentiate mesotheliomas from metastatic carcinomas (Fig. 75-1).

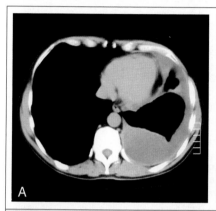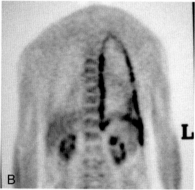

Figure 75-1. *A,* A left pleural mesothelioma, presenting with a large pleural effusion on computed tomography. *B,* Positron emission tomography scanning showed increased uptake along the serosal surface of the left pleural cavity. (Courtesy of Dr. Evaldo Marchi, São Paulo, Brazil.)

12. **What pleural (or peritoneal) fluid characteristics are typical in mesothelioma?**
    Thoracentesis should be performed in patients presenting with a pleural (or peritoneal) effusion in whom mesothelioma is suspected. The fluid is always exudative and is often bloody. No particular pleural fluid biochemical or tumor markers are reliable enough for diagnosing mesothelioma. Differentiating between benign reactive and malignant mesothelial cells is often difficult. The diagnostic yield of cytologic examination of pleural or peritoneal fluids varies widely (by 33–84%) and depends in part on the expertise of the cytopathologist. The diagnosis is by no means excluded, even in the presence of negative cytologic findings.

13. **What other disorders must be considered in the differential diagnosis?**
    Metastatic adenocarcinoma is probably the diagnosis most commonly confused with mesothelioma. Other diagnoses that should be considered include benign asbestos pleural effusion, pleural tuberculosis, collagen vascular disease, and pulmonary embolism.

14. **Is open or closed pleural biopsy useful for diagnosis?**
    In the early stage, the pleural surface affected may be small. Hence, closed pleural biopsies are subjected to sampling error and only modestly improve the diagnostic sensitivity. Pleural biopsy under direct vision during medical thoracoscopy or video-assisted thoracoscopy can establish the diagnosis in up to 98% of cases. Thoracotomy should only be reserved as a last resort in cases in which thoracoscopy is not technically feasible. It should be emphasized that mesothelioma often spreads along needle tracts from pleural aspiration or biopsy. Prophylactic radiotherapy to the pleural puncture sites is effective in preventing local tumor seeding and should be routinely provided for mesothelioma patients.

    Adams RF, Gray W, Davies RJ, Gleeson FV: Percutaneous image-guided cutting needle biopsy of the pleura in the diagnosis of malignant mesothelioma. Chest 120:1798–1802, 2001.

Boutin C, Rey F, Viallat JR: Prevention of malignant seeding after invasive diagnostic procedures in patients with pleural mesothelioma. A randomized trial of radiotherapy. Chest 108:754–758, 1995.

Boutin C, Rey F: Thoracoscopy in pleural malignant mesothelioma: A prospective study of 188 consecutive patients. Part 1: Diagnosis. Cancer 72:389–393, 1993.

KEY POINTS: DIAGNOSIS OF MALIGNANT PLEURAL MESOTHELIOMA

1. Most patients present with dyspnea, chest pain, or both, and a unilateral pleural effusion.

2. Individuals with asbestos exposure are at higher risk.

3. There are no pathognomic radiologic features for diagnosing mesothelioma.

4. Thoracentesis and (if thoracentesis is negative) pleural biopsy should be performed to establish the diagnosis.

5. A definitive diagnosis requires histologic or cytologic confirmation.

15. **Are there measures that can predict or prevent the development of mesothelioma in asbestos-exposed individuals?**
    There are no proven secondary prevention measures that can minimize the risk of mesothelioma development in individuals exposed to asbestos. Hence, the best strategy against mesothelioma is primary prevention against occupational and environmental exposure to asbestos. As there is no effective treatment for mesothelioma, screening of at-risk individuals for the disease has not attracted much attention. Soluble mesothelin-related (SMR) proteins have shown promise as a novel serum marker that may predict subsequent development of mesothelioma in exposed individuals, although the results need to be confirmed in larger series.

    Robinson BW, Creaney J, Lake R, et al: Mesothelin-family proteins and diagnosis of mesothelioma. Lancet 362:1612–1616, 2003.

16. **Are medicolegal issues involved in the diagnosis of mesothelioma?**
    Although differentiating between mesothelioma and metastatic adenocarcinoma may not always be clinically indicated, establishing a diagnosis of mesothelioma is important for medicolegal reasons. A firm tissue diagnosis may be desired, as most patients would pursue workers' compensation. A detailed occupational history is also essential to aid in establishing the likely source of asbestos exposure.

17. **What are the histologic subsets of mesothelioma and their implications on patient outcome?**
    Mesotheliomas are usually classified histologically into epithelioid (representing about 60% of cases) or sarcomatoid (10%) subtypes. The remainder show mixed epithelioid and sarcomatoid characteristics and are termed "biphasic" mesothelioma. In general, survival is longer with patients with epithelioid tumor (Fig. 75-2) than those with sarcomatoid mesothelioma.

18. **Is staging useful in mesothelioma? What is the most efficient approach?**
    There are no universally accepted staging systems for mesothelioma. The Butchart classification and the tumor-node-metastasis system from the International Mesothelioma Interest Group are among the most commonly used staging protocols in the literature. Both necessitate additional investigations not routinely required for patient care. Hence, staging is not justified in day-to-day practice but is useful in clinical trials to adequately characterize patients and to measure responses.

Rusch VW: A proposed new international TNM staging system for malignant pleural mesothelioma. From the International Mesothelioma Interest Group. Chest 108:1122–1128, 1995.

19. **What is the prognosis for patients with mesothelioma?**
    Mesothelioma remains a uniformly lethal malignancy. The reported survival varies from 4–18 months from diagnosis. Large population studies show no improvement in survival over the last decade, reflecting the lack of advances in its treatment. Better performance status, early-stage disease, younger age, less weight loss, an absence of chest pain, a shorter duration of symptoms before diagnosis, and an epithelioid histology are favorable prognostic factors for pleural mesothelioma.

    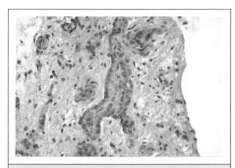

    Figure 75-2. Histology of the pleural tissue of a patient with epithelioid mesothelioma. (Courtesy of Dr. Colin Clelland, Oxford, UK.)

    A small number of patients will follow an indolent course irrespective of management strategies and may survive for many years. Why these patients behave differently from the rest remains unknown.

20. **Is there a role for surgical resection of mesothelioma?**
    Although widely practiced, surgery for mesothelioma is not supported by evidence-based medicine. The tumor tends to spread along the pleural surface and to infiltrate the underlying structures (e.g., lung and chest wall) early. This feature prohibits complete surgical resection. Extrapleural pneumonectomy (EPP) is an aggressive operation that involves removing the lung and pleura *en bloc*, as well as the hemidiaphragm and pericardium. Major postoperative complications occur in about 25% of patients, and the 30-day mortality is around 5%. Pleurectomy removes all gross tumor but seldom yields microscopically clear margins. Neither EPP nor pleurectomy is curative. There is no published evidence to suggest that surgery improves survival or quality of life in these patients over best supportive care.

21. **Is there a role for chemotherapy in mesothelioma?**
    Mesothelioma is resistant to most chemotherapy agents, and adequate drug delivery, either systemically or intrapleurally, to the pleural tumors is difficult. However, the combination regime of pemetrexed and cisplatin has demonstrated benefits in providing objective responses, delaying tumor progression, and improving median survival (12.1 vs. 9.3 months in those treated with cisplatin alone) in a large Phase III clinical trial, noteworthy as this is the only treatment to date that shows survival benefits for mesothelioma in a controlled clinical trial.

    Vogelzang NJ, Rusthoven J, Symanowski J, et al: Phase III study of pemetrexed in combination with cisplatin versus cisplatin alone in patients with malignant pleural mesothelioma. J Clin Oncol 21:2636–2644, 2003.

22. **Is there a role for radiotherapy in mesothelioma?**
    Mesothelioma is radiation sensitive, and prophylactic radiotherapy for preventing needle tract metastases after invasive pleural procedures was proven effective in a randomized controlled trial and is now routine practice in many centers. Palliative radiotherapy can be useful in patients with tumor invasion of the esophagus, superior vena cava, or spinal cord and in those with localized chest wall pain.

    However, radiotherapy with curative intent is not technically feasible. This is because administering curative doses over the entire ipsilateral visceral and parietal pleural surfaces produces unacceptable mortality and morbidity from major radiation toxicity to the underlying organs (e.g., the heart).

23. **What multimodality therapies are available for mesothelioma?**
As single modality treatments are ineffective, various combination therapies have been attempted, with disappointing results. Extrapleural pneumonectomy or pleurectomy and decortication followed by radiation and chemotherapy are practiced in selected centers. Such regimes offer cytoreduction but not cure. Disease inevitably relapses, after which the patients follow a rapid downhill course. There are high mortality and morbidity from EPP and further complications from subsequent chemoradiotherapy. The published data to date are uncontrolled and skewed by selection bias. A randomized controlled trial is now underway to investigate the role of surgery and adjunct chemoirradiation in mesothelioma, but the results will not be available for several years.

KEY POINTS: MANAGEMENT OF MALIGNANT PLEURAL MESOTHELIOMA

1. Sadly, there is no cure for malignant mesothelioma.

2. There is no clinical proof to date that surgery offers survival benefit or improves quality of life.

3. Treatment with pemetrexed and cisplatin prolonged survival in a randomized controlled trial.

4. Prophylactic radiotherapy to pleural puncture sites can prevent needle-tract metastases.

5. Successful pleurodesis can minimize dyspnea from recurrent pleural effusions.

6. Early referral to a multidisciplinary palliative care team is recommended.

24. **What is the role of pleurodesis in the palliation of mesothelioma?**
The primary aim is to provide maximum symptom relief and a minimum of adverse effects, preferably within the home. A multidisciplinary approach involving the palliative care team of physicians, nurses, social workers, and psychologists, together with active participation of the patient and his or her family, is strongly recommended. As dyspnea from recurrent pleural effusions is the most common presenting complaint, pleurodesis (by tube thoracostomy or thoracoscopy) should be considered early in the disease course.

BIBLIOGRAPHY

1. Jaklitsch MT, Grondin SC, Sugarbaker DJ: Treatment of malignant mesothelioma. World J Surg 25:210–217, 2001.

2. Lee YCG, Dean A, Thompson RI, Robinson BWS: Clinical and palliative care aspects of malignant mesothelioma. In Robinson BWS, Chahinian P (eds): Mesothelioma. London, Martin Dunitz, 2002, pp 111–126.

3. Lee YCG, De Klerk NH, Henderson DW, Musk AW: Malignant mesothelioma. In Hendrick DJ, Burge PS, Beckett WS, Churg A (eds): Occupational Disorders of the Lung. Recognition, Management and Prevention. London, W.B. Saunders, 2002, pp 359–379.

4. Lee YCG, Light RW, Musk AW: Management of malignant pleural mesothelioma: A critical review. Curr Opin Pulm Med 6:267–274, 2000.

5. Robinson BW, Creaney J, Lake R, et al: Mesothelin-family proteins and diagnosis of mesothelioma. Lancet 362:1612–1616, 2003.

6. Sterman DH, Albelda SM: Gene therapy in pleural diseases. In Light RW, Lee YCG (eds): Textbook of Pleural Diseases. London, Arnold Press, 2003, pp 526–535.

7. Vogelzang NJ, Rusthoven J, Symanowski J, et al: Phase III study of pemetrexed in combination with cisplatin versus cisplatin alone in patients with malignant pleural mesothelioma. J Clin Oncol 21:2636–2644, 2003.

PULMONARY MANIFESTATIONS OF SYSTEMIC DISEASE

Kamel Marzouk, MD, MS, and Om P. Sharma, MD, FRCP

CHAPTER 76

1. **Name some pulmonary manifestations of systemic disease.**
   See Table 76-1.

TABLE 76-1. PULMONARY MANIFESTATIONS OF SYSTEMIC DISEASE	
Disorder	**Lung Manifestation**
Endocrine	
Thyrotoxicosis	Dyspnea, increased oxygen consumption, increased carbon dioxide production, decreased lung compliance, weakness of respiratory muscles, pulmonary hypertension, and tracheal compression
Hypothyroidism	Decreased control of ventilatory response to hypoxia and hypercapnia, obstructive sleep apnea, pleural effusions, and weakness of respiratory muscle
Diabetes mellitus	Staphylococcal and gram-negative pneumonias and reactivation tuberculosis
Gastrointestinal	
Pancreatitis	Hypoxemia, pulmonary infiltrates, pleural effusions, and ARDS
Crohn's disease	Granulomatous lung involvement
Ulcerative colitis	Purulent bronchitis, bronchiectasis, BOOP, and tracheal stenosis
Cirrhosis or portal hypertension	Pleural: hepatic hydrothorax, chylothorax, and thoracobiliary fistula
	Parenchymal: bronchiectasis, bronchitis, BOOP, lymphoid interstitial pneumonia (LIP), nonspecific interstitial pneumonia (NSIP), and usual interstitial pneumonia (UIP)
	Pulmonary circulation: hepatopulmonary syndrome and portopulmonary hypertension
Gastroesophageal reflux	Cough
Hematologic	
Sickle-cell disease	Acute chest syndrome, rib infarctions, pneumococcal infections, and fat embolism
Bone marrow transplant	Pulmonary edema, cyclosporine lung toxicity, transfusion reactions, ARDS, BOOP, opportunistic infections, pulmonary embolism, veno-occlusive disease, and supraglottic airway obstruction

Continued

TABLE 76-1. PULMONARY MANIFESTATIONS OF SYSTEMIC DISEASE—CONT'D	
Disorder	**Lung Manifestation**
Paraproteinemias	Amyloidosis (tracheobronchial plaques, nodules, adenopathy)
	Multiple myeloma (pleural effusion, mediastinal mass, plasmacytoma of the lung, and pneumonias)
	Waldenström's macroglobulinemia (reticulonodular infiltrate, mass)
	Heavy chain disease (infiltrate, mediastinal adenopathy, recurrent pneumonias)
Cutaneous	
Hereditary hemorrhagic telangiectasia	Pulmonary arteriovenous fistulas
Ataxia–telangiectasia syndrome	Sinopulmonary infections
CREST syndrome	Interstitial fibrosis
Neurofibromatosis	Intrathoracic neurofibromas and diffuse interstitial fibrosis
Tuberous sclerosis	Interstitial fibrosis and spontaneous pneumothorax
Oculocutaneous albinism	Idiopathic interstitial fibrosis
Weber–Christian disease	Pulmonary panniculitis
Whipple disease	Nodular infiltrates and pleural adhesions
Yellow nail syndrome	Bronchiectasis and pleural effusions
Acanthosis nigricans	Bronchogenic carcinoma
Renal	
End-stage renal disease	Hypoxemia

CREST = calcinosis, Raynaud phenomenon, esophageal involvement, sclerodactyly, and telangiectasia syndrome.

2. **What are the pulmonary manifestations of amyloidosis?**

The lung is commonly involved in systemic amyloidosis. Thirty percent of patients with primary amyloidosis have cough and dyspnea, whereas, in secondary amyloidosis, respiratory symptoms are rare and the chest radiograph is usually normal. Four distinct patterns of lung involvement are seen in pulmonary amyloidosis:

1. Airway disease consists of localized nodular deposits of amyloid in the larynx, trachea, or bronchi. Initially, these patients are asymptomatic, but wheezing, recurrent pneumonia, and lung collapse can occur in some patients.
2. Single or multiple pulmonary nodules can occur infrequently. These nodules can calcify.
3. Diffuse parenchymal, alveolar–septal infiltration can occur in about 10% of patients.
4. Unilateral or bilateral hilar or mediastinal adenopathy has been described.

Howard M, Ireton J, Daniels F, et al: Pulmonary presentations of amyloidosis. Respirology 6:61–64, 2001.

3. **Name some of the common pulmonary–cutaneous syndromes.**
   Pulmonary arteriovenous fistulas occur in 60% of patients with hereditary hemorrhagic telangiecta-sia. Intrathoracic neurofibromas, neural tumors, and interstitial fibrosis are recognized pulmonary complications of neurofibromatosis. Bronchiectasis and pleural effusions are common manifestations of yellow nail syndrome. Interstitial fibrosis can occur in patients with tuberous sclerosis; calcinosis, Raynaud phenomenon, esophageal involvement, sclerodactyly, and telangiec-tasia (CREST) syndrome; and oculocutaneous albinism. Whipple's disease can cause pulmonary granulomas, nodular infiltrate, and pleural adhesion. Pulmonary panniculitis is associated with Weber–Christian disease. Acanthosis nigricans is a skin marker of bronchogenic carcinoma.

   Fuchizaki U, Miyamori H, Kitagawa S, et al: Hereditary haemorrhagic telangiectasia (Rendu-Osler-Weber disease). Lancet 362:1490, 2003.

   Iqbal M, Rossoff LJ, Marzouk KA, Steinberg HN: Yellow nail syndrome: Resolution of yellow nails after successful treatment of breast cancer. Chest 117(5):1516–1518, 2000.

KEY POINTS: PULMONARY EFFECTS OF LIVER CIRRHOSIS AND PORTAL HYPERTENSION

1. Pleural

   - Hepatic hydrothorax

   - Chylothorax

   - Thoracobiliary fistula

2. Parenchymal

   - Bronchiectasis, bronchitis

   - BOOP, LIP, NSIP, UIP

3. Pulmonary circulation

   - Hepatopulmonary syndrome

   - Portopulmonary hypertension

---

4. **Why is the diabetic patient susceptible to pulmonary infection?**
   The mechanisms for the increased susceptibility of the diabetic patient to infection are poorly understood. Impaired chemotactic, phagocytic, and bactericidal activities of the neutrophil are believed responsible for infections with staphylococci and gram-negative bacteria. Diabetes is the single most common predisposing condition in patients presenting with community-acquired pneumonia. Hyperglycemia decreases intracellular bactericidal activity of lymphocytes. Impaired phagocytic activity of monocytes may increase the risk of fungal infections, particularly mucormycosis. Tuberculosis reactivation occurs two to three times more often in diabetic patients with poor nutrition.

   Musher DM: Streptococcus pneumonia. In Mandell GL, Bennett JE, Dolin R (eds): Mandell, Douglas, and Bennett's Principles and Practice of Infectious Disease, 5th ed. Philadelphia, Churchill Livingstone, 2000.

5. **What structural changes are seen in the lungs of a diabetic patient?**
   In experimental animal models of diabetes mellitus, ultrastructural changes have been described in type 2 diabetes mellitus, affecting pneumocytes and nonciliated bronchiolar epithelial cells (i.e.,

Clara cells). Studies in humans are difficult, and most are based on postmortem specimens. The following changes have been described:

- Thickened alveolar epithelial and pulmonary capillary basal laminae is the most consistent change described. There is no significant correlation between the thickening of pulmonary basal laminae and the duration of diabetes mellitus.
- Microembolization of pulmonary arteries has been found.
- Some degree of centrilobular emphysema is also found in some studies in the lungs of diabetes subjects.

6. **What is the effect of diabetes mellitus on pulmonary physiology?**
   - The most consistent abnormality is reduced lung volumes, which is more common in children and adolescents and in patients who have limited joint mobility. This is attributed to impaired growth of the lungs and chest wall.
   - Decreased mobility of chest-wall joints and decreased compliance of the chest wall as a whole are common.
   - Reduced pulmonary elastic recoil has been described in both young and adult diabetic subjects.
   - The ventilatory increase in response to transient hypoxia is less in diabetics without autonomic neuropathy than in controls, but it is even weaker in diabetics with autonomic neuropathy. A similar pattern is seen in the ventilatory response to hypercapnia.

   No correlation has been found between the presence of abnormal ventilatory responses and the duration of diabetes mellitus. These changes are attributed to the altered functions of both the peripheral and the central chemoreceptors.

   Mancini M, Filippelli M, Seghieri G, et al: Respiratory muscle function and hypoxic ventilatory control in patients with type I diabetes. Chest 115(6):1553–1562,1999.

7. **What are the common respiratory symptoms of thyrotoxicosis?**
   Dyspnea is the most common complaint in thyrotoxicosis. Its cause is unclear, and its severity varies from patient to patient. Increased oxygen consumption, increased carbon dioxide production, increased minute ventilation, decreased vital capacity, impaired diffusion capacity, low lung compliance, and respiratory muscle weakness have all been implicated in causing dyspnea. Thyrotoxicosis patients also have high-output left ventricular failure. In some patients, tracheal compression by the enlarged thyroid gland may cause wheezing and stridor. Hyperactivity of the airways has also been observed.

   Ingbar DH: The pulmonary system in thyrotoxicosis. In Braverman LE, Utiger RD (eds): Werner and Ingbar's The Thyroid. A Fundamental and Clinical Text, 8th ed. Philadelphia, Lippincott Williams & Wilkins, 2000.

8. **How does hypothyroidism affect the respiratory system?**
   Hypothyroidism decreases central ventilatory sensitivity to hypoxia and hypercapnia. It can lead to respiratory failure and coma. An enlarged tongue or oropharyngeal narrowing due to soft tissue mucopolysaccharide and protein deposition and myopathic changes in the muscles of the upper airway can lead to obstructive sleep apnea. Pleural effusions, unilateral or bilateral, have been observed. Lastly, muscle weakness combined with obesity can decrease lung volumes and cause ventilation–perfusion mismatch leading to hypoxemia and carbon dioxide retention.

   Hattori H, Hattori C, Yonekura A, Nishimura T: Two cases of sleep apnea syndrome caused by primary hypothyroidism. Acta Otolaryngol Suppl 550:59–64, 2003.

9. **List the pulmonary effects of acute pancreatitis. What is their significance?**
   The lungs may be involved in 50–70% of patients with acute pancreatitis. The abnormalities include asymptomatic reduction in arterial oxygenation, significant hypoxemia with a normal chest radiograph, nonspecific infiltrates, pleural effusion, and acute respiratory distress syndrome (ARDS). The last occurs in about 15% of the patients with acute pancreatitis and carries a poor prognosis. The onset of pulmonary symptoms in the patient with acute pancreatitis likewise portends a poor prognosis. Sixty percent of deaths from acute pancreatitis that occur

during the first week are associated with respiratory failure. Only 25% of those who require mechanical ventilation survive. During and after the second week, pulmonary complications are usually the result of pancreatic infection or pseudocyst formation. Pleural effusions and ascites reflect the severity of the illness.

Maringhini A, Ciambra M, Patti R, et al: Ascites, pleural, and pericardial effusions in acute pancreatitis: A prospective study of incidence, natural history, and prognostic role. Dig Dis Sci 41:848–852, 1996.

Talaman G, Uomo G, Pezzilli R, et al: Renal function and chest x-rays in the assessment of 539 acute pancreatitis patients. Gut 41:A136, 1997.

10. **What is the association between Crohn's disease and sarcoidosis?**
Sarcoidosis (rarely) can present as a granulomatous colitis, and Crohn's disease has been reported to involve the lungs. Bronchoalveolar lavage fluid from patients with Crohn's disease and sarcoidosis shows that lymphocytes predominate with increased T4 subset during active disease. An elevated serum angiotensin-converting enzyme level may help differentiate sarcoidosis from Crohn's disease. A similar immunologic abnormality may be common to both disorders. The granulomatous lung involvement occasionally seen in patients with Crohn's disease improves, as does sarcoidosis, with corticosteroid therapy.

Dumot JA, Adal K, Petras RE, Lashner BA: Sarcoidosis presenting as granulomatous colitis. Am J Gastroenterol 93:1949–1951, 1998.

Nassar A, Ghobrial G, Romero C, et al: Culture of *Mycobacterium avium* subspecies paratuberculosis from the blood of patients with Crohn's disease. Lancet 363:1039–1044, 2004.

11. **Is there a relationship between ulcerative colitis and airway disease?**
In several series of patients with ulcerative colitis, concomitant bronchial disease, including both bronchiectasis and purulent bronchitis, has been described. These pulmonary manifestations appear to be unrelated to the activity of or therapy for the bowel disease. An exception may be that early treatment of the ulcerative colitis may avoid the development of bronchiectasis. In these patients, the chest radiograph may be normal, and pulmonary function testing has shown no consistent abnormality. Biopsies of lung tissue may show thickening of the epithelium and basement membrane, with inflammatory cell infiltration of the underlying connective tissue. A common abnormality in immune regulation affecting both bowel and bronchi has been postulated. High-dose corticosteroid therapy often leads to clinical improvement.

12. **What are the major differences between hepatopulmonary syndrome and portopulmonary hypertension?**
See Table 76-2.

13. **How does gastroesophageal reflux cause cough?**
Cough can be the sole presenting symptom of gastroesophageal reflux. It is caused by one of three mechanisms:
1. Reflux of stomach contents may irritate the esophageal mucosa and initiate the cough reflex through vagal sensory pathways.
2. Stomach contents may be aspirated, irritating sensory receptors of the tracheobronchial tree.
3. Stomach contents may reach the hypopharynx and larynx, irritating the afferent limb of the cough reflex without aspiration.
Diagnosis is certain only when the cough goes away in response to antireflux therapy.

14. **What is the "acute chest syndrome" of sickle-cell anemia?**
The combination of pleuritic chest pain, fever, cough, and parenchymal infiltrates on chest radiograph constitutes the acute chest syndrome. Infectious pneumonia and sickling of the abnormal red blood cells, either singly or in combination, are usually responsible. Rib infarctions, which are commonly observed radiologically, may also play a role in the pathogenesis. *In situ* thrombosis leading to pulmonary infarction may also occur. Infants and children commonly

TABLE 76-2. HEPATOPULMONARY SYNDROME VERSUS PORTOPULMONARY HYPERTENSION

	Hepatopulmonary Syndrome	Portopulmonary Hypertension
Definition	Triad of: 1. Intrapulmonary vascular dilatations 2. Liver dysfunction 3. Increased alveolar-to-arterial gradient	Criteria include: 1. Pulmonary capillary wedge pressure < 15 2. Mean pulmonary artery pressure (PAP) > 25 3. Portal hypertension 4. Absence of other causes of secondary pulmonary hypertension
Pathophysiology	Arteriovenous shunting in the lung, predominantly at the bases; "spider angiomata" in the lung	Vasoactive substances not filtered by the damaged liver cause intense vasoconstriction of pulmonary capillaries as well as remodeled, thickened pulmonary vasculature
Symptoms	Platypnea	Dyspnea on exertion, syncope, orthopnea, and chest pain
Physical findings	Hypoxemia, orthodeoxia	Loud pulmonic second sound (P2), right ventricular heave, and tricuspid regurgitation murmur; hypoxemia worsens with exercise
Diagnosis	Echocardiogram: positive bubble study	Echocardiogram shows elevated PAP; right heart catheterization confirms diagnosis
Treatment	Liver transplant, with 2–14 months to improvement	Same as primary pulmonary hypertension; if mean PAP is <40 mmHg, patient can undergo liver transplantation

present with symptoms of infection, whereas adults usually present with pain. Manifestations of the involvement of other organs—including hemiplegia, an altered mental status, renal failure, and petechiae—suggest fat embolism, which can occur in these patients. Recurrent episodes of acute chest syndrome may result in the development of chronic lung disease.

Taylor C, Carter F, Poulose J, et al: Clinical presentation of acute chest syndrome in sickle cell disease. Postgrad Med J. 80(944):346–349, 2004.

15. **How much oxygen should be administered to a patient with sickle-cell anemia who has acute chest syndrome?**
Hypoxemia is frequently a sequela of acute chest syndrome. Maintenance of an adequate level of oxygenation is necessary to reduce the adverse effects of hypoxia. Although oxygen may reduce the further sickling that occurs in these patients when the oxygen tension is reduced, it apparently does not alter the duration of the event, presumably because of the damage caused by vaso-occlusion before its administration. Administration of inspired oxygen at a high concentration, in excess of that necessary to maintain a safe level of saturation, traditionally has not been

KEY POINTS: ACUTE CHEST SYNDROME OF SICKLE-CELL ANEMIA

1. Pleuritic chest pain, fever, cough, and parenchymal infiltrates on chest radiograph

2. Infectious pneumonia (sickling of the abnormal red blood cells is usually responsible)

3. *In situ* thrombosis leading to pulmonary infarction may occur

4. Treatment includes oxygen, analgesics, hydration, transfusion of leukocyte-depleted red cells, antibiotics, and exchange transfusion in the setting of progressive infiltrates and hypoxemia

recommended on the basis that it suppresses erythropoiesis. However, the suppression of erythropoiesis in this situation is poorly defined. The hemoglobin level and reticulocyte count have been shown to fall in patients on oxygen therapy, and monitoring is advised, although the current belief is that oxygen concentrations of 50% or less are unlikely to do harm aside from the discomfort associated with the administration. One should keep in mind that pulse oximetry and oxygen saturation calculated from blood gas analyses may overestimate oxygen content due to the presence of abnormal hemoglobin.

Zipursky A, Robieux IC, Brown RT, et al: Oxygen therapy in sickle cell disease. Am J Pediatr Hematol Oncol 14:222–228, 1992.

16. **What pulmonary complications can occur after bone marrow transplantation?**
Patients undergoing bone marrow transplantation after aggressive salvage chemoradiation therapy are at high risk to develop pulmonary complications. Early in the course, within the first 100 days after transplantation, pulmonary edema from fluid overload or myocardial injury, diffuse alveolar hemorrhage from cyclosporine toxicity, and transfusion reactions are seen. ARDS may be caused by pneumonia and sepsis due to bacterial, fungal, and viral organisms. Interstitial pneumonitis from infection with *Pneumocystis jinovecii* or cytomegalovirus or due to chemotherapy, pulmonary embolism, or veno-occlusive disease is also probable during this period.

Late complications include bronchopneumonia from the aforementioned infections, fat embolism, veno-occlusive disease, interstitial pneumonitis of a nonspecific nature, bronchiolitis obliterans, bronchiolitis obliterans–organizing pneumonia (BOOP), lymphocytic interstitial pneumonitis, and graft-versus-host disease. Severe supraglottic airway obstruction due to Epstein–Barr virus lymphoproliferative disease has been reported in children.

Eikenberry M, Bartakova H, Defor T, et al: Natural history of pulmonary complications in children after bone marrow transplantation. Biol Blood Marrow Transplant 11(1):56–64, 2005.

Gosselin MV, Adams RH: Pulmonary complications in bone marrow transplantation. J Thorac Imag 17(2):132–144, 2002.

17. **What pulmonary complications can occur after liver transplantation?**
In the early days after transplantation, the right diaphragm is paralyzed and right lower lobe atelectasis is common. Pleural effusions occur in almost all patients, and pulmonary edema can result from excess fluids and blood products during the operation. Later complications may include bacterial infections, and fungal and cytomegalovirus infections are particularly common. Azathioprine and cyclosporine can cause interstitial pneumonitis and ARDS, respectively.

Saner F, Lang H, Fruhauf N, et al: Postoperative ICU management of liver transplantation patients. Eur J Med Res 8:511–516, 2003.

Sherlock S: The liver-lung interface. Sem Resp Med 9:247–253, 1988.

18. **Why does hypoxemia occur during hemodialysis?**

Transient hypoxemia is sometimes seen within 15 minutes of initiation of hemodialysis and is sometimes severe enough to be symptomatic or to exacerbate myocardial ischemia. The mechanism postulated to explain the fall in alveolar oxygen partial pressure (PaO_2) is acetate in the bath, causing hypoventilation and increased oxygen consumption. Dialysance of carbon dioxide and bicarbonate causes hypocapnia with a lag in bicarbonate regeneration from acetate metabolism. High-bicarbonate baths cause metabolic alkalosis. The compensating hypoventilation causes hypercapnia, which can be prevented by decreasing the bicarbonate concentration in the bath. Hypoxia can also result from complement activation by a bioincompatible dialyzer membrane, which can cause leukostasis and plugging of the pulmonary capillaries, with resulting hypoxemia. This effect can be reduced by use of synthetic membranes and citrate anticoagulation. In some cases, hypoxemia may persist after dialysis has ended or may develop in the postdialysis period.

Needleman JP, Setty BN, Varlotta L, et al: Measurement of hemoglobin saturation by oxygen in children and adolescents with sickle cell disease. Pediatr Pulmonol 28:423–428, 1999.

19. **Define postcardiac injury syndrome, or Dressler's syndrome.**

Postcardiac injury syndrome, or Dressler's syndrome, consists of pericarditis, pleuritis, and pneumonitis occurring 1–12 weeks after any one of several forms of cardiac injury. Although it occurs most frequently after cardiac surgery, it also can be seen after myocardial infarction, chest trauma, pacemaker implantation, or diagnostic left ventricular puncture. Fever, leukocytosis, auscultatory evidence of pleural and pericardial friction rubs, and a pronounced elevation of the erythrocyte sedimentation rate are common manifestations. The chest radiograph shows a pleural effusion, usually left-sided, often with accompanying infiltrate. Antimyocardial antibodies have been identified in patients with this syndrome. The diagnosis remains clinical.

Light, RW: Pleural effusions after coronary artery bypass graft surgery. Curr Opin Pulm Med 8(4):308–311, 2002.

Page numbers in **boldface type** indicate complete chapters.